An Introduction to th
Symptoms and Signs
of Surgical Disease

Third Edition

Norman L. Browse Kt, MD, FRCS, FRCP

Professor of Surgery, University of London

Honorary Consulting Surgeon, St Thomas' Hospital, London

Formerly, Chairman, London University MB BS and MS Examiners

Formerly, Member of Court of Examiners, Royal College of Surgeons of England

Formerly member of Council and Chairman of Examinations Committee and Academic Board, Royal College of Surgeons of England

Past-President, Royal College of Surgeons of England

ELBS with Arnold

Educational Low-Priced Books Scheme
funded by the British Government

The Education Low-Priced Books Scheme is funded by the Overseas Development Administration as part of the British Government overseas aid programme. It makes available low-priced, unabridged editions of British publishers' textbooks to students in developing countries.

Arnold
A member of the Hodder Headline Group,
338 Euston Road, London NW1 3BH

First published 1978
Reprinted 1979, 1980, 1981, 1982, 1983, 1984, 1985, 1986
1987 (twice), 1988
Second edition 1991
Reprinted 1992, 1993, 1995, 1996
Third edition 1997

ELBS edition first published 1979
Reprinted 1980, 1981, 1982, 1983, 1984, 1985, 1986, 1988
ELBS edition of second edition 1991
Reprinted 1992, 1993, 1995, 1996
ELBS edition of third edition 1997

ISBN 0 340 69145 X

Typeset in 10/11 pt Palatino by Scribe Design, Gillingham, Kent, UK
Printed and bound in Great Britain by Bath Press, Bath, UK

Contents

Preface to the First Edition

I believe that the main object of basic medical education is to train the student to talk to and to examine a patient in such a way that he can discover the full history of the patient's illness, elicit the abnormal physical signs, make a differential diagnosis and suggest likely methods of treatment. The object of further medical training is to amplify these capabilities in range and depth through practical experience and specialist training.

It is surprising, but a fact, that some students present themselves for their qualifying examination unable to take a history or to conduct a physical examination in a way that is likely to detect all the abnormal symptoms and signs. Even more are unable to interpret and integrate the facts they do elicit. I think there are two reasons for these deficiencies. First, and most important, students do not spend enough time seeing patients and practising the art of history taking and clinical examination. It is essential for them to realize at the beginning of their training that the major part of medical education is an **apprenticeship**, an old but well-proven system whereby the apprentice watches and listens to someone more experienced than himself and then tries it himself under supervision. The second reason is the lack of books which describe how to examine a patient and explain how the presence or absence of particular symptoms and signs lead the clinician to the correct diagnosis.

In this book I have attempted to describe, in detail, the relevant features of the history and physical signs of the common surgical diseases in a way which emphasizes the importance of the routine application of the techniques of history taking and examining.

The details of these techniques are fully described, and headings such as age, sex, symptoms, position, site, shape and surface are constantly repeated in an unobtrusive way. I hope that when you have finished reading the book you will have these headings so deeply imprinted in your mind that you will never forget them. If so, I will consider that the book has succeeded, for you will always take a proper history and perform a correct and complete examination.

Because the main object of the book is to emphasize the proper techniques of history taking and clinical examination, I have described only the common conditions that you are likely to see in a surgical clinic. Indeed the whole book is presented in a manner similar to that used by most teachers when they are in the presence of the patient. Special investigations and treatment are completely excluded because neither can be applied sensibly if you get the history and physical signs wrong.

To make the book useful for revision, I have put a number of the lists and classifications in special Revision Panels. The photographs are close to the relevant text but their legends contain enough information to make the picture-plus-legend a useful revision piece.

I hope this book will be more of a **teach-book** than a **text-book**, which will be read many times during your basic and higher medical training. There is a well-known saying 'A bad workman always blames his tools'. The doctor cannot make this excuse because his basic tools are his five senses. If he has not trained his senses properly in the manner described in this book and kept them finely honed by constant practice, he will practise bad medicine but he will have only himself to blame.

Preface to the Third Edition

The diseases and abnormalities described in this book have not changed for many thousands of years, nor have their symptoms and signs. Why then produce a third edition? The main reason is to improve and modernize the presentation of the information within the book in the belief that better presentation facilitates and improves learning.

Whereas the symptoms and signs of surgical disease have not changed in the past 20 years, methods of printing and publishing have. Computers graphics and colour printing now enable publishers to produce books of superb design, with infinite varieties of colour, at acceptable costs. The main changes in this new edition are therefore the introduction of colour into the general presentation and design, and the conversion of all 'blackboard-style' line drawings into coloured illustrations – still simple – but giving them the added impact on the memory provided by colour.

At the same time I have tried to illustrate all the clinical conditions with colour photographs – except for the few rare conditions, worthy of presentation, for which modern colour photographs are difficult to obtain. Unfortunately, the current trend is for patients to be unwilling to be photographed for illustrations to be used in books for teaching, thus making the compilation of a comprehensive library of clinical photographs far more difficult than it used to be.

I have also added a considerable number of new Revision Panels, now on a blue background, as students find them particularly helpful.

To remind students of their importance, the illustrations of methods of clinical examination (mostly black-and-white photographs) are outlined in Revision Panel blue.

I hope this revised presentation will give the book a new modern appearance and that it will continue to be attractive to new readers in the same way that it has been to the gratifyingly large number of students who have acquired it for their libraries over the past 20 years.

Sir Norman Browse
February 1997

Acknowledgements

I am extremely grateful to my friends and colleagues at St Thomas' Hospital and in surgical departments throughout the UK who have read and commented upon this edition and its predecessors. I am also indebted to Professor Fred Heatley, Mr Barry Jackson, Dr Clara Lowy, Dr Ralph Ross Russell, Mr Michael Sanders and Dr Colin Stern for providing some new illustrations for this latest edition.

Mr Graham Chambers of Oxford Illustrators has redrawn all my original line drawings and, by adding colour, has increased their impact and visual message.

My thanks to the staff at Arnold who have provided their traditional high-quality support and encouragement and Mrs Julia Hague has once again provided unstinting secretarial support.

Revising a book is not such a massive task as writing one, but without the constant understanding and support of my wife, Jeanne, this third edition would never have been completed.

History taking and clinical examination

1

You must be constantly *alert* from the moment you first see the patient, and employ your eyes, ears, nose and hands in a systematic fashion to collect the information from which you can deduce the diagnosis. The ability to appreciate an unusual comment or minor abnormality which may lead you to the correct diagnosis will only develop from the diligent and frequent practice of the routines outlined in this chapter. Always give the patient your whole attention and **never** *take short-cuts*.

In the outpatient clinic try to see the patient walk into the room rather than meet him undressed on a couch, in a cubicle. General malaise and debility, breathlessness, cyanosis, and difficulty with particular movements are much more obvious when the patient is exercising than when he is at rest.

It is also helpful to see the person accompanying the patient. A mother, wife or friend can often provide valuable information about changes in health and behaviour not noticed by the patient. However, remember that many patients are inhibited from discussing their problems by the presence of a third person.

Patients like to know to whom they are talking. They are probably expecting to see Mr Bloggs, the surgeon. If you are not Mr Bloggs, tell the patient your name and explain why you are deputizing for him. It is particularly important for medical students to do this.

Talk with the patient or, better still, let him talk to you. At first, *guide the conversation* but do not dictate it. Treat patients as the rational, intelligent human beings they are. They know more about their complaints than you, but cannot interpret their significance. Explain what you are doing, and why you are doing it, at all stages of their care.

Nowadays it is not uncommon to meet a patient who cannot talk your language. When conducting an interview through an interpreter, keep your questions short and simple, and have them translated and answered one at a time. You can never be certain that the translator understands your question or the patient's answer, or that there are words equivalent to yours in the patient's language.

All textbooks say that you should not ask leading questions; that is to say, questions which imply that there is only one answer. *All questions should leave the patient with a free choice of answers*. If you say, 'The pain moves to the right-hand side, doesn't it?' you imply that it should have moved in that direction and an obliging patient will answer 'Yes' to please you. The question should be, 'Does the pain ever move?' and if the patient answers 'Yes', you must then ask the supplementary question, 'Where does it go?' However, if communications are difficult you may have to suggest to the patient the possible answers so that he can confirm or reject them.

When a patient is having difficulty communicating with you, remember that a question which is not a leading one in your mind may be interpreted as one by the patient if he does not realize that there is more than one answer. For example, 'Has the pain changed?' can be a bad question. You may know of a variety of ways in which the pain can change – severity, nature, site, etc. – but the patient may be so disturbed by the intensity of the pain that he thinks only of its severity and forgets other features of it that may have changed. In such situations it often helps to include the possible answers in the question. For example, 'Has the pain moved to the top, bottom, or side of your abdomen or anywhere else?', 'Has the pain got worse, better or stayed the same?', or 'Can you walk as far, less far, or the same distance as you could a year ago?'

The patient will provide the true answer provided you ask the question in the right way; all that matters is that you discover the truth. So do not be over-concerned about the questions – worry about the answers, and accept that it will sometimes take a long time and a great deal of patience and perseverance to get them.

HOW TO TAKE THE HISTORY

The history should be taken in the order set out below. Do not write and talk to the patient at the same time – you will make mistakes.

Make sure you know, and **always record**, the patient's name, age, sex, ethnic group, marital status, occupation, and address; and always record **the date** of the examination.

1 The present complaint

It is customary to ask the patient 'What are you complaining of?' and to record the answer in the patient's own words.

It is currently fashionable to talk about 'problems' rather than 'complaints'. There is no difference, but problem-orientated management sounds more sympathetic.

If you ask 'What is the matter?' the patient will probably tell you his diagnosis, but it is better not to know the diagnosis made by the patient, or another doctor, because both might be wrong; so seek out the patient's complaints. If there is more than one complaint, list them in order of severity and, when possible, indicate why the patient is concerned with one complaint more than another.

2 The history of the present complaint

Next record the full details of the history of the main complaint or complaints. It is important to get right back to the beginning of the trouble. For example, a patient may complain of a sudden attack of indigestion. If further questioning reveals similar attacks some years previously, include their description in this section.

3 Remaining questions about the abnormal system

If the patient complains of indigestion it is sensible, after recording the history of the indigestion, to continue with the remainder of the alimentary system questions because many of the replies will throw light on the cause of the main complaint.

4 Systematic direct questions

These are direct questions that you must ask every patient, because the answers will not only amplify your knowledge about the main complaint, but often reveal the presence of other disorders of which the patient was unaware, or thought irrelevant. Negative answers are as important as positive answers.

The questions are described in detail because they are so important. It is essential to know them by heart because it is very easy to forget to ask some of them. When you have to go back to the patient to ask a forgotten question, you invariably find the answer to be very important. The only way to memorize this list is by taking as many histories as possible and writing them out in full, giving the answer to every question, whether it be positive or negative.

THE ALIMENTARY SYSTEM

Appetite Has the appetite increased, decreased, or remained unchanged? If it has decreased, is this caused by a lack of desire to eat, or is it due to apprehension because eating always causes pain? Has the patient developed any food fads; what are his special new likes or dislikes?

Diet What type of food does the patient eat? When does he eat his meals? How long do the meals take?

Weight Has the patient's weight changed? How much? How quickly? Many patients

Revision Panel 1.1

Synopsis of a history

1 *Names. Age and date of birth. Sex. Marital status. Occupation. Ethnic group. Religion. Hospital or practice. Record no.*

2 *Present complaints or problems* (PC, CO)
(In the patient's own words.)

3 *History of present complaint* (HPC)
Include the answers to the direct questions concerning the abdominal system.

4 *Systematic direct questions*

(a) *Alimentary system and abdomen* (AS)
Appetite. Diet. Weight. Taste. Nausea. Swallowing. Regurgitation. Flatulence. Heartburn. Vomiting. Haematemesis. Indigestion. Abdominal pain. Abdominal distention. Bowel habit. Nature of stool. Rectal bleeding. Jaundice.

(b) *Respiratory system* (RS)
Cough. Sputum. Haemoptysis. Dyspnoea. Hoarseness. Wheezing. Tachypnoea. Chest pain. Exercise tolerance.

(c) *Cardiovascular system* (CVS)
Dyspnoea. Paroxysmal nocturnal dyspnoea. Orthopnoea. Chest pain. Cough. Sputum. Dizziness. Headaches. Ankle swelling. Pain in limbs. Walking distance. Temperature and colour of hands and feet.

(d) *Urogenital system* (UGS)
Loin pain. Symptoms of uraemia: headache, drowsiness, fits, visual disturbances, vomiting. Oedema of ankles, hands or face. Frequency of micturition. Urgency. Precipitancy. Painful micturition. Polyuria. Thirst. Fluid intake. Colour of urine. Haematuria.
Problems with sexual intercourse: dyspareunia or impotence. Date of menarche or menopause. Frequency, quantity and duration of menstruation. Dysmenorrhoea. Previous pregnancies and their complications. Breast symptoms.

(e) *Nervous system*
Nervousness. Excitability. Tremor. Fainting attacks. Blackouts. Fits. Loss of consciousness. Muscle weakness. Paralysis. Sensory disturbances. Paraesthesiae. Changes of smell, vision, or hearing. Headaches. Changes of behaviour or psyche.

(f) *Musculoskeletal system*
Aches or pains in muscles, bones or joints. Swelling of joints. Limitation of joint movements. Weakness. Disturbances of gait.

(g) *Metabolism*
Change of weight. Appetite. General body build and appearance. Presence and time of development of secondary sex characteristics.

5 *Previous history* (PH)
Previous illnesses, operations or accidents. Diabetes. Rheumatic fever. Diphtheria. Bleeding tendencies. Asthma. Hayfever. Allergies. Tuberculosis. Syphilis. Gonorrhoea. Tropical diseases.

6 *Drug history*
Especially insulin, steroids, monoamine oxidase inhibitors and the contraceptive pill. Drug abuse.

7 *Immunizations*
BCG. Diphtheria. Tetanus. Typhoid. Whooping cough. Measles.

8 *Family history* (FH)
Cause of death of close relatives and presence of any serious familial illnesses.

9 *Social history* (SH)
Marital status. Sexual habits. Living accommodation. Occupation. Exposure to industrial hazards. Travel abroad. Leisure activities.

10 *Habits*
Smoking, drinking and eating habits.

never weigh themselves but will have noticed if their clothes have got tighter or looser, or friends may have told them of a change in physical appearance.

Teeth and taste Can the patient chew his food? Does he have his own or false teeth? Does he get odd tastes and sensations in the mouth? Does he get water brash or acid brash, the sudden filling of the mouth with watery or acid-tasting fluid (saliva and gastric acid respectively)?

Swallowing If the patient has difficulty in swallowing (dysphagia), ask about the type of food that causes difficulty, the level at which the food sticks, and the duration and progression of these symptoms. Is swallowing painful?

Regurgitation This is the effortless return of food into the mouth. It is quite different to vomiting, which is associated with a powerful although often involuntary contraction of the abdominal wall. Does the patient regurgitate? What comes up? How often does it occur and does anything, such as stooping or straining, precipitate it?

Flatulence Does the patient belch frequently? Does this affect any of his other symptoms?

Heartburn Patients may not realize that this symptom comes from the alimentary tract and they may have to be asked about it directly. It is a burning sensation behind the sternum caused by the reflux of acid into the oesophagus. How often does it occur? What makes it happen?

Vomiting How often does the patient vomit? Is the vomiting preceded by nausea? What is the nature and volume of the vomitus? Is it recognizable food from previous meals, digested food, clear acidic fluid or bile-stained fluid? Is the vomiting preceded by another symptom such as pain, headache or giddiness. Does it follow eating?

Haematemesis Always ask the patient if he has ever vomited blood because it is such an important symptom. Old, altered blood looks like 'coffee grounds'. Some patients have difficulty in differentiating between vomited or regurgitated blood and coughed-up blood (haemoptysis). The latter is usually pale pink and frothy. If the patient has had an haematemesis, ask if he has had a recent nose bleed.

Indigestion or abdominal pain Some people call all abdominal pains indigestion; the difference between a discomfort after eating and a pain after eating may be very small. Concentrate on the features of the pain, its site, time of onset, severity, nature, progression and duration, precipitating, exacerbating and relieving factors, radiation and course (see page 7).

Abdominal distension Has the patient noticed any abdominal distension? What brought this to his attention? When did it begin and how has it progressed? Is it constant or variable? What factors are associated with any variations? Is it painful? Does it affect respiration? Is it relieved by belching, vomiting or defaecation?

Defaecation How often does the patient defaecate? What are the physical characteristics of the stool?

- *Frequency of defaecation*?
- *Colour*: brown, black, pale, white or silver?
- *Consistence*: hard, soft or watery?
- *Size*: bulky, pellets, string- or tape-like?
- *Specific gravity*: does it float or sink?
- *Smell*?

Beware of the terms 'diarrhoea' and 'constipation'. They are lay words and mean different things to different people. Never use these words in your notes without also recording the frequency of bowel action and the consistence of the faeces.

Has the patient ever passed any blood? How much? Is the blood mixed with or on the surface of the stool, or does it appear after passing the stool? Is he passing more gas than usual? Has the patient ever passed mucus or pus? Is defaecation painful? When does the pain begin – before, during, after, or at times unrelated to defaecation?

Change of skin colour Has the patient's skin turned yellow (jaundiced)? When? How long did it last? Were there any other accompanying symptoms such as abdominal pain or loss of appetite? Did the skin itch? The melanin in the skin of the brown and black races masks most colour changes.

THE RESPIRATORY SYSTEM

Cough How often does the patient cough? Does the coughing come in bouts? When? Does anything, such as a change of posture, precipitate or relieve the coughing? Is it a dry or wet cough?

Sputum What is the quantity (teaspoon, dessertspoon, etc.), colour, taste, and smell of the sputum? Some patients only produce sputum in the morning or when they are in a particular position.

Haemoptysis Has the patient ever coughed up blood? Was it frothy and pink, red streaks in the mucus, or clots of blood? What quantity was produced? How often does the haemoptysis occur?

Dyspnoea Does the patient wheeze? Does he get breathless? How many stairs can he climb? How far can he walk on a level surface before the dyspnoea interferes with the exercise? Can he walk and talk at the same time? Is the dyspnoea present at rest? Is it present when sitting or lying down? How many pillows does the patient need at night? Does the breathlessness get worse if the patient slips off his pillows? Does the patient wake at night short of breath?

It is possible to grade dyspnoea numerically but it is better to describe the conditions that produce the dyspnoea rather than write down a number. Dyspnoea on lying flat is called **orthopnoea**. Is the dyspnoea induced or exacerbated by external factors such as allergy to animals, pollen or dust? Does the difficulty with breathing occur with both phases of respiration or just with expiration?

Pain in the chest Ascertain the site, severity and nature of the pain. Chest pains can be continuous, pleuritic (made worse by inspiration), constricting or stabbing.

THE CARDIOVASCULAR SYSTEM

Cardiac symptoms

Breathlessness Ask the same questions as those described under the 'respiratory system'

Orthopnoea (breathlessness when lying down) and **paroxysmal nocturnal dyspnoea** (sudden attacks of dyspnoea in the middle of the night that waken the patient). These are the forms of dyspnoea associated with heart disease.

Pain Cardiac pain begins in the mid-line and is usually retrosternal but may be epigastric. Its nature is often constricting, band-like or squeezing. It is usually related to exercise or excitement.

Does the pain radiate to the neck or to the left arm? Is the pain relieved by rest?

Palpitations These are episodes of tachycardia which the patient appreciates as a sudden fluttering or thumping of the heart in the chest.

Cough and sputum Ask the same questions as those asked for the respiratory system.

Dizziness and headaches These symptoms may be associated with a labile blood pressure, hypo- or hypertension.

Ankle swelling Do the ankles or legs swell? When? How much? What is the effect of bed-rest and/or elevation of the leg on the swelling?

Peripheral vascular symptoms

Does the patient get pain in the leg muscles on exercise (intermittent claudication)? Which muscles are involved? How far can he walk before the pain begins? Is the pain so bad that he has to stop walking? How long does the pain take to wear off? Can he walk the same distance again?

Is there any pain in the limb at rest? Which part of the limb is painful? Does the pain interfere with sleep? What analgesic drugs give relief? What positions relieve the pain? Are the extremities of the limbs cold? Are there colour changes in the skin, particularly in response to a cold environment? Does the patient experience any paraesthesiae in the limb, such as tingling or numbness?

THE UROGENITAL SYSTEM

Urinary tract symptoms

Pain Has there been any pain in the loin, groin or suprapubic region? What is its nature and severity? Does it radiate to the groin or scrotum?

Oedema Do any parts of the body, not just the ankles, swell?

Thirst Is the patient thirsty? Does he drink excessive volumes of water?

Micturition How often does the patient pass urine? Express this as a day/night ratio. How much urine is passed? Is micturition painful? What is the nature and site of the pain? Is there any difficulty with micturition, such as a need to strain or to wait? Is the stream good? Can it be stopped at will? Is there any dribbling at the end of micturition? Does the bladder feel empty at the end of micturition or does he have to pass urine a second time?

Urine What is the colour, smell and quantity of the urine? Has the patient ever passed blood in the urine? When and how often? Has he ever passed gas bubbles with the urine (pneumaturia)?

Other symptoms Also ask about headache, drowsiness, visual disturbance, fits and vomiting, because these are the symptoms of uraemia.

Genital tract symptoms

Scrotum and urethra Has the patient any pain in the penis or urethra, at rest, during micturition or intercourse? Is there any difficulty with retraction of the prepuce or any urethral discharge? Has the patient noticed any swelling of the scrotum? Can he achieve an erection and ejaculation?

Menstruation When did menstruation begin (menarche)? When did it end (menopause)? What is the duration and quantity of the menses? Is menstruation associated with pain (dysmenorrhoea)? When? What is the nature and severity of the pain? Is there any abdominal pain mid-way between the periods (mittelschmerz)?

Pregnancies Record details of the patient's pregnancies – number, dates and complications.

Dyspareunia Is intercourse painful?

Breasts Do the breasts change during the menstrual cycle? Are they ever painful or tender? Are there any swellings or lumps in the breasts? Did the patient breast-feed her children?

Secondary sex characteristics When did these appear?

THE NERVOUS SYSTEM

Mental state Is the patient placid or nervous? Has he noticed any changes in his behaviour or reactions to others? Patients will often not appreciate such changes themselves and these questions may have to be asked of close relatives. Does the patient get depressed and withdrawn, or excitable and extroverted?

Brain and cranial nerves Does the patient ever become unconscious or stuporous?

Does he ever have fits? What happens during a fit? It is often necessary to ask a relative or a bystander to describe the fit. Did the patient lie still or jerk about, bite his tongue, pass urine? Was he sleepy after the fit? Did he have any warning (an aura) that the fit was about to develop? Has there been any subsequent change in the senses of smell, vision and hearing?

Is the face ever weak or paralysed?

Peripheral nerves Are any limbs or part of a limb weak or paralysed? Is there ever any loss of cutaneous sensation – pain, light touch and temperature? Does the patient experience any paraesthesiae (tingling, 'pins and needles') in the limbs?

MUSCULOSKELETAL SYSTEM

Ask if the patient suffers from **pain, swelling, or limitation of the movement of any joint.** What precipitates or relieves these symptoms?

Are any limbs or groups of muscles weak or painful? Can he walk normally? Has he any congenital musculoskeletal deformities?

METABOLISM

Record the patient's weight and appetite, and any recent changes in either.

Ask if growth has been normal in rate and quantity. Has the patient noticed any abnormality of body growth and development?

5 Previous history of other illnesses, accidents or operations

Record the history of those conditions which are not directly related to the present complaint. Ask specifically about tuberculosis, diabetes, rheumatic fever, allergies, asthma, tropical diseases, bleeding tendencies, diphtheria, gonorrhoea, syphilis, and the likelihood of intimate contact with carriers of the human immunodeficiency virus (HIV).

6 Drug history

Ask the patient if he is taking any drugs. Specifically, enquire about steroids, monoamine oxidase inhibitors, insulin, diuretics, antihypertensives, ergot derivatives, hormone replacement therapy or the contraceptive pill.

Is the patient sensitive to any drugs or any topical applications such as adhesive plaster?

Patients usually remember about drugs prescribed by a doctor but often forget about drugs they have bought at a pharmacy.

7 Immunizations

Most children are now immunized against diphtheria, tetanus, whooping cough, measles, mumps, rubella and poliomyelitis. Ask about these, and smallpox, typhoid and tuberculosis vaccination.

8 Family history

Enquire about the health and age, or cause of death if not alive, of the patient's parents, grandparents, brothers and sisters, and children. If relevant, draw a family tree. If the patient is a child you will need information about the mother's pregnancy. Did she take any drugs during pregnancy? What was the patient's birth weight? Were there any difficulties during delivery? What was the rate of physical and mental development in early life?

9 Social history

Record the marital status and the type and place of dwelling. Ask about the patient's sexual life, the sex and variety of their sexual partners and the nature of their physical relationships. Ask about the patient's occupation, paying special regard to contact with hazards such as dusts and chemicals. What are the patient's leisure activities? Has the patient travelled abroad? List the countries he has visited and the dates of the visits.

10 Habits

Does the patient smoke? if so, cigarettes, cigar or pipe? Record the frequency, quantity and duration of smoking. Does the patient drink alcohol? Record the type and quantity consumed and the duration of the habit. Does the patient have any unusual eating habits?

HISTORY OF PAIN

We have all experienced pain. It is one of nature's ways of warning us that something is going wrong in our body. It is an unpleasant sensation of varying intensity. Pain can come from any of the body's systems but there are certain features common to all pains that should always be recorded.

Be careful of your use of the word 'tenderness'. Tenderness is pain which occurs in response to a stimulus, usually from the doctor, such as pressure by his hand, or forced movement. It is possible for a patient to be lying still without pain and yet have an area of tenderness. **The patient feels pain – the doctor elicits tenderness.** But although patients usually complain of pain, they may also have observed tenderness if they happen to have palpated a painful area or discovered a tender spot by accident. Thus tenderness can be both a symptom and a physical sign.

The history of a pain frequently betrays the diagnosis, so you must question the patient closely about each of the following features, some of which are depicted graphically in Fig. 1.1.

1 Site

Many factors may indicate the source of the pain but the most valuable indicator is its site.

It is of no value to describe a pain as 'abdominal pain', you must be more specific. Although the patient probably will not describe the site of his pain in anatomical terms, he can always point to the site of maximum intensity which you can convert into an exact description. If the pain is indistinct in nature and spread diffusely over a large area, you must describe the area in which the pain is felt and the point (indicated by the patient) of maximum discomfort.

It is also worthwhile asking about the **depth** of the pain. Patients can often tell you whether the pain is near to the skin or deep inside.

Revision Panel

The features of a pain that must be elicited

Site
Record the *exact* site

Time and mode of onset
Record the time and date of onset and the way the pain began.

Severity
Assess severity by its effect on the patient.

Nature
Aching, burning, stabbing, constricting, throbbing, distending, colic.

Progression of the pain
Describe the progression of the pain.

The end of the pain
Describe how the pain ended. Was the end spontaneous or brought about by some action by the patient or doctor?

Duration
Record the length of the pain.

Relieving factors

Exacerbating factors

Radiation
Record the time and direction of any radiation of the pain. Remember to ask if the nature of the pain changed at the time it moved.

Cause
Make a note of the patient's opinion of the cause of the pain.

2 Time and mode of onset

It may be possible to pinpoint the onset of the pain to the minute, but if this cannot be done record the part of the day or night when the pain began.

To make your notes exact you must record the calendar dates on which events occurred, but it is also very useful to add in brackets the time interval between each event and the current examination, because it is these intervals, not the actual dates, which are more relevant to the problems of diagnosis. For example, 'Sudden onset of severe epigastric pain on 16th September, 1973, at 11.00 a.m. (3 days ago)'; but remember that such comments are useless if you forget to record the date of the examination.

Whenever you write a note about a patient, whether it be a short progress note or his full history, make certain that you start by writing down the date.

Ask if the pain began insidiously or suddenly.

3 Severity

Individuals react differently to pain. A severe pain to one person might be described as a dull ache by another. Consequently you must be wary of the adjectives used by the patient to describe the severity of his pain. A far better indication of severity is the effect of the pain on the patient's life. Did it stop him going to work? Did it make him go to bed? Did he have to call his doctor or try proprietary analgesics? Did it wake him up at night, or stop him going to sleep? Did it force him to lie still or roll around?

The answers to these questions will give you a better indication of the severity of a pain

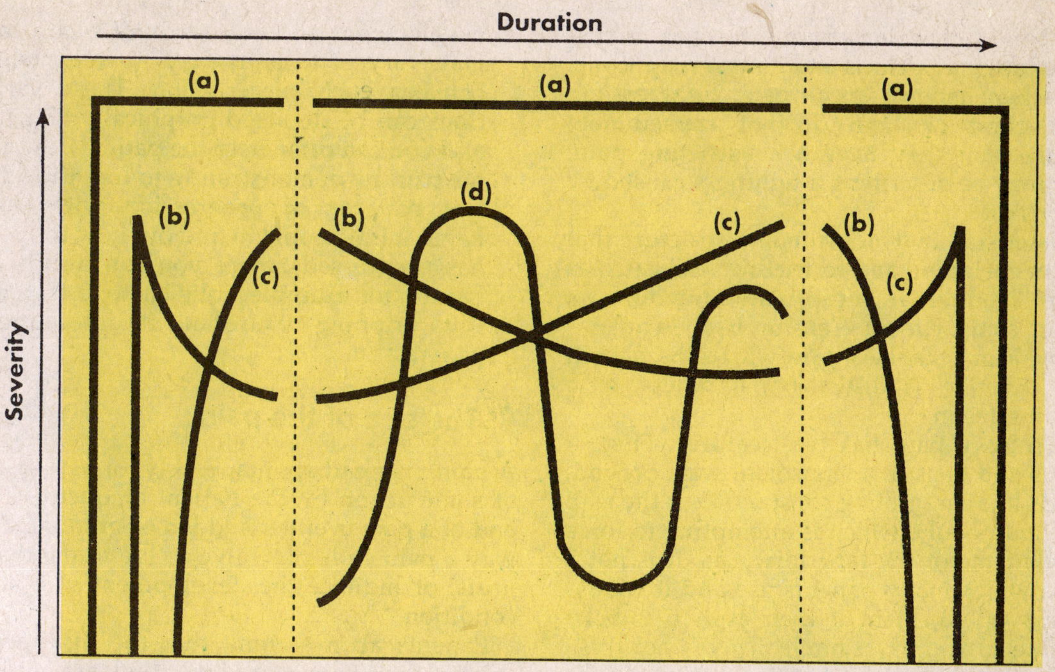

Onset	Progression	End
(a) Sudden onset at maximum severity	**(a)** Steady	**(a)** Sudden cessation
(b) Sudden onset and subsequent decline	**(b)** Gradual decline	**(b)** Gradual end
(c) Gradual onset	**(c)** Gradual worsening	**(c)** Crescendo and then sudden end
	(d) Fluctuating	

FIG. 1.1 The ways in which a pain can change (always record dates and calculate time intervals)

than words such as mild, severe, agonizing or terrible.

Your assessment of the way the patient responds to his pain, formed while you are taking the history, may profoundly affect your treatment.

4 Nature of the pain

Patients find it very difficult to describe the nature of their pain, but some of the adjectives which are commonly used, such as aching, stabbing, burning, throbbing, constricting, distending, gripping or colic, have a similar meaning to the majority of people.

Burning and **throbbing** sensations are within everyone's experience. We have all experienced a burning sensation from our skin following contact with intense heat, so when a patient spontaneously states that his pain is 'burning' in nature, it is likely to be so. We have all experienced a throbbing sensation at some time in our life so this description is also usually accurate.

A **stabbing** pain is sudden, severe, sharp, and short-lived.

The adjective **constricting** suggests a pain that encircles the relevant part (chest, abdomen, head or limb) and compresses it from all directions. A pain that feels like an iron band tightening around the chest is typical of angina pectoris and almost diagnostic, but when patients speak of a 'tightness' in their chest or limb do not immediately assume that they have a constricting pain; they may be describing a tightness caused by distension.

Distension may occur in any structure that has an encircling and restricting wall, such as bowel, bladder, an encapsulated tumour or a fascial compartment. Tension in the containing wall may cause a pain which the patient may describe as distension, tightness, or a bursting feeling.

A **colicky** pain has two features. First, it comes and goes in a sinusoidal way. Second, it feels like a migrating constriction in the wall of a hollow tube which is attempting to force the contents of the tube forwards. It is not a word which many patients use and it is dangerous to ask them if their pain is colicky without giving an example. This is not difficult because most of us have experienced colic during an episode of diarrhoea, and many women have suffered the colicky pains of labour. A recurring, intermittent pain is not necessarily a colic; it must also have a gripping nature.

'Just a pain, doctor.' Most pains have none of the features mentioned above and are described by the patient as 'a pain' which may vary in severity from a mild discomfort or ache to an agonizing pain that makes him think he is about to die. If the patient cannot describe the nature of his pain, do not press him. You will only make him try to fit his pain to your suggestions and ultimately mislead yourself.

5 Progression of the pain

Once begun, a pain may progress in a variety of ways.

It may begin at its maximum intensity and remain at this level until it goes.

It may increase steadily until it reaches a peak or a plateau, or conversely begin at its peak and decline slowly.

The severity of a pain may fluctuate. The intensity of the pain at the peaks and troughs of the fluctuations, and the rate of development and regression of each peak, may vary. The pain may go completely between each exacerbation. These variations can be depicted graphically (Fig.1.1) and you can often help the patient describe his pain by demonstrating to him the various patterns of progression with your hand. It is essential to find out how the pain has progressed before you can decide its nature; for example, colic has two features – its gripping nature and its intermittent progression.

6 The end of the pain

A pain may end spontaneously, or as a result of some action by the patient or doctor. The end of a pain is either sudden or gradual. The way a pain ends may give a clue to the diagnosis, or indicate the development of a new condition.

Patients always think that the disappearance of their pain means that they are getting better. They are usually right, but not always; their condition may have got worse.

7 Duration of the pain

The duration of a pain will be apparent from the time of its onset and end, but nevertheless it is worthwhile stating the duration of the pain in your notes. The length of any periods of exacerbation or remission should also be recorded.

8 Factors which relieve the pain

If there is anything, such as position, movement, a hot-water bottle, aspirins, food, antacids, etc., which relieves the pain, the patient is likely to know of it because the natural response to a pain is to search for a way to relieve it. Sometimes patients try the most bizarre remedies and many convince themselves that some minor change in habit or a personal remedy has been helpful, so accept their replies to this question with caution.

9 Factors which exacerbate the pain

Anything that makes the pain worse is also likely to be known to the patient. The type of stimulus which exacerbates a pain will depend upon the organ from which the pain emanates, and the cause of the pain. For example, alimentary tract pains may be made worse by eating particular types of food; musculoskeletal pains are affected by joint movements, muscle exercise and posture. If the initial description of the pain gives an idea of its source, it is acceptable to ask direct questions about those stimuli which you think might affect the pain.

10 Radiation

Radiation is the extension of the pain to another site whilst the initial pain persists. For example, a patient with a posterior penetrating duodenal ulcer will have a persistent pain in the epigastrium but sometimes the pain spreads through the abdomen to his back. The extension of the pain usually has the same character as the initial pain.

A pain may occur in one site and then reappear in another. This is not radiation: it is a new pain in another place.

If both pains are caused by the same condition, the second pain is called a **referred pain.** Thus referred pain is a pain which is felt at a distance from its source. For example, inflammation of the diaphragm will cause a pain which is felt at the tip of the shoulder. A referred pain is caused by the inability of the central nervous system to distinguish between visceral and somatic sensory impulses. From the patient's viewpoint the pain is where he feels it – the fact that the source is some distant organ does not concern him.

11 Cause

It is worthwhile asking the patient what he thinks about the cause of his pain. Even if he is hopelessly wrong you will get some insight into his worries. Sometimes a patient will be obsessed with the cause of his complaint and careful questioning may reveal that he will gain or lose compensation or insurance money as the result of your opinion.

Always listen to the patient's views with care and tolerance.

HISTORY OF A LUMP

When you examine a lump you attempt to discover its site, shape, size, surface, edge, consistence, tenderness, temperature and reducibility. However, your findings at the time of examination will not necessarily be typical of the lump when it was first noticed. Most patients with a lump feel it frequently and should be able to tell you about the history of its clinical features. Therefore you should seek answers to the following questions.

1 When was the lump first noticed?

It is important to be precise with dates and terminology. Do not write 'the lump first appeared 6 months ago', when you mean 'the lump was first noticed 6 months ago'. Many lumps may exist for months, even years, before the patient notices them.

2 What made the patient notice the lump?

There are three common answers to this question:

'I felt/saw it when washing.'

'I had a pain and found the lump when I felt the painful area.'

'Someone else noticed it and told me about it.'

The presence or absence of pain is important, particularly if it is the presenting feature. In very general terms, pain is usually associated with inflammation, not neoplastic change. Most patients expect cancer to be painful – and do themselves irreparable harm by ignoring a lump just because it does not hurt them.

3 What are the symptoms of the lump?

The lump may be painful. If so, you must take a careful history of the pain, its duration, progression, nature, etc., as described earlier in this chapter. The characteristic feature of pain associated with acute infection is its throbbing nature.

A lump may be disfiguring or interfering with movement, respiration or swallowing. Describe the history of each symptom carefully.

4 Has the lump changed since it was first noticed?

This is where you use the patient's own knowledge of his physical signs. The feature most apparent to the patient is the size of the lump. He should be able to tell you if it has got bigger, smaller, or fluctuated in size. If the patient has noticed a change in size he may also have appreciated a change in shape, a change in consistence, or a change in the nature of the surface and the edge of the lump. Another feature he will have observed closely is tenderness, which may have altered in any of the ways that a pain can change.

5 Does the lump ever disappear?

A lump may disappear on lying down, or during exercise, and yet be irreducible at the time of your examination. The patient should always be asked if the lump ever goes away, because this physical characteristic is peculiar to only a few varieties of lump.

6 Has the patient ever had any other lumps?

You must ask this question because it might not have occurred to the patient that there could be any connection between his present lump and a previous lump, or even a coexisting one.

7 What does the patient think caused the lump?

Lumps occasionally follow injuries or systemic illnesses known to the patient.

Revision Panel 1.3

The history of a lump or an ulcer

Duration
When was it first noticed?

First symptom
What brought it to the patient's notice?

Other symptoms
What symptoms does it cause?

Progression
How has it changed since it was first noticed?

Persistence
Has it ever disappeared or healed?

Multiplicity
Has (or had) the patient any other lumps or ulcers?

Cause
What does the patient think caused it?

HISTORY OF AN ULCER

An ulcer is a break in the continuity of an epithelium. Unless it is painless and in an inaccessible part of the body, the patient will notice it from the moment it begins, and if he has dressed it each day he will know a great deal about its clinical features.

The questions to be asked concerning an ulcer follow a pattern similar to those for a lump.

1 When was the ulcer first noticed?

Ask the patient if he thinks he noticed the ulcer when it began or whether it could have been present for some time before he noticed it. The latter often occurs with neurotrophic ulcers on the sole of the foot.

2 What drew the patient's attention to the ulcer?

The commonest reason is pain. Occasionally, the presenting feature is bleeding, or a purulent discharge which may be foul smelling.

3 What are the symptoms of the ulcer?

The ulcer may be painful. It may interfere with daily activities such as walking, eating or defaecation. Record the history of each symptom.

4 How has the ulcer changed since it first appeared?

The patient's observations about changes in size, shape, edge, depth, base, discharge and pain are likely to be detailed and accurate. If the ulcer has healed and broken down, record the features of each episode.

5 Has the patient ever had a similar ulcer on the same site, or elsewhere?

Obtain as complete a history of any previous ulcer as for the present one.

6 What does the patient think caused the ulcer?

Most patients believe they know the cause of their ulcer, and are often right. The commonest initiating cause is trauma. If so, try to assess the severity and type of injury. A large ulcer following a minor injury suggests that the skin was abnormal before the injury.

THE CLINICAL EXAMINATION

Each chapter of this book deals with a specific region of the body and its surgical diseases. Those methods of examination peculiar to each region are described in detail in the relevant chapter. The emphasis in this introductory chapter is on the importance of taking an *exact and full history*, but it would not be complete without a description of the basic plan of a physical examination, with particular reference to those regions not discussed in later chapters, such as the heart, the lungs and the nervous system. As this is a thumb-nail sketch of clinical examination, your knowledge will need to be enlarged by additional reading, but your understanding and ability to solve the practical problems of clinical examination can only be clarified by frequent bedside practice. Examine as many patients as you can. Nothing can be learnt without frequent practice. *Repetition is the secret of learning*. This axiom applies as much to the doctor as it does to the sportsman or the concert pianist. You will become confident of your interpretation of your visual, tactile and aural appreciation of the patient's body only by repeatedly exercising these senses.

An experienced clinician rarely begins the routine physical examination without some suspicions about the diagnosis suggested by the history. Consequently, he often modifies the impartial systematized examination described in textbooks by specifically looking for signs which will confirm or refute his tentative diagnoses. If he detects a sign that denies his suspicions, he returns to the textbook routine. *Students must not do this*. Although it is a practical and time-saving method in a busy clinic, and acceptable from someone with years of clinical experience who can pick out those patients to whom it can be applied, it is fundamentally wrong. Bad habits grow fast without encouragement. Unless the student disciplines himself to use the standard textbook routine for every physical examination, he will surely make many mistakes and, as time passes, completely forget some parts of the examination, with serious consequences.

The easiest way to ensure that you perform a complete examination is to learn the routine by heart and repeat it to yourself during the examination. Whilst looking at a lump, say to yourself, 'position, shape, size', etc. If you do not do this you will find, when you sit down to write your notes, that you have forgotten to elicit some of the lump's physical features and will have to go back to the patient. Always keep to the basic pattern of looking, feeling, tapping and listening (inspection, palpation, percussion, auscultation), whatever you are examining. However, whilst keeping to the routine it is often best to examine first the part of body which is the source of the patient's complaint.

General assessment

The first part of the physical examination is performed when taking the history. While you are talking to the patient you can observe his general demeanour, his intellectual ability and intelligence, and his attitudes to his disease, to you, to his treatment, and to society in general. These observations affect the manner in which you conduct the examination. Your instructions will need to be extremely simple if the patient is unintelligent, or coaxing and gentle if the patient is shy or embarrassed. Record your views on these features at the beginning of the history.

Record, especially in emergency circumstances, both medical and surgical, the patient's level of consciousness by using the Glasgow Coma Scale (Revision Panel 1.4).

Make a note of the patient's general mental state, his memory and use of words. There is a whole vocabulary used by the neurologists to describe various speech and communication disorders. Some of the common ones are:

Dysarthria: impaired speech caused by muscle weakness.
Dysphasia or **aphasia**: impaired or absent ability to speak caused by a neurological abnormality.
Dysgraphia or **agraphia**: impaired or absent ability to write.
Dyspraxia or **apraxia**: impaired or absent ability to perform purposeful movements *in the absence of paralysis*.

You can also observe a number of physical characteristics when taking the history, such as **posture, mobility, weight, colour of skin, facial appearance** and **general body build**.

Revision Panel 1.4
The Glasgow Coma Scale

	Score
Eyes	
Open spontaneously	4
Open to command	3
Open to pain	2
Do not open	1
Speech	
Sensible / orientated	5
Confused	4
Inappropriate words	3
Incomprehensible sounds	2
None	1
Motor responses	
Obeys commands	6
Localizes stimuli	5
Withdraws from stimuli	4
Flexion responses	3
Extension responses	2
None	1
Total	

Hold the patient's hand and examine it

Make physical contact with the patient early in the examination by holding his hand and counting the pulse. It is very important for the patient to feel that you are willing to get physically as well as mentally close to him. The physical contact that is essential for the examination forges an intimate bond between you and the patient. It is an extraordinary privilege granted to you by the patient and must never be abused.

The features of the hands to be observed are as follows.

Revision Panel 1.5
Some common causes of weight loss

In the young
- Malnutrition
- Diabetes
- Malabsorption
- Anorexia nervosa
- Tuberculosis

From middle age onwards
- Diabetes
- Thyrotoxicosis
- Chronic hypoxia
- Chronic heart failure
- Malignant disease
- Senile cachexia
- Neglect

Pulse See details on page 23.

Nails Look at the colour and shape of the nails. Spoon-shaped nails (koilonychia) are associated with anaemia, clubbing of the nails occurs in pulmonary and cardiopulmonary disease, and splinter haemorrhages under the nails are caused by small arterial emboli. Pits and furrows are associated with skin diseases such as psoriasis. Bitten nails may indicate nervousness and anxiety.

Temperature Observe the temperature of the hands – but remember that it will be affected by room temperature and the duration of exposure.

Moisture Are the patient's palms sweating excessively?

Colour Pallor of the skin of the hands, especially in the skin creases of the palm and in the nail beds, suggests anaemia. Reddish-blue hands occur in polycythaemia and cor pulmonale. The fingers may be stained with nicotine.

Callosities The position of any callosities may reflect the patient's occupation.

Examine the head and neck

Eyes Test the reaction of the pupils to light and accommodation. Examine the eye movements. Look for exophthalmos and corneal or lens opacities. Test the visual acuity and the visual fields. Inspect the fundi with an ophthalmoscope.

Ears and nose Do not forget to look into the ears to inspect the external auditory canal and the ear-drum. Look up the nose. The ears and nose are often forgotten during routine examination but they are important, particularly if there is any possibility of disease in the head and neck.

Mouth Note the colour and state of the lips. Ask to see the patient's tongue; observe its movement, symmetry and surface.

Look at the teeth and gums. Use a spatula to inspect the soft palate, tonsils and posterior wall of the oropharynx.

Neck The important features to examine in the neck are the jugular veins, the trachea, the thyroid gland and the lymph nodes.

Examine the cranial nerves

'On Old Olympus Towering Tops A Finn And German Picked Some Hops' is the most-used mnemonic for the names of the cranial nerves.

I Olfactory nerve

Ask the patient about his sense of smell and test it with bottles containing cloves, peppermint, etc.

II Optic nerve

Test the **visual acuity**, i.e. the ability to read or recognize known objects at varying distances. Test the **visual fields** – sit directly in front of the patient, ask him to close one eye and look straight at you with the other eye. Keeping your hand mid-way between you and the patient, extend your arm so that your hand is beyond your own peripheral vision. Then gradually move it towards the mid-line until it appears in your visual field. If you and the patient have normal visual fields you will both see your finger at the same time. Test **colour vision** with Ishihara charts.

III Oculomotor nerve

This nerve supplies all but two of the extrinsic **eye muscles**, and the **levator palpebrae superioris** and the **muscle of accommodation**. If it fails to function, the eye will turn downwards and outwards, the upper lid will droop (ptosis) and the pupil will be fixed. Sometimes individual muscles supplied by the third nerve can be paralysed. To test the superior rectus ask the patient to 'look up'; inferior rectus – 'look down'; medial rectus – 'converge'; and inferior oblique – 'look up and out'.

IV Trochlear nerve

This nerve supplies the **superior oblique muscle**, which turns the eye downwards and outwards. If the nerve is damaged and the patient cannot perform this movement, his eye will look inwards and he will have diplopia below the horizontal plane.

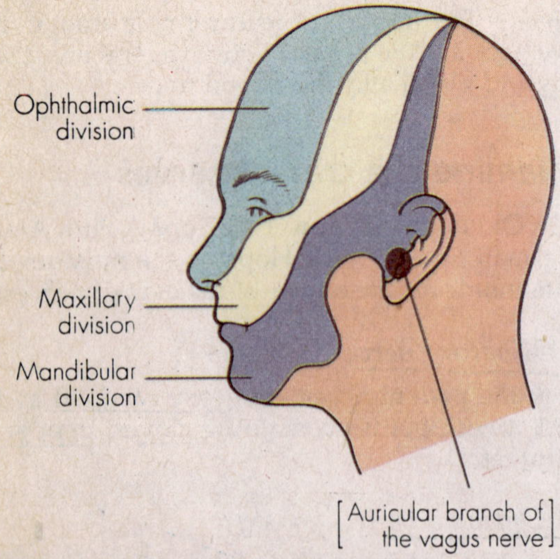

FIG. 1.2 The distribution of the three sensory divisions of the trigeminal nerve

V Trigeminal nerve

This nerve has sensory and motor functions. It is **sensory** to the whole of the side of the face. The cutaneous distribution of its three sensory divisions – ophthalmic, maxillary and mandibular – is shown in Fig. 1.2.

The trigeminal nerve is also the sensory nerve of the conjunctiva and the inside of the mouth, so elicit the conjunctival reflex (ophthalmic division), the sensitivity of the mucous membrane of the nose, pharynx, roof of mouth, soft palate and tonsil, and elicit the palatal reflex (maxillary division) and test the sensitivity of the tongue, lower teeth and mucous membrane over the mandible (mandibular division).

The taste fibres of the anterior two-thirds of the tongue travel with the lingual nerve, one of the branches of the mandibular division of the trigeminal nerve, after leaving the geniculate ganglion as the chorda tympani. Taste can be tested with sweet, sour, salt and bitter substances, such as sugar, acid, salt and quinine.

The **motor fibres** of the trigeminal nerve run with the mandibular division to the muscles of mastication – masseter, temporalis and the pterygoid muscles. Ask the patient to clench his teeth and feel if the masseter contracts.

VI Abducens nerve

This nerve supplies the **lateral rectus muscle**, which turns the eye outwards. If the patient attempts to look sideways, the eye will not move and he will get diplopia.

VII Facial nerve

This is the motor nerve of the muscles of facial expression. When a facial nerve fails to function, the affected side of the face is flabby, the eyelids cannot be closed properly and the mouth becomes asymmetrical when the patient tries to bare his teeth. He cannot whistle. The nucleus of the seventh nerve is in the pons varolii. Any lesion in the tract or nerve distal to the nucleus causes paralysis of the whole of the side of the face; but a lesion above the nucleus misses those fibres coming from the opposite hemisphere to the upper part of the face so that the function of the forehead and eyelid muscles is preserved. To test the facial nerve ask the patient to look up (the forehead should wrinkle), to close his eyes tightly (test the strength of the orbicularis oculi by trying to part the eyelids) and to show you his teeth (lips should part symmetrically).

VIII Auditory nerve

This nerve innervates the hearing mechanism in the cochlear and the position sense organs in the semicircular canals. Hearing can be tested very easily by speaking softly and asking the patient to repeat your words, or by asking him if he can hear your thumb and finger rubbing lightly together close to his ear. If the nerve is normal and the deafness is caused by inadequate conduction through the bones of the middle ear, a **conduction deafness**, the note of a tuning fork will be heard clearly if its base is placed firmly on the mastoid process but not when it is held in the air close to the ear. This is called Rinne's test. If the tuning fork is placed on the centre of the forehead, the ear with a conduction deafness will appreciate a louder sound. This is Weber's test. When there is nerve deafness the sound cannot be heard whatever the position of the tuning fork.

The sensitivity of the vestibular apparatus is tested by assessing the response to changes in temperature in the external meatus – the caloric test. This must be done under careful supervision in the Ear, Nose and Throat Department.

IX Glossopharyngeal nerve

This nerve is the sensory nerve of the posterior third of the tongue, including taste, and the mucous membrane of the pharynx. It is motor to the middle constrictor of the pharynx. You can test the sensory integrity of this nerve by stroking the back of the oropharynx, so causing the pharyngeal gag reflex.

X Vagus (pneumogastric) nerve

This is the motor nerve of the soft palate, pharynx and larynx, and the sensory nerve of the heart, lungs and gut. Ask the patient to open his mouth wide and say 'Aarrh'. The soft palate should arch upwards symmetrically. If one side of the palate is paralysed, it will not move and the uvula will be pulled over towards the functioning side. Loss of function of the recurrent laryngeal nerves (branches of the vagus) should be suspected if there is a change in the patient's voice or an inability to cough. The vocal cords must be examined with a laryngeal mirror to make a definite diagnosis.

XI Spinal accessory nerve

This nerve supplies the trapezius and sternomastoid muscles. The function of these muscles is tested by asking the patient to shrug his shoulders, and to press the point of his chin downwards on your hand.

XII Hypoglossal nerve

This is the motor nerve of the tongue. When one hypoglossal nerve is paralysed, the tongue will deviate to that side when the patient tries to push the tongue forwards. The weak side will also be wasted.

Examine the chest wall and lungs

Inspection

The colour of the patient and his respiratory rate will give some indication of the adequacy of ventilation. Cyanosis caused by a cardiopulmonary abnormality is most easily seen in the inner aspect of the lips. Cyanosis of the nail beds and the tip of the nose and ears may be caused by a peripheral or a central abnormality. If these areas are a deep reddish-purple colour and the patient's face is also red and plethoric, he may be polycythaemic, not cyanotic. Cyanosis is difficult to detect if the patient is anaemic.

Count the rate of respiration and notice the rhythm A regular fluctuation of respiratory rate and volume with periods of apnoea between episodes of tachypnoea is called Cheyne–Stokes or periodic respiration. It is caused by variations in the sensitivity of the respiratory centre to normal stimuli, and occurs commonly in heart failure and following severe cerebrovascular accidents. Notice if respiration seems to require voluntary effort and compare the duration of inspiration with expiration. Watch the chest during inspiration to see if there is any inward movement of the intercostal spaces (paradoxical movement).

Record any abnormality in the shape of the chest. The two common deformities are funnel chest (pectus excavatum) and pigeon chest (pectus carinatum) (see Fig. 8.29, page 219).

Revision Panel 1.6

Common causes of pleuritic pain

- Pneumonia
- Pulmonary infarction (thromboembolic)
- Neoplasia (primary and secondary)
- Fractured ribs
- Muscle strains
- Pre-rash herpes zoster
- Bornholm disease

Revision Panel 1.7

Common causes of haemoptysis

- Acute respiratory tract infection
- Lung cancer
- Tuberculosis
- Pulmonary infarction (thromboembolic)
- Bronchiectasis

Palpation

Trachea Check the position of the trachea at the suprasternal notch.

Chest expansion Spread your hands around the chest so that the thumbs just meet in the mid-line. Ask the patient to take a deep breath. Your thumbs will be dragged apart to a distance roughly equivalent to half the chest expansion. If the expansion is asymmetrical it will be felt and seen. Chest expansion is the difference between the circumference of the chest at full inspiration and after a full expiration, measured at the level of the nipples.

Apex beat The apex beat is the lowest and most lateral point at which you can feel the cardiac impulse. It will move laterally if the heart enlarges but may move medially or laterally if the **mediastinum shifts**. The mediastinum (and the trachea) will move to one side if it is pulled over by a collapsed, contracting lung or pushed over by air or fluid in the opposite pleural cavity.

Tactile vocal fremitus Place your whole hand firmly on the chest and ask the patient to say '99'. The vibrations which you can feel with your hand are called the vocal fremitus. Compare the strength of these vibrations on either side of the chest, front and back, and over the apical, middle and basal zones.

To feel vocal fremitus the sound waves must be conducted through the air in the bronchi, bronchioles and alveoli to the chest wall. A blocked bronchus or a layer of fluid or air between the visceral and parietal layers of the pleura will suppress the conduction of the sound waves and reduce the intensity of the palpable fremitus. A stiffening of the substance of the lung tissue with patent air passages – as in very early pneumonia – increases conduction through the lung, and tactile vocal fremitus is increased.

Axillae Palpate both axillae.

Percussion

The whole of the surface of the lungs must be percussed. The surface markings of the lungs

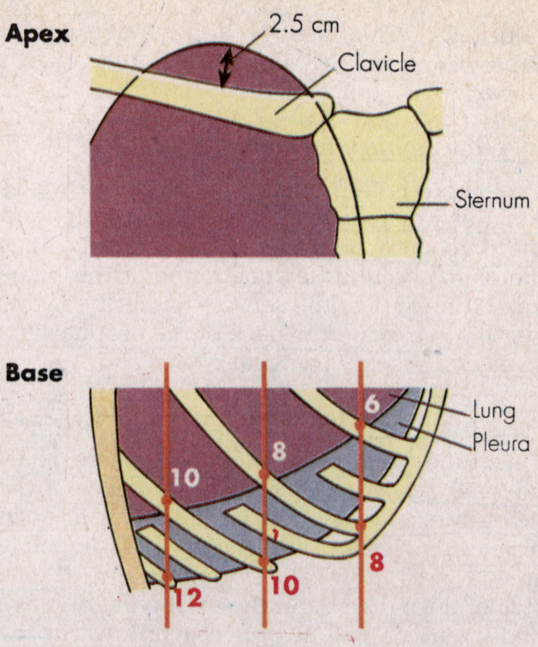

	Edge of erector spinae	Mid-axillary line	Mid-clavicular line
Lung	**10**	**8**	**6**
Pleura	**12**	**10**	**8**

FIG. 1.3 The surface markings of the lung and pleura

are shown in Fig. 1.3. Place one hand flat on the chest wall, keeping the finger you intend to strike straight and firmly applied to the underlying skin. Tap the centre of the middle phalanx of this finger with the tip of the middle finger of the other hand. Listen carefully to the sound and compare it with the sound produced by percussing the same area on the other side of the chest.

The two areas most often forgotten when percussing the chest are the lateral zones high in the axillae, and the anterior aspect of the apices behind the clavicles. Percuss this latter area by striking the clavicle directly with the percussing finger.

The normal chest gives a resonant sound when percussed; a sound which is, to some extent, felt by the percussing finger as well as being heard. Anything solid in the pleural space or in the substance of the lungs will

TACTILE VOCAL FREMITIS

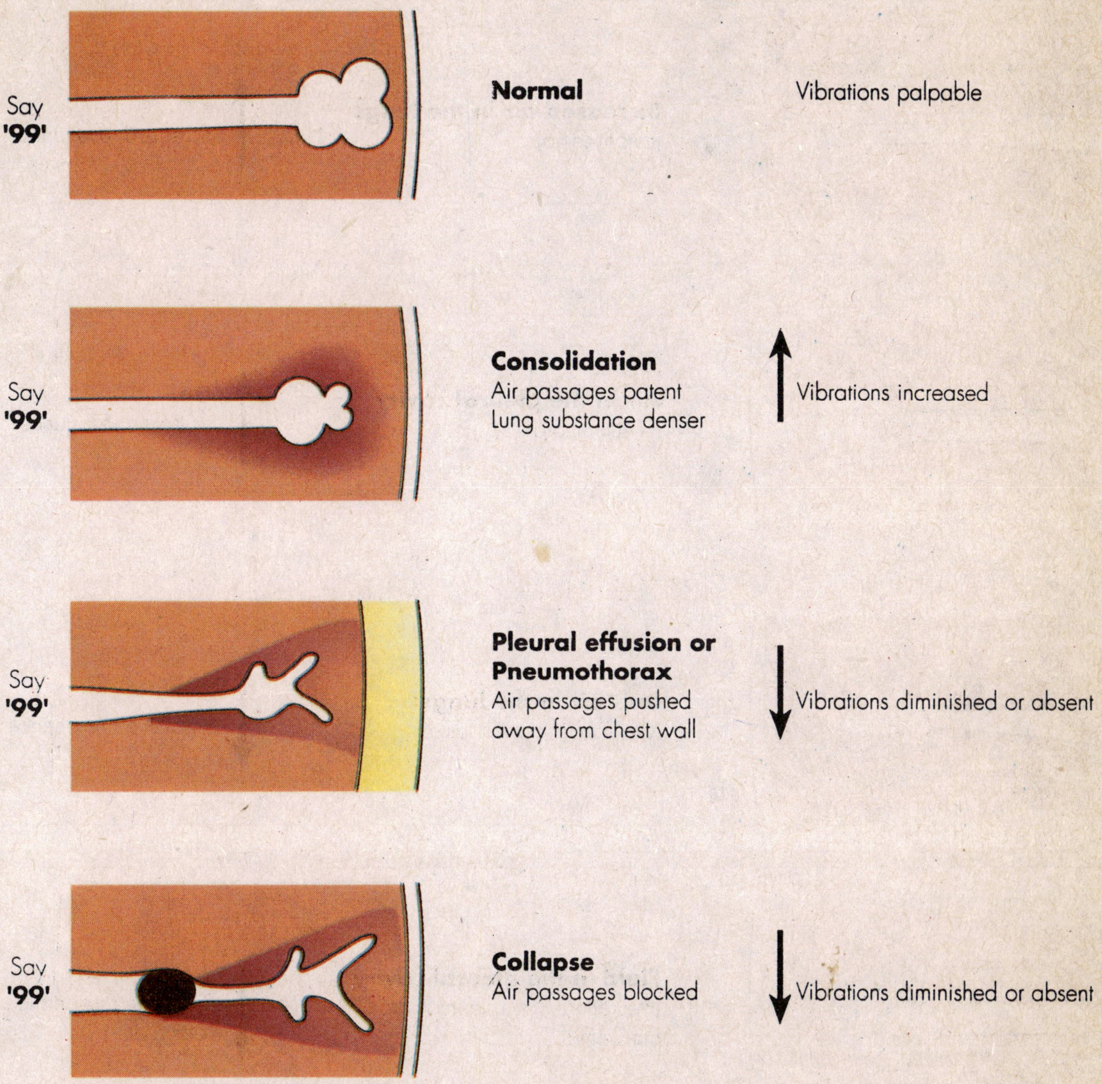

FIG. 1.4 Tactile vocal fremitus can only be felt if there are patent air passages right out to the chest wall

decrease the resonance and sound dull. Any extra air, whether in the pleural space (pneumothorax) or in the lung substance (emphysematous bullae), will make the sound more resonant (hyper-resonance) (see Fig. 1.5).

A sign peculiar to a large pneumothorax is the ringing resonance heard through a stethoscope when the percussion is performed by tapping a coin held against the chest wall with a second coin.

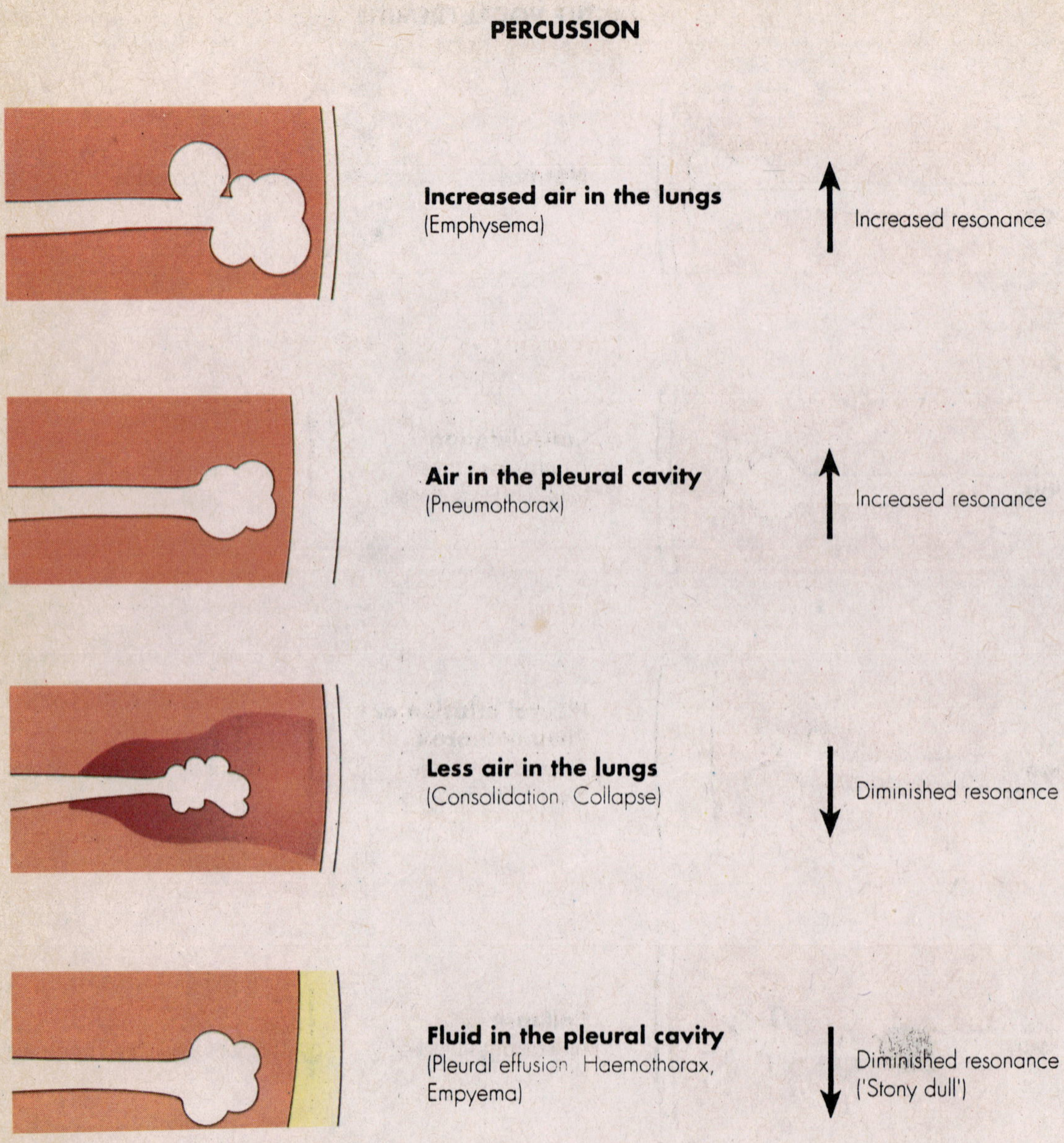

FIG. 1.5 The causes of change in lung resonance

Auscultation (see Figs 1.6 and 1.7)

The **normal sounds** of breathing can be heard all over the chest except over the heart and spine. They consist of an inspiratory sound followed immediately by a shorter, softer, expiratory sound. There is **no gap** between the two phases. This sound is known as **vesicular breathing** and is caused by the movement of air in and out of the smaller bronchioles and alveoli.

If the periphery of the lung is solid, as in pneumonia, you hear the sound of air moving in the larger bronchioles and main bronchi.

BREATH SOUNDS

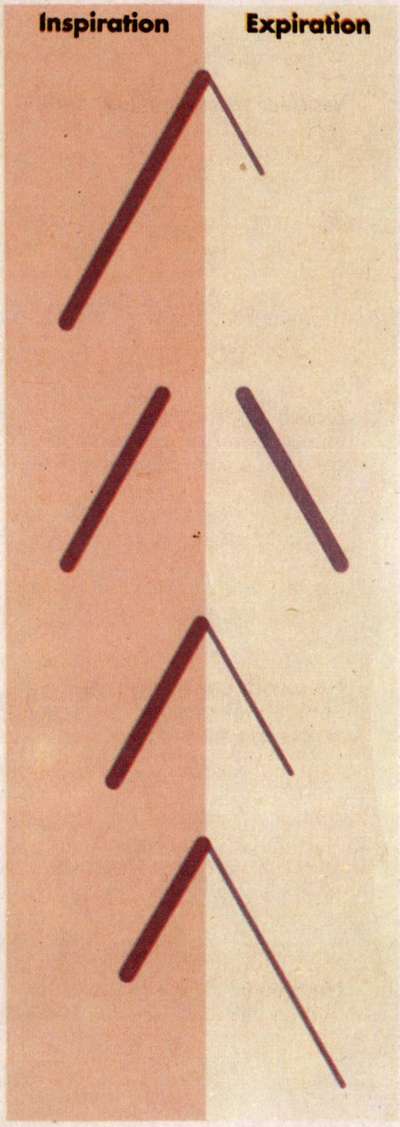

Vesicular	Expiration much shorter and softer than inspiration **No gap** between each phase
Bronchial	Inspiration and expiration of equal length and quality (harsh and loud) **Gap** between the two phases
Bronchovesicular	Inspiration and expiration of equal length but expiration is softer and smoother **No gap** between each phase
Asthmatic	Prolonged expiration, usually associated with inspiratory and expiratory rhonchi

FIG. 1.6

This sound is harsher and louder than vesicular breathing. **The inspiratory and expiratory phases are of equal length and separated by a short, silent gap**. This is called **bronchial breathing**. The quality of the sound and the gap are the two distinguishing features.

The pitch of bronchial breathing may be high or low. The high-pitched variety is sometimes called **tubular** bronchial breathing. The low-pitched variety, which sounds like the noise produced by blowing across the mouth of a jar, is called **amphoric** bronchial breathing. Amphoric sounds are heard when air is

EFFECT OF LUNG DISEASE ON THE BREATH SOUNDS

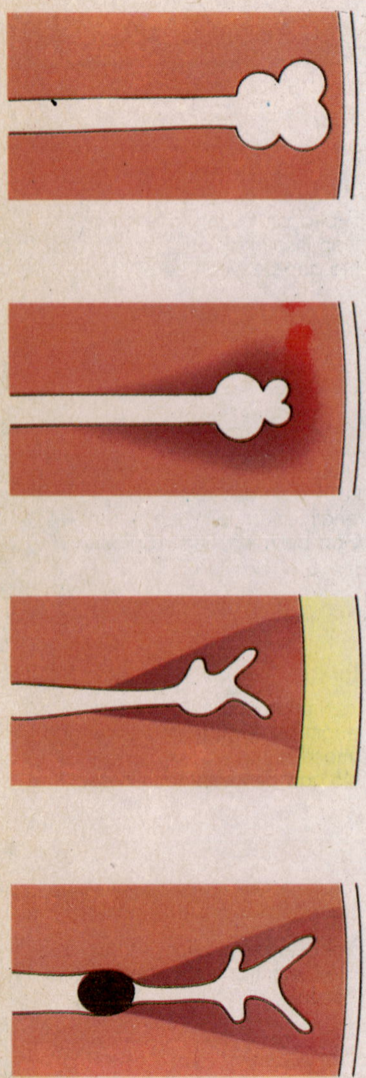

Normal	**Vesicular** sounds audible
Consolidation	**Bronchial** sounds audible, caused by increased sound conduction from large bronchi
Pleural effusion or Pneumothorax	**No sounds** audible as layer of fluid or air prevents conduction of sound to the surface
Collapse	**No sounds** audible as obstruction of bronchus stops sound conduction

FIG. 1.7 The causes of abnormal breath sounds

passing in and out of a cavity in the lung such as a tuberculous cavity.

There is a type of breath sound mid-way between vesicular and bronchial breathing, known as **bronchovesicular** breathing. In this variety the inspiratory and expiratory sounds are of equal length and slightly harsher than vesicular breathing, but there is **no gap** between the two phases. Bronchovesicular breathing is often heard in normal people over the anterior aspect of the upper lobes where there are large bronchi near the surface of the lung.

Breath sounds are abolished or diminished by any process which reduces the normal conduction of sound through the lung substance and chest wall. The two common causes are bronchial obstruction (producing collapse of the distal part of the lung) and pleural effusion or pneumothorax (see Fig. 1.7).

When the lung substance is thickened (consolidation) but the air passages stay patent, the thickened lung transmits the sound from the larger bronchi. Thus bronchial breathing is heard over an area of consolidated lung but there are no breath sounds over an area of collapsed lung.

Added sounds

There are three varieties of added sounds: rhonchi, râles and crepitations.

Wheezes (rhonchi) These are the whistling noises made by air passing through narrowed air passages. They are commonly heard in patients with asthma or chronic bronchitis. Their pitch depends upon the velocity of air flow, and the diameter of the bronchioles from which they originate. They are unmistakable.

Coarse crackles (râles) These are the coarse bubbling noises caused by air passing through bronchioles containing water, mucus or pus. The sound is identical to that made by air bubbling through water. Moving the fluid may abolish the noise, so ask the patient to take a deep breath and cough, and then listen again. If the bubbling sounds have gone, they must have been râles because crepitations cannot be abolished in this way.

Fine crackles (crepitations) These are fine crackling sounds similar to the noise you hear if you roll a lock of your hair between your thumb and index finger. They are said to be produced as the alveoli and their ducts pop open to allow air entry when there is interstitial oedema. Crepitations are heard over areas of consolidation, such as pneumonia, and often provide important evidence of left ventricular failure. They are not abolished by coughing.

Some authorities do not distinguish râles from crepitations and use the term **moist sounds** for either variety.

Pleural rub If the pleura is inflamed, its visceral and parietal layers cannot slide easily over one another. As the roughened pleural surfaces rub together they produce a noise similar to the sound heard when a finger is pressed hard onto a pane of glass and then slid across it. It is a mixture of grating and squeaking sounds. A pleural rub can only be heard when the chest is moving, i.e. during inspiration or expiration. The patient often complains of pleuritic pain over an area where there is an audible rub.

Examine the heart and circulation

Much will have been learnt about the circulation from your initial observations of the patient's colour, rate of respiration and activity. It is easiest, and common practice, to feel the pulse when you take the patient's hand at the beginning of the examination.

The pulse

The following features should be observed and recorded.

Rate Express the rate in beats/minute. Do not count the pulse for 5 seconds and multiply by 12; always count for at least 15 seconds, longer if the beat is irregular.

Rhythm The pulse beat may be regular or irregular. If it is irregular it may have a regular recurring pattern or be totally irregular. The latter is sometimes called an irregularly irregular pulse and indicates atrial fibrillation. Some varieties of irregular pulse are shown in Fig. 1.8.

Volume The examining fingers can appreciate the expansion of the artery with each beat and consequently get an impression of the amount of blood passing through the artery. A patient with a high cardiac output will have a strong pulse. A patient suffering from haemorrhagic shock will have a weak, thin, 'thready' pulse.

Nature of the pressure wave Every pressure wave has definable characteristics such as the rate of increase and decrease of pressure, height, and possibly regular irregularities.

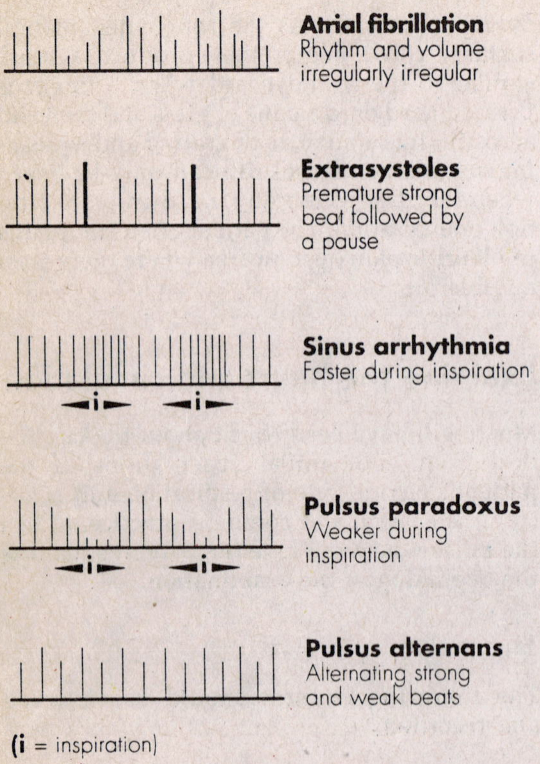

FIG. 1.8 Common variations of the rhythm and volume of the pulse

The shape of the pulse wave can be appreciated with the fingers, often more easily over the carotid than the radial artery. A steep rise followed by a rapid fall, with a large pulse pressure (high peak), is called a 'collapsing' or 'water-hammer pulse' and is typical of aortic regurgitation. Conversely, aortic stenosis causes a slow rise and fall. Figure 1.9 shows the common types of pulse wave.

Nature of the artery It is quite easy to estimate the diameter of the radial artery and guess the thickness of its wall, but the presence or absence of thickening of the radial artery gives no indication of the thickness of other vessels in the body.

Measure the blood pressure

The blood pressure is usually measured in the brachial artery with a sphygmomanometer.

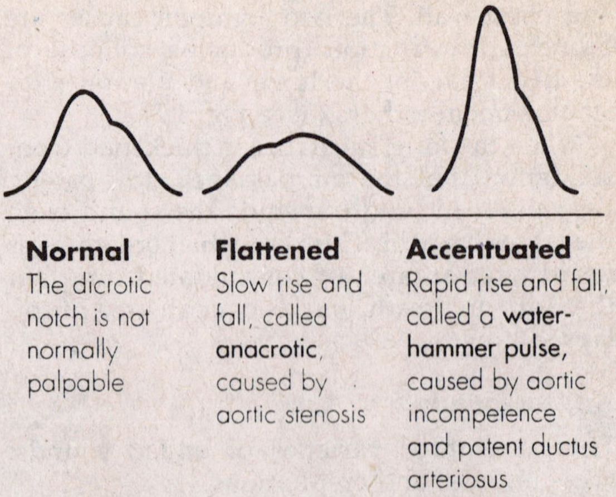

FIG. 1.9 Variations of the pulse wave

The cuff should be firmly wrapped around the middle of the upper arm. The commencement of flow below the cuff, as the cuff is deflated, is detected by listening over the brachial artery at the elbow with a stethoscope or palpating the pulse at the wrist. The sounds which can be heard over the artery below the cuff when the blood flow begins are caused by turbulent blood flow. They were first described by Korotkoff and are known as Korotkoff sounds.

Pump up the cuff to a high level (250 mmHg) and then let it down slowly until the sounds begin. This point is the systolic pressure. Continue to lower the cuff pressure and note the pressure at which the Korotkoff sounds suddenly diminish or, more often, disappear. This is the diastolic pressure. The cuff must fit snugly and be at least 10 cm wide. A narrow cuff gives false readings. If the arm is very fat the readings will be falsely high by as much as 10 mmHg.

Whenever there is the possibility of disease of the aorta and its branches, **measure the blood pressure in both arms.**

Inspect the head and neck again

You will already have looked at the patient's skin, face and general demeanour. Look again for the signs particularly indicative of cardiovascular disease – **cyanosis, plethora and dyspnoea.**

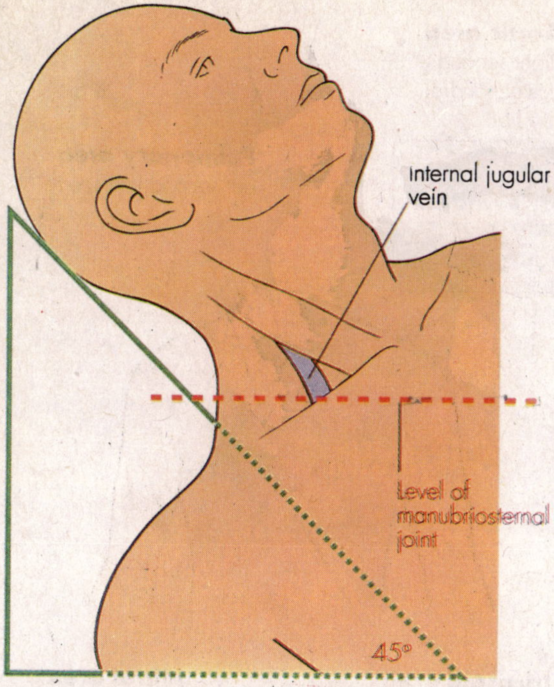

FIG. 1.10 The measurement of the jugular venous pressure

Xanthoma These are grey-yellow plaques of lipid in the skin. They often occur in the skin of the upper eyelid. Their presence may indicate an abnormal lipid metabolism such as hyperlipidaemia, but they are not uncommon in patients with normal blood lipids.

Arcus senilis This is a white ring at the junction of the iris and sclera. It is said to be more common in people with advanced arteriosclerosis, but in practice it is not a reliable indicator of the presence of vascular disease. If it is present in a patient less than 40 years old, it may indicate the presence of a hyperlipoproteinaemia.

Jugular venous pressure The pressure in the great veins is slightly greater than the pressure in the right atrium. The pressure in the right atrium is one of the most important controlling mechanisms of cardiac activity. An increase of right atrial pressure raises cardiac output by stimulating an increase of cardiac contractility and rate. Thus it can be said that the right atrial pressure 'drives' the heart. The pressure in the right atrium can be estimated clinically from the pressure in the internal jugular veins. In a normal person, reclining at 45°, the great veins in the neck are collapsed. There should be no visible venous pulsations above the level of the manubriosternal joint which, when the patient is reclining at 45°, is at the same level as the mid-point of the clavicles (see Fig. 1.10).

If there are visible pulsations in the internal jugular veins when the patient is reclining at 45°, the right atrial pressure is raised. The vertical distance between the upper limit of the venous distension and the level of the clavicle should be estimated by eye and expressed and recorded in centimetres.

Obstruction of the great veins in the superior mediastinum will also cause distension of the neck veins but there will not be a visible venous pulse wave.

Neck arteries Feel the pulses in the neck and listen along their whole length, especially over the sternoclavicular joints, in the supraclavicular fossae, and at the level of the hyoid bone just below the angle of the jaw. These sites correspond to the origins of the subclavian, vertebral and internal carotid arteries, respectively (see Fig. 1.11).

The trachea Deviation of the trachea from the mid-line can be detected by palpating the position of its anterior surface just above the suprasternal notch.

Examine the heart

Inspection The heart may be seen to be beating rapidly or to be heaving up the chest wall with each beat. **Dyspnoea** and **tachypnoea** may be caused by heart disease.

Palpation Place your whole hand firmly on the chest wall, just below the left nipple, and ascertain the strength of the **cardiac impulse.** It may be weak, normal or heaving in nature. The apex beat is the lowest and most lateral point at which the cardiac impulse can be felt. It should be in the fifth intercostal space, near the mid-clavicular line (an imaginary vertical line which passes through the middle of the clavicle). If the heart is enlarged, the apex beat

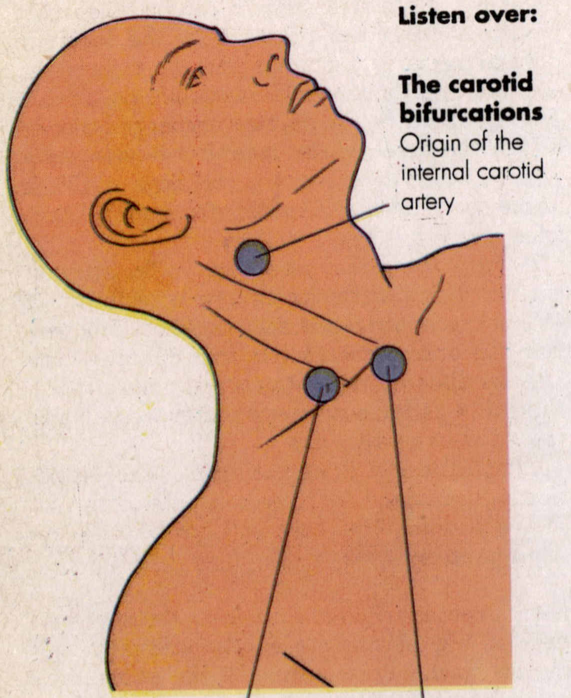

FIG. 1.11 The sites of auscultation for vascular bruits on the neck

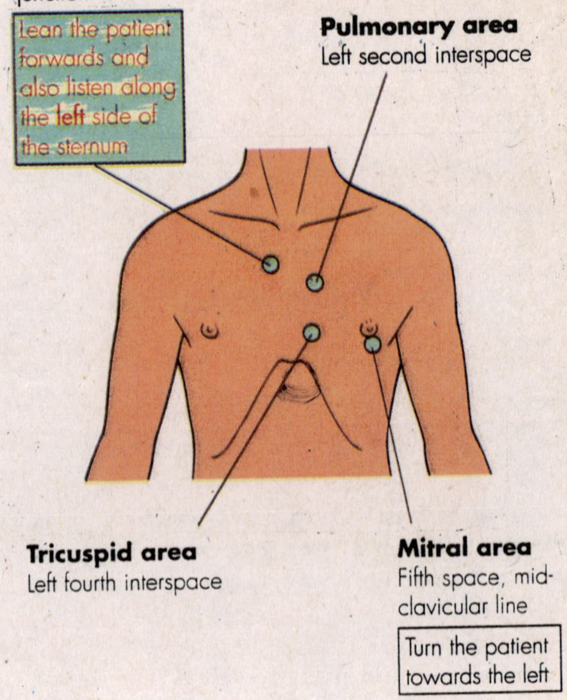

FIG. 1.12 Areas of cardiac auscultation

moves laterally and may be felt as far out as the mid-axillary line. In addition to the cardiac impulse it may be possible to feel vibrations, called **thrills**, which correspond to audible heart murmurs. Thrills may be felt during systole, diastole or throughout the whole cardiac cycle.

Remember to palpate the back of the chest. Thrills from abnormalities of the aorta, such as a patent ductus arteriosus or coarctation, are conducted posteriorly as well as anteriorly.

Feel the femoral pulses.

Percussion The area of cardiac dullness should be delineated by percussion. Enlargement of the atria may cause the cardiac dullness to extend to the right of the sternum.

Auscultation The whole of the anterior aspect of the heart must be examined with the stethoscope, but the areas where the sounds from the four valves are best heard are shown in Fig. 1.12.

Begin by listening at the apex of the heart – the mitral area. First, identify the first and second heart sounds. The heart sounds are traditionally described as sounding like the words *lub-dub*; that is to say, the first sound is slightly longer and softer than the second sound. As this is not always the case, it is wise to confirm that the sound you believe to be the first sound corresponds to the beginning of the cardiac impulse or the subclavian or carotid pulse. Having decided which sound is which, listen carefully to the second sound. It

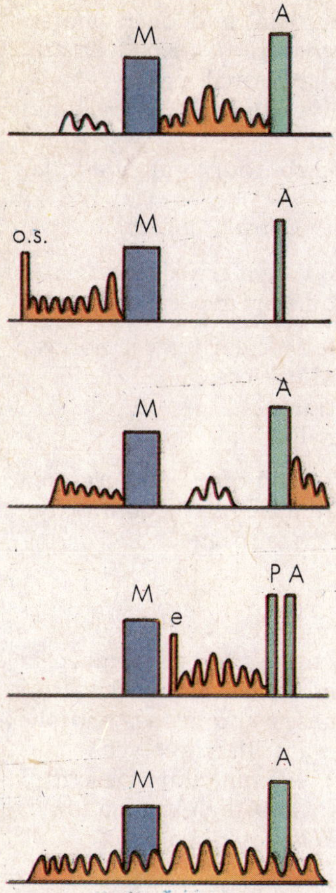

Mitral incompetence	Pansystolic murmur Soft first sound May be a short mid-diastolic murmur preceded by a third sound
Mitral stenosis	Diastolic murmur with a presystolic crescendo preceded by an opening snap (o.s.) Loud first sound
Aortic incompetence	Early diastolic murmur May be a soft mid-diastolic murmur
Aortic stenosis	Systolic murmur preceded by an ejection click (e) Split second sound
Patent ductus arteriosus	'Machinery' murmur Continuous throughout systole and diastole

FIG. 1.13 The sounds of some common cardiac abnormalities (M = 1st heart sound, A = 2nd heart sound)

may be sharper and shorter than usual – almost a click – or it may be split. A double, or split, second sound occurs when the aortic and pulmonary valves close asynchronously. A double sound can be heard when the sounds are 0.2 or more seconds apart.

Next, listen carefully to the intervals between the two main sounds, diastole and systole, for any additional heart sounds or murmurs.

Murmurs are due to turbulent flow and the vibration of parts of the heart. They may vary in nature from a low-pitched rumble to a high-toned swish. Try to decide whether the murmur occupies the whole or part of diastole or systole and whether its intensity changes.

Think of the way you are going to record your findings (see Fig. 1.13): two blocks for the main heart sounds (M_1 and A_2) and a zig-zag line for the murmur. Imagine your drawing as you listen to the sound and you will find it easier to define the timing of the murmur. A detailed description of the many heart sounds and their interpretation is beyond the scope of this book. The student must refer to a textbook of cardiology, but Fig. 1.13 illustrates the common types of murmur and their likely causes.

The exercise just described must be repeated over the other three areas where the aortic, pulmonary and tricuspid valve sounds are best heard. Some murmurs will be audible in more than one area. Find the murmur's site of maximum intensity by 'inching' the stethoscope over the chest wall between each area. The same technique should be used to see if, and how far, aortic murmurs are conducted into the neck.

The sounds at the apex, from the mitral valve, can be made louder by asking the patient to turn over onto his left side; the aortic valve sounds can be amplified by asking the patient to lean forwards.

Always listen to the heart sounds at the *back* of the chest. The murmur of a patent ductus or coarctation can often be heard all down the line of the aorta, posteriorly, just to the left of the mid-line.

Look for oedema

Oedema commonly appears first in the feet and lower third of the legs but may be more apparent in the sacral and buttock regions if the patient has been bedridden for some time.

Cardiac oedema is very soft, 'pits' easily and often gives the skin a pale, waxy, transparent appearance.

Examine the abdomen

Examination of the abdomen is described in detail in Chapter 16. It has been put there in the hope that you will read it whenever you refer to other parts of the chapter.

A large amount of the surgical disease presenting to a surgical clinic is intra-abdominal and so a good technique of abdominal examination is essential.

Examination of the abdomen follows the standard pattern:

- *Inspection* for asymmetry, distension, masses, visible peristalsis and skin discolouration.
- *Palpation* for superficial and deep tenderness, the normal viscera (liver, spleen and kidneys) and any abnormal masses.
- *Percussion* of the liver and splenic areas and any other masses.
- *Auscultation* for bowel sounds and vascular bruits.
- *Rectal examination; vaginal examination.*

There are four things which are easy to forget, so do them before you start general palpation:

1 Palpate the supraclavicular lymph glands.
2 Palpate the hernial orifices.
3 Feel the femoral pulses.
4 Examine the genitalia.

Two further things which often get forgotten are auscultation and the rectal examination, but you must leave these to the end.

Revision Panel 1.8

Common causes of ankle swelling

Dependency/immobility
Pregnancy
Heart failure
Low plasma proteins
Chronic venous insufficiency
Deep vein thrombosis
Lymphatic insufficiency

Examine the limbs

There are four main tissues to be examined in a limb: the bones and joints, the muscles and soft tissues, the arteries and veins, and the nerves. The first three are often involved in surgical disease and their examination is described in Chapters 4 and 7. Only the examination of the peripheral nerves is described here.

Musculoskeletal system See Chapter 4, page 92.

Arteries and veins See Chapter 7, page 162.

Peripheral nerves The nerves in the limbs serve three functions: motor, sensory and reflex. Examine each of these functions in turn.

Motor nerve function

Voluntary movement Ask the patient to move each joint in all directions, as far as possible. This will reveal any loss of voluntary muscle function and the presence of any musculoskeletal abnormalities, such as arthritis or muscle contractures, which might limit movement.

Strength of the muscles Check in a systematic way the strength of the muscles which move each joint. Strength is assessed by asking the patient to move the joint against a resistance, or by asking him to keep the joint fixed while you try to move it. The latter is the simplest method because the patient only needs to be instructed to keep the limb still.

It is customary to grade muscle strength as follows:

5: Normal.
4: Good, but not full strength.
3: Can work against the force of gravity but not against a greater resistance.
2: Cannot work against gravity, but the muscles contract.
1: Barely perceptible contractions.
0: Complete paralysis.

However, it is better to describe the strength of the muscles than use a numerical code.

The segments of the spinal cord and the nerves which control each joint are listed in Revision Panel 1.10.

Sensory nerve function

The peripheral nerves serve the sensations of light touch, deep touch and pressure, pain, temperature, vibration sense, position sense, and muscular coordination.

The appreciation of light touch This is tested with a wisp of cotton wool. Make sure

Revision Panel 1.9
Classification of muscle strength

	Score
Normal	5
Weak but can overcome gentle resistance	4
Cannot overcome gentle resistance but can overcome gravity	3
Cannot overcome gravity but muscle contracts	2
Barely perceptible muscle contractions	1
No contractions	0

Revision Panel 1.10
The nerves and spinal segments which innervate the major muscle groups

Muscle groups		*Spinal segments*	*Nerves*
Shoulder:	Flexion	C5, 6	Nerve to pectoralis major, circumflex nerve
	Extension	C5, 6	Subscapular nerve
	Abduction	C5, 6	Circumflex nerve
Elbow:	Flexion	C5, 6	Musculocutaneous nerve
	Extension	C6, 7, 8	Radial nerve
Wrist:	Flexion	C6, 7, 8	Median nerve and ulnar nerve
	Extension	C6, 7, 8	Radial nerve
Intrinsic hand muscles:		C8, T1	Median nerve and ulnar nerve
Hip:	Flexion	L2, 3, 4	Lumbar and femoral nerves
	Extension	L5, S1, 2	Inferior gluteal nerve
	Abduction	L4, 5, S1	Superior gluteal nerve
	Adduction	L2, 3, 4	Obturator nerve
	Rotation	L5, S1, 2	–
Knee:	Flexion	L4, 5, S1, 2	Sciatic nerve
	Extension	L2, 3, 4	Femoral nerve
Ankle:	Flexion	L5, S1, 2	Medial popliteal and posterior tibial nerves
	Extension	L4, 5, S1	Anterior tibial nerve
Foot:	Inversion	L4, 5	Anterior and posterior tibial nerves
	Eversion	L5, S1	Musculocutaneous nerve

THE IMPORTANT DERMATOMES
(the others can be estimated if you remember these)

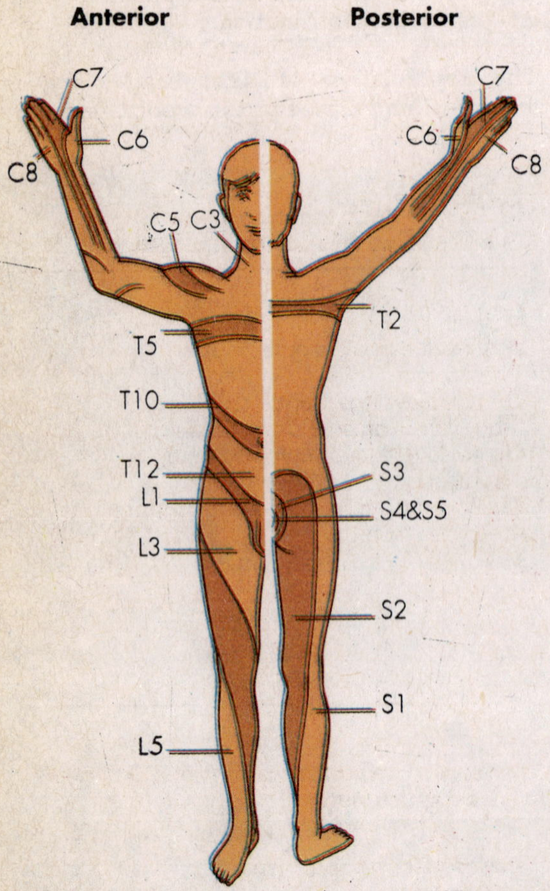

FIG. 1.14

that the patient cannot see you touching him. Move over the limb in a random manner, but when mapping out an area of hypoaesthesia, move from the normal to the abnormal. The important dermatomes are shown in Fig. 1.14.

Deep touch and pressure sensation This is tested by pressing firmly on the skin with a blunt object. It is unlikely to be abnormal if the response to light touch is normal.

Pain The best test of pain sensibility is the response to a pinprick. Use a normal pin and ask the patient to differentiate between pressure from its point and its head by indicating whether he feels it to be 'sharp' or 'blunt'.

Temperature Ask the patient to differentiate between a hot and a cold object. The simplest way of providing such objects is to fill two test tubes with hot and cold water.

Vibration sense Strike a tuning fork firmly. Place its base on a bony protuberance, such as the malleolus at the ankle, and ask the patient to describe the sensation he can feel. If he has normal vibration sense he will describe a 'buzzing' or 'vibrating' sensation. Do not put these words into the patient's mind by using them in a leading question.

Position sense The proprioceptive nerve endings in a joint tell the brain about the joint's spatial orientation. Test this ability by moving the great toe or thumb into different positions of flexion or extension and ask the patient to identify them. It is easier to ask the patient to state the direction in which the digit is pointing (e.g. up or down) than to use unfamiliar anatomical terms. The patient must keep his eyes shut.

Muscle coordination Test the coordination of the upper limbs by asking the patient to touch your upheld finger with his index finger and then to touch the tip of his nose. If you ask him to do this a second time with his eyes shut, you will also be testing joint position sense. Coordination in the lower limbs is tested by asking the patient to slide the heel of one foot up and down the shin of the other leg. This should also be done with the eyes open and then shut.

Reflex function

The limb reflexes are all stretch reflexes and test the integrity of the spinal segments, and the motor and sensory nerves which innervate the muscles being stretched.

To stimulate a good stretch reflex you must stretch the tendon suddenly by striking it with a rubber hammer. If a reflex is weak, it can be reinforced by asking the patient to clench his teeth or interlock his fingers and try to pull them apart.

The spinal segments involved in the common stretch reflexes are given in Revision Panel 1.11.

Clonus The increase in muscle tone that occurs with an upper motor neurone lesion increases the susceptibility of the tendons to the stretch reflex. Sudden and persistent stretching can cause repeated contractions known as **clonus**.

The plantar reflex Scraping the lateral aspect of the sole of the foot causes a withdrawal reflex and **flexion of the great toe**. If there is an upper motor neurone lesion, the toe will extend. This reflex involves the L5, S1 and 2 spinal segments.

Abdominal reflexes Stroking the upper and lower abdomen causes the rectus abdominis muscle to contract. This tests the T8, 9 and 10, and T11 and 12 segments, respectively.

Cremasteric reflex Stroking the inner side of the thigh makes the cremaster contract, so testing the L1 segment.

Test the urine, faeces and sputum

It is important to note the volume, colour and smell of a patient's urine even though there are a multitude of simple modern methods for testing the urine for sugar, blood, acetone and protein. Whilst using these methods it is a good idea to learn the standard chemical laboratory techniques from a textbook of medicine or chemical pathology.

Do not forget to measure the **specific gravity** and inspect any precipitate, after centrifugation, under the microscope.

Revision Panel 1.11

The segments involved in the common stretch reflexes

Biceps jerk	C5, 6
Triceps jerk	C6, 7
Finger jerk	C8
Knee jerk	L2, 3, 4
Ankle jerk	S1, 2

Look at the **faeces**, especially if the patient complains that they are abnormal.

Look at the **sputum**.

EXAMINATION OF A LUMP

Many of the points made in the ensuing paragraphs will be reiterated throughout the book because lumps, bumps and ulcers form an important part of surgical practice. This section will give the general outline of examination. Repeatedly revise this list of physical signs.

Position

The location of a lump must be described in exact anatomical terms, using distances measured from bony points. Do not guess distances; use a tape-measure.

Colour and texture of overlying skin

The skin over a lump may be discoloured and become smooth and shiny or thick and rough.

Temperature

Is the lump hot or of normal temperature? There is no difference between the sensitivity of the palm of your hand and the back of your hand to temperature changes, but the dorsal surfaces of your fingers are usually dry (free of sweat) and cool, so you will find it easier to assess the skin temperature with this surface than with the palm of the hand or fingers.

Tenderness

Is the lump tender? Which parts are tender? Always try to feel the non-tender part before feeling the tender area, and watch the patient's face for signs of discomfort as you feel.

Shape

Remember that lumps have three dimensions. You cannot have a circular lump because a circle is a plane figure. Many lumps are not regular spheres, or hemispheres, but have an asymmetrical outline. In these circumstances, it is permissible to use descriptive terms such as pear shaped or kidney shaped.

Size

Once the shape is established, it is possible to measure its various dimensions. Again, remember that all solid objects have at least three dimensions: width, length, and height or depth. Asymmetrical lumps will need more measurements to describe them accurately; sometimes a diagram will clarify your written description.

Revision Panel 1.12

The examination of a lump or ulcer

Local examination
- Position
- Colour
- Temperature
- Tenderness
- Shape
- Size
- Surface
- Edge [*Ulcer:* Edge, Base, Depth, Discharge]
- Composition:
  - Consistence, Fluctuation, Fluid thrill, Translucency, Resonance } Solid or Fluid or Gas
  - Pulsatility, Compressibility, Bruit } Vascular
- Reducibility
- Relations to surrounding structures
- Regional lymph glands
- State of local tissues:
  - Arteries
  - Nerves
  - Bones and joints

General examination

Surface

The first feature of the lump that you will notice when you feel it will be its surface. It may be smooth or irregular. An irregular surface may be covered with smooth bumps, rather like cobblestones, which can be called bosselated; or be irregular or rough.

There may be a mixture of surfaces if the lump is large.

Edge

The edge of a lump may be clearly defined or indistinct. It may have a definite pattern.

Composition

Any lump must be composed of one or more of the following:

- Cells which make it solid.
- Extravascular fluid, such as urine, serum, CSF, synovial fluid, or extravascular blood, which make the lump cystic.
- Gas.
- Intravascular blood.

The physical signs which help you decide the composition of a lump are: consistence, fluctuation, fluid thrill, translucency, resonance, pulsatility, compressibility, and bruits.

Consistence

The consistence of a lump may vary from very soft to very hard. As it is difficult to describe hardness, it is common practice to compare the consistence of a lump to well-known objects. A simple scale for consistence is as follows:

Stony hard: not indentable.
Rubbery: hard to firm, but slightly squashable, similar to a rubber ball.
Spongy: soft and very squashable, but still with some resilience.
Soft: squashable and no resilience.

The consistence of a lump depends not only upon its structure but also on the tension within it. Some fluid-filled lumps are hard, some solid lumps are soft; therefore the final decision about composition (i.e. whether it is fluid or solid) rarely depends upon an assessment of the consistence. Other features peculiar to fluid are more important.

Fluctuation

Pressure on one side of a fluid-filled cavity makes all the other surfaces protrude. This is because an increase of pressure within a cavity is transmitted equally and at right-angles to all parts of its wall. If you press on one aspect of a solid lump, it may or may not bulge out in another direction, but it will not bulge outwards in every other direction.

Fluctuation can only be elicited by feeling at least two other areas of the lump whilst pressing on a third. If two areas on opposite aspects of the lump bulge out when a third area is pressed in, the lump fluctuates and contains fluid. This examination is best carried out twice, the second at right-angles to the first.

Fluid thrill

A percussion wave is easily conducted across a fluid but not across a solid. The presence of a fluid thrill is detected by tapping one side of the lump and feeling the transmitted vibration when it reaches the other side. If a swelling is large, a percussion wave can be transmitted along its wall. This is prevented by placing the edge of the patient's or an assistant's hand on the lump mid-way between your percussing and palpating hands.

Percussion waves cannot be felt across small lumps because the wave moves so quickly that the time gap due to conduction cannot be appreciated, or distinguished from the mechanical shaking of the tissue caused by the percussion. The presence of a fluid thrill is a diagnostic and extremely valuable physical sign.

Translucency

Light will pass easily through clear fluid but not through solid tissues. If a lump transilluminates then it must contain water, serum, lymph or plasma, or highly refractile fat. Blood and other opaque fluids do not transmit light. Transillumination requires a bright pinpoint light source and a darkened room. Attempts at transillumination with a poor-quality flashlight in a bright room are bound to fail and mislead.

Resonance

Solid and fluid-filled lumps sound dull when percussed. A gas-filled lump will sound hollow (resonant).

Pulsatility

Many lumps pulsate but the majority do so because they are near to an artery and so get moved by its pulsations. Always let your hand rest still for a few seconds on every lump to see if it is pulsating. If it does, you must find out whether the pulsations are being **transmitted** to the lump from elsewhere or are caused by the **expansion** of the lump itself. Place a finger of each hand on opposite sides of the lump and feel if they are being pushed apart – true expansile pulsation; or pushed in the same direction (usually upwards) – transmitted pulsation. The two common causes of expansile pulsations are aneurysms and very vascular tumours.

Compressibility

Some fluid-filled lumps can be compressed until they disappear. When the compressing hand is removed the lump re-forms. Such a sign is common with venous vascular malformations where the intravascular pressure is low. Compressibility should not be confused with reducibility (see below). A lump which is reducible – such as a hernia – can be pushed away into another place but will not reappear spontaneously without the application of an opposite force such as that produced by coughing or gravity.

Bruits

Always listen to a lump. Vascular lumps may have a systolic bruit; lumps containing bowel may have audible bowel sounds.

Reducibility

You should always see if a lump is reducible by gently compressing it. Reducibility is a feature of herniae. The lump will be felt to move into another place. If you ask the patient to cough the lump may return, expanding as it does so. This is called a **cough impulse** and is also a feature of herniae and some vascular lumps. In some ways the differences between compressibility (see above) and reducibility are semantic.

Relations to surrounding structures

By careful palpation it is usually possible to decide which structure contains the lump, and its relation to overlying and deeper structures. The attachment of skin and other superficial structures to a lump can easily be determined because both are accessible to the examiner and any limitation of their movement easily felt. Attachment to deeper structures is more difficult to decide. Underlying muscles must be tensed to see if this reduces the mobility of an overlying lump or makes it less easy to feel, a sign which indicates that the lump is within or deep to the contracting muscle.

State of the regional lymph glands

Never forget to palpate the lymph nodes that would normally receive lymph from the region occupied by the lump. The skin, muscles and bones of the limbs and trunk drain to the axillary and inguinal nodes; the head and neck to the cervical nodes; and the intra-abdominal structures to the pre- and para-aortic nodes.

State of the local tissues

It is important to examine the overlying and nearby skin, subcutaneous tissues, muscles and bones, and the local circulation and nerve supply. This is particularly relevant when examining an ulcer; but some lumps may be associated with a local vascular or neurological abnormality, or cause an abnormality of these systems, so this part of the examination must not be forgotten.

General examination

It is often tempting to examine the lump about which the patient is complaining and then do no more. This will cause you to make innumerable misdiagnoses. **You must always examine the whole patient.**

EXAMINATION OF AN ULCER

The examination of an ulcer follows the same pattern as the examination of a lump. When an ulcer has an irregular shape which is difficult to describe, draw it on your notes and add the dimensions. When an exact record of size and shape is needed, press a piece of sterile gauze onto the ulcer and get its imprint, and then cut around it or trace it. Alternatively, place a thin sheet of sterile transparent polythene over the ulcer and trace around its edge with a felt-tipped pen.

After recording the **position, colour, tenderness, temperature, shape** and **size** you must examine the base, edge, depth, discharge and surrounding tissues, the state of the local lymph glands, local tissues, and complete the general examination.

Base

The base, or floor, of an ulcer usually consists of slough or granulation tissue, but recognizable structures such as tendon or bone may be visible. The nature of the floor occasionally gives some indication of the cause of the ulcer.

Solid brown or grey dead tissue indicates full-thickness skin death. Syphilitic ulcers have a slough that looks like a wash-leather. Tuberculous ulcers have a base of bluish unhealthy granulation tissue. Ischaemic ulcers often contain no granulation tissue, and tendons and other structures may lie bare in their base.

The redness of the granulation tissue reflects the underlying vascularity and indicates the ability of the ulcer to heal.

Edge

There are five types of edge (see Fig. 1.15).

A flat, sloping edge This indicates that the ulcer is shallow and that epithelium is growing in from the edge in an attempt to heal it. This type of ulcer is usually superficial, often only half-way through the skin. Venous ulcers are a typical example. The new skin around the edge is red-blue and almost transparent.

A square-cut or punched-out edge This follows the rapid death and loss of the whole thickness of the skin without much attempt by the body to repair the defect. This form of

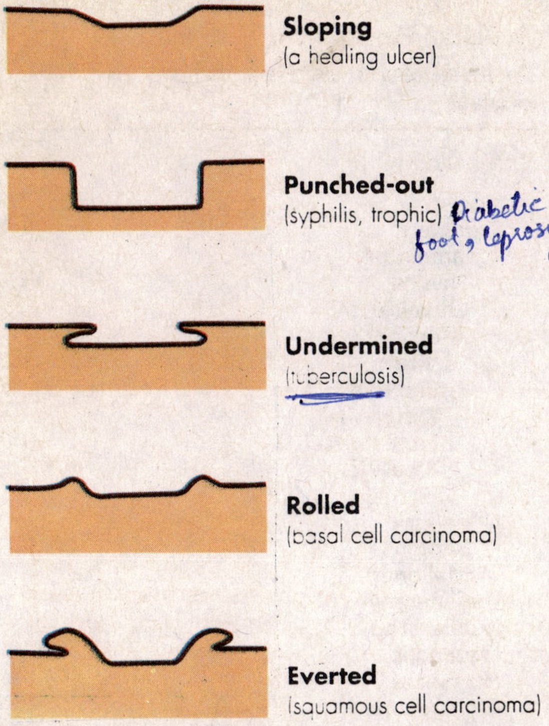

FIG. 1.15 The varieties of ulcer edge

ulcer is most often seen in the foot due to pressure on an insensitive piece of skin, i.e. a trophic ulcer secondary to a neurological defect. The classic textbook example of a punched-out ulcer is the ulcer of tertiary syphilis, but these lesions are rare today in Europe. Most of the punched-out ulcers that you will see will be secondary to the neuropathy of diabetes or, outside Europe and North America, leprosy.

An undermined edge When an infection in an ulcer affects the subcutaneous tissues more than the skin, the edge becomes undermined. This type of ulcer is commonly seen in the buttock as a result of pressure necrosis, because the subcutaneous fat is more susceptible to pressure than the skin; but the classic textbook example is the tuberculous ulcer – also uncommon in modern Europe.

A rolled edge This develops when there is slow growth of tissue in the edge of the ulcer. The edge looks like the heaped-up mound around an ancient Roman earthwork. A rolled edge is typical, and almost diagnostic, of a **basal cell carcinoma** (rodent ulcer). The edge is usually pale pink or white, with clumps and clusters of cells visible through the paper-thin superficial covering of squamous cells.

An everted edge This develops when the tissue in the edge of the ulcer is growing quickly and spilling out of the ulcer to overlap the normal skin. An everted edge is typical of a **carcinoma** and is seen wherever carcinomata occur, on the skin, in the bowel, in the bladder and in the respiratory tract.

Depth

Record the depth of the ulcer in millimetres, and anatomically by describing the structures it has penetrated or reached.

Discharge

The discharge from an ulcer may be serous, sanguinous, serosanguinous, or purulent. The quantity of discharge may be large and easy to see or you may have to inspect the dressings to see it.

Always take a **bacteriological swab** of an ulcer.

You may not be able to see the edge, the base or the discharge if the ulcer is covered with dried discharge (a scab). It is then necessary **to remove the scab** to examine the ulcer properly. Students should not do this without the permission of the doctor in charge of the patient.

Relations

Describe the relations of the ulcer to the surrounding tissues, particularly those deep to it. It is important to know if the ulcer is adherent to deep structures.

Local lymph glands

Examine the local lymph nodes carefully. They may be enlarged because of secondary infection or secondary tumour deposits and they may be tender.

State of the local tissues

Pay particular attention to the local **blood supply** and **innervation** of the adjacent skin. Many ulcers in the lower limbs are secondary to vascular and neurological disease.

There may be evidence of previous ulcers which have healed.

General examination

This is very important because many systemic diseases present with skin lesions and ulcers. Conversely, many primary skin diseases present with ulcers. Examine the whole patient with care.

Revision Panel 1.13

Remember the four basic techniques

Inspection *Palpation* *Percussion* *Auscultation*	All four can always, and should always, be applied whatever part you are examining. The third and fourth are often forgotten when examining parts outside the chest.

Revision Panel 1.14

A classification of the aetiology of disease

Congenital

Acquired
- Traumatic
- Inflammatory
  - Physical
  - Chemical
  - Infection:
    - Viral
    - Bacterial
    - Rickettsial
    - Spirochaetal
    - Parasitic
    - Fungal
- Neoplastic
  - Benign
  - Malignant
- Degenerative
- Proliferative
- Metabolic
- Hormonal
- Collagenosis
- Autoimmunopathy
- Psychosomatic
- Iatrogenic

The skin

2

There are many lesions of the skin that require surgical treatment and form an important part of general surgical practice. This chapter describes only the common or dangerous lesions.

It is difficult to draw up a set of simple diagnostic pathways suitable for all skin lesions, because they have such varied features. For example, a basal cell carcinoma can be a raised nodule, a flat plaque, or an ulcer; and can be skin coloured, pearly white, brown or pink. The solution is to learn the physical features of each lesion and the best way to do this is by examining as many as possible.

When you are familiar with the physical features of the common skin lesions do not use this knowledge to indulge in the game of 'spot diagnosis' – instant diagnosis after one brief glance. This is a dangerous game and likely to lead to mistakes. However familiar the lesion, always examine it fully before making a diagnosis.

Lesions in the skin have two basic distinguishing features: their colour and their relationship to, and effect on, the overlying epidermis.

If the abnormal tissue is in the superficial part of the dermis, the overlying epidermis is likely to be raised and look abnormal. If the epidermis is destroyed, the lesion becomes an ulcer. When the abnormal tissue is deep in the dermis the overlying epidermis may be stretched but be otherwise normal. It is possible, therefore, to subdivide all skin lesions into three categories: those with the epidermis intact but abnormal, those with the overlying epidermis destroyed (ulcers), and those covered with a normal epidermis. In the latter case the bulk of the lesion is likely to be in the subcutaneous tissues, and even though it may be derived from a skin structure (e.g. a sebaceous gland) it is usually classified as a subcutaneous lesion. Such lesions are discussed in the next chapter.

The colour of the lesion may be more helpful. Skin lesions may be black, brown, yellow, red, or normal skin colour.

The following classification, based on the condition of the overlying epidermis and its colour, gives some idea of the multitude of lesions that you must learn to recognize but, as a classification and an aid to diagnosis, it is of little practical use.

Epidermis intact but abnormal

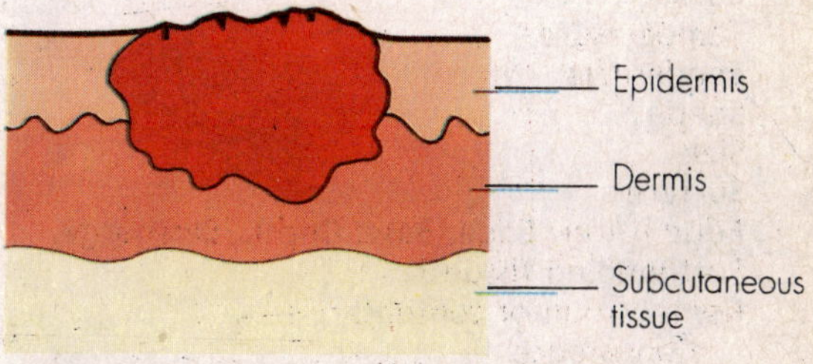

FIG. 2.1 Epidermis intact but abnormal

- *Black* Gangrenous skin. Early pyoderma gangrenosum. Early anthrax pustule.
- *Brown* Freckles. Moles of all varieties. Malignant melanoma. Pigmented basal or squamous cell carcinoma. Café au lait patch. Pigmentation following a bruise, thrombophlebitis, or venous hypertension. (The epidermis may be normal in the last three conditions.)

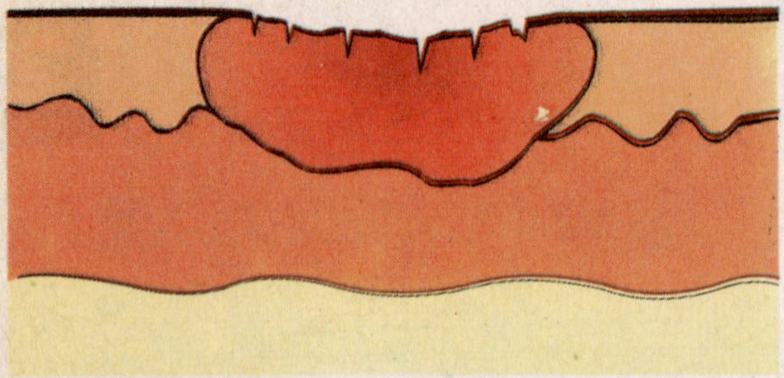

FIG. 2.2 Destruction of the overlying epidermis – ulceration

Revision Panel 2.1

The features of the history and examination of a lump or skin lesion that must be elicited

History
- Age. Sex. Ethnic group. Occupation
- First local symptom
- Other symptoms
- Duration of symptoms
- Development of symptoms
- Persistence of symptoms
- Multiple or single lesions
- Cause
- Systemic symptoms (direct questions)
- Family history
- Social history

Local examination
- Position
- Colour
- Temperature
- Tenderness
- Shape
- Size
- Surface
- Edge [*Ulcer:* Edge, Base, Depth, Discharge, Surrounding tissues]
- Composition or contents
  - Consistence
  - Fluctuation
  - Resonance
  - Fluid thrill
  - Translucency
  - Pulsatility
  - Compressibility
  - Bruit
- Reducibility
- Relations to surrounding structures
- Lymph drainage
- State of local tissues (arteries, nerves, bones and joints)

General examination

- *Greyish-brown* Wart. Seborrhoeic keratosis. Keratoacanthoma. Callosities.
- *Yellow–white* Xanthoma. Lymphangioma. Pustules of furunculosis and hidradenitis.
- *Red–blue* Strawberry naevus. Port-wine stain. Spider naevus. Campbell de Morgan spot. Telangiectases. Pyogenic granuloma.
- *Skin colour* Papilloma. Early basal and squamous cell carcinoma. Keloid scar. Keratoacanthoma. Pyogenic granuloma.

Destruction of the overlying epidermis: ulceration

- *Sloping edge* A healing ulcer.
- *Punched-out edge* Ischaemic, trophic, or syphilitic ulcer.
- *Undermined edge* Chronic infection. (Tuberculosis, carbuncle.)
- *Rolled or everted edge* Malignant ulceration.

Overlying epidermis normal

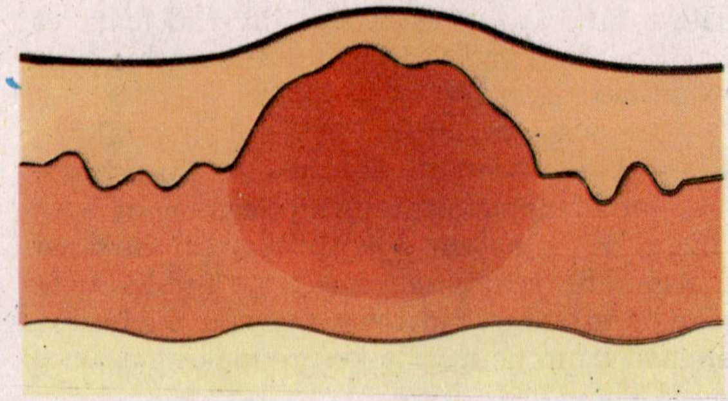

FIG. 2.3 Overlying epidermis normal

Although these lesions may have arisen from a skin structure, their mass is beneath the skin and does not affect its structure. They are usually classified as subcutaneous conditions and are described in the next chapter.

Throughout this book each disease will be described using the standard plan of history taking and examination presented in Chapter 1. I make no apologies for the repetitious manner in which the headings appear – repetition is the secret of learning. Revise the plan of history taking and clinical examination that you should use from Revision Panel 2.1.

Benign papilloma

A benign papilloma of the skin is a simple overgrowth of all layers of the skin. The word papilloma suggests that this lesion is a benign neoplasm but this is not the case; it would be better classified as a hamartoma, or even called a skin tag.

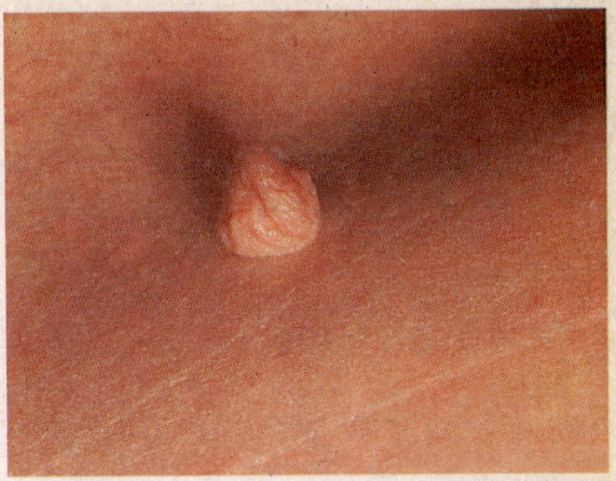

A smooth papilloma with a narrow pedicle, almost a fibrolipomatous polyp

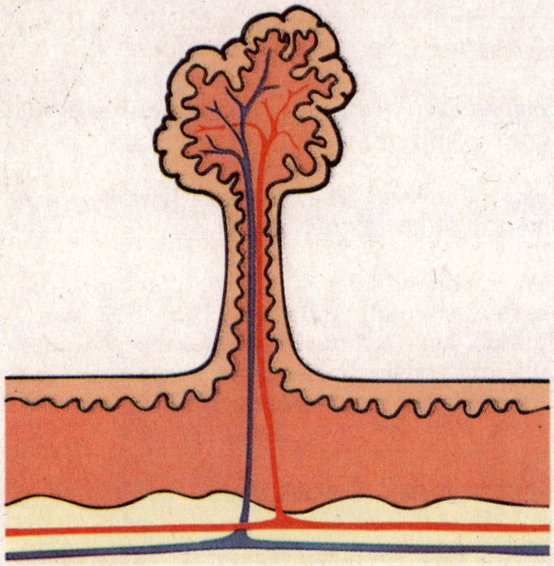

FIG. 2.4 A papilloma is an overgrowth of all layers of the skin with a central vascular core

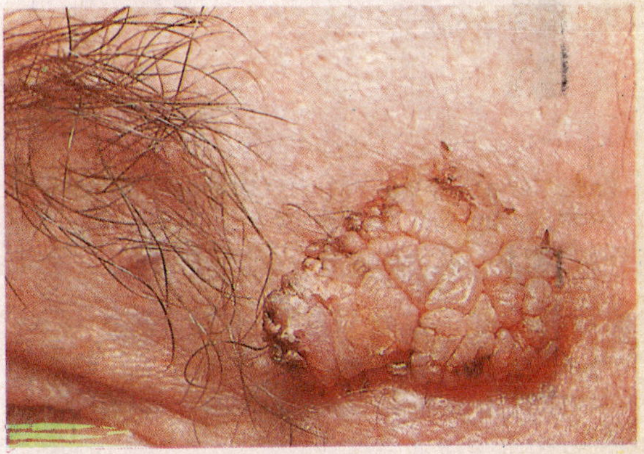

A sessile polyp with excess epithelium covering the clefts and corrugations

HISTORY

Age Papillomata can appear at any age. A few are congenital.

Symptoms The commonest complaint is that the pedunculated swelling catches on clothes or rubs against another part of the body. If it is injured it can become red and swollen and ulcerate, or even infarct. Spontaneous ulceration is rare. The skin that forms a papilloma contains sweat glands, hair follicles and sebaceous glands. All of these structures can become infected and make the papilloma swollen and tender. If the granulation tissue that forms in response to the infection becomes exuberant, the swelling can look like a carcinoma.

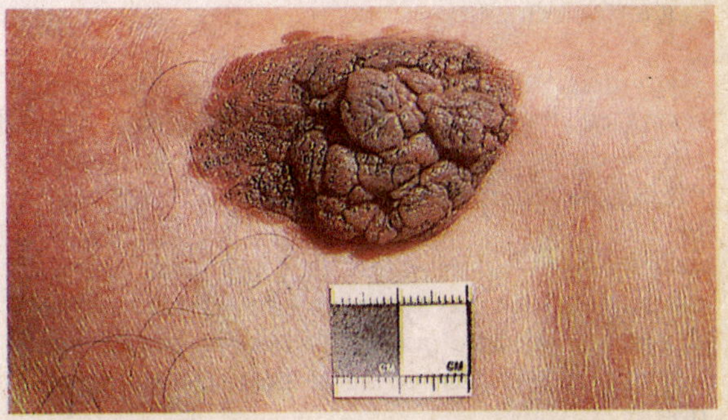

Papillomata may be deeply pigmented

FIG. 2.5 PAPILLOMATA

EXAMINATION

Position Papillomata occur anywhere on the skin.

Colour They are the colour of normal skin.

Shape and size Their shape can vary from a smooth, raised plaque to a papilliferous, pedunculated polyp. The size is equally variable.

Composition Papillomata are soft, solid and not compressible.

Lymph nodes The regional lymph glands should not be enlarged.

Local tissues The local nerves and blood vessels are normal.

Warts

Warts are patches of hyperkeratotic overgrown skin, whose growth has been stimulated by the presence of a papilloma virus.

HISTORY

Age Warts occur at any age but are most common in children, adolescents and young adults.

Duration They grow to their full size in a few weeks but may be present for months or years before the patient complains to his doctor about them, because he has usually made his own diagnosis and decided that there was no cause for concern.

Symptoms Warts are disfiguring. Multiple warts on the fingers can interfere with fine movements. They are only painful if they are rubbed or become infected.

Progression Once present, they may persist unchanged for many years or regress and disappear spontaneously. 'Kiss lesions' may appear on adjacent areas of skin that make frequent contact.

Family history Other members of the family may have warts.

EXAMINATION

Position Warts are commonly found on the hands, but they may appear on other exposed areas which are frequently touched by the hands, such as the face, arms and knees.

Colour and shape Warts are greyish-brown and hemispherical.

Surface Their surface is rough and hyperkeratotic, and often covered with fine filiform excrescences.

Composition Warts are usually hard and not compressible.

Lymph drainage The regional lymph nodes should not be enlarged.

Warts on the soles of the feet (plantar warts) are fundamentally the same as any other wart, but they have a different appearance, because they are pushed into the skin. They are described in Chapter 6, page 157.

Seborrhoeic keratosis

This lesion is also called a senile wart, seborrhoeic wart, verruca senilis, or basal cell papilloma. It is a benign overgrowth of the basal layer of the epidermis containing an excess of small dark-staining basal cells, which raise it above the level of the normal epidermis and give it a semi-transparent, oily appearance.

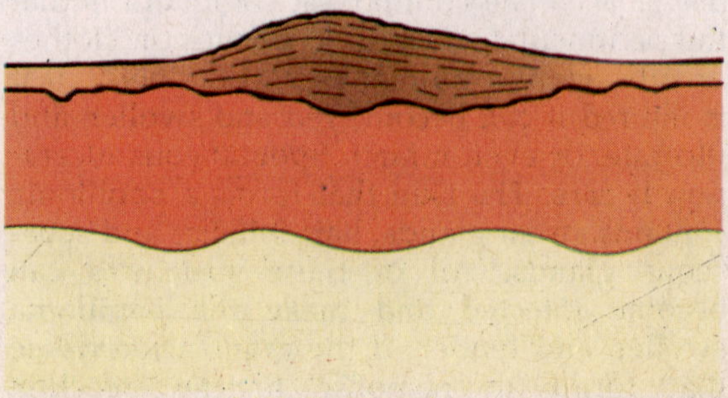

FIG. 2.6 A seborrhoeic keratosis. The plaque consists of an excess number of basal cells and will peel off

HISTORY

Age Senile warts occur in both sexes but, as the name implies, they become more common with advancing years. Most people over the age of 70 years have got one or two of these lesions.

Duration They are slow growing, beginning as a minute patch which gradually increases in area. The patient does not notice the early changes in the skin and has invariably had the lesion for months or years before complaining about it.

Symptoms As the lesion gets bigger, it becomes **disfiguring** and may start to **catch on clothes**. It seldom bleeds but may get infected. Sometimes there is sufficient melanin in the lesion to make the patient think it is a mole.

Progression Senile warts gradually increase in area, but not in thickness. They can suddenly fall off, uncovering a pale pink patch of skin.

They are more likely to become prominent if the skin is not regularly and firmly washed; hence seborrhoeic warts are more common on the back of the trunk.

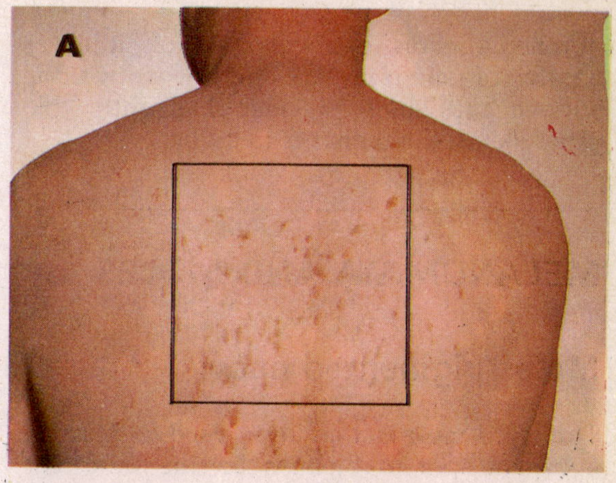

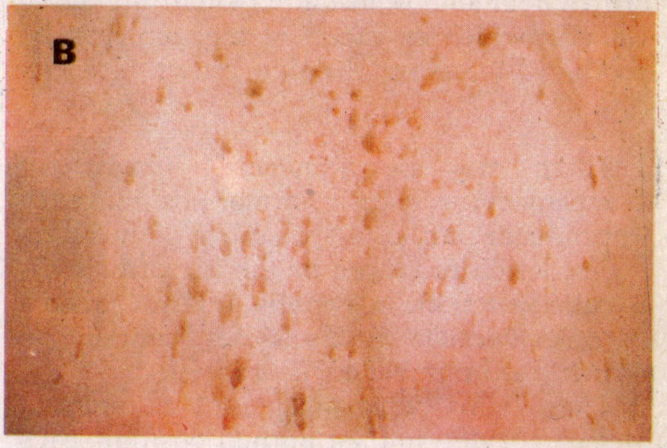

FIG. 2.7 A patient whose back was covered with seborrhoeic keratoses. The area outlined in (A) is enlarged in (B)

EXAMINATION

Position Seborrhoeic keratoses occur on any part of the skin except those areas subjected to regular abrasion, such as the palms of the hands and the soles of the feet. The majority are found on the back of the trunk (see Fig. 2.7).

Colour Their colour varies from normal skin colour through grey to brown, depending on the thickness of the epithelium and the quantity of melanin in the underlying skin.

Shape, size and surface They form a raised plateau of hypertrophic, slightly greasy skin, with a square cut and distinct edge. They have a rough, sometimes papilliferous surface and vary in size from a few millimetres to 2–3 cm in diameter.

Bleeding into a senile keratosis caused by trauma makes the lesion swell and turn brown – changes that may be confused with malignant change in a melanoma.

An infected keratosis also becomes swollen and tender and can be confused with a pyogenic granuloma or an epithelioma.

Consistence Senile warts are a little harder and stiffer than normal skin. The surrounding tissues are healthy but there may be other seborrhoeic warts nearby. The regional lymph nodes should not be enlarged.

Special diagnostic feature Because seborrhoeic keratoses are patches of thick squamous epithelium, **they can be picked off**. If you are sure of the diagnosis, you may try to pick off the edge of the plaque with blunt forceps, but **never pick hard at the edge of any lesion** for fear of damaging it. Interfering in this way with a malignant tumour may hasten its local spread.

When a seborrhoeic wart peels off, it leaves a patch of pale pink skin and one or two fine surface capillaries that bleed slightly. No other skin lesion behaves like this.

MELANOMATA AND MOLES

Moles/pigmented naevi

The word mole is a lay term used to describe a brown spot or blemish on the skin. The brown pigment is melanin. There are three ways in which an excess of melanin may be produced to colour the skin brown (see Fig. 2.8).

1 There may be a normal number of melanocytes, in their normal position, each producing an excess quantity of melanin. The lesion produced by this abnormality is called a **freckle** or **ephelis**. It is not called a mole because it does not contain an increased number of melanocytes.
2 There may be an increased number of melanocytes, in their normal position, each producing normal quantities of melanin. The lesion produced by this abnormality is called a **lentigo**.
3 There may be an increased number of melanocytes, in abnormal clusters at the dermo-epidermal junction, producing normal or excess quantities of melanin. The lesion produced by this abnormality is called a **mole** or **pigmented naevus**.

If the cells of a mole invade adjacent tissues or show signs of abnormal and excessive multiplication, the mole has become a **malignant melanoma**. If there is no invasion but some nuclear abnormalities it is called a **dysplastic naevus**.

Because the three benign pathological entities described above often have similar macroscopic features, it is safest to be non-committal and call all benign melanin-producing lesions 'moles' or 'pigmented naevi' (until you are expert enough to distinguish freckles and lentigo) and malignant melanin-producing lesions 'malignant melanoma'

PATHOLOGY

Whereas the clinical appearance of pigmented naevi is infinitely variable and almost unclassifiable, moles can be defined according to their microscopic appearance (see Fig. 2.8).

Melanocytes are normally found in small numbers among the cells of the basal layer of the epidermis. If they proliferate, they first cluster in the basal layer of the epidermis and then migrate into the dermis.

The mature adult mole consists of clusters of melanocytes in the **dermis** and is therefore called an **intradermal naevus**. Macroscopically, the intradermal mole can be flat or raised, smooth or warty, and hairy or non-hairy. Most of the moles on the arms, face and trunk are of this variety. They hardly ever turn malignant.

If the growth and movement of the melanocytes stop before they have all migrated into the dermis, there will be clusters of cells at various stages of maturity in the epidermis and the dermis. This lesion is called a **compound cellular naevus**.

If the melanocytes remain around the junction between the epidermis and dermis, the naevus is called a **junctional naevus**. Junctional naevi are immature and unstable and can turn malignant. The majority of malignant melanomata begin in junctional moles.

Many of the moles on the palms of the hands, the soles of the feet and the external genitalia are of the junctional variety.

Melanocytes which have never reached the epidermis and therefore lie in the deep dermis or subcutaneous tissues may still proliferate and produce excess melanin. The resulting lesion has a blue appearance and is called a **blue naevus**.

Although some may think it unfortunate that the clinical appearance does not reflect the microscopic features, such an association would cause problems of clinical management, because it would be wrong to assume, for example, that all junctional moles will become malignant. The only practical clinical approach is to excise any mole that you suspect might be undergoing malignant change.

THE HISTOLOGICAL VARIETIES OF PIGMENTED SPOTS OR BLEMISHES

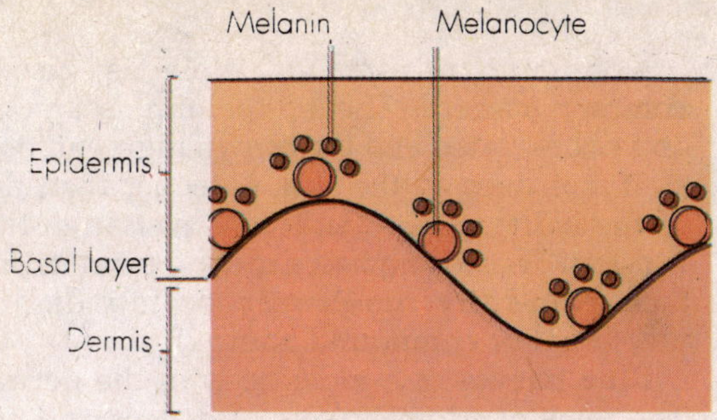

Normal skin

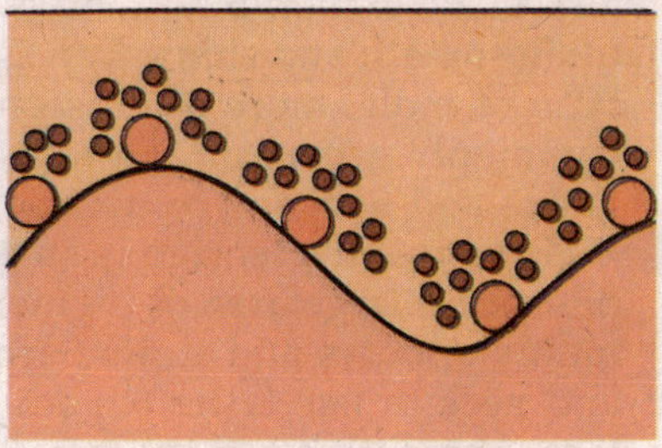

Freckle (Ephelis)
Normal number of melanocytes, in normal position, producing excess melanin

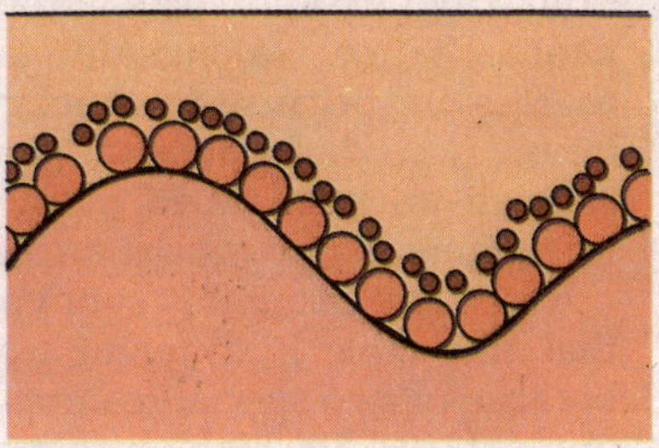

Lentigo
Excess melanocytes, in normal position producing normal amount of melamin

Pigmented naevus/mole

Excess melanocytes, in clusters, variable but usually excess melanin production

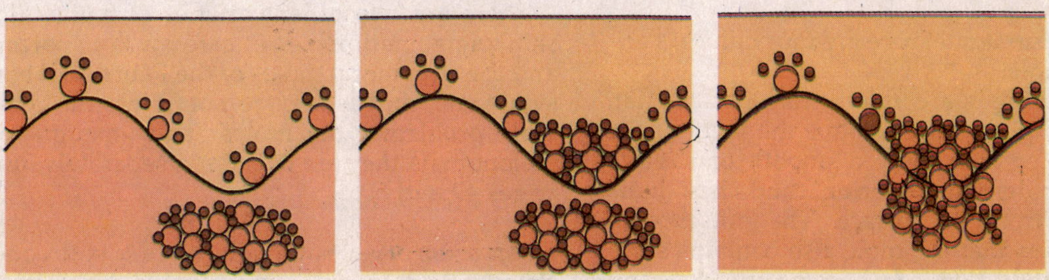

Intradermal naevus **Compound naevus** **Junctional naevus**

FIG. 2.8

HISTORY

Age Everyone (except albinos) has a few moles at birth but the number increases during life. It has been estimated that most Caucasians have 15–20.

During childhood and adolescence, moles may become more pigmented or completely regress. When enlarging and getting darker, a mole on a child may be clinically and histologically difficult to distinguish from a malignant melanoma, but true malignant (invasive) change is uncommon before puberty.

Ethnic group Moles are more common in Caucasians living in hot countries, such as Australia, because the skin is exposed to a greater quantity of ultraviolet light. Moles occur in Negroes, particularly in the less pigmented areas (soles of feet and of hands), but, overall, malignant change is less common.

Symptoms Moles rarely cause any serious symptoms. They may be **disfiguring, protrude** above the skin surface and **catch on clothes**.

EXAMINATION

Position Although moles can occur on any part of the skin, they are most common on the limbs, face, neck and trunk.

Colour Their colour varies from light brown to black. Amelanotic naevi do occur, but without their pigment they are unlikely to be recognized. The colour does not fade with pressure.

Size Most moles are 1–3 mm in diameter.

Shape and surface There are four clinical varieties of mole.

Hairy mole is a common variety. It is flat, or very slightly raised above the level of the surrounding skin, with a smooth or slightly warty epidermal covering, and has hairs growing from its surface. The presence of hairs means that the mole also contains sebaceous glands that can become infected and cause changes such as swelling and tenderness, which may be indistinguishable from malignant change. Hairy moles are always intradermal naevi.

Non-hairy or smooth mole is also a common variety. The epithelium is smooth and not elevated and the brown pigment looks as if it is deep in the skin – deeper than that of the hairy mole – but this is just an optical illusion. There is no hair growing from its surface. Non-hairy moles may be intradermal, junctional or compound naevi.

Blue naevus is a mole deep in the dermis. The thick overlying layers of dermis and epidermis mask the brown colour of the melanin and make it look blue. The overlying skin is often smooth and shiny. This is an uncommon type of mole, more often seen in children. It commonly occurs on the face, dorsum of the hands and feet, and buttock.

Hutchinson's lentigo is an eponym used to describe a large area of pigmentation. It commonly appears and slowly grows on the face and neck in late (after 60) adult life. The surface is smooth but there may be raised, rough nodules which correspond to areas of junctional activity and become the sites of malignant change, alongside pale areas of regression. Because the background pigmentation is so dark, areas of malignant change causing an increase in pigmentation but no thickening may pass unnoticed.

It is worth using this eponym to remind you that this mole is different from other moles because of two special features – its late development and its high incidence of malignant change. Some pathologists believe that it is precancerous or even malignant from its beginning, an example of malignant change *'in situ'*.

Pigmented naevi may regress. A mole surrounded by a white halo of regression is known as a **halo naevus**.

There are two other varieties of melanotic skin pigmentation – the 'café au lait' patch, and the circumoral moles of the Peutz–Jeghers syndrome – but as they do not fit into the general problems of moles and malignant melanomata they are discussed separately, on pages 49 and 50.

Composition Moles usually have a soft consistence and are indistinguishable, by palpation, from the surrounding tissues.

Lymph nodes The local lymph nodes should not be enlarged.

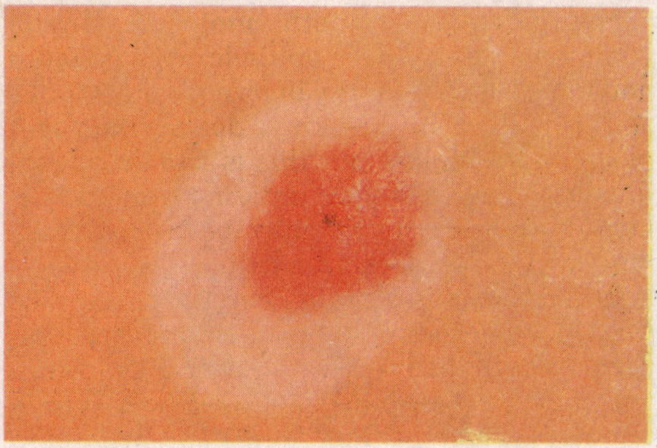

A 'halo' mole. This mole is regressing. It has faded and the skin around it has become depigmented

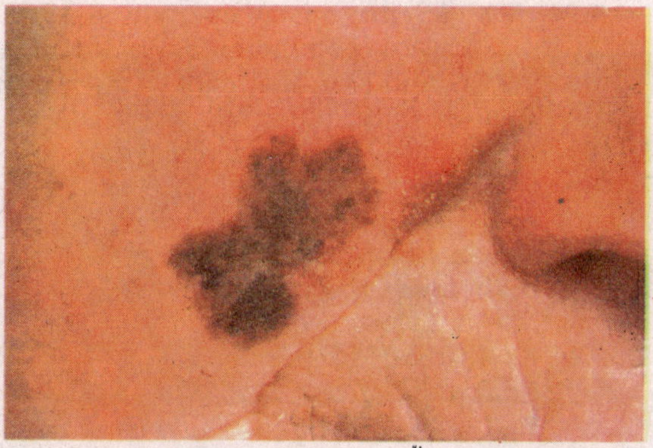

Hutchinson's lentigo on the face (see text)

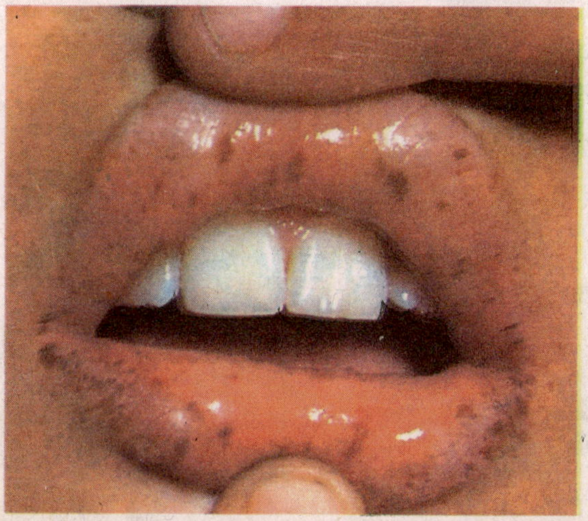

The circumoral pigmented naevi of the Peutz–Jeghers syndrome

FIG. 2.9 VARIOUS PIGMENTED NAEVI

Malignant melanoma

Because of the confusion which has arisen from using the word 'melanoma' to describe a benign lesion and 'malignant melanoma' to describe a malignant one, use the terms **mole** or **pigmented naevus** for benign lesions and **malignant melanoma** for malignant lesions.

The melanocyte originates from the neural crest and so is neuro-ectodermal in origin. It could be argued that malignant change in melanocytes should be called a carcinoma, but terms such as 'melanocarcinoma' or even 'melanosarcoma' only add to the confusion. It is best to use the well-established descriptive term 'malignant melanoma'.

Cardinal symptoms of malignant change in a mole

Change in surface One of the earliest changes associated with malignant change is loss of the normal skin markings (creases) over the mole. The skin may also become rough and scaly.

Itching This is an early and significant symptom, often associated with a pale pink halo around the mole.

Increase in size, shape or thickness The patient usually complains that a long-standing mole, or a recently developed brown spot, has grown steadily over a period of a few weeks or months. Rapid growth in a few days is atypical.

Malignant growth occurs in all directions. The mole or part of the mole may become wider and thicker, often changing from a flat plaque to a nodule, or simply change in outline.

Change in colour Malignant melanocytes usually produce more melanin, so the mole gets darker. The colour change is often patchy with some areas becoming almost black, others turning blue–purple with the increased vascularity, and some areas not changing at all. Very occasionally the malignant melanocytes do not produce melanin so that the new growth is colourless.

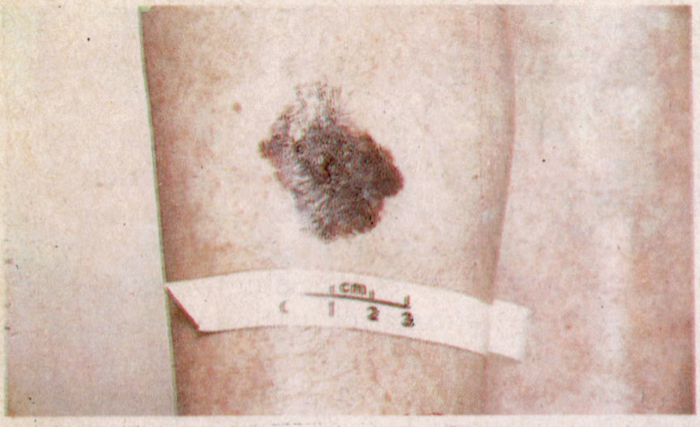

A superficial spreading melanoma. The lesion is thin, with an irregular edge and varying degrees of pigmentation

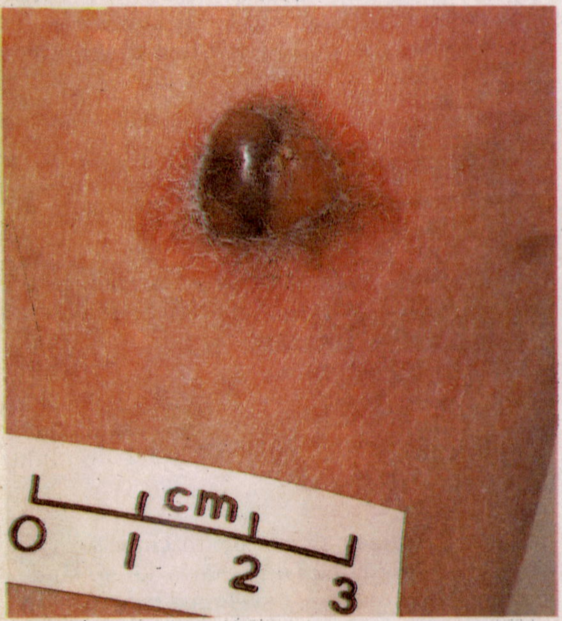

A nodular melanoma arising in a long-standing benign mole (pigmented naevus)

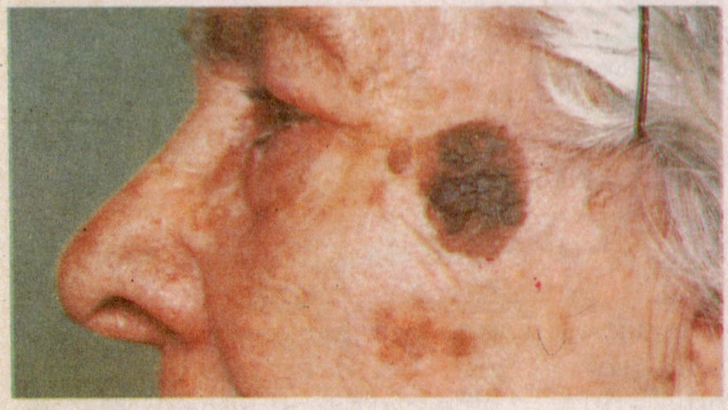

Nodules of malignant melanoma arising in a patch of Hutchinson's lentigo which had been present for many years

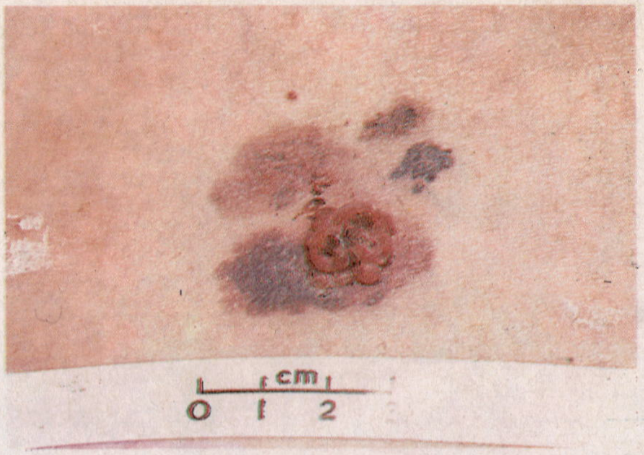

A superficial spreading melanoma with an amelanotic nodular area. The nodule had appeared within the previous month and had itched and bled

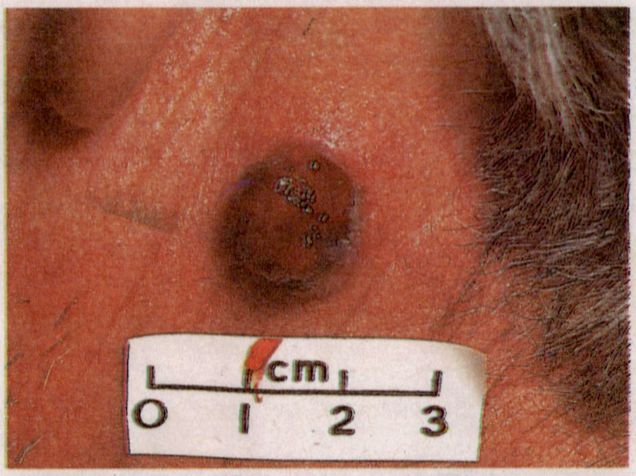

A large nodular melanoma which arose in previously normal skin

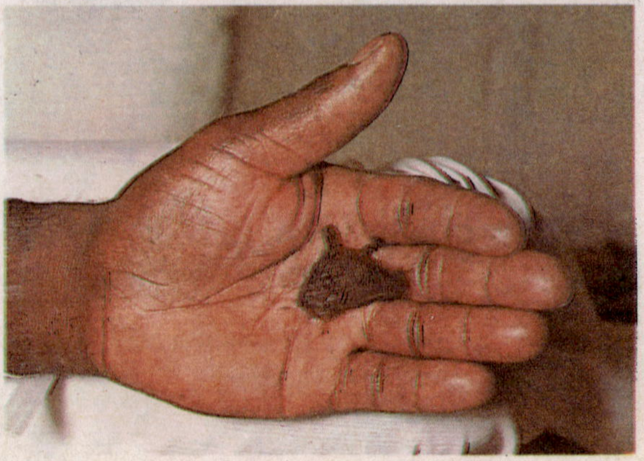

A malignant melanoma in the palm of the hand of a black-skinned manual worker

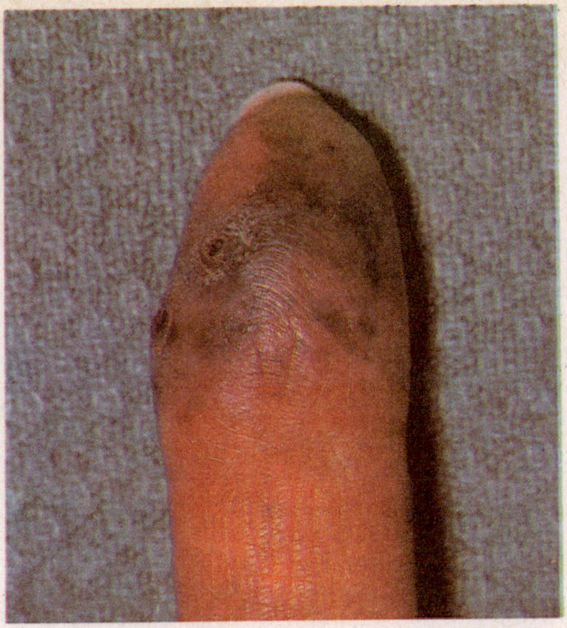

An acral lentiginous melanoma of the pulp of the index finger

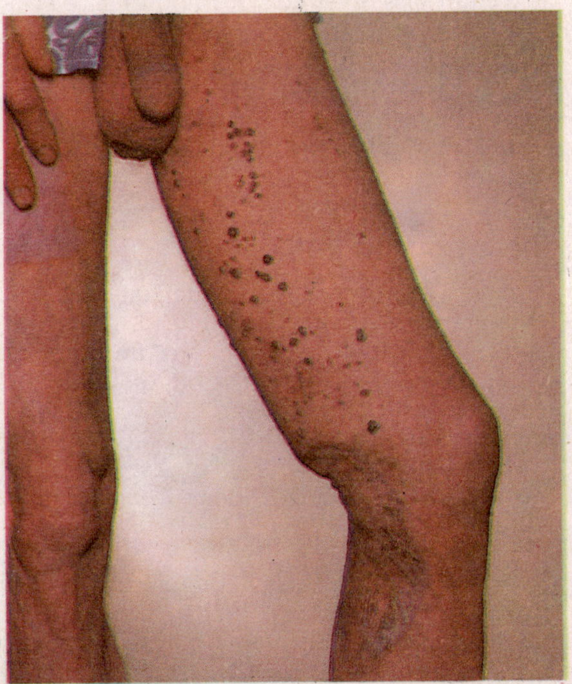

Multiple metastatic nodules of melanoma that appeared 4 years after the primary lesion, which was behind the knee, had been excised

FIG. 2.10 MALIGNANT MELANOMATA

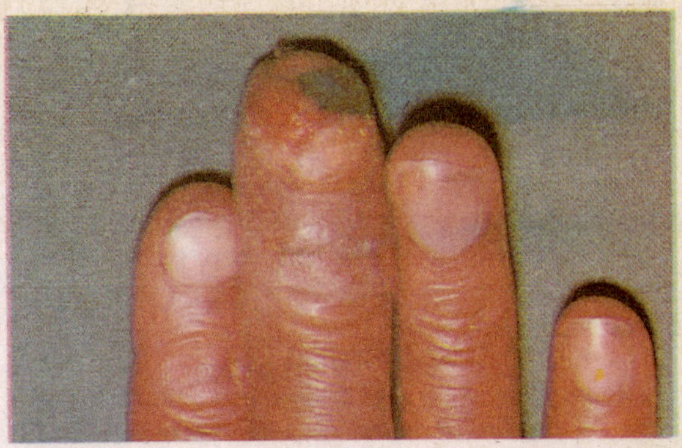

An ulcerated melanoma on the tip of the middle finger. The ulceration and lack of pigmentation caused the referring physician to think it was a chronic pulp space infection

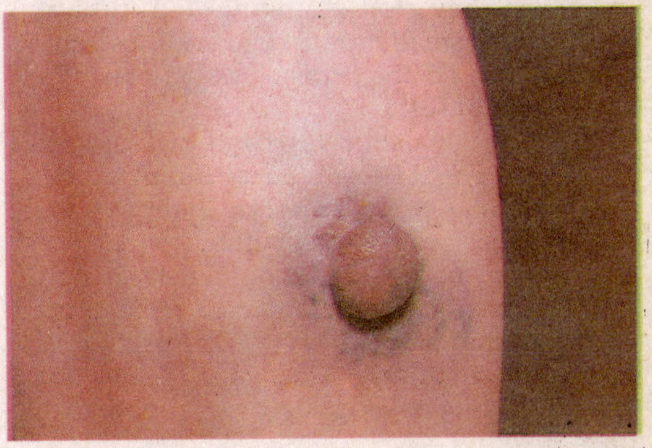

Satellite nodules of tumour cells around a nodular melanoma

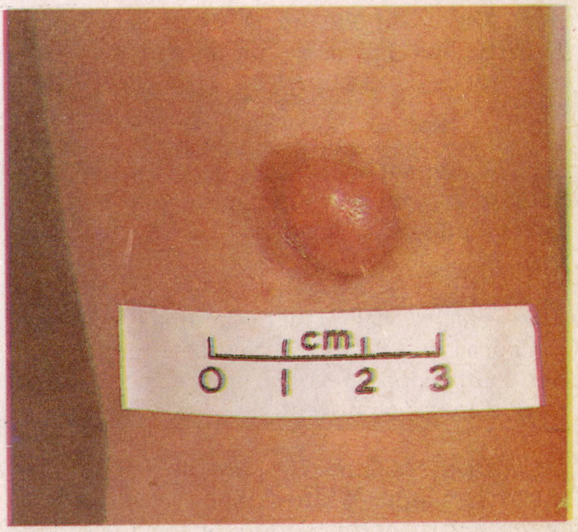

A nodular amelanotic melanoma. This arose in normal skin and was at first thought to be an histiocytoma

Bleeding As the tumour cells multiply, the overlying epithelium becomes anoxic and either ulcerates spontaneously or breaks down after a very minor injury. The subsequent bleeding is slight but recurs each time the scab is rubbed off. Bleeding is a late sign.

Evidence of local or distant spread The pigment produced by the malignant melanocytes may spread diffusely into the surrounding skin to produce a **brown halo** around the primary lesion.

The malignant cells may also spread through the skin in the intradermal lymphatics. When they stop migrating and multiply they become small intradermal nodules. Small nodules around the primary lesion are called **satellite nodules**.

Malignant melanocytes commonly spread by the lymphatics to the **local lymph nodes**. The combination of enlarged lymph nodes and changes in a mole within the area of drainage of those nodes is highly significant.

Not all malignant melanomata arise in pre-existing pigmented naevi. All the changes listed above can develop in a lesion that appeared quite quickly a few weeks or months previously.

HISTORY

Age Malignant melanoma is very rare before puberty, but it can occur in children. The majority develop in patients aged 20–30 years or more.

Sex Malignant melanoma occurs equally in both sexes, but is found more often in the lower limbs in women and on the trunk in men.

Ethnic group Malignant melanoma is common in Caucasians and rare in Negroes. People with fair complexions, red hair and a tendency to freckle are more susceptible.

Occupation Melanocytes are stimulated by ultraviolet light. White-skinned people living in those parts of the world which enjoy excess sunlight, such as Australia and the west coast of America, have a high incidence of malignant melanoma. Those who work out of doors in these regions, especially those with a history of repeated episodes of sunburn, are particularly susceptible.

Symptoms The cardinal features, which may be symptoms or signs, have already been described – a change of size or colour, bleeding and the appearance of a brown halo or satellite nodules. It is usually the **cosmetic disfigurement** caused by the enlarging lesion that brings the patient to the doctor (examples are shown in Fig. 2.10). More than 25% arise *de novo*, i.e. in normal skin not in a pre-existing lesion.

Malignant melanomata **often itch** but are **not painful**.

Sometimes the patient will have observed the changes in the mole herself, but if the mole is on the sole of the foot or the back of the trunk she may be unaware of its existence and present with lymph gland enlargement or symptoms caused by distant metastases, such as **weight loss, dyspnoea**, or **jaundice**.

Multiplicity Multiple malignant melanomata are very rare. Although there are often multiple secondary nodules around a primary lesion, two concurrent primary lesions are very uncommon.

LOCAL EXAMINATION

Position The majority of malignant melanomata are found on the limbs, head, neck and trunk. Within the limbs they are uncommon on the palms of the hands and the soles of the feet (except in African Negroes) and the subungual tissues.

Malignant melanomata may also occur at the muco-cutaneous junctions – the mouth and the anus.

Colour They may be any colour from a pale pinkish-brown to black. If they have a rich blood supply they develop a purple hue.

Temperature and tenderness A malignant melanoma is no warmer than the surrounding skin, in spite of its vascularity and cellular activity, and is not tender.

Shape and size When first noticed, the area of malignant change is usually quite small,

0.5–2 cm in diameter, but the mole in which the change has begun may be any size. If a malignant melanoma is neglected it will become a large florid tumour, protruding from and overlapping the surrounding skin.

Surface When the tumour is small it is covered by smooth epithelium. When the epithelium dies, from ischaemic necrosis, the resulting ulcer is covered with a crust of blood and serum. Bleeding and subacute infection may make the surface of the tumour wet, soft and boggy.

Composition The primary tumour has a firm, solid consistence. Small satellite nodules feel hard.

Clinical types Although the above description indicates that a malignant melanoma may have many forms, there are four common clinical types.

Superficial spreading melanoma is the most common type. It may occur on any part of the body, is usually palpable but thin, with an irregular edge and a variegated colour.

Nodular melanoma is a variety of melanoma that is thick, protrudes above the skin, has a smooth surface and a regular outline, and may arise *de novo*. It is often bleeding and ulcerated by the time of presentation.

Lentigo maligna melanoma is a malignant melanoma arising in a Hutchinson's lentigo. The malignant areas are thicker than the surrounding pigmented skin, usually darker in colour, but seldom ulcerate.

Acral lentiginous melanoma is a rare type but important to remember because it is often misdiagnosed as a chronic paronychia or a subungual haematoma. It presents as an irregular expanding area of brown or black pigmentation on the palm, sole or beneath a nail.

Relations The malignant tissue is within the skin, but rarely attached to deeper structures.

Lymph drainage The local lymph nodes may be enlarged.

Surrounding tissues There may be a **halo** of brown pigment in the skin around the tumour and **satellite nodules** in the skin and subcutaneous tissue between the primary tumour and the nearest lymph nodes. It is important to feel all the subcutaneous tissues along the course of the lymphatics which drain the lesion.

GENERAL EXAMINATION

Malignant melanoma first spreads through the lymphatics to the regional lymph nodes. It may then spread via the blood stream to the lungs, liver and brain. Pleural effusions, hepatomegaly, jaundice and neurological abnormalities are indications of distant metastases. Blood-borne secondary deposits in the skin and subcutaneous tissues are not uncommon.

Skin pigmentation associated with other diseases

Café au lait patch

Café au lait patches are areas of pale brown pigmentation. They are present at birth and often associated with neurofibromatosis and sometimes with phaeochromocytoma. The pale brown, milk-coffee colour is a reflection of the small amount of melanin in the lesion. Histologically they can be freckles or lentigo. This lesion does not undergo malignant change.

Revision Panel 2.2

The changes which suggest that a mole has turned malignant

Loss of normal surface markings (e.g. skin creases)

Change in size, shape or thickness

Change in colour

Itching

Bleeding/ulceration

Halo
- Pink (inflammatory reaction) – early
- Brown (pigment) – late

Satellite nodules

Distant spread: lymphadenopathy

Multiple circumoral moles associated with the Peutz–Jeghers syndrome

The Peutz–Jeghers syndrome is multiple polyposis of the mucosa of the stomach and small intestine and multiple small moles on the skin of the face, particularly around the mouth, on the lips and in the buccal mucous membrane. Histologically these are patches of lentigo. They do not turn malignant.

HAEMANGIOMATA AND LYMPHANGIOMATA

There are many forms of cutaneous haemangioma, such as strawberry naevus, port-wine stain, spider naevus, vin rosé patch, and Campbell de Morgan spots. All are various shades of pink or red but each one has distinctive features. Once you have seen these lesions you will always be able to recognize them. Their obvious common feature is their red colour.

Strawberry naevus

The name is an accurate description because this bright red lesion, which sticks out from the surface of the skin, looks just like a strawberry. The term 'naevus' is correctly used because strawberry naevi are present at birth. From a pathological point of view, they are congenital intradermal haemangiomata.

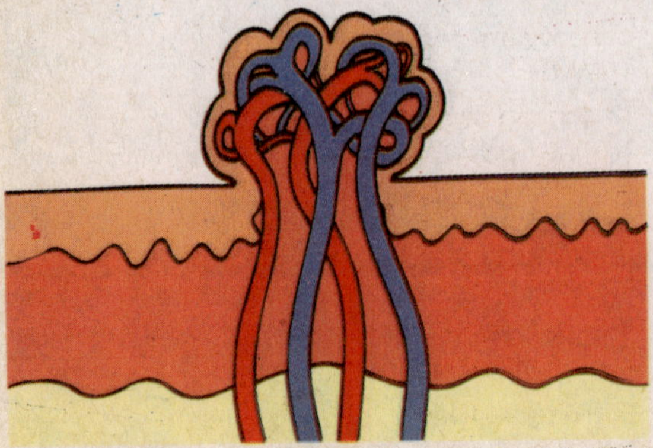

FIG. 2.11 A strawberry naevus is an intradermal and subdermal collection of dilated blood vessels

HISTORY

Age Strawberry naevi are present at birth.

Sex They occur equally in both sexes.

Duration They often regress spontaneously, a few months or years after birth.

Symptoms The child is brought to the doctor by its parent for diagnosis and because the red lump is disfiguring or a nuisance. Naevi in places likely to be rubbed or knocked may ulcerate and bleed. Lesions on the buttocks get wet and infected.

A child may have more than one strawberry naevus.

EXAMINATION

Position Strawberry naevi can occur on any part of the body but are most common on the head and neck.

Colour They are bright or dark red.

Shape They protrude from the skin surface. Small naevi are sessile hemispheres, but as they grow they can become pedunculated.

Size Strawberry naevi are usually 1–2 cm in diameter, but they can become quite large (5–10 cm).

Surface Their surface is irregular, but covered with a smooth, pitted epithelium. There may be small areas of ulceration covered with scabs.

Consistence The strawberry naevus is soft and **compressible but not pulsatile**. Gentle sustained pressure will squeeze most of the blood out of the lesion leaving it collapsed, crinkled and colourless. The rate of refilling depends upon the number of feeding arteries.

Relations These naevi are confined to the skin and are freely mobile over the deep tissues.

Lymph drainage The regional lymph glands should not be enlarged.

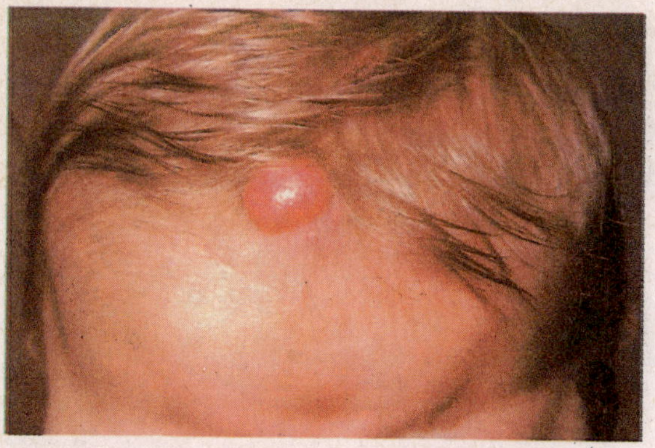

A large sessile strawberry naevus on the forehead

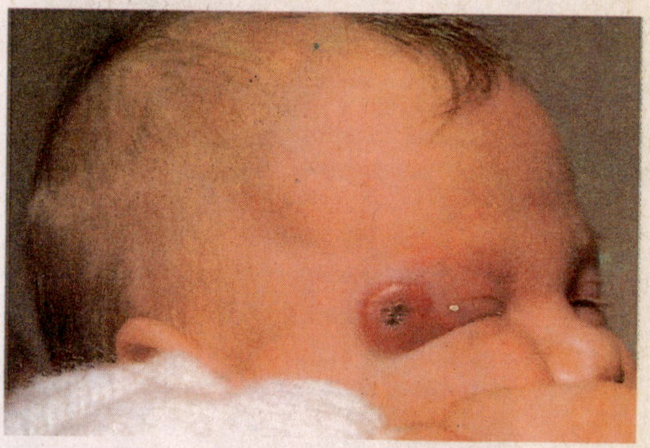

A regressing cavernous haemangioma

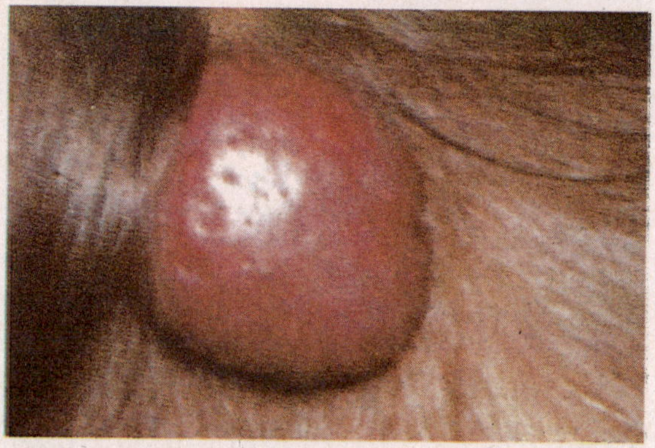

A close-up view of a strawberry naevus on the forehead showing the smooth epithelial covering and little pits which, with the red colour, make the lesion look like a strawberry

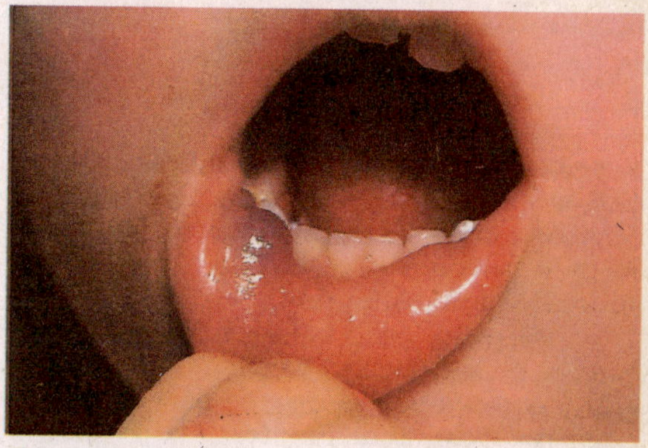

A haemangioma on the inside of the lower lip. These lesions are similar to strawberry naevi of the skin but are smooth and usually dark purple in colour

FIG. 2.12 HAEMANGIOMATA

Surrounding tissues The blood supply of the surrounding skin is absolutely normal. This congenital condition is not associated with any other congenital vascular abnormality.

Port-wine stain

This is an extensive intradermal haemangioma, mostly venous but involving all types of skin blood vessels. It discolours the skin, giving it a deep purple–red colour; hence its name.

HISTORY

Age Port-wine stains are present at birth and do not change in size thereafter, relative to the size of the rest of the body, but their colour may alter.

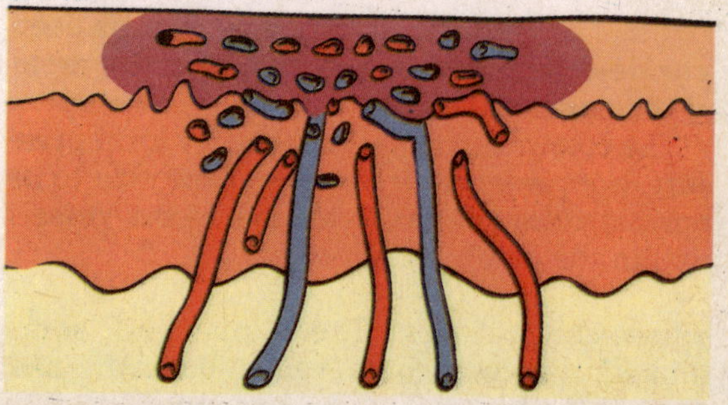

FIG. 2.13 A port-wine stain is a collection of dilated venules and capillaries just below the epidermis

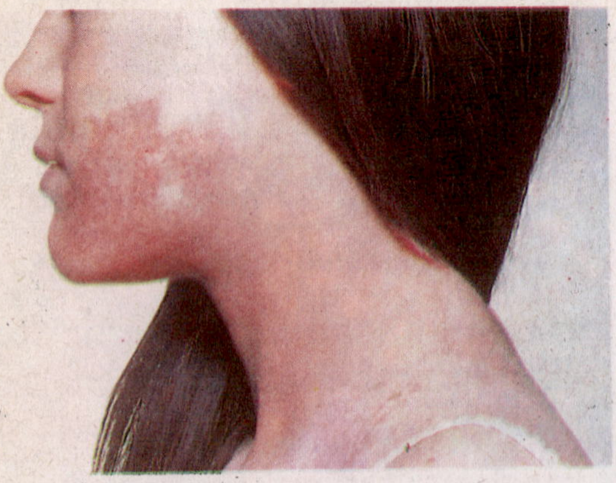

An extensive port-wine stain of the lower face and neck

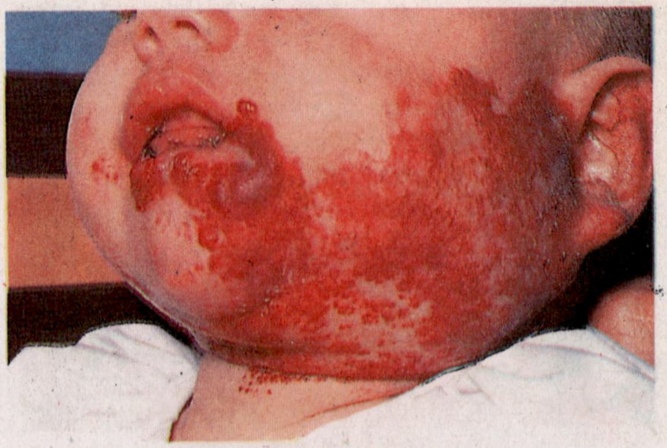

A mixture of strawberry and port-wine-stain naevi of the face which is beginning to regress

FIG. 2.14 HAEMANGIOMATA

Symptoms The distress these stains cause the patient's parents and, later on, the patient is entirely related to their colour and position. As they are common on the face they are very noticeable and disfiguring.

Occasionally, small vessels within the stain become prominent and bleed.

The port-wine stain may be part of a more extensive vascular deformity.

EXAMINATION

Position Port-wine stains are common on the face and the junctions between the limbs and the trunk; i.e. the shoulders, neck and buttocks. Sometimes they seem to be confined to a single dermatome, especially when they are part of a generalized vascular deformity, but there are never any associated neurological abnormalities.

Colour Their distinctive feature is their deep purple–red colour. There may be paler areas at the edge of the patch.

The colour can be diminished by local pressure, but pressure rarely returns the skin to its normal colour because all the blood vessels within the patch are abnormal.

Surrounding tissues There may be some dilated subcutaneous veins beneath and around the lesion. The sensory innervation of the stain is normal.

Spider naevus

The spider naevus is a solitary dilated skin arteriole feeding a number of small branches which leave it in a radial manner. It is an **acquired** condition and may be associated with a generalized disease.

HISTORY

Spider naevi are not noticed by the patient except when they are in a prominent position on the face. They cause no symptoms. They are multiple and tend to increase in number over the years. It is important to enquire about the patient's consumption of alcohol because they may be associated with chronic liver disease.

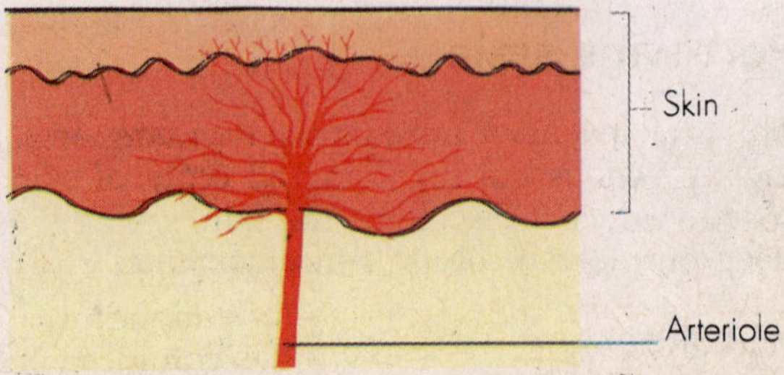

FIG. 2.15 A spider naevus is a solitary dilated arteriole with visible radiating branches

EXAMINATION

Position Spider naevi appear on the upper half of the trunk, the face and the arms. It has been observed that this is the area of drainage of the superior vena cava, but it is doubtful if this is a significant observation.

Colour The central arteriole is bright red and the vessels radiating from it are of a similar colour but not so red or so noticeable.

Temperature Spider naevi do not cause a change of skin temperature and are not tender.

Size The central arteriole is 0.5–1.0 mm in diameter. The radiating vessels spread for a varying distance, usually 1–2 mm.

Compressibility Spider naevi fade completely when compressed with the finger, or preferably a glass slide, and refill as soon as the pressure is released. Compression of the central arteriole with the head of a pin makes the radiating 'legs' fade.

Local tissues There should be no other abnormalities of the local circulation.

GENERAL EXAMINATION

The general examination is important because spider naevi may be associated with serious diseases such as hepatic cirrhosis, tumours destroying the liver, and tumours producing oestrogen.

Vin rosé patch

This is a congenital intradermal vascular abnormality in which mild dilatation of the vessels in the subpapillary dermal plexus gives the skin a pale pink colour. It is often associated with other vascular abnormalities such as extensive haemangiomata, giant limbs due to arteriovenous fistulae and lymphoedema.

The vin rosé patch can occur anywhere and causes no symptoms. It is not dark enough to be disfiguring and the patient has commonly accepted its presence as a minor birthmark and forgotten about it.

Campbell de Morgan spot

This lesion is a bright red, clearly defined spot caused by a collection of dilated capillaries fed by a single or cluster of arterioles. The cause of these spots is unknown and they are not associated with any other disease.

HISTORY

Age Campbell de Morgan spots increase in number as the patient gets older. They are uncommon in people under 45 years of age.

Duration They appear suddenly, usually one at a time, but sometimes a cluster of spots will appear in one area of the skin.

Symptoms They are not painful or tender, and not disfiguring unless they are multiple and extensive.

EXAMINATION

Position Campbell de Morgan spots appear on both aspects of the trunk, more on the upper half than the lower half. They occasionally appear on the limbs and rarely on the face.

Size and shape They vary from 1 to 3 mm in diameter. They are circular and have a sharp edge which is sometimes slightly raised.

Colour Their colour is their diagnostic feature. They have a uniform deep red or purple colour which makes them look like drops of dark red paint or sealing wax just under the epidermis.

Compressibility Although they are a collection of dilated capillaries, they do not always empty when compressed, but always fade slightly.

Lymphangioma

(Lymphangioma circumscriptum)

This is a circumscribed cluster of many small dilated lymph sacs in the skin and subcutaneous tissues which **do not** connect into the

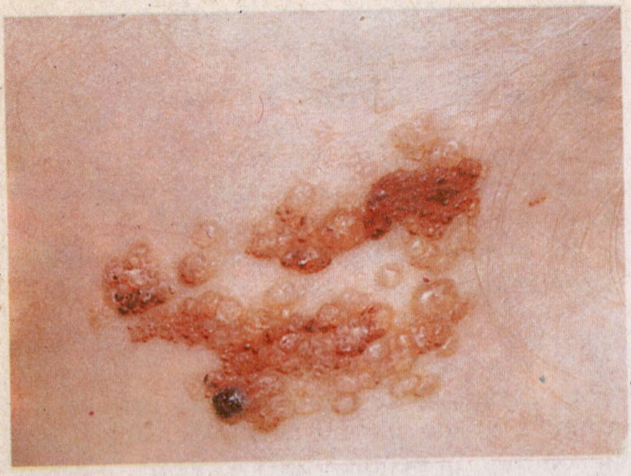

In this small localized lesion many of the vesicles are red, black or brown because they contain old blood

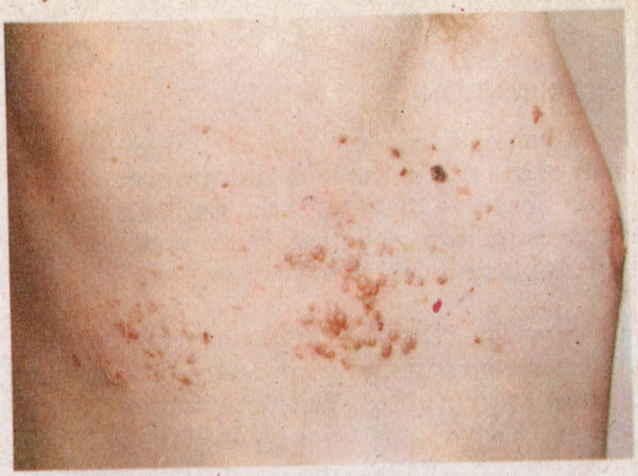

This extensive lesion spreads across the whole of the side of the chest just below the axilla. The swelling deep to the posterior part of the lesion is caused by the subcutaneous cysts

FIG. 2.16 LYMPHANGIOMA CIRCUMSCRIPTUM

normal lymph system. The aetiology of these blind sacs is unexplained but, as they are congenital, it is likely that they are clusters of lymph sacs that failed to join into the lymph system during its development. Large, translucent lymph cysts confined to the subcutaneous tissues are called cystic hygromata (see page 266).

HISTORY

Age Lymphangiomata are present at birth but may not be noticed until the skin vesicles appear a few years later.

Symptoms They are usually noticed by the child's parents, who consult the doctor because they are concerned about the diagnosis and the disfigurement. Occasionally, the skin vesicles contain clotted blood which turns them brown. Sometimes the vesicles leak clear fluid. When very prominent, the vesicles become rubbed by the clothes and may get infected and painful.

Development As the years pass, the subcutaneous cysts fill with fluid and become prominent and the number and extent of the skin vesicles increases.

EXAMINATION

Position Lymphangiomata circumscriptum are found at the junction of the limbs and the neck with the trunk; i.e. around the shoulder, axilla, buttock and groin.

Colour The skin vesicles contain clear fluid which looks watery or yellow. Blood in the vesicles turns them red-brown or even black.

Overall appearance The subcutaneous cysts make the abnormal area bulge slightly but the edges of this swelling are indistinct. The skin contains vesicles of varying sizes and colour, ranging from 0.5 to 3 or 4 mm in diameter.

Size A large area of skin may be involved, the whole of the buttock or shoulder may be abnormal; but most lymphangiomata are 5–20 cm across when they present for treatment.

Composition The whole lesion is soft and spongy. If there are multiple cysts the swelling will not fluctuate. If there are just one, or two, large cysts then the signs of fluid (fluctuation, fluid thrill and translucency) will all be present. The mass is not compressible. The dark red or brown vesicles **do not** fade with pressure.

Lymph drainage The local lymph nodes are usually normal unless the cysts have been infected.

State of local tissues The blood and nerve supplies to the area of a lymphangioma circumscriptum are normal. The tissues between the cysts and vesicles have a normal lymph drainage, so they are not oedematous.

Pyogenic granuloma

All skin wounds heal by the development of small capillary loops which knit the wound together and form a base for the overgrowth of epithelium. In the base of a healing ulcer these capillary loops form a layer of bright red tissue known as **granulation tissue**. If the capillary loops grow too vigorously they may form a protruding mass of tissue which becomes covered with epithelium. This mass usually becomes infected and is called a pyogenic granuloma.

Thus the infection is a secondary event, not the initiating stimulus. The cause of this abnormality of tissue repair is not known.

HISTORY

Age Pyogenic granulomata are uncommon in children.

Symptoms There may be a history of a minor injury, usually a cut or scratch, but the patient cannot always remember the initial injury. Pyogenic granulomata sometimes occur in response to chronic infections such as paronychiae.

The patient complains of a **rapidly growing lump** on the skin, which bleeds easily and discharges a serous or purulent fluid. So rapid is the growth of the lump (it may double in size in a few days) that most patients think it is a tumour. When it is completely covered with epithelium the bleeding and weeping stops.

Pyogenic granulomata are not painful.

EXAMINATION

Position Pyogenic granulomata are most common on those parts of the body likely to be injured, such as the hands and face (see Fig. 2.17).

Colour At first they have the bright red colour of healthy granulation tissue but as they get bigger and less vascular they fade to a pale pink. When they become covered with epithelium they turn skin colour or white.

Tenderness Although they are not painful, they are sometimes slightly tender.

Shape and size They begin as a hemispherical nodule which grows upwards and outwards. The lump is rarely more than 1 cm across because beyond this size the blood supply becomes inadequate. The growth from a few millimetres to full size can occur in a few days.

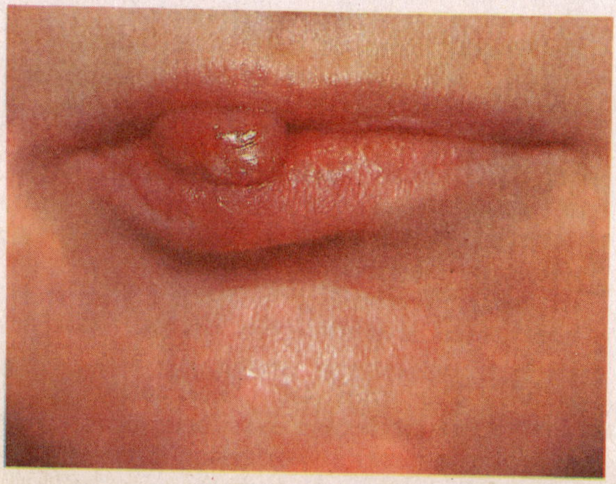

A pyogenic granuloma on the lip. This lump grew in 6 days following a minor injury to the lip. By the time this photograph was taken the lump was covered with epithelium

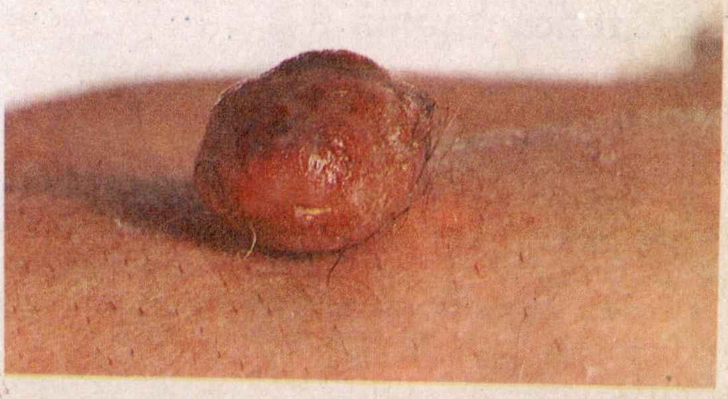

A pyogenic granuloma on the skin of the chest that appeared 4 days after a deep scratch

FIG. 2.17 PYOGENIC GRANULOMATA

Surface Before the surface is epithelialized it has a covering of dried blood or plasma. It may bleed when rubbed.

Composition Pyogenic granulomata are soft and slightly compressible but do not pulsate.

Relations They are usually confined to the skin, because the skin is the commonest structure to suffer minor injury. The base is always fixed to the tissue which is producing the granulations.

Lymph drainage The local lymph nodes will only be enlarged when the granuloma is heavily infected.

Complications The lump bleeds easily when knocked. Very rough handling may break it off at its base with only slight bleeding. It may then reform in the next few days, or heal normally.

Natural history Once the granulations have become completely covered with epithelium, the nodule begins to shrink, but it rarely goes completely.

Differential diagnosis The important conditions to exclude are squamous carcinoma, non-pigmented melanoma and, in some parts of the world, Kaposi sarcoma (see page 88). A history of trauma and the very rapid growth are the peculiar features of a pyogenic granuloma but an excisional biopsy is often necessary to confirm the diagnosis.

Keratoacanthoma

(Adenoma sebaceum, molluscum pseudo-carcinomatosum)

This is a self-limiting overgrowth and subsequent spontaneous regression of hair follicle cells. Because it grows rapidly it is often mistaken for a squamous cell carcinoma.

HISTORY

Keratoacanthomata occur in adults. The patient complains of a rapidly growing lump in the skin, which develops a central dark brown core. It is not painful but can be very unsightly. The lump takes 2–4 weeks to grow and 2–3 months to regress.

The cause is unknown. It may be a self-limiting benign neoplasm or an unusual response to a viral infection.

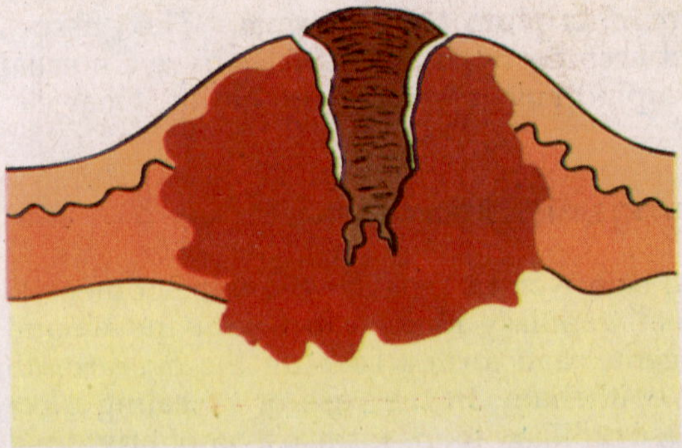

FIG. 2.18 A keratoacanthoma is an overgrowth of hair follicle cells which produce a central plug of keratin. When the plug separates, the lesion usually undergoes spontaneous regression

EXAMINATION

Position Keratoacanthomata are usually found on the face but they can occur anywhere where there are sebaceous glands. It is unusual to have multiple lesions.

Colour The lump has a normal skin colour, but the necrotic centre is brown or black.

Size By the time the centre of the lump begins to necrose, the nodule is 1–2 cm in diameter.

Shape The lump is hemispherical or conical and, when the central slough appears and retracts, looks like a volcano.

Consistence The bulk of the lesion is firm and rubbery, but the central core is hard.

Relations The lump is confined to the skin and is freely mobile over the subcutaneous tissues. There is never any extension beyond the skin into the surrounding tissues.

Lymph drainage The local lymph nodes should not be enlarged.

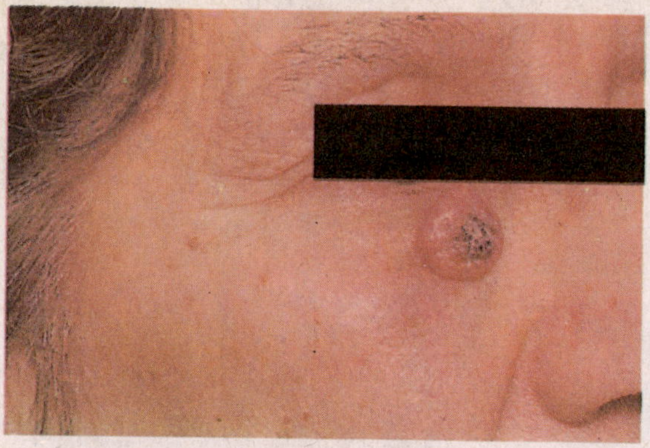

A large keratoacanthoma on the face

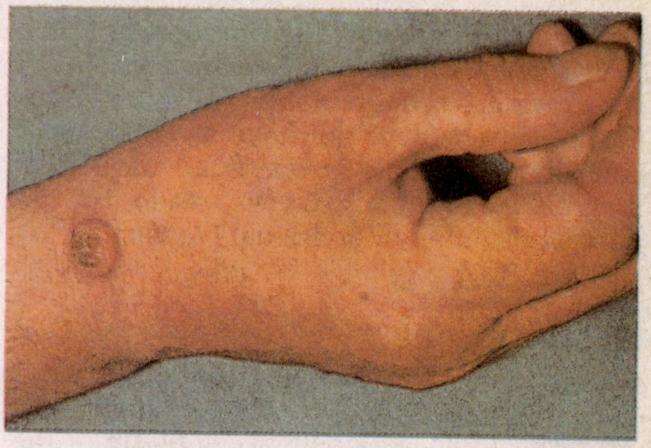

A keratoacanthoma on the wrist. The slough is just beginning to separate

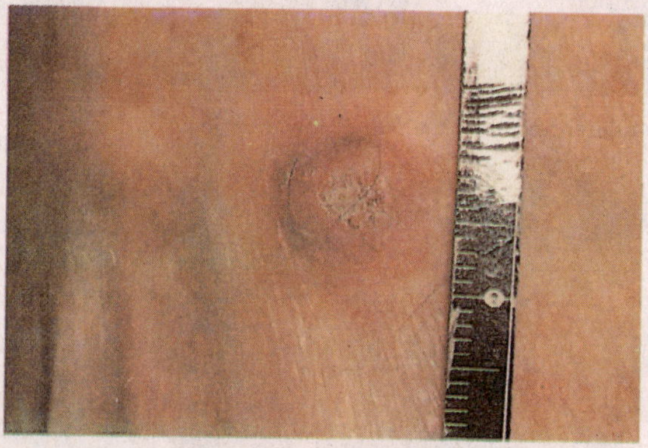

A keratoacanthoma that is beginning to collapse, the slough having separated

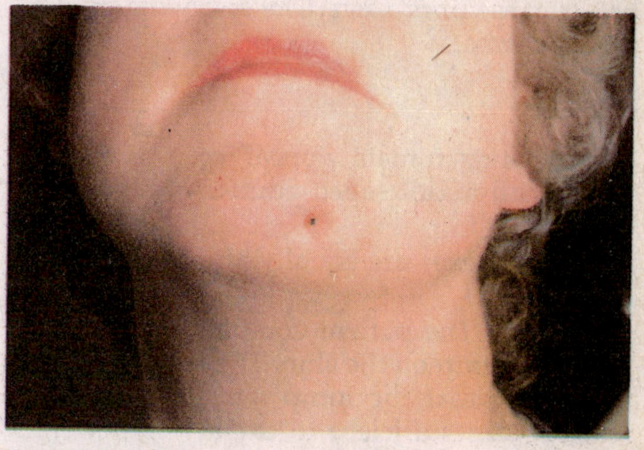

The end result if the lesion is not excised – a deep, puckered scar

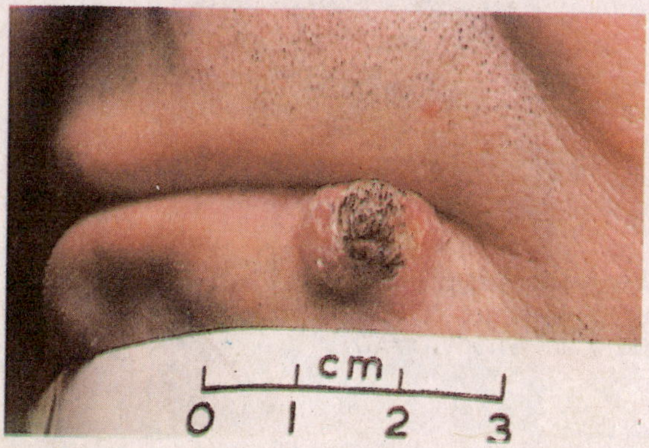

A close-up view of the slough

FIG. 2.19 KERATOACANTHOMATA

Natural history If a keratoacanthoma is left alone the central core eventually separates and the lump collapses, leaving a deep indrawn scar. In spite of this self-limiting natural history, keratoacanthomata are usually excised to confirm the diagnosis, and to prevent the development of the disfiguring scar.

Differential diagnosis The important lesion that is often similar to a keratoacanthoma is the squamous cell carcinoma. The latter grows a little slower, does not have a central dead core and eventually becomes an ulcer. The diagnosis should always be made by the pathologist after an excisional biopsy.

Hystiocytoma

(Dermatofibroma, sclerosing angioma)

An histiocytoma is a benign neoplasm of the fibroblasts of the dermis. Its name is derived from the many histiocytes which are present between the fibroblasts. The overlying epidermis is normal.

HISTORY

Age Histiocytomata appear on the skin of young and middle-aged adults.

Sex Both sexes are equally affected.

Symptoms The patient complains of a **slow-growing lump** on the skin. The rate of growth is so slow that the lump may take years to reach a size sufficient to excite the patient's curiosity or get in the way of clothing.

There are no associated general symptoms.

EXAMINATION

Position Histiocytomata can occur anywhere, but are slightly more common on the skin of the limbs.

Colour They are covered by normal-coloured epidermis which may contain sufficient haemosiderin to give them a brown colour and therefore the appearance of a mole.

Tenderness They are not tender.

Shape As they grow, they form a hemispherical lump which then flattens into a thick disc. The edges of the disc may overhang its base.

Size Most patients complain of these tumours when they are 1–2 cm across but they can grow to a considerable size if they are neglected.

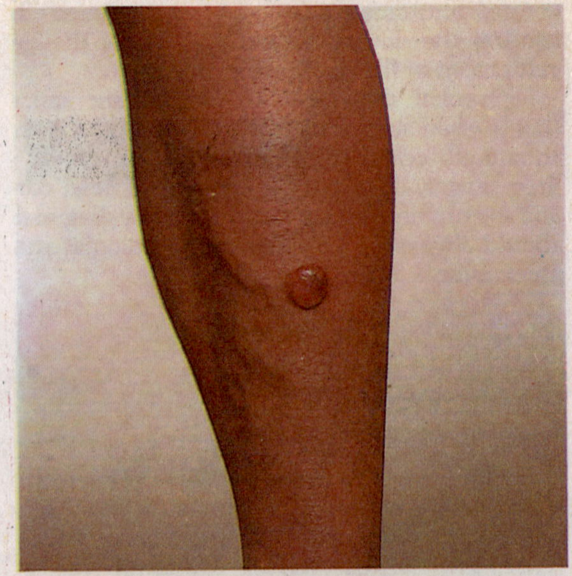

An histiocytoma of the skin of the lower leg

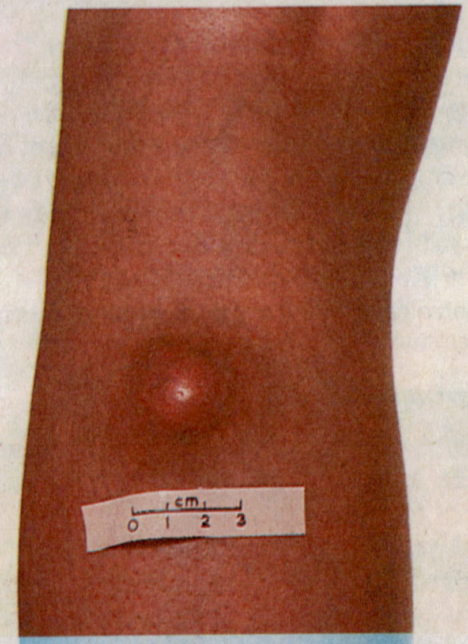

A large histiocytoma on the calf

FIG. 2.20 HISTIOCYTOMATA

Surface The skin covering the lump is often loose and slightly crinkled, even though it is inseparable from the lump.

Composition These tumours usually have a soft-solid consistence, almost spongy. They do not fluctuate or transilluminate.

Relations They are in the skin, separate from and freely mobile over the deep tissues.

Lymph drainage The local lymph glands should not be enlarged.

State of local tissues The surrounding tissues are normal.

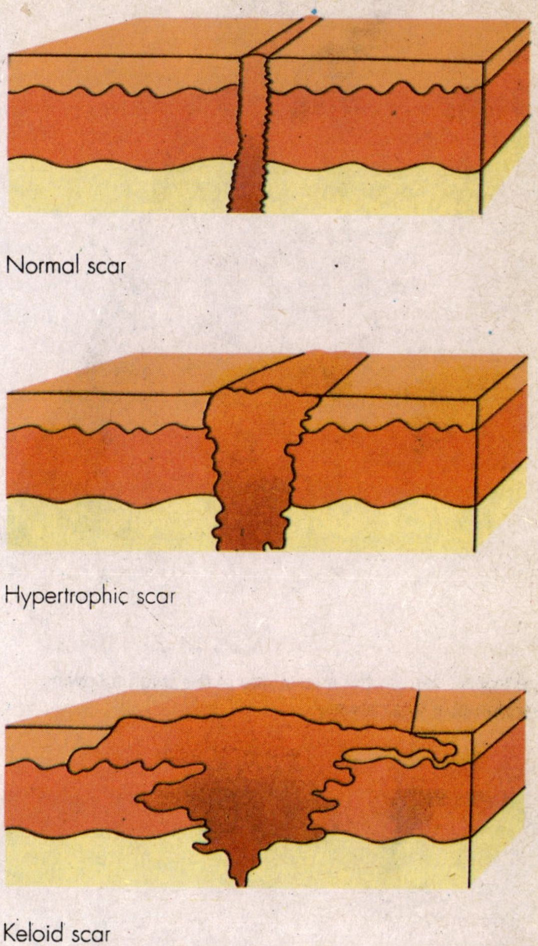

FIG. 2.21 Normal, hypertrophic and keloid scars

Keloid and hypertrophic scars

A wound heals in three stages. First, the gap in the tissue is filled by blood and fibrin. This is then replaced by collagen and fibrous tissue which knits the tissues together. Finally, the fibrous tissue is organized to give the wound the maximum strength. This process is remarkably well controlled. Most scars in the skin are thin lines containing the minimum amount of scar tissue. However, sometimes the fibrous tissue response is excessive and the result is a hypertrophic or keloid scar.

In a **hypertrophic scar** there is an excessive amount of fibrous tissue but it is confined to the scar; i.e. it is between the skin edges. Hypertrophic scars are quite common, particularly if there has been some extra stimulus to fibrous tissue formation during healing, such as infection or excessive tension. Scars crossing skin creases are particularly susceptible to both these complications. Hypertrophic scars grow only for 2–3 months.

In a **keloid scar** the hypertrophy and overgrowth of the fibrous tissue extends *beyond* the original wound into normal tissues. This means that the scar has some of the characteristics of a locally malignant neoplasm. The tendency to produce keloid scars is a congenital trait, common in Negroes. Some tribes exploit the trait for the production of decorative scars on the face and trunk. Keloid scars continue to enlarge for 6–12 months after the initial injury.

As a keloid scar grows it can become exceedingly **unsightly**, is often **tender** to touch and may **itch**. Although the cosmetic disfigurement of a hypertrophic scar may be as great as that of a keloid scar, it is important to try to distinguish the two abnormalities because hypertrophic scars will not recur after they have been excised if the causative factors are eliminated, whereas keloid scars are highly likely to recur whatever you do.

Callosities and corns

These conditions are known to everyone. They are areas of skin thickening and hyperkeratosis secondary to pressure and repeated minor trauma (see also page 156). If the thickened skin is pushed inwards by constant pressure, e.g. on the sole of the foot, it becomes painful and is known as a corn.

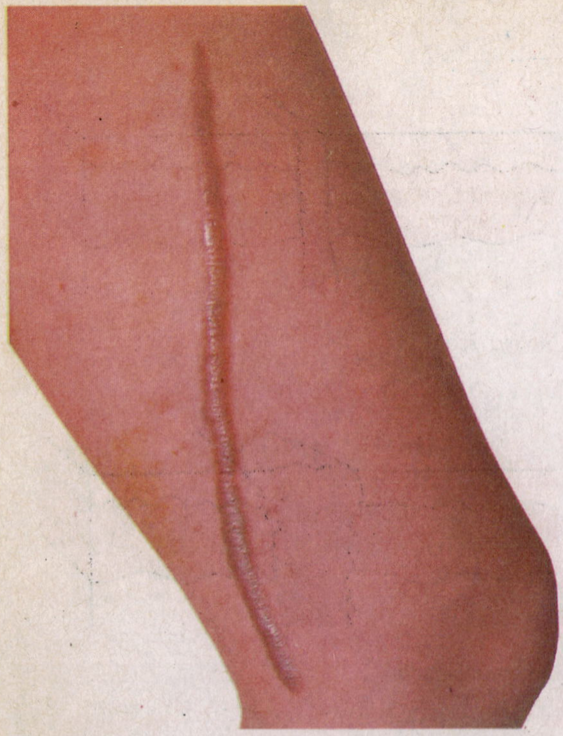

A hypertrophic scar on the medial side of the thigh following the excision of a large lipoma

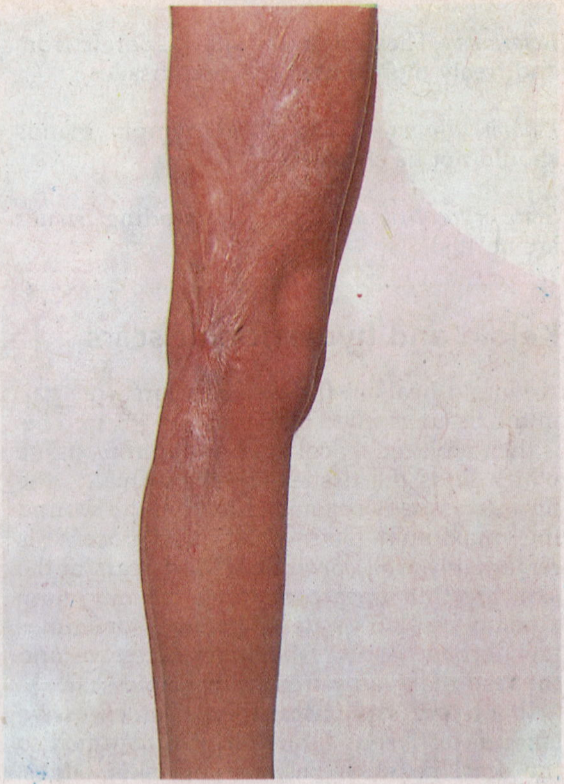

Hypertrophic scars after a burn

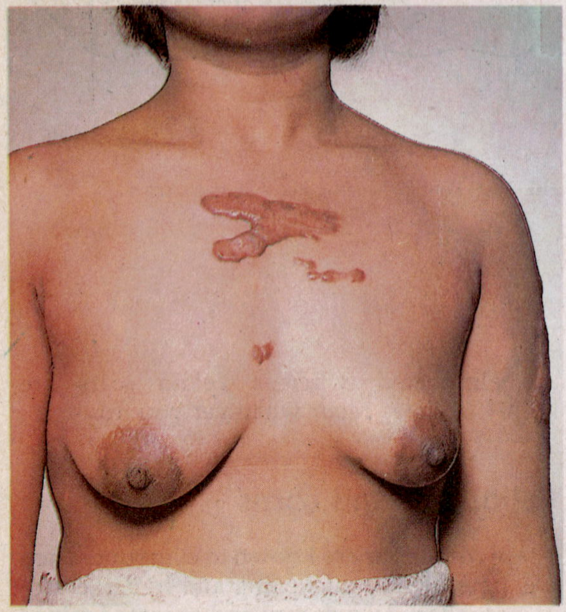

Keloid scars after tribal marking

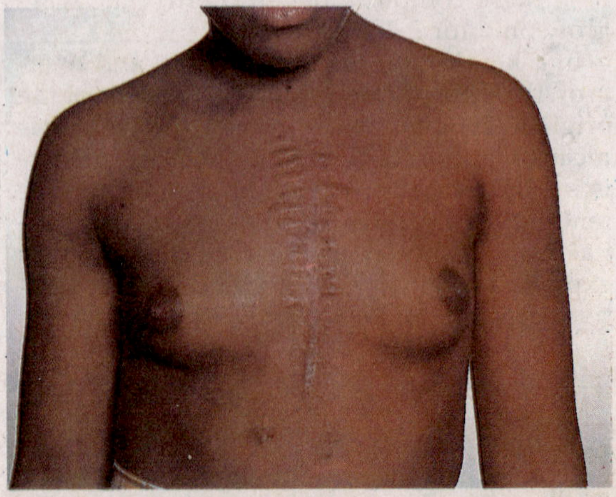

Keloid scars after a median sternotomy

FIG. 2.22 HYPERTROPHIC AND KELOID SCARS

HISTORY

Age Corns and callosities are more common in the elderly, not because their skin growth changes but because changes of the skeleton cause redistribution and maldistribution of weight bearing.

Symptoms Callosities may get rubbed and sore but are not usually painful. Corns are painful, when pressed, because they are narrow and deep.

EXAMINATION

A **callosity** is a raised, thickened patch of greyish-brown hyperkeratotic skin over an area of excessive wear and tear. Thus they are common on the hands and feet, and their site varies with the patient's occupation and skeletal structure.

As they exercise a protective function, they are best left alone; but the diagnosis can be confirmed by carefully paring away the top layer of roughened skin to expose the homogeneous, shiny, translucent layers of dead skin beneath.

A **corn** is a similar but smaller lesion that is pushed into the skin. Thus it forms a palpable nodule with a central yellow-white core of dead cornified epidermal cells. Corns are found on the soles of the feet, the tips of the toes and over the dorsal surface of the interphalangeal joints. The main *differential diagnosis* is the **plantar wart**. These two lesions are identified by paring away the top layers of skin with a knife to expose either the corn's core of dead translucent tissue, or the verruca's soft filiform processes.

Solar keratosis

Prolonged exposure of the skin to sunlight can cause areas of hyperkeratosis of the skin, which may undergo malignant change.

HISTORY

The patient notices the gradual appearance of thickened patches of skin. They are not painful but can become unsightly. If they become prominent they may catch on clothing and interfere with hand function.

Natural history Solar keratoses grow slowly and the patients, usually elderly men who have worked out of doors for many years, ignore them. These lesions must be watched carefully for any change in size or appearance.

EXAMINATION

Site The common sites to find solar keratoses are the backs of the fingers and hands, the face and the rim of the ears.

Colour The thickened patches of skin have a yellow-grey, or sometimes brown, colour.

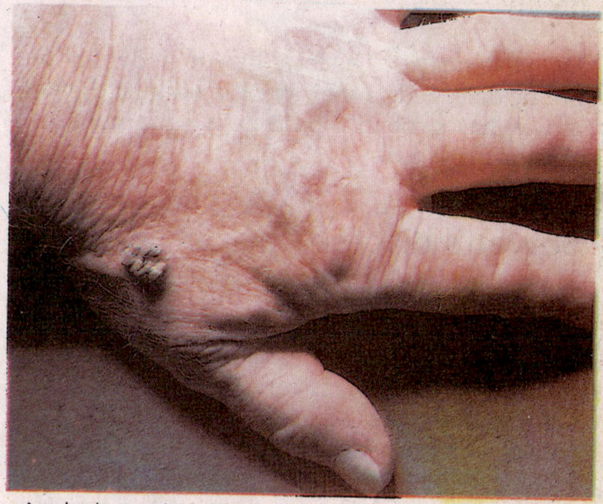

A solar keratosis on the back of the hand

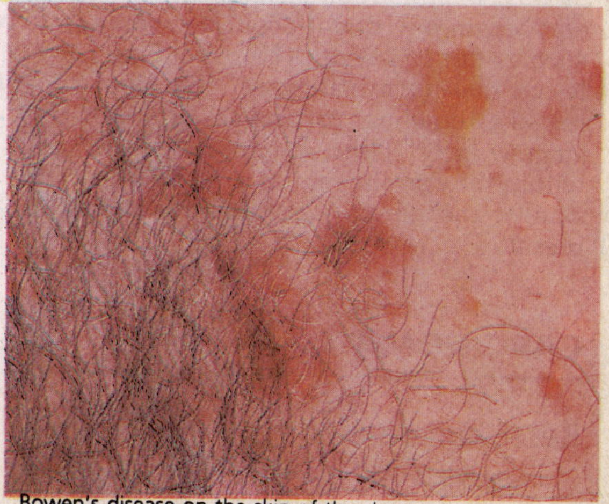

Bowen's disease on the skin of the chest

FIG. 2.23 PRECANCEROUS CONDITIONS OF THE SKIN

Shape and size Beneath their horny surface layer there is a raised plaque of skin which may vary in diameter from a few millimetres to 1 cm, and protrude above the skin surface. The whole of the strip of skin along the rim of the pinna may be affected.

Composition The keratinous layer is very hard and clearly part of the underlying skin.

Relations Solar keratoses are confined to the skin. If a nodule or patch is tethered to the underlying structures then it has turned into a squamous carcinoma and is infiltrating deeply.

Lymph drainage The local lymph nodes should not be enlarged. If they are, then one of the keratoses has probably become a squamous cell carcinoma.

Bowen's disease

This is a rare condition but is mentioned because it is precancerous.

It presents as a cluster of flat, pink, papular patches which are covered with crusts. The patches and the adjacent skin have a pale brown, thickened appearance. The patient usually believes he has a patch of eczema.

When the crusts are removed the papules can be seen to have a wet, oozy, slightly bloody, papilliferous surface.

When in any doubt about a chronic lesion such as this it is wise to biopsy it because this lesion may turn malignant. The biopsy may reveal a squamous carcinoma, or, in the early stages, large clear carcinoma-in-situ cells within the dermis, similar to those seen in the skin of the nipple in Paget's disease of the breast.

CARCINOMATA

Basal cell carcinoma

(Rodent ulcer)

This is a locally invasive carcinoma (also known as a **rodent ulcer**) of the basal layer of the epidermis. It does not metastasize but nevertheless can kill by local infiltration. It is common in exposed skin, especially in regions where there is a high incidence of ultraviolet irradiation, i.e. bright sunlight.

HISTORY

Age The incidence of basal cell carcinoma increases with age because it is related to the duration of exposure of the skin to ultraviolet light.

Geography They are more common in countries that have much bright sunlight.

Ethnic group They are rare in dark-skinned races.

Sex Males are affected more than females.

Duration Basal cell carcinomata grow very slowly and have usually been present for months or years before the patient seeks advice.

Symptoms The principal complaint is of a persistent **nodule or an ulcer with a central scab** that repeatedly falls off and then reforms, sometimes with a little bleeding. The lesion grows slowly but eventually becomes disfiguring and annoying. It may **itch**. If it is neglected and becomes a deep ulcer it may cause pain, bleed and become infected. The large, neglected rodent ulcer destroying one side of the face, commonly displayed in textbooks, is nowadays fortunately rare.

Development The lesion grows very slowly and may have been present for months or years before the patient bothers to complain about it. This long history gives the patient a false impression that the lesion is benign and unimportant. They often think that they have a patch of chronic dermatitis.

Persistence Some basal cell carcinomata spread laterally through the skin, leaving a central scar. This may make the patient think that it has healed spontaneously.

Multiplicity Basal cell carcinomata are often multiple.

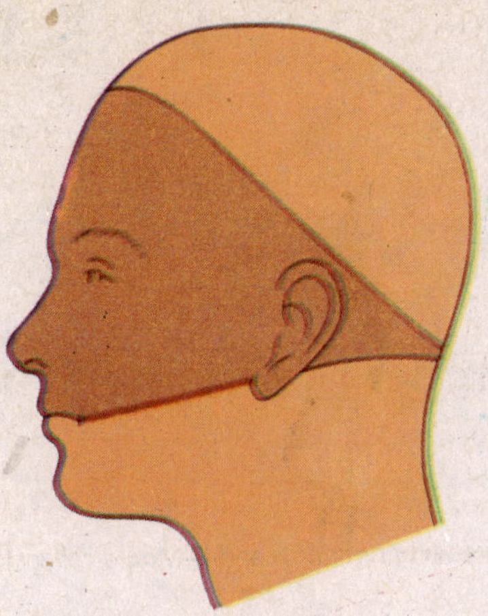

FIG. 2.24 Basal cell carcinomata commonly appear in the shaded area

Predisposing factors Skin that has been treated with arsenic is liable to develop basal cell carcinomata. Arsenic was once a common ingredient of skin ointments.

EXAMINATION

Position Rodent ulcers are commonly found on the face above a line drawn from the angle of the mouth to the lobe of the ear. This does not mean that they do not occur in other sites; all skin is susceptible, particularly the skin of the scalp, neck, arms and hands.

Colour The raised portion of the lesion – that is to say, its edge if it is annular, or its centre if it is a nodule – is smooth, glistening and slightly transparent. This gives the impression that there are pearl-white nodules of tissue just below the epidermis. These nodules also give the ulcerating variety its typical 'rolled edge', but the term 'pearly edge' can be confusing because the term 'epithelial pearls' is also used to describe the histological appearance of the nodules of a squamous carcinoma.

The surface of the nodular variety is covered by fine, distinct blood vessels which may give it a pink hue.

The whole lesion may be coloured brown by excess melanin.

Size Most patients come and complain of the ulcer or nodule when it is quite small, but basal cell carcinomata can grow to a considerable size if they are neglected. A few grow outwards from the skin to become a fungating mass on the skin surface, but the majority erode deeply, destroying the underlying tissues and forming a deep cavity.

Shape Figure 2.25 shows some of the macroscopic appearances of rodent ulcer. Only two are true ulcers, so it is better to use the term 'basal cell carcinoma', not 'rodent ulcer'.

The tumour always starts as a nodule. When the centre dies the resulting ulcer has a **rolled edge**. This means that the edge is raised up and rounded **but not everted**. If the centre of the tumour does not necrose and ulcerate, the nodule can become quite large and look like a cyst. It is not cystic because it is solid and non-fluctuant, but the bad and contradictory term 'cystic rodent ulcer' is sometimes used to describe this appearance.

Edge When the nodule first ulcerates, the rolled edge is circular, but, as the malignant cells spread, the shape of the ulcer becomes irregular. If the ulcer heals, the raised edge may be the only clue to the diagnosis. An irregular raised edge around a flat white scar is sometimes called a **geographical** or **forest fire** basal cell carcinoma. When the ulcer erodes into deeper structures the edge becomes more prominent and florid but does not become everted.

Base The base of a small rodent ulcer is covered with a coat of dried serum and epithelial

Revision Panel 2.3

The clinical appearances of basal cell carcinomata

Nodule

'Cystic' (a large seemingly transparent nodule)

Ulcer

Deeply eroding ulcer, 'rodent ulcer'

Pigmented nodule

Geographical (advancing edge, healing centre)

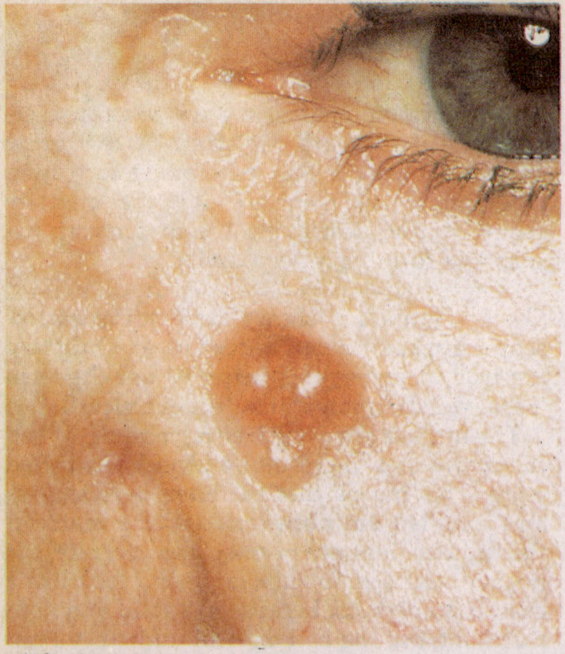

An early nodule (sometimes mistakenly thought to be cystic) just below the eye

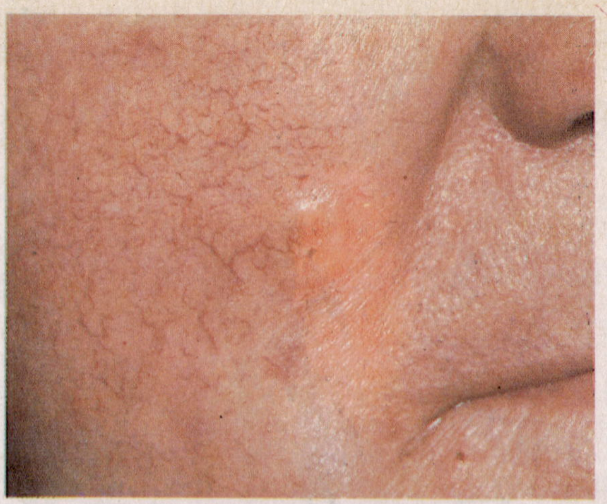

A nodular lesion spreading outwards and leaving a collapsed, scarred centre

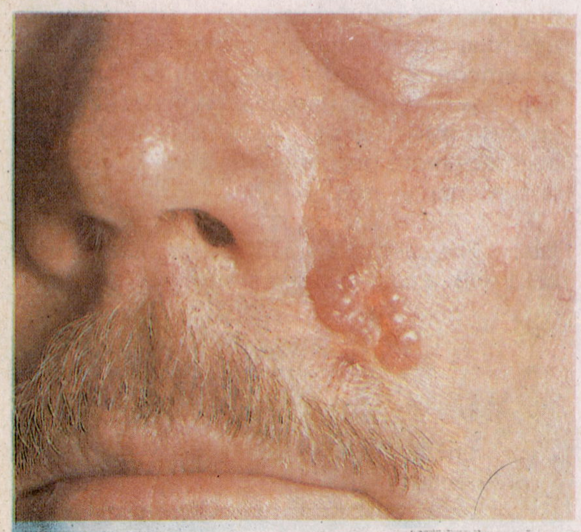

A slow-growing lesion on the cheek – difficult to see and often ignored by the patient who notices only a small scab, which periodically appears and then falls off, at the centre of a slightly thickened area of the skin

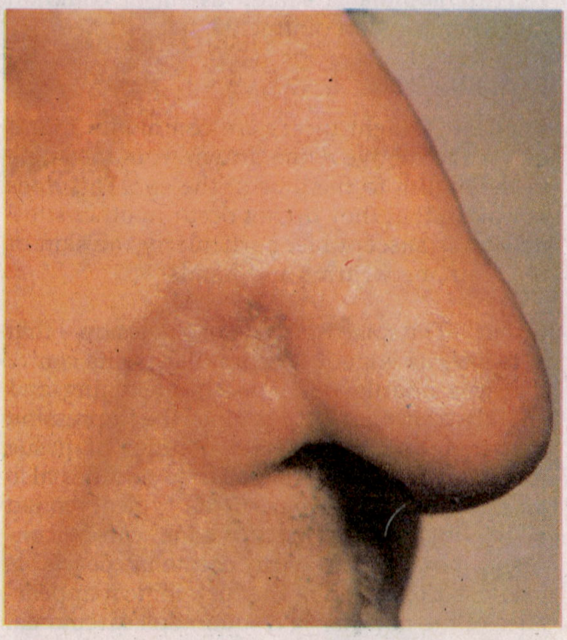

A lesion with a deep, scarred centre without a noticeably raised edge

FIG. 2.25 BASAL CELL CARCINOMATA

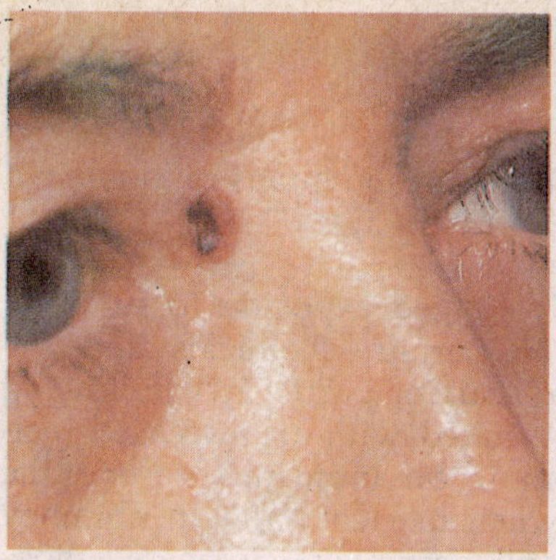

A pigmented basal cell carcinoma

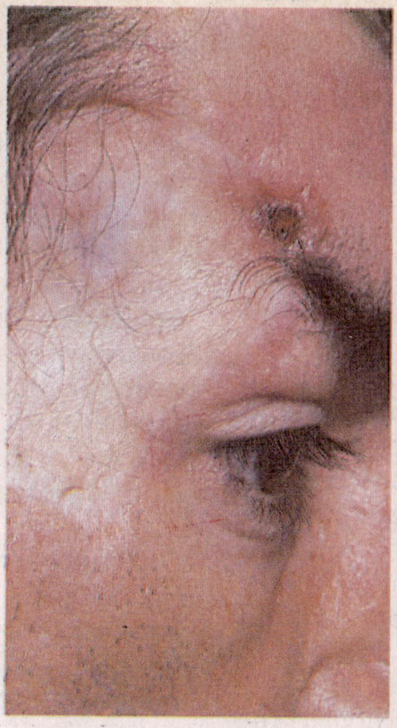

A recurrent basal cell carcinoma at the edge of a skin graft placed to cover the skin defect of a previous excision 7 years earlier

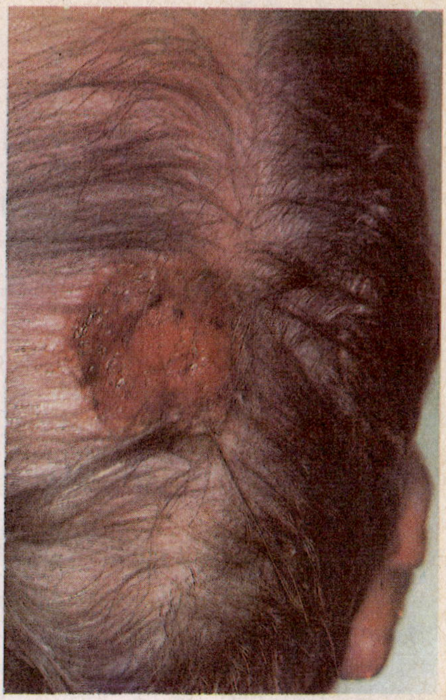

A raised, wet, weeping basal cell carcinoma that was thought, by the patient, to be a patch of eczema

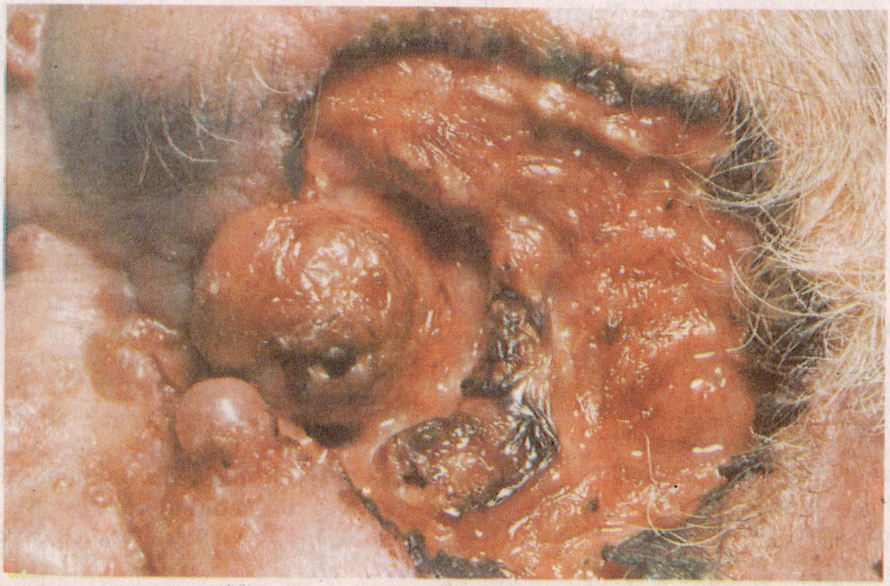

A true 'rodent ulcer'. The basal cell carcinoma has destroyed the orbit and the eye

FIG. 2.25 *Continued*

cells. If this is picked off, the base will bleed slightly.

The base of eroding ulcers consists of the tissue into which the tumour is eroding (fat, bone, muscle, or eye) covered with poor-quality granulation tissue. The base of a deep ulcer is not usually tender.

Depth Long-standing ulcers may erode deep into the face, destroying skin and bone and exposing the nasal cavity, air sinuses and even the eye. Such extensive lesions are uncommon. Most basal cell carcinomata are superficial and confined to the skin.

Lymph drainage The local lymph nodes **should not be enlarged**.

Relations The early lesion is confined to the skin and is freely movable over the deep structures. Fixation of the ulcer indicates that it has invaded deeply.

Important differential diagnoses A rodent ulcer can resemble a squamous cell carcinoma. The long history and the rolled edge are the clinical features which indicate its basal cell origin. A keratoacanthoma (see page 56) just beginning to slough at its centre can also look like an early rodent ulcer, but the short history and the deep slough should suggest the correct diagnosis.

In every instance the final diagnosis must be made by the pathologist.

Squamous cell carcinoma

(Epithelioma)

This is a carcinoma of the cells of the epidermis that normally migrate outwards to the surface to form the superficial keratinous squamous layer. The tumour cells infiltrate the epidermis, the dermis and adjacent tissues. Microscopic examination reveals tongues of tumour cells spreading in all directions and clusters of cells with concentric rings of flattened squamous cells at their centre. These onion-like clumps of cells are often called 'epithelial pearls', but this is a histological metaphor, not a macroscopic clinically detectable appearance.

HISTORY

Age The incidence of squamous carcinoma of the skin increases with age.

Occupation Prolonged exposure to sunlight, solar keratoses, certain chemicals and the presence of old scarring particularly following burns, are associated with an increased incidence of squamous carcinomata. Cancer of the scrotal skin was once common in chimney sweeps and still occurs in engineers whose clothes become soaked in oil.

Duration The lesion has usually been growing steadily for 1 or 2 months before the patient complains of it. If it is in an inaccessible part, such as in the middle of the back, it may be quite big before being noticed.

Symptoms The patient complains of a **lump**, or of **bleeding and discharge from an ulcer**. Bleeding is more common with squamous cell than basal cell carcinomata.

The tumour may become **painful** if it invades deep structures.

The patient may complain of **enlarged lymph glands** and be unaware of the primary lesion.

Development The lesion enlarges steadily and inexorably. Ulcers get larger, in area and in depth, and the edge becomes more prominent and florid.

Multiplicity There may be multiple tumours in an area affected by precipitating factors such as exposure to ultraviolet light or chemicals.

Systemic effects There are no systemic effects while the tumour is confined to the skin. Dissemination of tumour cells throughout the body is a late event. If the ulcer becomes heavily infected there may be general malaise and fever.

LOCAL EXAMINATION

Position Squamous cell carcinomata can occur on any part of the skin, but are more common on exposed skin, (head and neck, hands, forearms and upper trunk) and skin

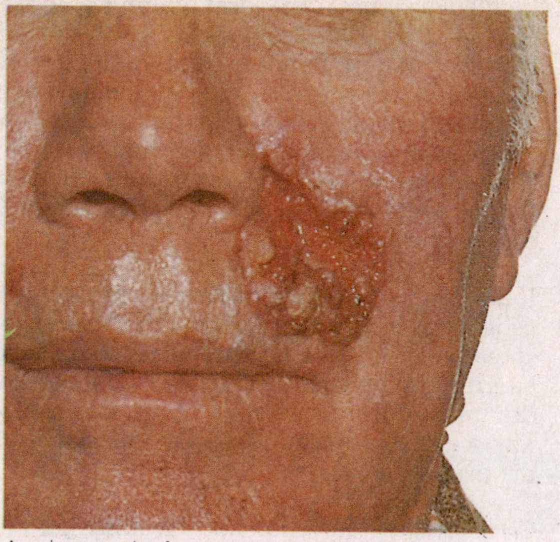

An ulcer, on the face, with an everted edge and a necrotic base

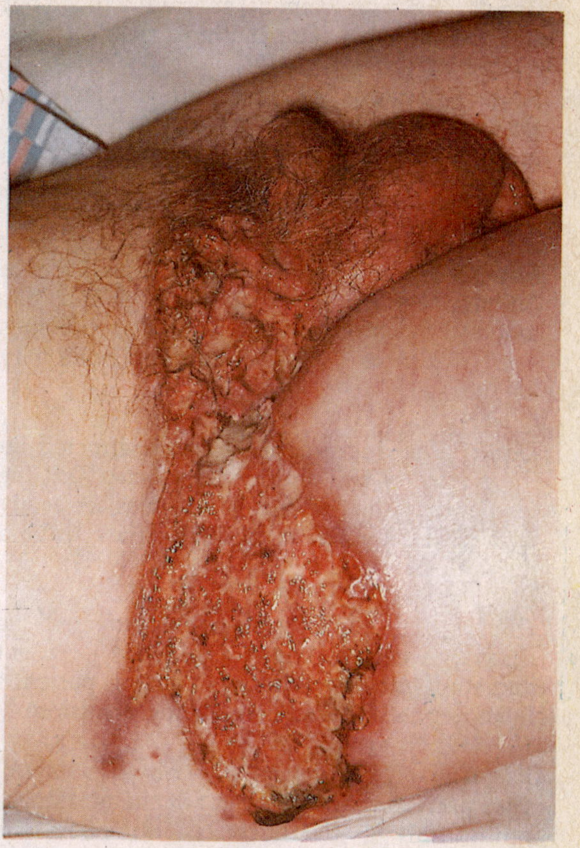

An extensive squamous carcinoma of the skin of the groin and scrotum

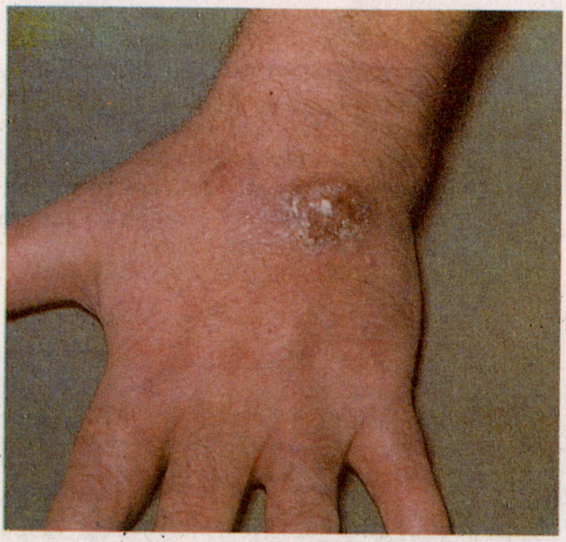

An ulcer, on the hand, whose edge is not yet everted but is raised and almost everted on the proximal side

FIG. 2.26 SQUAMOUS CELL CARCINOMATA

subjected to repeated chemical or mechanical irritation.

Colour The everted edge of a carcinomatous ulcer is usually a dark red–brown colour because it is very vascular. The whole ulcer may be covered with old coagulated blood or serum.

Tenderness The ulcer is not usually tender and has a normal temperature.

Shape and size Squamous carcinomata begin as small nodules on the skin. As they enlarge the centre becomes necrotic, sloughs, and the nodule turns into an ulcer, which is initially circular with prominent everted edges, but can become any shape as it enlarges.

Edge Squamous cell carcinomata have an everted edge because the excessive tissue growth raises it **above and over** the normal skin surface.

Base The base of the ulcer consists of necrotic tumour covered with serum and blood. There is usually some granulation tissue but this tends to be pale and unhealthy. Other tissues such as fibrous tissue, tendon and bone may be exposed.

Depth The depth of the ulcer is affected by the nature of the underlying tissues and the virulence of the tumour. Soft tissues are easily invaded and when they slough they leave a deep ulcer.

Discharge If the ulcer becomes infected the discharge can be copious, bloody, purulent and foul smelling. This is often the patient's most depressing and debilitating symptom.

Relations The relations to nearby tissues will vary according to the extent of the malignant infiltration. If the ulcer is immobile the tumour has spread beyond the skin and subcutaneous tissues into deeper structures.

Local lymph nodes The local lymph nodes are often enlarged, but this does not always mean that they contain tumour. About one-third of patients with palpable lymph glands have lymphadenopathy caused by infection which subsides after treatment of the primary lesion. However, until it is proved otherwise, it should be assumed that palpable lymph nodes contain metastases.

Local tissues The surrounding tissues may be oedematous and thickened. Subcutaneous spread may involve nearby nerves and cause neuritis. Involvement of local blood vessels can cause thrombosis and tissue ischaemia. These events are features of the late stages of the disease.

Complications Infection and bleeding are the common complications. If the ulcer erodes into a large blood vessel the bleeding can be massive and fatal.

GENERAL EXAMINATION

All the lymph glands between the primary lesion and the great veins in the neck should be examined. All types of distant metastases are uncommon; nevertheless examination of the chest may reveal areas of collapse, or a pleural effusion, caused by pulmonary metastases. There may be hepatomegaly.

Revision Panel 2.4
The diagnostic features of the four common surgical skin lesions

	Duration of growth	*Physical features*
Squamous cell carcinoma	Few months	Nodule, or ulcer with everted edge Occasional bleeding
Basal cell carcinoma	Many months or years	Nodule, or ulcer with rolled edge and permanent scab No bleeding
Keratoacanthoma	Few weeks	Nodule with central hard necrotic core No bleeding Spontaneous regression
Pyogenic granuloma	Few days	Soft red nodule that becomes covered with epithelium Bleeds easily

Differential diagnosis The common skin lesions similar to squamous cell carcinoma are the basal cell carcinoma, keratoacanthoma, malignant melanoma, solar keratosis, pyogenic granuloma and infected seborrhoeic wart.

Marjolin's ulcer

(Squamous cell carcinoma)

Marjolin's ulcer is an eponym reserved for a **squamous carcinoma** which arises in a long-standing benign ulcer or scar. The commonest ulcer to become malignant is a long-standing venous ulcer. The scar that is most often associated with malignant change is the scar of an old burn.

These carcinomata have characteristics similar to those of the ordinary squamous carcinoma, except that they may not be so florid.

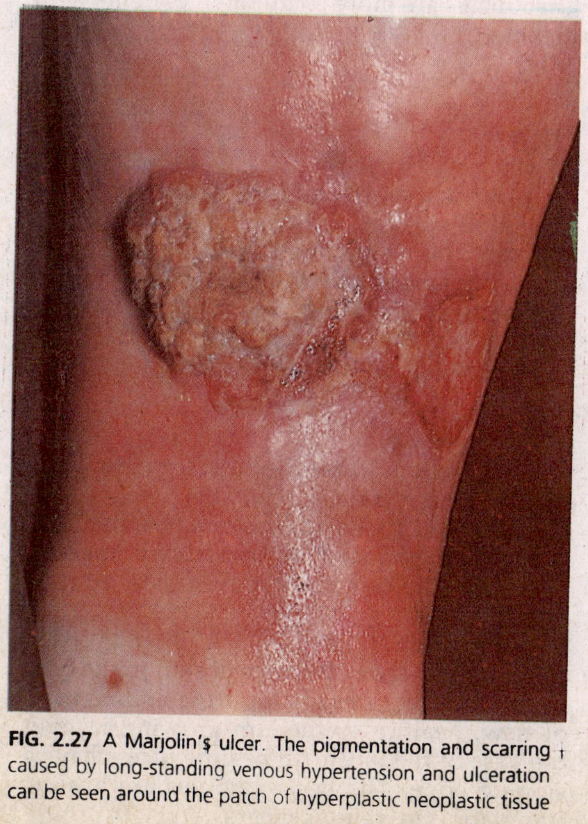

FIG. 2.27 A Marjolin's ulcer. The pigmentation and scarring caused by long-standing venous hypertension and ulceration can be seen around the patch of hyperplastic neoplastic tissue

Their edge is not always raised and everted, and other features may be masked by the pre-existing chronic ulceration or scarring. Unusual nodules or changes in a chronic ulcer or a scar should be viewed with suspicion.

This type of carcinoma is not so invasive, slower growing and slightly less malignant than the spontaneous squamous carcinoma, but must be treated as vigorously.

Mycosis fungoides

This is a rare skin lesion but occasionally it presents in a surgical clinic. It begins as a patch of thickening and reddening of the skin which enlarges, rises up above the surrounding skin as a plaque and then ulcerates. The lesions may be multiple.

It is a cutaneous manifestation of a lymphomatous condition and may indicate the presence of a generalized lymphoma or reticulosis. Hence it is important to recognize it.

SKIN INFECTIONS

Furunculosis (boils)

Furuncles and boils are manifestations of infection in a hair follicle. The infection first produces pus and then forms a central core.

When the lesion contains only pus it is called a furuncle; when it contains a solid core it is called a **boil**.

Boils are often multiple and associated with general debility, or an underlying disease such as **diabetes**. They can occur on any part of the body but are common in the skin of the head and neck, axillae and groins. They begin as a hard, red, tender area which gradually enlarges and causes a throbbing pain. Eventually the tissue in the centre of the infected area dies and forms a thick yellow slough which will not separate from the adjacent tissue until it is surrounded by pus. When this happens the lump becomes fluctuant, the centre of the covering skin sloughs and the pus and necrotic core are discharged.

Squeezing a boil before the slough has separated will do more harm than good because it will not evacuate the slough, but may spread the infection.

Hidradenitis suppurativa

Whereas boils are infections in the hair follicles, hidradenitis is an infection of the apocrine sweat glands. It is most often seen in the axillae and groins of Caucasians living in tropical countries.

The patient presents with multiple tender swellings in the axillae or groins, which enlarge and then discharge pus. The condition is made worse if there is an underlying systemic disease, such as diabetes. The site and the chronic recurring nature of this condition make it unpleasant and disabling.

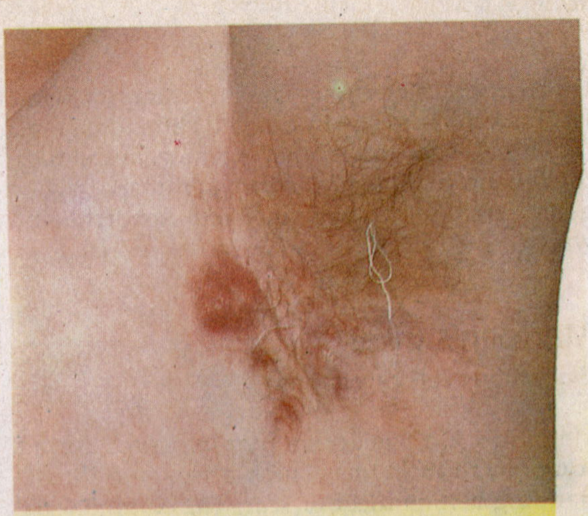

FIG. 2.28 Hidradenitis suppurativa. One set of infected apocrine glands has already been excised from this man's left axilla but another cluster has become red, swollen and tender

Erysipelas and cellulitis

Erysipelas is an infection of the skin and subcutaneous tissues by a pathogenic streptococcus. Whereas the staphylococcus commonly causes a localized infection and pus formation, the streptococcus spreads easily through the skin and produces a diffuse cellulitis. The erythrotoxins produced by the streptococcus make the infected area red, hot, tender and oedematous. Oedema of the reddened skin gives the involved area a **raised border** – a diagnostic clinical appearance. The patient has a high temperature, tachycardia and general debility. If the centre of a patch of erysipelas is mistakenly incised, the incision will exude a thin serum. Streptococcal infections rarely form thick pus.

Careful examination may reveal a source of entry for the organism, such as a small cut or a scratch. Erysipelas is especially common when there is pre-existing oedema caused by venous or lymphatic insufficiency.

Infection of the skin and subcutaneous tissues caused by other organisms, without the bright red discolouration of the skin and the raised border, is called **cellulitis**. A patch of cellulitis may necrose and suppurate.

A spreading, necrotizing infection of the subcutaneous tissues with multiple openings onto the skin is called a **carbuncle**. The skin between the openings may become gangrenous as the tissues beneath it die. Carbuncles are more common in patients with diabetes.

Ulcers

An ulcer is a solution of the continuity of an epithelial surface.

Ulcers follow traumatic removal, or death and desquamation by disease, of the whole or part of an epithelium.

An ulcer has a number of features that should be examined (see also Chapter 1).

THE EDGE

The edge of an ulcer is the most important feature because it is the junction between healthy and diseased tissue and takes a characteristic form according to the underlying disease. There are five common types of ulcer edge.

Sloping edge (Fig. 2.29) A sloping edge slopes gently from the normal skin to the base of the ulcer. It is reddish-purple and consists of new, healthy epithelium growing in over the base of the ulcer. All healing ulcers have a sloping edge. The best examples are healing traumatic and venous ulcers.

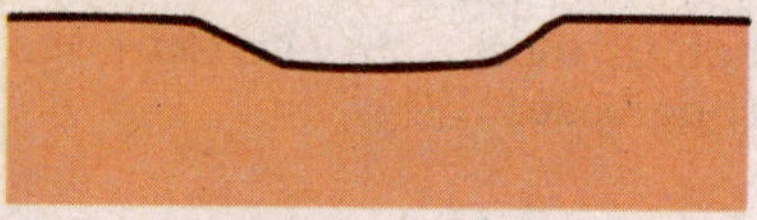

FIG. 2.29 Sloping edge

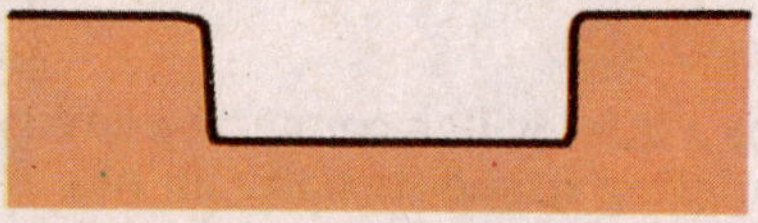

FIG. 2.30 Punched-out edge

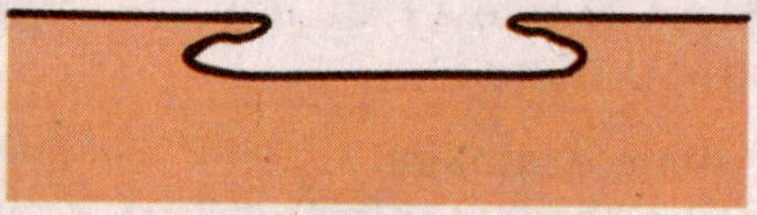

FIG. 2.31 Undermined edge

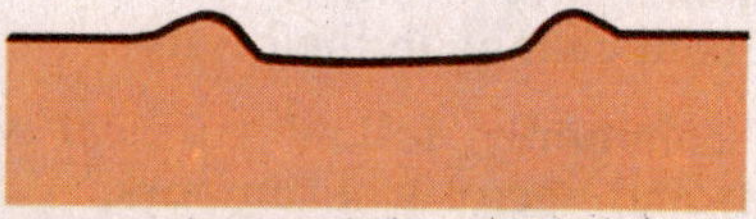

FIG. 2.32 Rolled edge

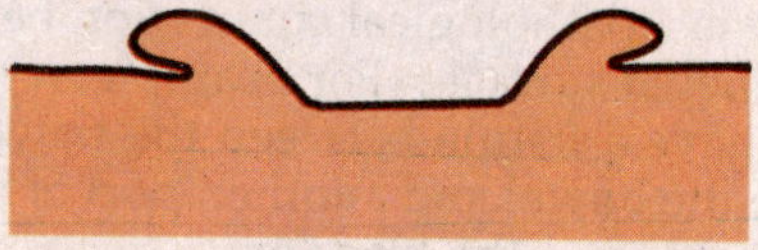

FIG. 2.33 Everted edge

Punched-out edge (Fig. 2.30) This edge drops down at right-angles to the skin surface to make the ulcer look as if it has been cut out of the skin with a punch. It indicates a localized, usually full-thickness, area of skin loss surrounded by healthy tissue. The best examples of this type of ulcer are the deep trophic ulcer, and the ulcer left after a patch of gangrenous skin has sloughed. The condition causing the ulcer is limited to the ulcer and is less severe in the surrounding tissues but prevents healing.

Undermined edge (Fig. 2.31) The disease causing this type of ulcer spreads in and destroys the subcutaneous tissues faster than it destroys the overlying skin. The overhanging skin is usually reddish-blue, friable and unhealthy. Tuberculous ulcers are usually undermined.

Rolled edge (Fig. 2.32) A rolled ulcer edge develops when an invasive cellular disease becomes necrotic at its centre, but grows quite quickly at its periphery so that it rises above the surface of the skin. A rolled edge ulcer is typical of a basal cell carcinoma. 'Rolled' is a poor description, but it is the best we have. The edge of this type of ulcer looks like the circular mound of earth found around an ancient fortification.

Everted edge (Fig. 2.33) When an ulcer is caused by a fast-growing infiltrating cellular disease the growing portion at the edge of the ulcer heaps up and, in its malignant exuberance, spills over the normal skin to produce an everted edge. This appearance is typical of the squamous cell carcinoma, and the ulcerated adenocarcinoma.

THE BASE

The base of the ulcer should be examined carefully. It may be necessary to remove the slough before this can be done. The base is likely to consist of three types of tissue.

Granulation tissue This is a red sheet of delicate capillary loops and fibroblasts covered by a thin layer of fibrin or plasma. It is the first stage of the healing process.

Revision Panel 2.5

The causes of chronic ulceration of the skin

- Infection
- Repeated trauma
- Anoxia
- Oedema
- Denervation
- Malignant change

Dead tissues A piece of dead tissue is called a **slough**. When a slough separates it may expose healthy tissues, which then become covered with granulation tissue, or further involved in the ischaemic process.

Tumour The base of a squamous cell carcinoma is the malignant tissue itself. It may be slightly vascular or necrotic but does not develop healthy granulation tissue.

DISCHARGE

The discharge from an ulcer may be serous or serosanguinous, purulent, offensive, copious, or so slight that it dries into a scab.

The discharge should be cultured to ascertain the nature of any infecting organisms.

Venous ulcers

Venous ulcers are found in the lower medial third of the lower limb. Their site is a diagnostic feature. They are described in detail in Chapter 7.

Ischaemic ulcers

Arterial insufficiency is usually manifest at the ends of the limbs. It is rare to see ulcers caused by arterial disease at the base of the limbs or on the trunk. Ischaemic ulcers are described in detail in Chapters 6 and 7.

Trophic ulcers

A trophic ulcer is an ulcer which has developed as the result of the patient's insensitivity to repeated trauma. They are commonly associated with those forms of neurological disease which cause loss of pain and light touch sensation in weight-bearing areas. They are described in Chapter 6.

Neoplastic ulcers

The ulcers caused by basal and squamous cell carcinomata are described in detail earlier in this chapter.

When metastases from distant or underlying cancers appear in the skin, they may ulcerate and have features similar to a primary carcinomatous ulcer – an everted edge and a proliferating base.

Sinuses and fistulae

Sinus

A sinus is a tract which connects a cavity lined by granulation tissue (usually an old abscess) with an epithelial surface.

A sinus produces a serous or purulent discharge and continues to do so until the deep cavity closes. However, an abscess cavity will fail to close if there is:

- Inadequate drainage.
- A specific chronic infection (e.g. actinomycosis, tuberculosis, syphilis).
- A foreign body (e.g. stitch material).
- Epithelialization of the cavity.
- Malignant change in the cavity.

Sinuses commonly follow surgical wound infections and necrosis of tumours.

Fistula

A fistula is a pathological connection between two epithelial surfaces. For example, it is possible to have a fistula between the bowel and the skin, the bowel and another loop of bowel, or the bowel and the bladder.

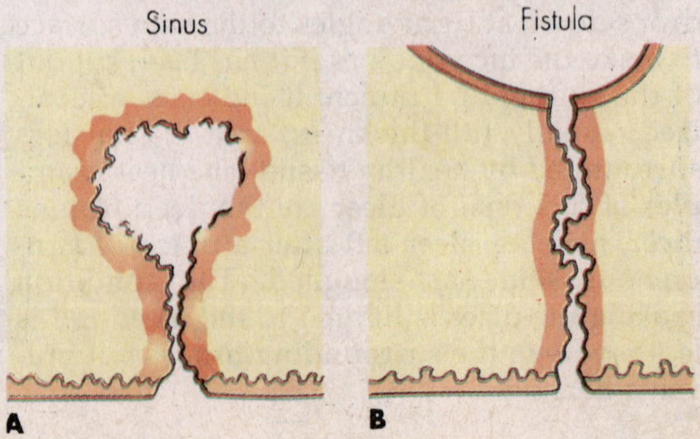

Fig. 2.34 A: A sinus is a connection between a cavity lined with granulation tissue and an epithelial surface. **B**: A fistula is a connection between two epithelial-lined surfaces

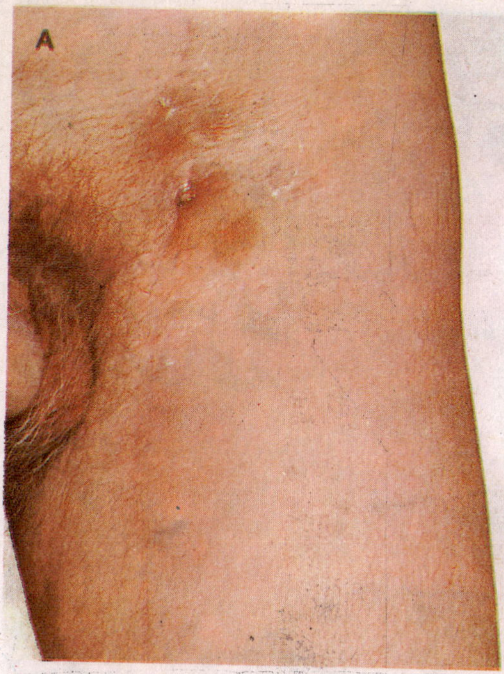

A discharging sinus at the centre of a groin wound

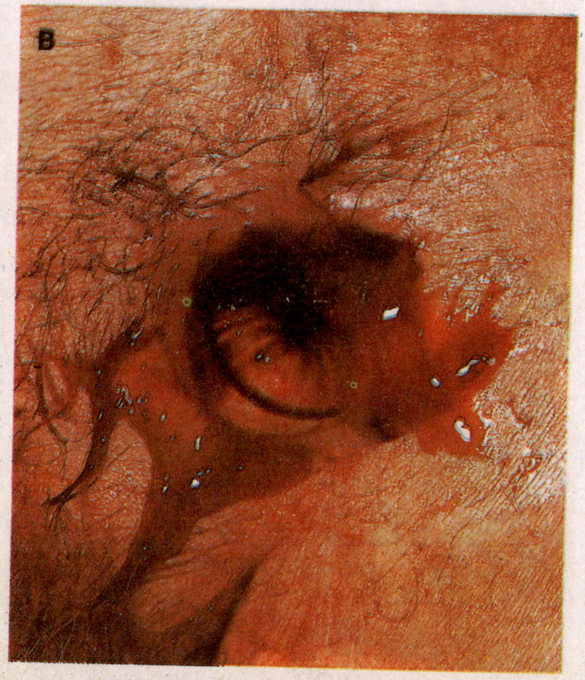

The wound above 3 weeks later. The sinus has opened widely to reveal its cause, an infected Dacron arterial graft

FIG. 2.35

Fistulae are usually lined with granulation tissue but they can become epithelialized.

They form when a chronic abscess bursts in two directions and so connects two epithelial surfaces. They persist if they have to conduct the contents of one of the epithelial-lined cavities because its normal outflow is obstructed.

They will not resolve until the cause of the abscess is eradicated (see above for the factors which delay abscess closure) or the obstruction to the emptying of the viscus is removed.

The common fistulae seen in surgical practice are between the anal canal and the perianal skin and the bowel.

Sweating

All skin contains sweat glands. If these glands secrete an excessive quantity of sweat (hyperhidrosis) the skin becomes soggy, white and moist.

Hyperhidrosis of the hands is a distressing condition. The sweat may drip off the fingers, and everything the patient touches gets wet.

Axillary hyperhidrosis is also embarrassing because the clothes become saturated with sweat and thus become offensive.

Revision Panel 2.6

The causes of a chronic abscess or persistent sinus

- Inadequate drainage
- Specific chronic infection (tuberculosis, actinomycosis)
- Foreign body (stitch material)
- Epithelialization of the cavity
- Malignant change in wall of the cavity or sinus

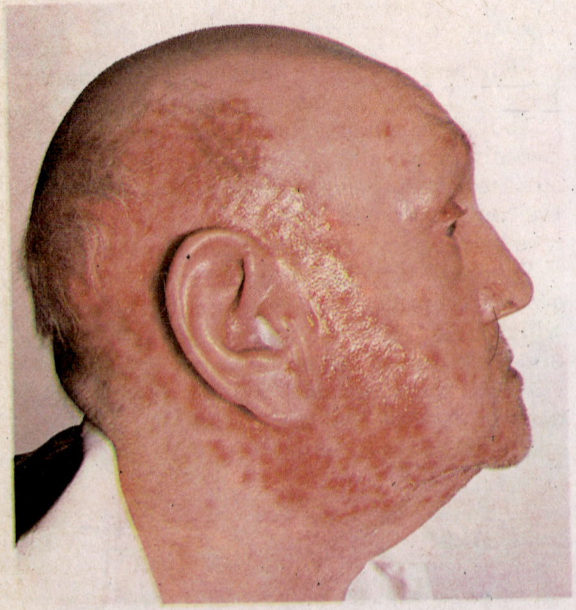

Herpes zoster (shingles) of Mandibular V

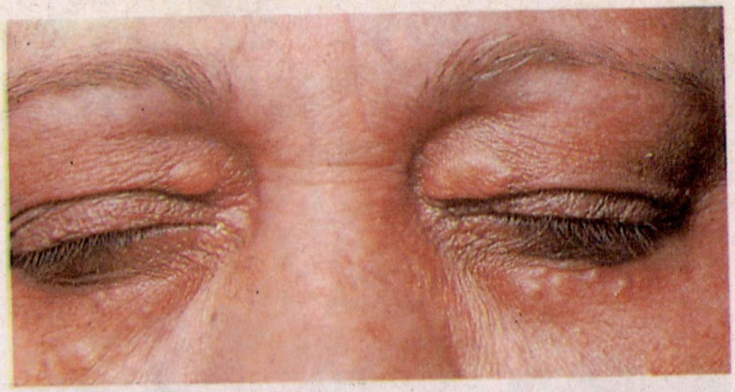

Xanthoma of the upper eyelid

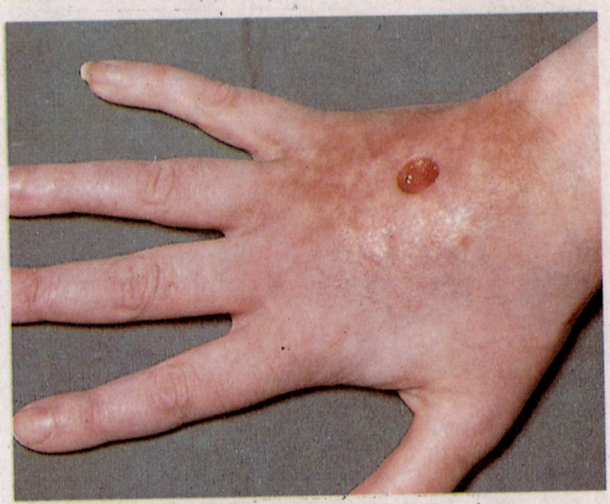

An injection ulcer on the back of the hand

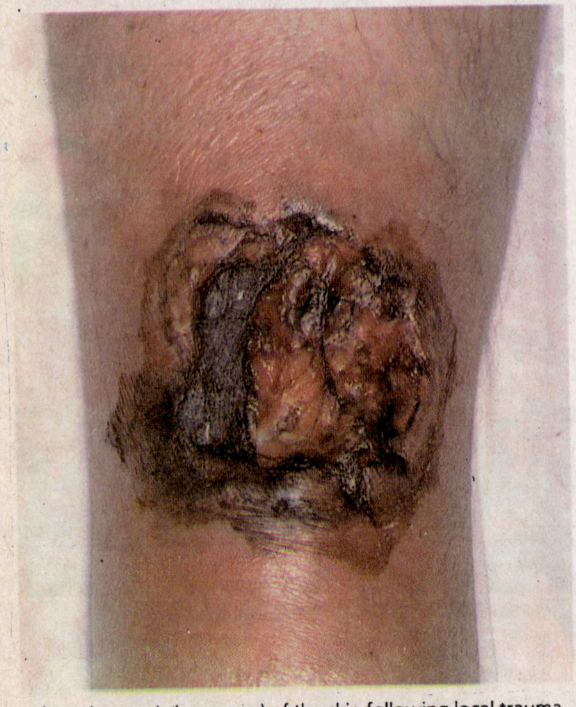

Infected necrosis (gangrene) of the skin following local trauma on a patient taking steroids

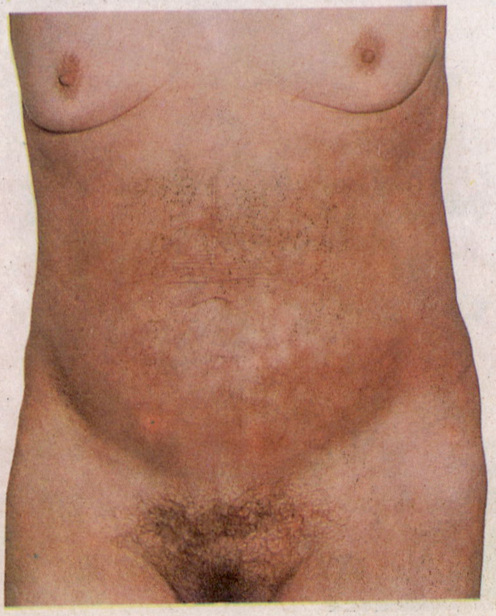

Erythema ab igne caused by the constant application of a hot water bottle to relieve abdominal pain

FIG. 2.36 SOME MORE SKIN LESIONS

The subcutaneous tissues

3

This chapter is concerned with lumps deep to the skin but superficial to the deep fascia and the muscles, but includes those lumps which arise from skin structures but which lie within the subcutaneous tissues.

Lipoma

A lipoma is a cluster of fat cells which have become over-active and so distended with fat that they have become palpable lumps. They never turn malignant. Liposarcomata, which most often arise in the retroperitoneal tissues, probably arise *de novo* and not in a benign lesion.

HISTORY

Age Lipomata occur at all ages but are not common in children.

Duration It is usually difficult to discover the age of a lipoma because it has probably been present for months or years before being noticed.

Symptoms Most patients come to the doctor because they have noticed a lump and want to know what it is. The lump may be **unsightly** or interfere with movement, especially if it becomes pedunculated. If a lipoma is knocked repeatedly it may swell and **become hard and painful** because of **fat necrosis**. Repetitive friction can cause the overlying skin to ulcerate.

Development Lipomata grow slowly over many years. They rarely regress.

Multiplicity Patients often have many lipomata, or a history of having had others excised in the past.

Multiple contiguous lipomata cause enlargement and distortion of the subcutaneous tissues. This condition is called **lipomatosis.** It usually occurs in the buttocks and sometimes in the neck.

Multiple lipomatosis is a condition in which the limbs and sometimes the trunk are covered with lipomata of all shapes and sizes. It is not very common. The lipomata in this condition are no different, macro- or microscopically, from solitary lipomata.

EXAMINATION

Position Lipomata are most common in the subcutaneous tissues of the upper limbs, especially the forearm, but can occur anywhere where there is fat.

Colour The skin that overlies the lump is normal, but may be a little stretched and have a glazed, transparent appearance. The veins crossing the lipoma may be visible as faint blue streaks.

Tenderness Lipomata are not tender and can be palpated firmly without discomfort to the patient, provided they have not been recently injured.

Temperature The temperature of the overlying skin is normal.

Shape The shape is often the most obvious diagnostic feature. Unrestricted, lipomata are

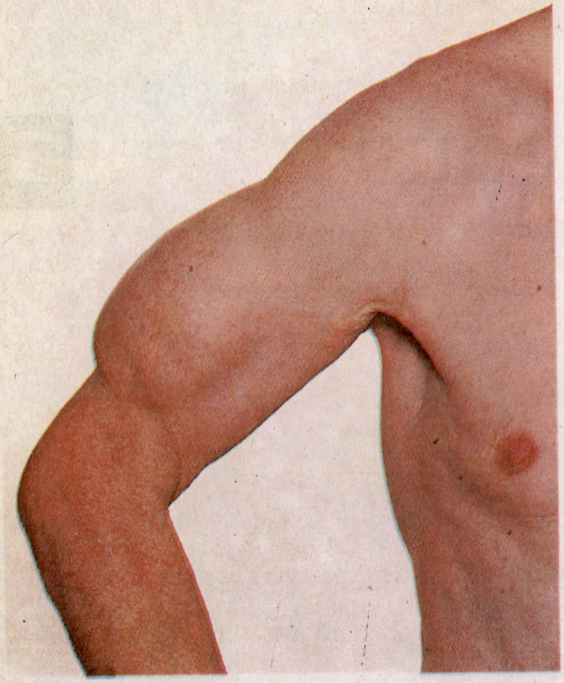

A lipoma in the subcutaneous tissues of the upper arm. Note the lobulation

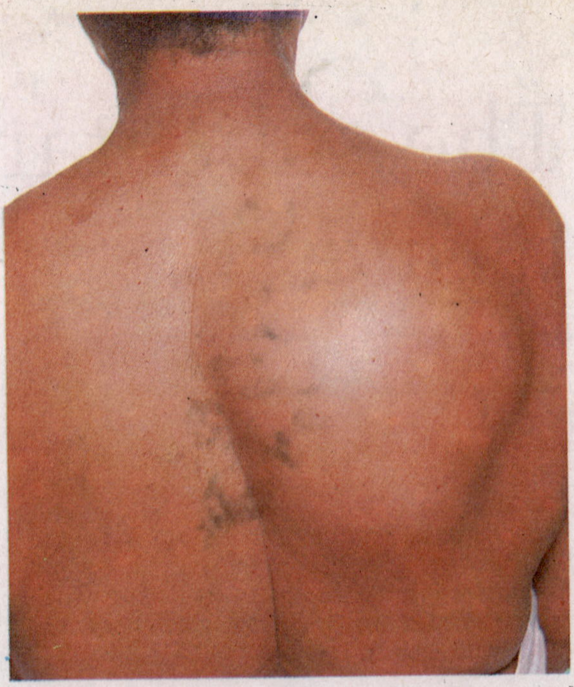

A large lipoma overlying the scapula

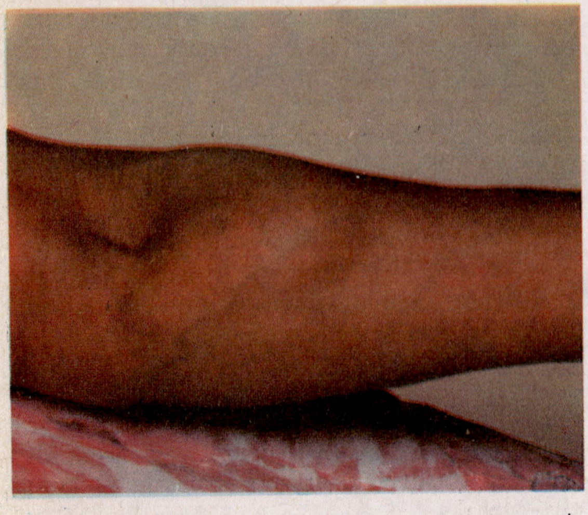

A lipoma in the forearm. This swelling became more prominent and fixed when the forearm muscles were contracted, showing that it was superficial to the muscle but attached to its fascia

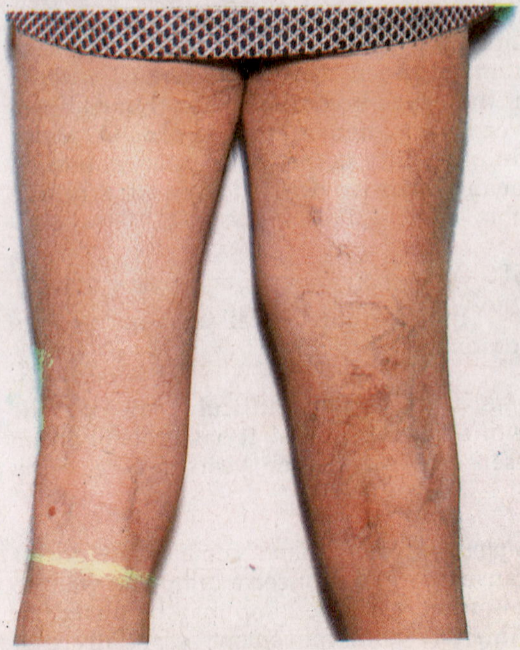

A large lipoma in the right thigh which became less distinct when the hamstring muscles were contracted, showing that it was deep to the muscles. Note the distended veins caused by compression of the superficial femoral vein by the mass

FIG. 3.1 LIPOMATA

spherical, but subcutaneous lipomata which are caught between two resistant tissues, the skin and the deep fascia, become flattened. They are therefore usually discoid or hemispherical.

Still more significant is the fact that, because most lipomata are a collection of overgrown fat cells not one solitary cell, they are **lobulated**. The lobules can be seen and felt on the surface and at the edge of the lump.

Size Lipomata come in all sizes.

Surface The surface feels smooth, but gentle pressure reveals that it is bosselated, the bosses being individual lobules. The lobules become more prominent with firm palpation because the increased pressure within the lipoma makes each lobule bulge out between the fine strands of fibrous tissue which surround it.

Edge The edge is not circular but a series of irregular curves corresponding to each lobule. Because the edge is soft, compressible, and sometimes quite thin, it slips away from the examining finger. This has been described as the 'slip sign'. It is not a very useful or a diagnostic feature. Evidence of lobulation on the surface and at the edge is the most significant physical sign.

Composition Students often argue about the composition of a lipoma; is it solid or is it liquid? The answer is that it can be either, depending on the nature of the fat and the temperature at which it liquefies. Most lipomata contain a soft but solid jelly-like fat if they are cut open immediately after removal. The fat hardly ever runs out of the lump in liquid form. Consequently, most small lipomata feel soft but do not fluctuate. Because they are so soft they give the impression of fluctuating but careful examination will reveal that they are just yielding to pressure and spreading out in all directions, not becoming more tense and prominent in the plane at right angles to the palpating finger. Large, more rounded lipomata do fluctuate.

Lipomata will transilluminate with the light from an ordinary torch only if they are sufficiently large and prominent to permit the light to be shone right across them. They do not have a fluid thrill and are dull to percussion. They are not reducible unless they have herniated out of a muscle. They do not pulsate.

The equivocal responses to fluctuation and transillumination occasionally make students think that a lipoma is a soft cyst. This emphasises the diagnostic importance of the soft consistence and the **lobulation**.

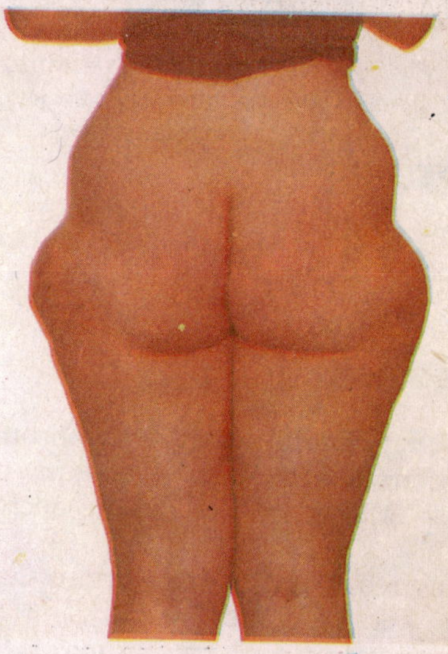

FIG. 3.2 Diffuse lipomatosis over both hips

Relations Lipomata may arise within deep structures, such as muscles, and bulge out into the subcutaneous tissues. These lipomata are fixed deeply and may become more prominent if they are pushed out of the muscle, or disappear if they are drawn into the muscle, when it contracts. Apart from this special variety, subcutaneous lipomata are not usually attached superficially or deeply and can be moved in all directions.

Lymph drainage The regional lymph nodes should not be enlarged.

Local tissues The surrounding tissues should be normal, but there may be other lipomata nearby.

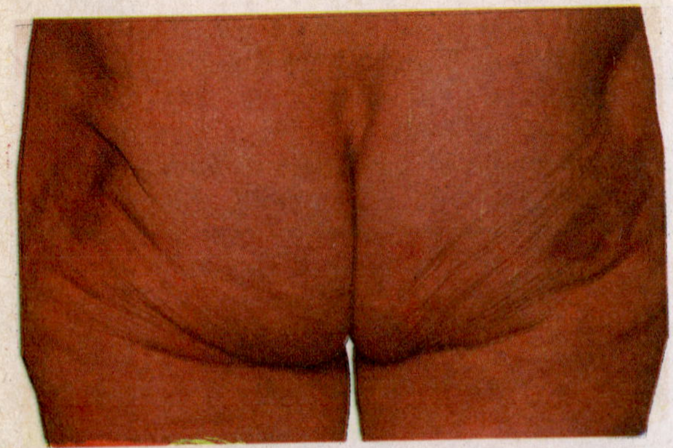

FIG. 3.3 Fat necrosis of the buttock fat caused by repeated injections of insulin. Note the tethering, indrawing, and pigmentation of the skin. Beneath these areas were hard, indistinct lumps of necrotic fat

Fat necrosis

Necrotic fat becomes hard and fibrous. If the necrotic area is close to the skin, the skin becomes tethered or fixed to the necrosis and indrawn.

In the breast, which is an organ that is frequently knocked and bruised, fat necrosis may be mistaken for a carcinoma.

The buttock is a common site to find fat necrosis, particularly in patients who have frequent subcutaneous injections, such as diabetics.

Sebaceous cysts

The skin is kept soft and oily by the sebum secreted by the sebaceous glands. The mouths of these glands open into the hair follicles. If the mouth of a sebaceous gland becomes blocked, the gland becomes distended by its own secretion and ultimately becomes a sebaceous cyst.

HISTORY

Age Sebaceous cysts occur in all age groups, but as they are slow growing they rarely present before adolescence.

Sometimes they appear suddenly during adolescence because the skin gland secretions change at puberty, but most sebaceous cysts present in early adulthood and middle age.

Duration They are slow growing and have usually been present for some years before the patient asks a surgeon to remove them.

Symptoms Sebaceous cysts are most frequently found on the scalp and the commonest complaint is of a **lump** that gets scratched when the patient is combing his hair. Such scratches may get infected. If the cyst becomes infected it enlarges rapidly and becomes acutely painful.

A slow discharge of sebum from a wide punctum sometimes hardens to form a **sebaceous horn**.

Infection of the cyst wall and the surrounding tissues produces a **boggy, painful, discharging swelling** known as **Cock's peculiar tumour**. This only happens if an infected cyst is neglected.

Development Sebaceous cysts usually enlarge as the years pass by, but the increase in size is accelerated if the cyst becomes infected. Sometimes a cyst will discharge its contents through its punctum and then regress or even disappear.

Multiplicity Sebaceous cysts are commonly multiple.

EXAMINATION

Position Most sebaceous cysts are found in the hairy parts of the body. The scalp, scrotum, neck, shoulders and back are the common sites, but they can occur wherever there are sebaceous glands. There are no sebaceous glands on the palms of the hands and soles of the feet.

Colour The skin over the cysts is usually normal.

Tenderness Uncomplicated sebaceous cysts are not tender. Pain and tenderness indicate infection.

Temperature The temperature of the skin over a cyst is normal except when the cyst is inflamed.

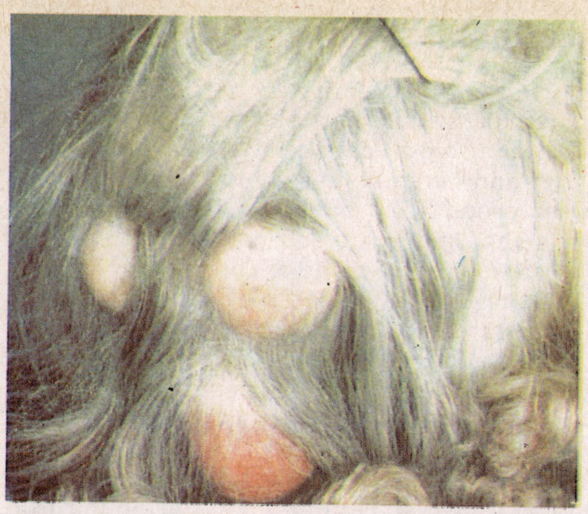

Three sebaceous cysts of the scalp. Note that you cannot see a punctum, a common finding

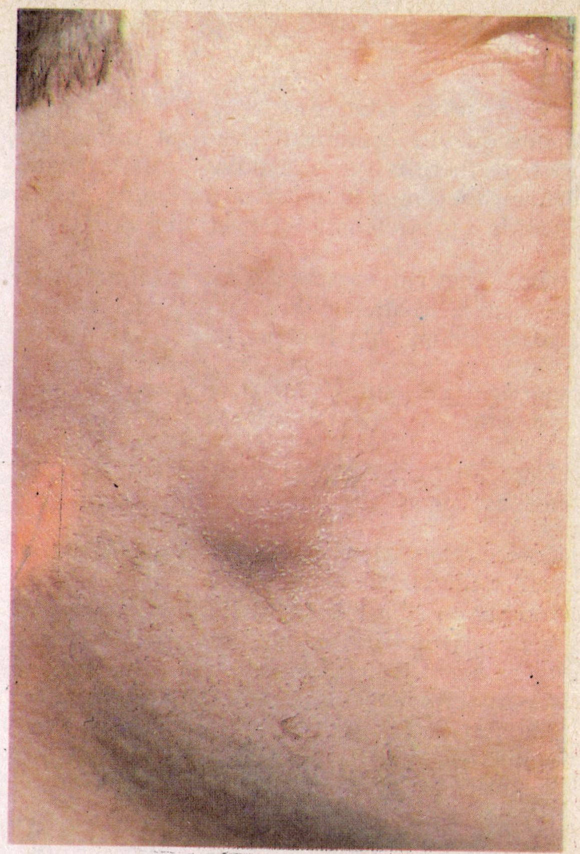

A small sebaceous cyst on the skin. The slight erythema is the residue of a recent infection in the cyst

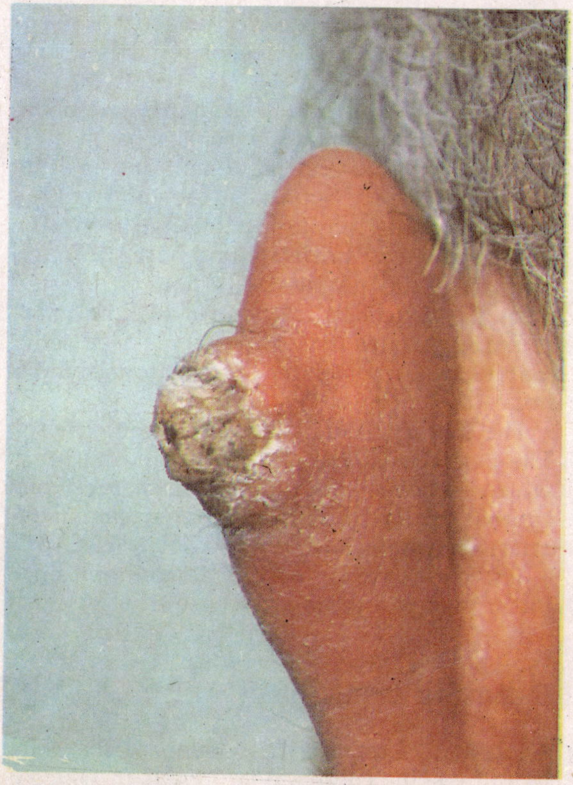

A sebaceous horn on the ear. The 'horn' is simply the hardened sebaceous material (epithelial cells and sebum) extruding from the cyst

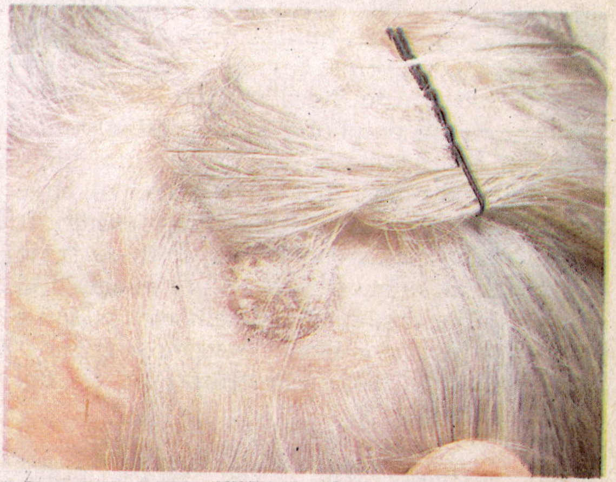

'Cock's peculiar tumour'. This is a mass of granulation tissue protruding from the base of a previously infected and ruptured sebaceous cyst

FIG. 3.4 SEBACEOUS CYSTS

Shape Most sebaceous cysts are tense and consequently **spherical**. Even on the scalp, where there is the unyielding skull beneath them, they remain spherical by bulging outwards and stretching the overlying skin.

Size They can vary from a few millimetres to 4–5 cm in diameter, but most patients seek advice before they become very large.

Surface The surface of a sebaceous cyst is smooth.

Edge The edge is well defined and easy to feel as it is usually lying in subcutaneous fat.

Composition Most sebaceous cysts feel hard and solid. Occasionally they are so tense that it is not possible to elicit fluctuation, especially if there is no firm underlying tissue to press them against. On the scalp the resistance of the underlying skull usually enables one to fix the cyst and press it firmly enough to elicit some degree of **fluctuation**.

Sebaceous cysts are dull to percussion and do not have a fluid thrill, even when large, because their contents are like thick cream. They are not compressible or pulsatile.

Relations Although they arise from what is basically a skin structure, they lie in the subcutaneous tissues. Their point of discharge is usually along a hair follicle, or through a fine duct which, in normal circumstances, is invisible, directly on to the skin. However, as the cyst grows this point of fixation is often pulled inwards to become a **small punctum**. Only one-half of the cysts that you will see will have a visible punctum, but when it is present it is a useful diagnostic sign. Even if there is no punctum, **all sebaceous cysts are attached to the skin**. The area of attachment may be quite small but it prevents the cyst moving independently of the skin. Sebaceous cysts are not attached deeply.

Lymph drainage The local lymph nodes should not be enlarged.

Sebaceous horn

A sebaceous horn arises from a sebaceous cyst.

If the sebum in a sebaceous cyst exudes slowly from a large central punctum it may dry and harden into a conical spike. This is a sebaceous horn. Normally the friction from clothes, and soap and water, removes the secretions of the gland as soon as they appear. A horn can only grow if the patient is unaware of its presence or fails to wash the skin over the cyst. The tendency to form a horn is greater if there is a wide opening into the cyst, as sometimes occurs after an infected cyst has ruptured or been incised.

Sebaceous horns can be broken off or pulled out of the cyst, because they have no intrinsic living structure.

Cock's peculiar tumour

This eponym is still used by surgeons for sentimental and aesthetic reasons – it is a nice name.

Cock's peculiar tumour is an infected, open, granulating, oedematous sebaceous cyst. It looks angry, sore and malignant and is often mistaken for a squamous cell carcinoma of the scalp. Granulation tissue arising from the lining of the cyst heaps up and bursts through onto the skin, giving the lesion an everted edge. The infection in the cyst wall and surrounding tissues makes the whole area oedematous, red and tender. The regional lymph nodes may be enlarged.

The history usually betrays the diagnosis. The patient will tell of a long-standing lump which became painful and discharged pus spontaneously or was treated by an inadequate incision.

This condition has become uncommon since the advent of antibiotics.

Dermoid cysts

A dermoid cyst is a cyst, deep to the skin, lined by skin. There are two ways in which a piece of skin can become trapped deep to the normal skin: as an accident during antenatal development, and following an injury which implants some skin into the subcutaneous tissue. Dermoid cysts are therefore **congenital** or **acquired**.

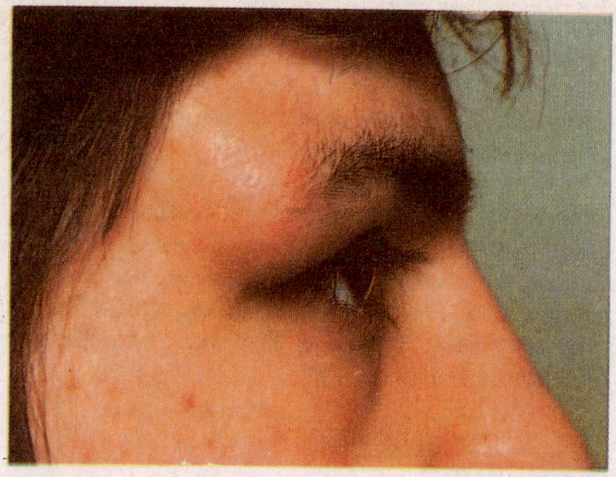

A right external angular dermoid cyst, so called because it lies beneath the outer end of the eyebrow over the external angular protuberance of the skull. This is a congenital dermoid cyst

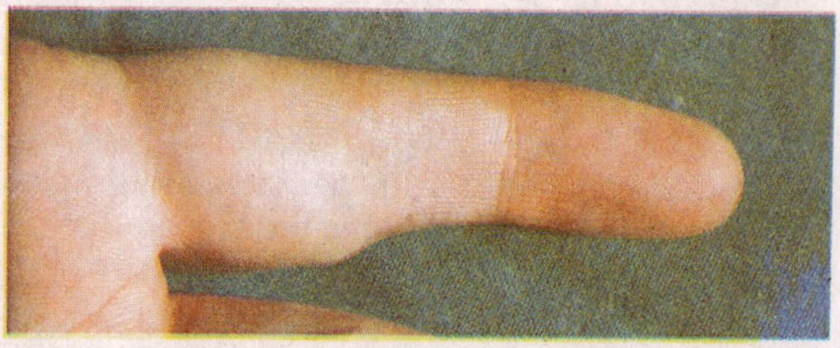

An inclusion dermoid cyst. This cyst appeared 2 years after a small stab wound at the base of the finger

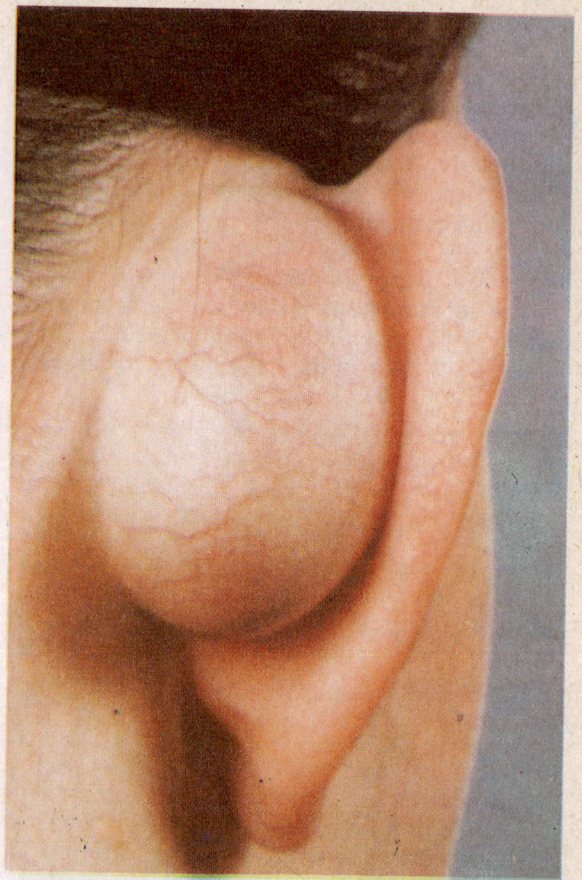

A dermoid cyst behind the ear. A congenital postauricular dermoid

FIG. 3.5 DERMOID CYSTS

Congenital dermoid cysts

HISTORY

Duration The cyst may have been noticed at birth but it is more often first noticed a few years later when it begins to distend.

Symptoms The principal symptom is parental distress at the cosmetic disfigurement because most congenital dermoid cysts occur in the head and neck, or parental concern about the diagnosis. Dermoid cysts rarely become big enough to cause any serious mechanical disability and rarely become infected.

Multiplicity Congenital dermoid cysts are not usually multiple.

EXAMINATION

Position Congenital dermoid cysts are formed in intrauterine life when the skin dermatomes fuse. Consequently, they can occur at any point in the mid-line of the trunk, but are particularly common in the neck and face, along the lines of fusion of the ophthalmic and maxillary facial processes, and at the inner and outer ends of the upper eyebrow.

Shape and size They are usually ovoid or spherical and 1–2 cm in diameter.

Surface Their surface is smooth.

Composition Cysts on the face often feel soft, not tense and hard. They fluctuate, but will only transilluminate if they happen to contain clear fluid instead of the usual thick opaque mixture of sebum, sweat and desquamated epithelial cells. Large cysts will conduct a fluid thrill and are dull to percussion. They are not pulsatile, compressible or reducible.

Relations Dermoid cysts lie deep to the skin, in the subcutaneous tissue. Unlike sebaceous cysts they are not attached to the skin. They are not attached to the underlying structures.

Acquired 'implantation' dermoid cysts

HISTORY

These cysts follow the survival of a piece of skin forcibly implanted into the subcutaneous tissues by an injury – often a small deep cut or stab injury. The patient may not remember the initial injury.

Symptoms Implantation dermoid cysts are usually small and tense. Because they usually occur in areas subject to repeated trauma, they may be painful and tender. Cysts on the fingers may interfere with the grip and touch.

EXAMINATION

Position Implantation dermoid cysts are commonly found beneath skin liable to be injured, such as that of the fingers. Surprisingly, surgical incisions are very rarely affected.

Shape and size The cysts are spherical, smooth and small, 0.5–1.0 cm in diameter.

Composition Implantation dermoid cysts feel hard and tense, sometimes stony hard. Their size makes detection of their cystic nature – fluctuation and fluid thrill – almost impossible. The deduction that they are cystic often depends solely on their shape.

Relations The overlying skin is often scarred. The cyst may be tethered to the deep aspect of the scar or even be within it. The deeper structures should be normal and the cyst freely mobile over them unless they were also injured.

Lymph drainage The regional lymph nodes should be normal.

Complications Implantation dermoid cysts rarely become infected.

Differential diagnosis The cyst commonly confused with the implantation dermoid cyst is the sebaceous cyst. The history of an old injury and the presence of a scar closely related to the cyst are the most significant diagnostic features.

Ganglion

A ganglion is a cystic, myxomatous degeneration of fibrous tissue. Consequently, ganglia can occur anywhere in the body, but they are common where there is a lot of fibrous tissue, i.e. around the joints.

Ganglia are *not* pockets of synovium protruding from joints.

HISTORY

Age Ganglia are seen in patients of all ages. The majority present between the age of 20 and 60 years. They are rare in children.

Duration They grow slowly and have usually been present for months or years before the patient seeks advice.

Symptoms A ganglion is not painful. Most patients seek advice because they wish to know the diagnosis or because the lump is disfiguring.

Persistence Some ganglia slip away between neighbouring bones, so giving the false impression that they are reducing into the joint, but a true ganglion should not connect with or empty into a joint.

Ganglia may rupture into the subcutaneous tissue and so seem to disappear suddenly. If the patient is lucky it will not reappear, but it usually refills in a few months.

EXAMINATION

Position Most ganglia are found near the capsule of a joint but they can occur anywhere. At

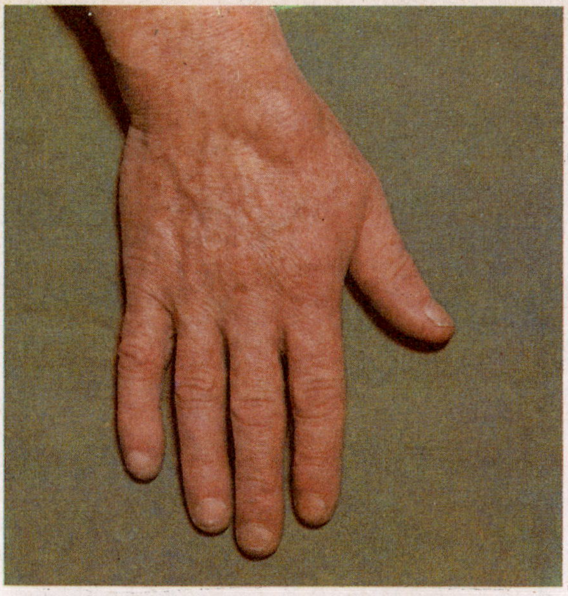

A soft multilocular ganglion on the back of the wrist

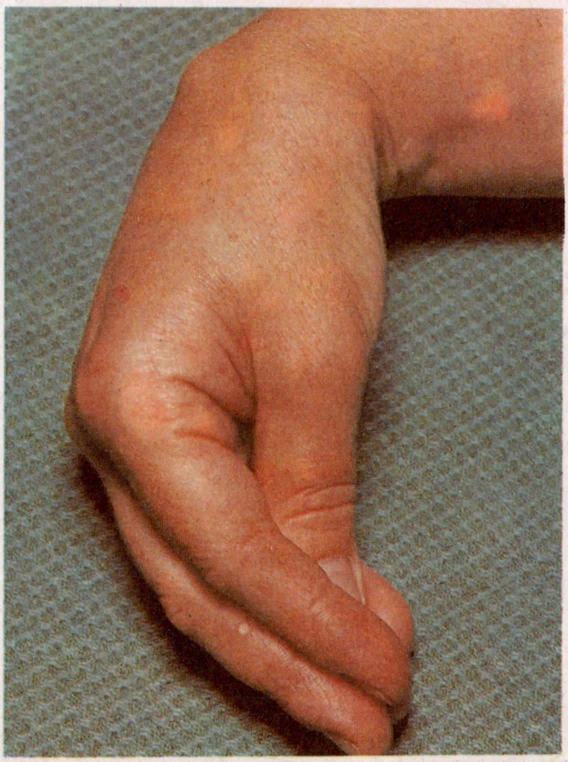

A small tense ganglion on the back of the wrist which was only clearly visible and palpable when the wrist was flexed

FIG. 3.6 GANGLIA

least 90 per cent arise on the dorsal and ventral surfaces of the wrist joint and hand.

Shape and surface Ganglia are spherical and have a smooth surface. Some are multilocular and feel like a collection of cysts.

Size They come in all sizes. Small ones (0.5–1.0 cm) tend to be tense and spherical. Large ones, which can be up to 5–6 cm across, are flattened and soft.

Composition Ganglia feel solid but the consistence varies from soft to hard. The gelatinous material within them is very viscous but most ganglia fluctuate, provided they are not very small and very tense.

Reducibility A ganglion may slip away between deeper structures when pressed, giving the false impression that its contents have reduced into the joint.

Relations Ganglia are usually attached to the fibrous tissue from which they originate. They are not attached to the overlying skin, which should be freely mobile over them. The mobility of a ganglion depends on the extent and nature of its deep attachment. If the tissue of origin is part of a joint capsule, tendon sheath or intramuscular septum, the ganglion will become less mobile when these structures are made tense. Therefore remember to palpate ganglia in all positions of the underlying joint and with the surrounding muscles relaxed and tense.

Local tissues The surrounding tissues should be normal.

Differential diagnosis The three common swellings found close to joints are bursae, cystic protrusions of the synovial cavity of arthritic joints, and ganglia. The first two are usually soft; the ganglion is tense. With the first and third, the joint is normal.

Subcutaneous bursae

Bursae are fluid-filled cavities, lined with a flattened endothelium similar to synovium, that develop between tendons, bones and skin to allow easier movement between them. There are a considerable number of bursae which are always present and described in anatomical textbooks, but others may develop wherever there is friction between two layers of tissue. These are called **adventitious bursae**.

HISTORY

Age Bursae are uncommon in the young unless they have a skeletal deformity. They usually appear in middle and late life as a result of prolonged friction between skin and bone associated with the patient's occupation or a deformity produced by injury or arthritis.

Symptoms Pain, discomfort and an enlarging swelling at the site of repeated trauma are the common symptoms. A severe throbbing pain and a rapid increase in size indicate the presence of infection. **Crepitus** – a grating sensation – may be noticed by the patient if the lining of the bursa is rough or if the fluid contains small loose fibrinous particles.

When the bursa is an occupational hazard – such as housemaid's knee – it may stop the patient working.

Development The growth of the swelling is usually rapid even though the bursa has probably been present in its normal, almost empty, state for many years. The sudden increase in the quantity of bursa fluid which makes the swelling enlarge is usually secondary to minor infection or trauma.

Multiplicity Bursae are often symmetrical, e.g. on both knees or elbows.

Cause The patient often knows the cause of the swelling (prolonged friction or a skeletal deformity) and may have had a similar complaint before.

EXAMINATION

Position Subcutaneous bursae occur where there is friction between skin and bone. The common sites are:

- Between skin and olecranon – student's elbow.

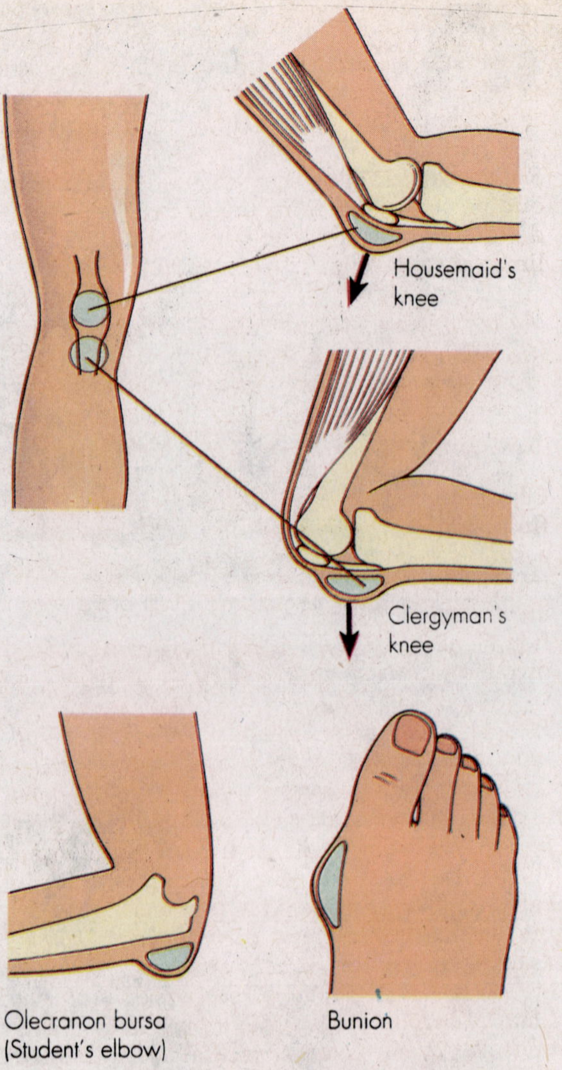

FIG. 3.7 The common adventitious bursae

- Between skin and patella – housemaid's knee.
- Between skin and patellar ligament – clergyman's knee.
- Between skin and head of first metatarsal – bunion.

Colour They are covered with skin that has been repeatedly rubbed and worn, so it is always thickened, shiny, white and cracked.

Tenderness Bursae are only tender if they are very tense or inflamed. When they become inflamed the overlying skin turns red and hot.

Shape and size Bursae are usually circular in outline with an indistinct edge, but their depth, or thickness, can vary from a few millimetres to 3–4 cm.

Surface The texture of the surface of a bursa is difficult to assess because it is intimately attached to the overlying skin. When the skin is not attached to the bursa the surface feels smooth.

Composition Bursae contain a clear viscous fluid, similar to synovial fluid, that gives them a soft or spongy consistence. They fluctuate, transilluminate, may have a fluid thrill and are dull to percussion. These signs may be difficult to elicit if the wall of the bursa is thick or the quantity of fluid small.

Relations As subcutaneous bursae develop between two moving tissue planes to reduce the amount of friction between them, the deep and superficial surface of a bursa is usually firmly attached to the two tissues it separates, so that the friction occurs between the lubricated inside surfaces of the bursa. This makes the bursa immobile and the walls impalpable as separate entities, except at their edge.

State of local tissues The bones and joints beneath the bursa must be carefully examined because a bursa may have developed to ease the movement of the skin over a skeletal abnormality such as an exostosis or deformed joint. The overlying skin is usually grey, horny and cracked.

Complications Bursae can become inflamed by repeated trauma and by conditions which cause inflammation of synovial surfaces, such as rheumatoid arthritis and gout. They also get infected from organisms in the blood stream. Sometimes they become so large that they are a mechanical hindrance.

GENERAL EXAMINATION

Even though the patient complains of only one lump, examine the same spot on the other limb because it is quite likely that he has symmetrical lesions. Also look for other skeletal abnormalities and joint diseases.

Neurofibroma

Neurofibromata are benign tumours which contain a mixture of neural (ectodermal) and fibrous (mesodermal) elements. There is much argument amongst pathologists about their origin. Tumours which are derived purely from the fibrocytes (fibromas), or from the sheaths of nerves (neurilemmomas and schwannomas), are very rare. Neurofibromata are often multiple. If they are **multiple, congenital** and **familial**, the condition is known as **Von Recklinghausen's disease** (see below).

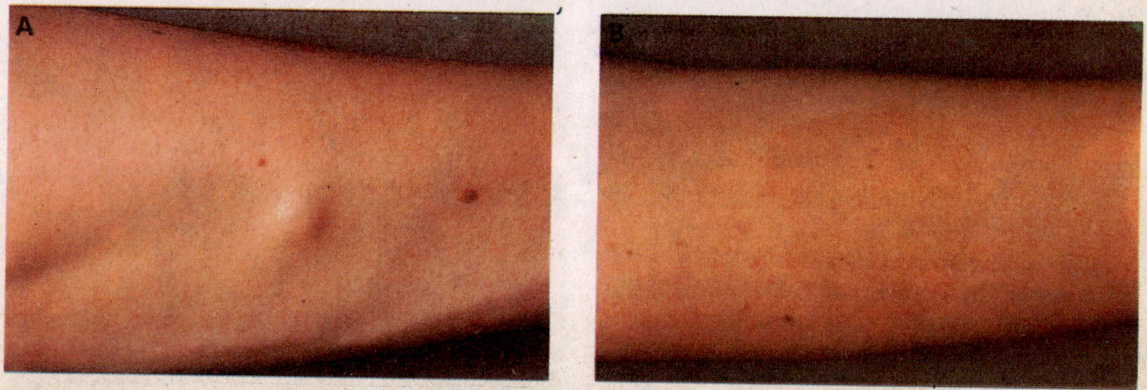

FIG. 3.8 A: A neurofibroma on the leg of a patient with five other similar lesions. **B**: A 'café au lait' patch on the forearm of the same patient

HISTORY

Age Neurofibromata can appear at any age but usually present in adult life.

Symptoms Most neurofibromata cause no discomfort and are rarely big enough to be disfiguring. If they are related to a nerve trunk they may be tender and the patient may get tingling sensations in the distribution of the affected nerve.

Multiplicity Neurofibromata are often multiple.

EXAMINATION

Position They can occur anywhere in the subcutaneous tissues and in the skin. The forearms seem to be most often affected, perhaps because they are the part of the body most frequently palpated by the patient.

Shape and size Neurofibromata are usually fusiform, with their long axes lying along the length of the limb. They are rarely more than a few centimetres in length.

Composition They have the consistence of firm rubber and are dull to percussion.

Relations The surrounding structures are normal. Subcutaneous neurofibromata are mobile within the subcutaneous tissues but move most freely in a direction at right-angles to the course of the nerve to which they are connected.

Multiple neurofibromatosis

(Von Recklinghausen's disease)

Multiple, congenital, familial neurofibromatosis is known as **Von Recklinghausen's disease** and is associated with a number of related abnormalities:

- Fibroepithelial skin tags.
- Patches of light brown discolouration of the skin – the '**café au lait**' patch.
- Neuromas on major nerves, particularly on the acoustic nerve (**acoustic neuroma**) and the sensory roots of the spinal nerves – often a **dumb-bell neuroma**.
- **Malignant change** (neurofibrosarcoma) in 5 per cent of cases.
- **Phaeochromocytoma**.

HISTORY

Most of the neurofibromata are present at birth, but they increase in size and number during life. The disease is inherited through a dominant gene, so one of the patient's parents and some of his brothers and sisters will be affected.

EXAMINATION

The patient is covered with nodules of all sizes from minute lumps, a few millimetres across, to large subcutaneous nodules. Some are in the

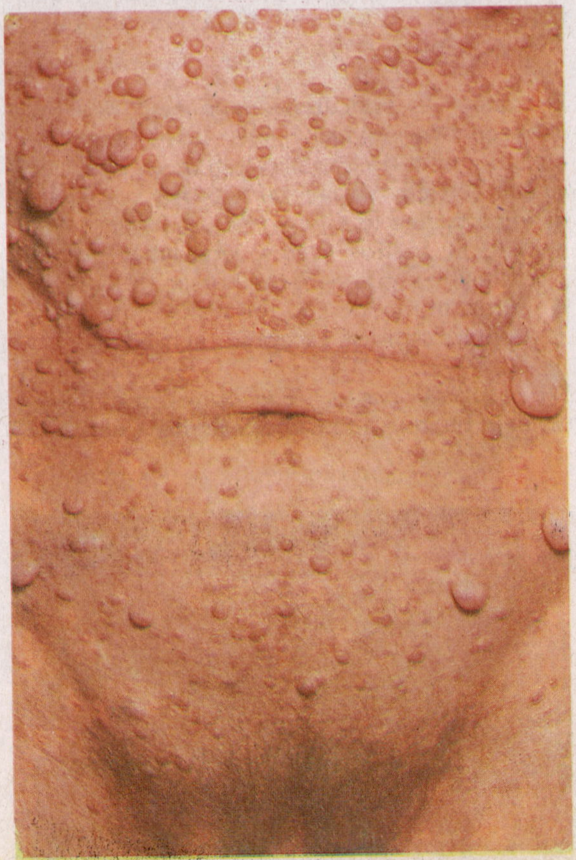

FIG. 3.9 Multiple neurofibromatosis of Von Recklinghausen's disease. The patient did not have a 'café au lait' patch within the area of this photograph

skin, some tethered to it, some in the subcutaneous tissues, and some become pedunculated. The nodules vary in consistence from soft to hard but each one is discrete with clear-cut edges. The disease is extremely disfiguring.

Neurological abnormalities are uncommon. It is important to test hearing and examine the spinal nerves to exclude the presence of major nerve damage caused by true neuromas.

Careful examination of the skin will nearly always reveal irregular patches of pale brown pigmentation. The pigment is melanin and the patches are known as **café au lait** patches. They are a diagnostic feature of Von Recklinghausen's disease. The blood pressure should be checked, as a coexisting phaeochromocytoma may cause persistent hypertension.

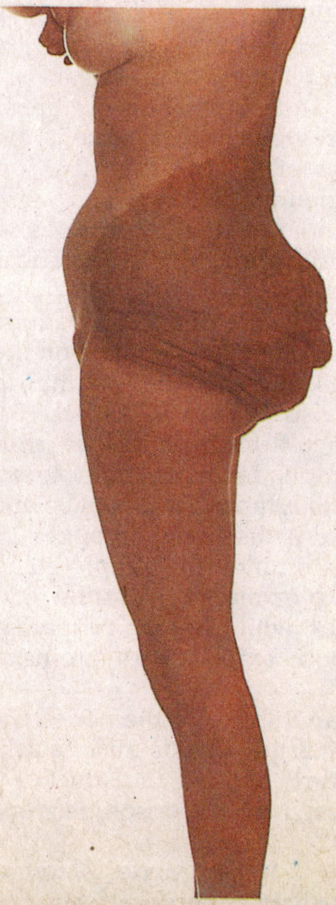

FIG. 3.10 A very dark brown area of pigmentation over an extensive mixed plexiform neurofibroma and haemangioma

Plexiform neurofibromatosis

Although this is a very rare condition, it is mentioned because it is one of those conditions which causes considerable diagnostic confusion if the doctor has never heard of it.

It is an excessive overgrowth of neural tissue in the subcutaneous fat and makes the tissues look oedematous. The resemblance to oedema is so great that the disease is also called elephantiasis neurofibromatosis. It is often diagnosed as lymphoedema but the lymphatics are normal. Remember it when presented with a child with an apparent overgrowth of the soft tissues of his hand or foot. The diagnosis can only be made by the histologist.

Hidradenoma

This is a benign tumour of a sweat gland and is rare. The cells are spindle shaped and arranged in regular alveolar patterns.

HISTORY

Age These tumours occur in middle and late life.

Symptoms They are not painful, just awkward and disfiguring.

Multiplicity They are frequently multiple. Multiple tumours of this kind on the scalp have been likened to a turban, and so this lesion is sometimes called a **turban tumour** (see page 214).

EXAMINATION

Site Although hidradenomata can occur anywhere that sweat glands exist, they are most often seen on the scalp.

Shape and size They are spherical or slightly flattened and vary from a few millimetres to 4–5 cm in diameter.

Surface They are smooth, but the edge may be difficult to feel because they are soft.

Composition Hidradenomata are so soft that the examining fingers get the feeling that they are soft cysts, but they **do not fluctuate**. When they form a large mass they may be less dense than the surrounding tissue and appear to transilluminate. This latter sign and their softness often lead to a mistaken diagnosis of multiple cysts, but hidradenomata are **solid** tumours. They are dull to percussion and not compressible.

Complications Malignant change, causing rapid growth and ulceration, is a rare complication.

Kaposi sarcoma

Kaposi sarcoma is a cutaneous sarcoma which, before the appearance of HIV infection, was a rare sporadic condition in Europe, but not uncommon and endemic in sub-Saharan Africa, particularly Zäire and Western Uganda.

The variety not associated with HIV infection runs a slow, indolent course and is only very rarely associated with spread to the intestine or generalized malignant lymphoma.

The variety associated with HIV infection and the acquired immune deficiency syndrome (AIDS) runs an aggressive course and is commonly associated with systemic tumour infiltration of lymph nodes, intestine, mucous membranes, lungs and other organs.

HISTORY

The patients complain of the presence of painless nodules or plaques in and beneath the skin. They often appear first in the legs. There may also be a multitude of systemic symptoms if the patient has the acquired immune deficiency syndrome.

EXAMINATION

The nodules are red, hemispherical, and painless. They lie in the subcutaneous tissues but the overlying skin is often red, adherent to and involved in the disease process. The overlying skin may break down into an ulcer.

The lymph glands

The lymph glands which receive lymph from the skin and the limbs lie in the subcutaneous tissues of the groin and axilla. The epitrochlear lymph gland in the arm and the popliteal lymph gland in the leg are present in most adults and may enlarge before the axillary or groin glands when there is disease in the hand or foot.

Lymph glands are enlarged and made tender by inflammatory conditions, and enlarged by infiltration with metastatic and primary tumours.

The diagnosis of axillary and inguinal lymphadenopathy depends as much on the **site** of the swellings as the presence of multiple firm lumps in the subcutaneous tissues.

It is difficult to misdiagnose axillary or inguinal lymphadenopathy, but enlargement of the cervical lymph glands can be difficult to diagnose and is discussed on pages 256–263.

When examining the lymph glands it is important to examine all sites containing lymph nodes which might be palpable; i.e. the neck, both axillae, both groins and the abdomen.

The size and shape of the nodes should be recorded. Enlarged glands may be solitary, or multiple; clearly defined, indistinct or 'matted' together; hard, rubbery, or soft; tender or painless.

Whenever a lymph node is found to be enlarged, the area of tissue it drains should be carefully examined.

> Revision Panel 3.1
>
> **The causes of enlargement of lymph nodes**
>
> *Infection*
> - Non-specific
> - Glandular fever
> - Tuberculosis
> - Syphilis
> - Lymphogranuloma
>
> *Metastatic tumour*
>
> *Primary reticuloses*
> - Lymphoma
> - Lymphosarcoma
> - Reticulosarcoma
>
> *Sarcoidosis*

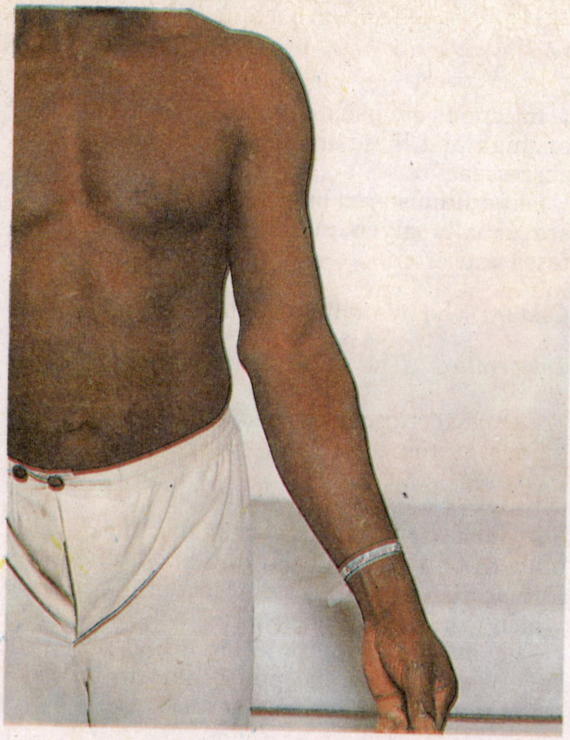

An enlarged epitrochlear lymph gland. The patient had a non-Hodgkin's lymphoma

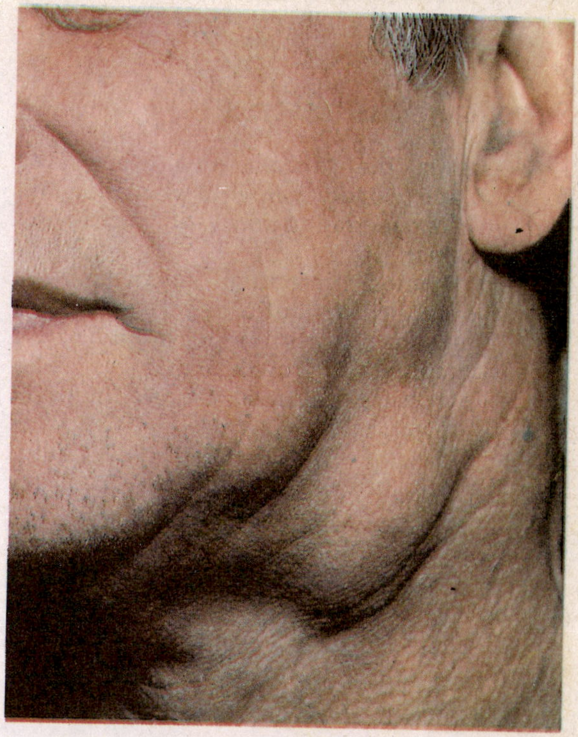

Multiple enlarged upper cervical lymph glands. The patient had a carcinoma of the nasopharynx

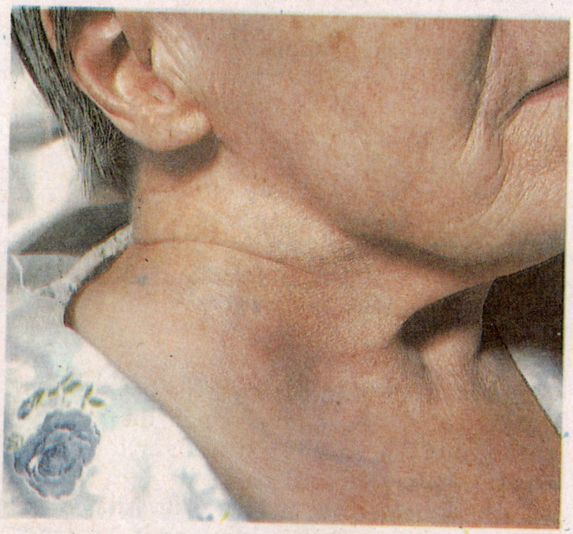

An enlarged right supraclavicular lymph gland. The patient had a carcinoma of the breast

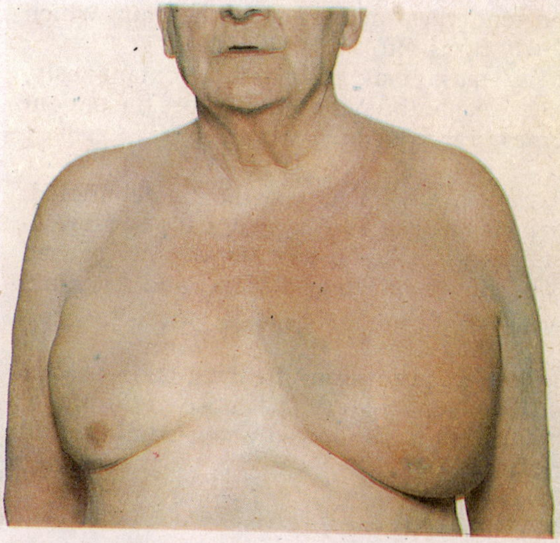

Enlarged left supraclavicular and axillary lymph glands causing oedema of the arm and chest wall. The patient had a lymphosarcoma

FIG. 3.11 ENLARGED LYMPH GLANDS

Subcutaneous abscess

Abscesses in the subcutaneous tissue are common and usually follow implantation of bacteria by a penetrating injury, or infection in a haematoma.

The common infecting organism is *Staphylococcus aureus*, but almost any organism can cause an abscess if the local conditions are favourable to its growth. An abscess is a pocket of pus surrounded by granulation tissue.

HISTORY

Age Subcutaneous abscesses occur in all ages and both sexes.

Hygiene Poor social conditions and bodily hygiene will increase the chances of an infection following a minor injury such as a pinprick.

Symptoms The principal complaint is of a **throbbing pain** which gets steadily worse and keeps the patient awake at night.

The patient notices an area of thickening and tenderness at the site of the pain, which slowly turns into a hard mass.

The mass may discharge spontaneously, with relief of the symptoms, before the patient comes to the doctor.

Previous history Patients who are debilitated, diabetic or drug addicts may have had previous abscesses because of the debility caused by their underlying disease and frequent injections.

Habits Enquire about the drug-taking habits of the patient if you have cause to think that the abscess has followed a self-administered injection.

EXAMINATION

The four classical signs of an abscess (the signs of Celsus) are tumor, rubor, calor and dolor (swelling, redness, heat and pain).

Position Areas subjected to trauma are more susceptible. The hands are common sites for subcutaneous infection (see page 150).

Injections are usually given into the buttock or thigh and these are also common sites for abscesses.

Self-administered injections by drug addicts are usually given into veins in the cubital fossa and groin.

Colour The overlying skin is red.

Temperature The skin over an abscess is hot.

Tenderness Abscesses become increasingly tender as the tension in the pocket of pus increases.

Shape and size The initial change is the development of a patch of induration. As the pus forms, this patch turns into a definite mass which is basically spherical.

The mass may become large and lose its spherical shape if the pus begins to spread through the subcutaneous tissues.

Surface The inner surface of an abscess is a layer of granulation tissue which is inseparable from the indurated inflamed tissues around it. Thus an abscess does not have a definable outer surface even though its contents may be easy to feel.

Edge The edge is not palpable as the induration and oedema gradually merge into the normal tissues.

Composition In the early stages an abscess feels hard and solid. As the pus forms, the centre of the area becomes soft and, if it is not too tender to press, fluctuant. It is dull to percussion and not reducible.

Relations The skin over a subcutaneous abscess is invariably involved in the inflammatory process, so it is red, oedematous and fixed to the underlying mass.

If the pus points to the skin, the skin becomes white and then black as it dies and sloughs away. When the dead skin separates the pus can escape from the abscess.

Deep fixation depends upon the size and direction of spread of the abscess.

Local lymph nodes The lymph nodes which receive lymph from the infected area are likely to be **enlarged and tender**. They may even become abscesses themselves.

Local tissues The local tissues should be normal, apart from those close to the abscess which are involved in the inflammation. There may be scars from previous abscesses.

GENERAL EXAMINATION

A large abscess can cause considerable systemic disturbance. The patient looks pale and ill but may be sweating and having rigors and episodes of flushing. The temperature and pulse are elevated.

4 Muscles, tendons, bones and joints

It is essential that all doctors have a sound basic knowledge of orthopaedic disease, because so many of the patients who come to the general surgical and medical clinics have abnormalities of their musculoskeletal system. You must be able to examine the muscles, bones and joints properly. This chapter describes the examination of each of these structures and then their common abnormalities and diseases.

GENERAL PLAN FOR EXAMINING THE BONES, MUSCLES AND JOINTS OF A LIMB

The basic approach still applies: **inspection** followed by **palpation**, including movement, followed when indicated by **percussion** and **auscultation**. Although moving the limb is part of inspection and palpation, it is such an important part of the examination that it is presented as a separate exercise. The basic plan is therefore Inspection, Palpation and Movement, or in simple English:

LOOK, FEEL AND MOVE

Always begin by looking at both limbs and examining the good limb first.

Always ask the patient to perform active movement before you perform passive movements.

Inspection and movement should be performed with the patient supine and standing.

Inspection

Skin Is the skin discoloured? Look for scars and sinuses. Are there any abnormal or asymmetrical skin creases?

Shape Is there any swelling, deformity or wasting?

Length Compare the length of each part of the limb with the other side, by eye.

Palpation

Skin Feel the temperature of the skin. Is there any oedema – local or dependent? Feel any scars or areas of thickening and find their relation to the bones and joints. Is any part of the limb tender?

Shape Define the cause of any swelling, e.g. fluid in a joint, thickening of the synovium, muscle or bony swellings. You must elicit all the physical characteristics, described on page 31, of any swelling or lump.

Define the cause of any deformity by palpating the bones and joints.

Record any deformity of alignment, in degrees, on a diagram.

Length Measure the **real length** of each limb and of each bone and the **apparent length** of the limb (see page 102).

Movement

Active Ask the patient to move each joint through its full range of movements and show you any trick or abnormal movements. Watch the limb working: standing, walking, lifting, etc.

Passive Move all the joints of the limb through their full range. Test the strength of each movement against resistance. Test for abnormal movements by testing the integrity of the ligaments of each joint.

Arteries and nerves

It is essential to examine the structures that keep the limb alive and make it work – the arteries and nerves.

Arteries Palpate all the pulses. Note the temperature and colour of the limb (see page 162).

Nerves Test the motor, sensory and reflex innervation.

Motor You will already have obtained some information on the ability of the muscles to contract during your examination of movement and strength. Work out which muscles cannot contract properly and their nerve root innervation.

Sensory Check the appreciation of light touch, pinprick, temperature changes, deep pain, vibration sense and position sense.

Reflex Test all the limb's reflexes.

MUSCLES AND MUSCLE DISEASE

Examination of a muscle

If a muscle appears to contain a definite lump, begin by examining the lump to ascertain its physical characteristics, as described in Chapter 1. If there is doubt about the presence of a lump or its relation to the whole muscle,

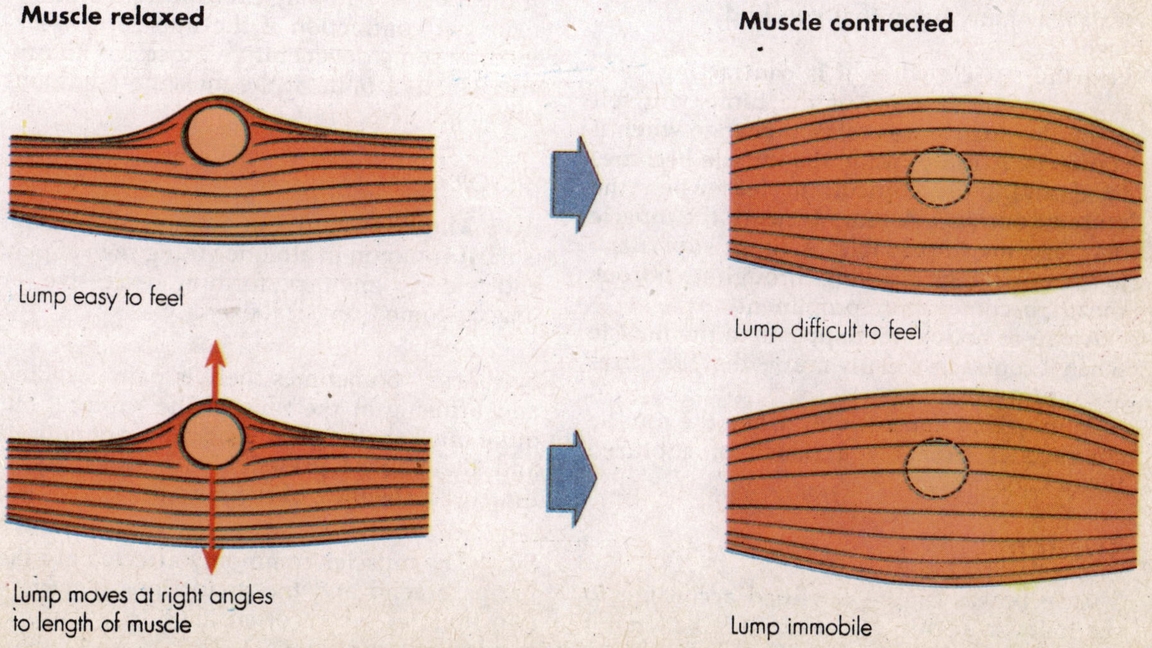

FIG. 4.1 PRINCIPAL FEATURES OF AN INTRAMUSCULAR LUMP

then it is better to examine the muscle first and the lump second.

Inspection

Observe the shape of the muscle at rest Note any wasting, hypertrophy or irregularity of shape caused by a lump, or displacement of the muscle. Always compare the abnormal muscle with the normal muscle of the other limb.

Observe the shape of the muscle when it is contracting Alterations in shape that appear when the muscle contracts are caused by either a lump being concealed or made more prominent by the contracting muscle, or by knotting-up or parting of ruptured muscle fibres.

Look at the neighbouring bones and joints

Palpation

Feel the muscle at rest Put the limb in a comfortable position so that the muscle is relaxed. Assess the texture of the muscle.

Try to decide whether there is a localized swelling or an abnormal muscle. Elicit all the features of any lump that you find.

Feel the muscle when it is contracting See if any of the features of the lump you felt when the muscle was relaxed change when it contracts. A lump inside the muscle becomes fixed and more difficult to feel when the muscle contracts. A lump beneath the muscle may become impalpable. A lump superficial to the muscle, or breaking through its fibrous sheath, becomes more prominent.

A gap or hollow that appears in the muscle when it contracts usually means that the fibres are ruptured.

A lump that appears only when the muscle contracts is probably a bunch of ruptured fibres knotting-up.

Strength

Muscle power can be classified according to the following scale. However, it is better not to use numbers but to describe the strength.

0: Completely paralysed.
1: Barely perceptible contractions.
2: Cannot lift the limb against the pull of gravity.
3: Can move the limb against the pull of gravity only.
4: Fairly strong but not full strength.
5: Full strength.

Innervation and blood supply

You know if the muscle is innervated because you have tested its motor function; but you must examine the integrity of the whole nerve and the spinal segment supplying the muscle by testing all of its other motor, sensory and reflex functions. This means that you must know which nerves and which spinal segments innervate the main muscle blocks in the body (see Revision Panel 1.10 on page 29).

Examine the pulses in the limb.

Ruptured muscle fibres

Muscle fibres usually rupture during an excessively strong or unusually sudden contraction of the muscle. Pathological rupture can follow a normal contraction if the muscle is weakened by some degenerative process. The rupture usually occurs at the musculo-tendinous junction.

HISTORY

Age Muscle rupture can occur at all ages but is most common in athletic young men at play and elderly men performing excessive or unaccustomed physical exercise.

Symptoms Sometimes there is pain, swelling and bruising at the time of the rupture, but quite often the original incident is not noticed and the patient presents with weakness, a limp, or a swelling of the muscle.

Site The muscles commonly affected are the biceps brachii and the quadriceps femoris – two muscles which often have to withstand sudden severe strains.

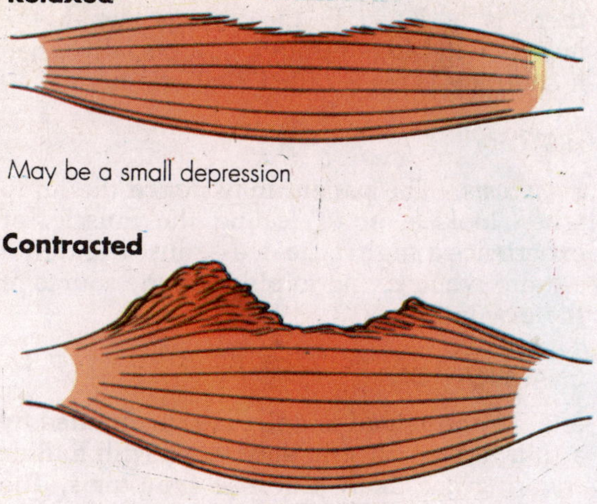

FIG. 4.2 The clinical features of ruptured muscle fibres

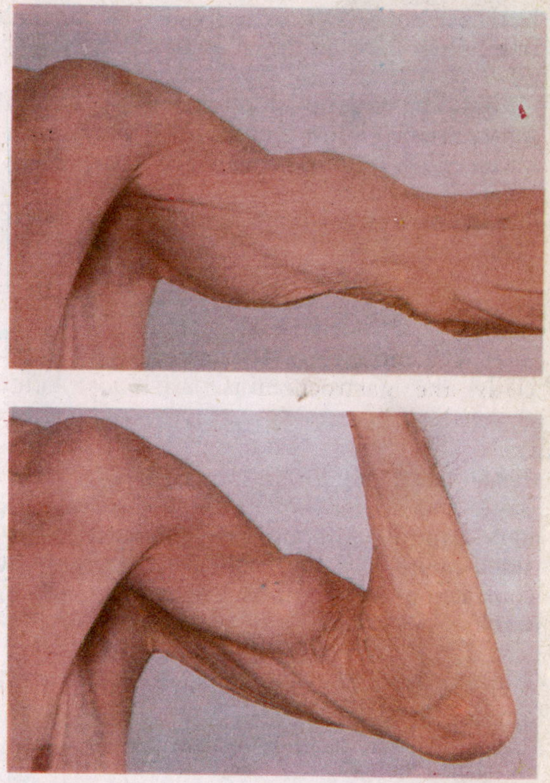

FIG. 4.3 A rupture of the long head of the biceps. In the upper photograph the muscle is relaxed and its contours are normal. In the lower photograph the muscle is contracting and the ruptured fibres are bunched up into a firm mass in the middle of the arm

EXAMINATION

The diagnostic feature of a bundle of ruptured muscle fibres is the appearance of a lump in the muscle on one or both sides of a depression, when the muscle contracts. The lumps are the bunched-up free ends of the contracted ruptured fibres.

The lumps cannot be felt when the muscle is relaxed because they have the same consistence as the adjacent muscle, but the hollow between the broken fibres may be palpable and visible.

The lump (or lumps) which appears when the muscle contracts is firm in consistence, has indistinct edges and cannot be moved independently of the muscle.

The local arteries, nerves, bones and joints are normal unless the rupture is due to attrition or a chronic musculoskeletal disease such as rheumatoid arthritis.

Do not forget to examine the neighbouring bones and joints.

If a significant number of fibres are ruptured the strength of the muscle will be reduced. If all the fibres are ruptured, the movement normally produced by the muscle will be absent.

Intramuscular haematoma

This condition follows a direct injury or a tear of the muscle fibres and the intramuscular blood vessels. It can follow a severe cramp or a violent sudden muscle contraction. Although some of the muscle fibres are ruptured, not enough are divided to produce the physical signs of a ruptured muscle.

HISTORY

Symptoms The two main symptoms are **pain** and **swelling** in the muscle. The pain is present at rest but is exacerbated by any movement of the muscle, passive or active. The patient may also have noticed a diffuse swelling of the limb or a tender lump in the muscle.

Cause The patient can often recall the initial injury. Trivial injuries only cause intramuscular bleeding if there is a haematological or vascular abnormality.

Ask the patient if he is taking anticoagulants.

EXAMINATION

Site The muscles of the lower limbs, especially the gastrocnemius, are most often affected.

Tenderness The lump is tender for a few days, and all movements of the muscle are very painful. Although the tenderness subsides quite quickly, the pain caused by contraction of the muscle may persist for weeks.

Size The size of the lump depends upon the amount of bleeding. It is not always easy to assess because the edge of the lump is usually indistinct.

Shape Haematomata are usually ovoid, with their long axis parallel to the muscle fibres.

Composition The composition of a haematoma depends upon the state of the blood within it. The blood in most haematomata is coagulated, so the lump feels hard. But sometimes the central portion stays fluid, making the lump soft and fluctuant.

Local tissues The surrounding tissues, including the adjacent muscle, should feel normal, but contraction of the muscle causes pain and makes the lump more difficult to feel.

Lymph nodes The lymph nodes at the root of the limb should not be enlarged.

Muscle hernia

When a muscle contracts it becomes shorter and thicker. If it is contained by a fibrous sheath the tension within the sheath rises. If there is a defect in the fibrous sheath the muscle will bulge through it, especially when it contracts. This is called a muscle hernia.

HISTORY

Symptoms The patient may notice the lump when looking at or feeling the muscle, or experience a slight ache in the muscle and find a lump when trying to pinpoint the source of the discomfort.

EXAMINATION

Site Although all muscles are surrounded by a thin fibrous sheath, only those with a thick covering are likely to cause symptoms. The commonest muscle hernia is through the thick fascia which covers the anterior compartment of the lower leg.

Size and shape Muscle herniae can be of any size. Their characteristic feature is that they **change in size** according to the tension in the muscle. When the muscle contracts it bulges through the fascial defect. When the muscle is relaxed there is no lump – just a hole.

Occasionally these signs are reversed. The muscle may bulge through the defect when relaxed but be pulled back into its compartment when it retracts. Do not be confused by this variation. Provided the lump comes and goes as the muscle tension changes and there is a palpable defect in its covering fascia, it is a muscle hernia.

Intra- and intermuscular lipomata

There is not much fat inside a muscle, but there are often small collections of fat around the nutrient blood vessels and in the loose areolar tissue which separates the different sections of a group of muscles. Lipomata can develop in this fat. Histologically they are no different from any other lipomata, but the site gives them some distinctive physical signs.

HISTORY

Symptoms An intra- or intermuscular lipoma may interfere with the function of the muscle and cause pain when the muscle is being used, but it rarely makes the muscle weak.

The patient may have felt a lump, or seen a lump appear during exercise. If an intramuscular lipoma suddenly bursts out of a muscle during exercise, the patient experiences a sharp pain and notices the sudden appearance of the lump. He will then believe that the exercise caused the lump. The lump may change in size and shape as the muscle contracts.

Muscle lipomata are rarely multiple.

EXAMINATION

Site Any muscle can be affected. There is more fat between the flat muscles of the trunk than between the muscles of the limbs, so deep lipomata are more common on the back of the trunk.

Shape If there is only a thin layer of muscle or fascia covering the lipoma, its typical multilobular shape will be palpable.

Size These lipomata are often quite large (5–10 cm in diameter) because they grow unnoticed within or between the muscles for many years. They may become larger, smaller or disappear when the muscle contracts according to their relation to the main bulk of the muscle (see Fig. 4.1).

Edge Their edge is difficult to feel. When a lipoma has herniated through a thick layer of fibrous tissue you may feel a sharp edge, corresponding to the defect in the muscle, but there is usually a lot more of the lipoma deep to this edge which you cannot feel.

Composition The consistence varies with the tension in the muscle. When the muscle is relaxed, the lipoma has its typical soft consistence and may seem to fluctuate. When the muscle contracts, the lipoma, if it is still palpable, becomes hard and tense.

Relations Inter- and intramuscular lipomata are tethered to their site of origin and usually become fixed when the muscle contracts. An intermuscular lipoma may become impalpable when the muscle overlying it contracts.

Myositis ossificans

This is calcification, and sometimes ossification, of part of a muscle. It is an uncommon condition that may follow an injury that has caused extensive intramuscular haemorrhage and a fracture of the adjacent bone. The muscles most often affected are the brachialis, after a supracondylar fracture of the humerus; and the quadriceps femoris, after a fracture of the femur, or a direct blow such as a kick.

HISTORY

Previous injury The patient will know about his previous fracture or, when not associated with a fracture, remember a previous major soft tissue injury.

Symptoms The principal symptoms are caused by an inability of the muscle to relax. The nearby joint becomes **stiff** because there is a reduction of all the movements normally permitted by relaxation of the affected muscle (e.g. myositis of the quadriceps femoris restricts knee flexion but there is full extension). All forced movements are **painful**. If the intramuscular ossification is extensive the joint may become completely fixed.

EXAMINATION

Site The common sites for myositis ossificans are the lower part of the brachialis muscle and the lower part of the quadriceps femoris muscle.

Tenderness The mass of ossified muscle is not normally tender but forced passive movements may cause pain.

Temperature The mass has a normal temperature.

Shape The ossification takes the shape of the muscle in which it is occurring. It is usually an elongated mound filling the muscle and **fixed to the underlying bone.**

Surface The surface is smooth but irregular.

Composition The mass is bony hard and dull to percussion.

Relations In most cases the ossification in the muscle is continuous with the callus that developed around the fracture. Thus the mass is often mistaken for a bony swelling.

The muscles over a callous can usually work normally whereas ossifying muscles cannot work properly and cannot be moved over the callus. The muscle fibres can be felt running into the mass.

Local tissues There may be other evidence of the previous trauma – bone and joint deformities, or nerve and artery damage – so it is important to examine the whole limb very carefully.

Myosarcoma

True tumours of muscle are rare. If they arise from smooth muscle they are called **leiomyosarcomata**. If they arise from striated muscle they are called **rhabdomyosarcomata**. Almost all of the sarcomata that you will see will actually be fibrosarcomata arising from the inter- and intramuscular fibrous septae or the fibrous tissue at the origin or insertion of the muscles. Fibrosarcomata are described in the next section.

The diagnostic features of a tumour arising in or from a muscle are:

- It moves freely when the muscle is relaxed, especially in a direction at right-angles to the length of the muscle.
- It becomes immobile when the muscle contracts and its physical features may change. It may become more or less prominent, harder or softer, and change shape (see Fig. 4.1).

FIBROUS TISSUE

The fibrous tissue that covers muscles and links them to bone in the form of tendons, fibrous insertions, aponeuroses, tendon sheaths, etc., is tough, durable and stable. It causes little trouble during life but is sometimes the site of malignant change.

Three tumours can arise from this tissue. The pure benign fibroma is very rare and can be forgotten, but the fibrosarcoma is one of the commonest mesodermal malignant tumours. The third variety is a less common, locally invasive and recurrent fibrous tumour known by various names, but most often as Paget's recurrent desmoid tumour.

Fibrosarcoma

This is a malignant tumour of fibrous tissue. It is locally invasive and also spreads via the blood stream to the lungs and liver. Spread to the lymph nodes is an uncommon, but not unheard of, event. Distant spread is a late event and the primary will often grow locally for years before metastasizing.

HISTORY

Age Fibrosarcomata are more common in elderly patients but they can occur at any age.

Duration The patient has often known of the existence of a lump for months – sometimes years – before he comes to the doctor to complain of it.

Symptoms The reasons for complaint include:

- Growth of the lump, causing disfigurement or interference with muscle movements.
- Pain in the lump itself or from invasion of nearby structures.
- Muscle weakness caused by infiltration of nearby muscles.
- General debility, from multiple metastases.

EXAMINATION

Site Fibrosarcomata can occur anywhere in the body but more occur in the limbs than elsewhere.

Colour If a large vascular tumour is near the skin it may make the skin shiny and pink.

Temperature Sarcomata, even slow-growing ones such as fibrosarcomata, have an abnormal blood supply and usually feel warmer than the surrounding tissue.

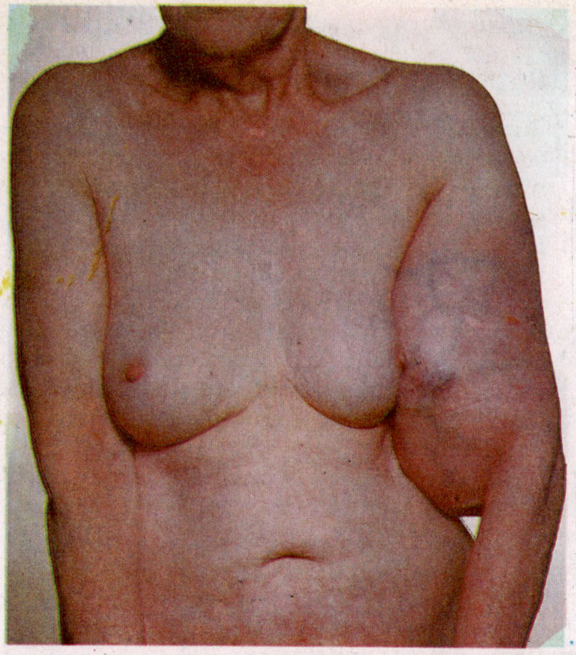

FIG. 4.4 A slow-growing fibrosarcoma of the arm. The overlying skin is stretched and many distended subcutaneous veins are visible. There was no ischaemia or paralysis in the arm or forearm

Shape Their shape depends upon their site of origin. If a tumour grows in the middle of a soft tissue it will be roughly spherical. If it arises close to a bone it will be hemispherical with its deep surface fixed to the bone.

Surface The surface is usually smooth.

Edge The edge of slow-growing tumours is well defined. Fast-growing and invasive tumours have an indistinct edge.

Composition The consistence of fibrosarcomata is firm or hard. They are rarely stony hard because they do not ossify and their vascularity keeps them soft. They may be so vascular that they pulsate, have an audible bruit and a palpable thrill.

Relations The relations of the tumour to the surrounding tissues depend entirely on its site of origin, size and invasiveness. It is likely to be firmly fixed to nearby structures and may invade neighbouring bones, nerves and arteries.

Lymph drainage On rare occasions the local lymph nodes may be enlarged by secondary deposits.

State of local tissues Take particular care to test the integrity of any nerves running close to the mass of the tumour. A nerve deficit is more likely to indicate infiltration than stretching and is almost diagnostic of a locally malignant lesion.

Paget's recurrent desmoid tumour

This condition is mentioned because it is an interesting variety of sarcoma. It occurs most often in the fascia covering the abdominal muscles – the rectus sheath and the external oblique aponeurosis – of middle-aged women. However, it can occur in other sites such as the plantar fascia of the foot or the palmar fascia in the hand. The malignant change affects a wide area because after an extensive and apparently adequate excision of the presenting lump, new lesions may appear years later, in fascia that was apparently healthy at the time of operation.

The lump has the same features as a fibrosarcoma except that it is less vascular and very slow growing.

TENDONS AND TENDON SHEATHS

Ruptured tendons

When the tendon of a muscle is divided the muscle becomes ineffective. To assess the integrity of a tendon you must know its site of insertion and the movement that contraction of its parent muscle would normally produce.

Tendons can be ruptured by direct violence, especially if they have been weakened by rubbing over a fracture callus or the osteophytes and new bone produced by arthritis – a process called **attrition**; but in most cases tendons rupture at a site that has been weakened by avascularity and degeneration (e.g. the Achilles tendon and long head of the biceps) or ischaemic pressure necrosis, such as that caused by a haematoma in the fibro-osseus sheath of the extensor pollicis longus. The tendon of the biceps brachii, the Achilles tendon, and various tendons in the hands are the tendons most often ruptured.

Ruptured biceps tendon

If the long, thin tendon of the long head of the biceps muscle ruptures, the muscle belly retracts into the middle of the arm where it can be seen as a lump, and be made more prominent by asking the patient to flex his elbow against a resistance. This condition is common in the elderly. It does not cause any significant weakness of the shoulder joint. (see Fig. 4.3.)

Ruptured Achilles tendon

Rupture of the Achilles tendon follows a sudden contraction of the gastrocnemius muscle during exercise. The patient feels a sudden severe pain and cannot walk properly. If the rupture happens during walking or running the patient may fall down.

Examination reveals an inability to plantar flex the foot and to stand on the toes of the affected leg. The gap in the tendon is easy to feel, even though there is often a considerable amount of oedema around the tendon and the ankle joint.

The rupture may be bilateral or the patient may have ruptured the other side in the past.

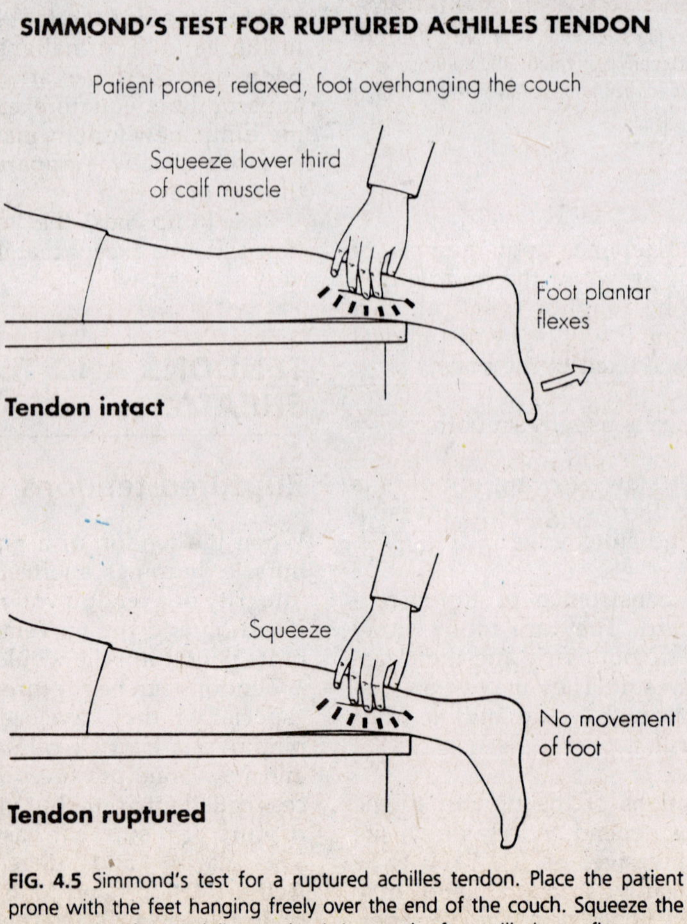

FIG. 4.5 Simmond's test for a ruptured achilles tendon. Place the patient prone with the feet hanging freely over the end of the couch. Squeeze the calf muscles. If the Achilles tendon is intact, the foot will plantar flex

Rupture of the Achilles tendon is easy to miss but easy to detect with Simmond's test. Lie the patient prone with the feet beyond the edge of the couch, fully relaxed. Squeeze the calf. The foot will plantar flex if the Achilles tendon is intact but will not move if it is ruptured.

Ruptured patellar tendon

This is an avulsion of the tendinous insertion of the quadriceps femoris from the upper border of the patella. It usually occurs in elderly people and is uncommon. There is a loss or reduction of knee extension and a visible and palpable gap between the quadriceps muscle and the upper border of the patella.

Ruptured patellar ligament

This rare event is caused by an excessively strong contraction of the quadriceps femoris muscle in athletic young men. The obvious abnormality is an inability to extend the knee joint. The patella lies high in the supracondylar groove of the femur with a visible and palpable gap below it, in the area normally occupied by the hard tense patellar ligament.

Ruptured extensor pollicis longus

Any of the finger tendons can get cut, but these present an acute emergency with a definite history of trauma. It is important to check which finger movements are lost and confirm that this is due to the tendon injury and not to muscle paralysis caused by an associated nerve injury.

Some tendons, especially the tendon of the extensor pollicis longus, lie in a position which makes them liable to constant friction if arthritic changes (rheumatoid or osteoarthritic) occur in the underlying joint, or to pressure from their surrounding fibro-osseus sheath. When the tendon ruptures there is no pain, just a sudden loss of movement. In the case of the extensor pollicis longus the patient cannot extend the distal phalanx of the thumb. Palpation will reveal the absence of tension in the tendon during extension of the thumb and the loss of the ulnar border of the anatomical 'snuff box'- at the base of the thumb.

Mallet finger

This is a rupture of the extensor tendon of a finger just proximal to its insertion. It is described on page 141.

Trigger finger

The movement of a tendon through its sheath can be impeded in two ways: by thickening of the tendon or by thickening of the sheath.

A trigger finger is a finger which gets fixed in flexion and can only be extended by excessive voluntary effort or sometimes physical assistance from the other hand. When extension begins it does so with a jerk, just as the trigger of a gun moves when the resistance of its spring is overcome. The cause of this abnormality is a thickening of the tendon or the tendon sheath just where the tendon enters the sheath, which stops the tendon sliding freely into the sheath during extension.

Stenosing tenovaginitis

(of de Quervain)

This is an example of the restriction of tendon movement by thickening of the tendon sheath and/or the paratenon (i.e. a tenovaginitis or a tenosynovitis). The tendons involved are the extensor pollicis brevis and the abductor pollicis longus where they lie in their fibrous sheath on the lateral side of the wrist, just above the styloid process of the radius. The cause of the inflammation is usually repeated excessive movement of the tendons, e.g. typing.

All movements of the proximal phalanx of the thumb, especially abduction, become painful and crepitus may be felt as the tendons move through their sheath.

Palpation reveals a tender, sausage-shaped swelling just above the styloid process of the radius.

BONES AND BONE IRREGULARITIES

The basic plan – inspection, palpation including measurement and movement, and percussion – should be followed.

Inspection

The overlying skin may give an indication of the underlying pathology. An old tethered scar or a discharging sinus may indicate old or active osteomyelitis.

Redness and oedema of the skin may be caused by underlying infection or malignant growth.

If there is a bony deformity, record its site and angle.

Palpation

If there is a localized swelling, you must elicit all the physical signs pertaining to a swelling, described on page 31.

Feel the whole length of the bone to assess its shape and compare it to the normal side.

Note the temperature of the skin. Conditions which increase bone blood flow, such as infection, tumours and Paget's disease, may raise the temperature of the surrounding tissues.

Measurement

Measure the length of the bone and the length of the limb. There are three measurements which you can obtain:

1 The true length of individual bones.
2 The **apparent** length of the whole limb.
3 The **real** length of the whole limb.

The methods and principles of measurement are best described with respect to the lower limb, but they apply equally to the upper limb.

1 *Bone length*

This is a simple measurement because you are not measuring across any joints. Choose recognizable anatomical points at either end of the bone and measure between them. Do the same on the other side.

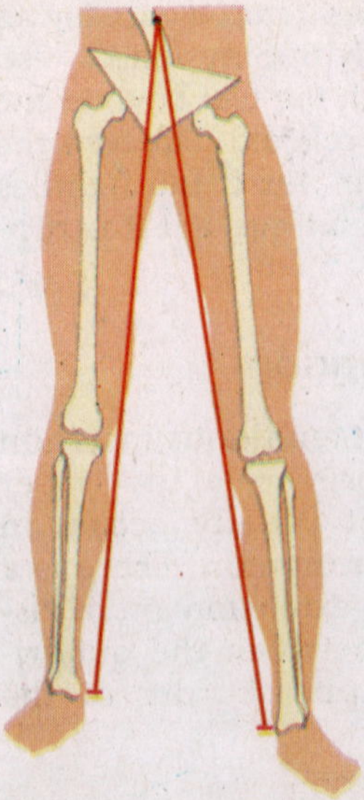

FIG. 4.6 The apparent length of the limbs is measured from a central point with the patient lying comfortably straight. It is not possible with this measurement to tell whether any difference in limb length is caused by a bone or a joint abnormality

Bony points have to be felt through the overlying skin and muscle and it is difficult to get the end of the tape measure on exactly identical points on both sides. The easiest method is to hold the measure firmly between thumb and index finger and then press the back of the index finger firmly up against the bony point or edge that you are using as a landmark.

2 *Apparent length of the limb*

When a patient lies flat and 'straight' on a couch the limbs may appear to be of different length. This may be caused by a bone or joint abnormality. It is customary to record the apparent length, because when it is compared with the true length it gives some indication of the degree to which the skeleton has adapted its position to keep both legs parallel and both feet flat on the ground when the patient stands up, or alternatively an indication of the effect of a joint deformity on the length of the limb.

Method Ask the patient to lie straight on the bed. (Ask a child to lie like a soldier standing to attention.) Choose a point in the mid-line of the trunk – the umbilicus or xiphisternum – and measure from this central point to the tips of both medial malleoli.

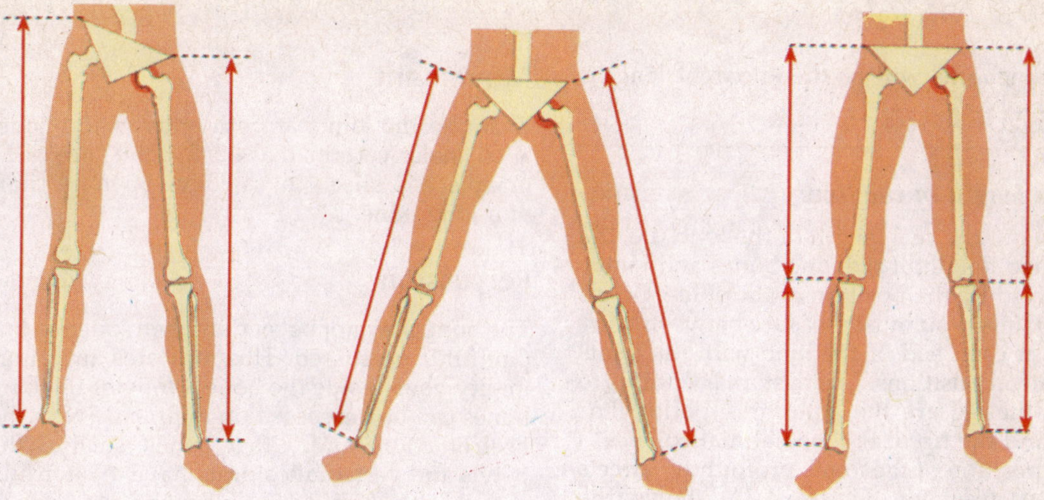

A

No

You cannot detect the real length of the limbs like this because the joints are in different positions

B

Yes

To measure the true lengths of the limbs you must put the joints in identical positions. This patient has a fixed abduction of the left hip so the right hip was abducted to the same degree before measuring

C

To detect the site of bone shortening you must measure the length of each bone

D

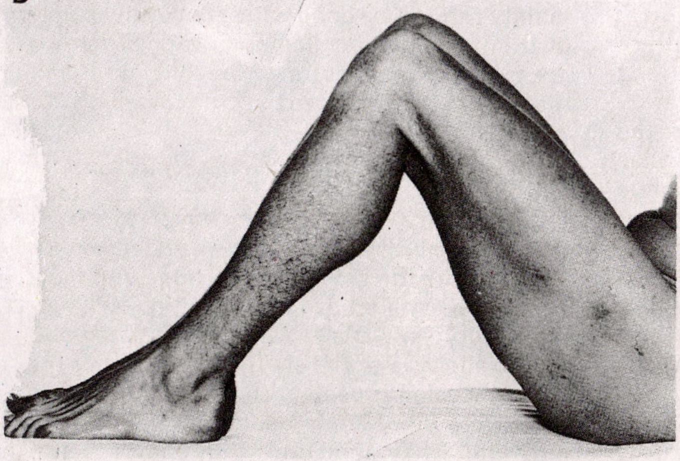

E

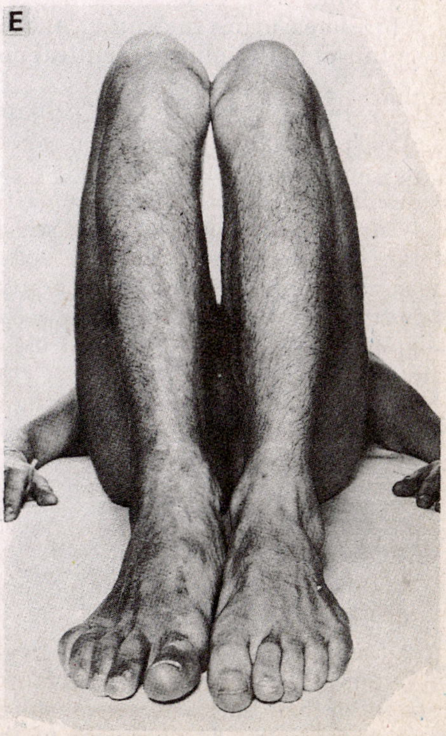

FIG. 4.7 A: You cannot compare these two measurements because the joints are in different positions. **B**: To measure *true length* you must put the joints of both limbs in identical positions. **C**: To detect the exact site of any difference in length you must measure the length of each bone. **D** and **E**: A quick method of detecting difference in bone length is to put the heels together, with the knees flexed, and look from the side and the end of the bed. This patient has shortening of the left tibia

These lengths will be the apparent lengths of the limbs.

3 *Real length of the limb*

To find out the real length of the limb (i.e. the combined length of the limb bones and joints, unaffected by the position of the spine, pelvis or hip joints) you must measure between bony points at each end of the limb with the joints in identical positions. The customary points to use in the leg are the anterior superior iliac spine and the tip of the medial malleolus.

The position of the joints profoundly affects this measurement. Figure 4.7A shows the measurements between the iliac spine and the medial malleolus in a patient, lying straight in bed, with disease of the left hip which has caused some fixed abduction. In order to lie straight in the bed the patient has tilted his pelvis and adducted the other hip. If you measure between the iliac spine and malleolus in this position you are bound to get different measurements, because one hip is abducted and the other adducted.

Before measuring real limb length, place the joints of both limbs in identical positions (Figs 4.7B and C).

Begin by getting the pelvis square to the sagittal plane by checking that both iliac spines are in the same plane at a right-angle to the line of the spine. After doing this you may find the femur on the diseased side abducted or adducted. Place the good leg in the same position. Check that the position of the knee joints is identical – if one has some fixed flexion then flex the good side to the same degree.

Now you can measure on both sides, from iliac spine to medial malleolus, and get a true comparison of real leg lengths.

4 *Joint deformities*

Record the deformity of a joint in terms of the angle by which the distal bone is deviated from the sagittal plane (i.e. the angle of varus or valgus – see page 116). Bones may also be **rotated** on their long axis. Assess the angle of rotation from the displacement of the bony protuberances.

Movement

Examine the joints at both ends of the bone. Also make certain that each bone moves as one piece. A false joint can develop in the shaft of a long bone.

Percussion

The bone may not be tender when touched but painful if percussed. This indicates an abnormality deep inside the bone. Many of the long bones can be percussed on their ends with the heel of your hand. Other bones, such as the pelvis and vertebral column, have to be firmly struck with the side of a clenched fist to elicit deep tenderness. Percussion is seldom indicated and need not be part of a routine examination.

Exostosis

As the word implies, an exostosis is a lump which sticks out from the bone. The lump is mainly cancellous bone with a covering of cortical bone and a cartilaginous cap. Exostoses are usually single but may be congenital and multiple.

Solitary (diaphyseal) exostosis

Exostoses are derived from small pieces of metaphyseal cartilage which were not remodelled during the growth of the bone and have become separated from the main cartilaginous epiphyseal plate. Although isolated and left on the side of the shaft (diaphysis) of the bone, they continue to grow and ossify and so produce a bony knob just above the epiphyseal line. They sometimes have an adventitious bursa over their cap. They are not neoplasms.

HISTORY

Age Exostoses present when they are large enough to cause symptoms – usually in teenage and early adult life.

Symptoms The patient may have felt the lump or it may have become noticeable and cosmetically disfiguring.

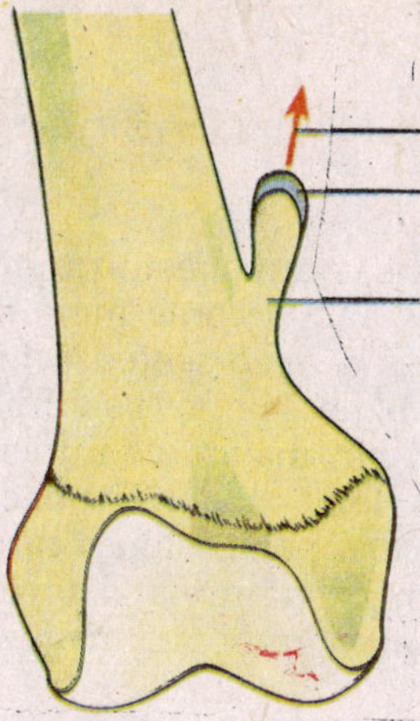

FIG. 4.8 The features of a solitary exostosis

Because exostoses are near joints they sometimes interfere with the movement of the joint and its tendons. Patients may find the movements of the joint limited or associated with 'clicks' or 'jumps' as the tendons slip over the lump.

The overlying bursa, if present, may become enlarged and inflamed.

EXAMINATION

Position Exostoses are adjacent to the epiphyseal line of the bone, just on the diaphyseal side. The majority occur at the lower end of the femur and upper end of the tibia.

Shape Initial palpation gives the impression of a sessile, smooth, hemispherical protuberance, but with careful palpation it is often possible to feel that the base is quite narrow and that the exostosis leans away from the joint.

Size Exostoses are usually 1–2 cm in diameter when they are first noticed, but if they are not removed they may enlarge until all their cartilaginous cap is ossified and become so large (4–5 cm across) that they interfere with joint movement.

Surface Their surface is smooth.

Composition Exostoses are bony hard but their consistence may be masked by a soft fluctuant bursa overlying their cap.

Relations They are fixed to the underlying bone. It is important to palpate the lump while the adjacent joint is moving to feel which muscles and tendons lie close to the lump and to measure the range of joint movement.

Local tissues The rest of the bone and the nearby joint should be normal.

Multiple exostoses (diaphyseal aclasis)

This is a hereditary condition. It is carried in an autosomal dominant manner, so half the patient's children can be expected to have the abnormality. Boys are more susceptible than girls. All the bones that ossify in cartilage can be affected, with the exception of the spine and skull. Because this condition is caused by a widespread generalized abnormality of bone remodelling at the epiphyseal line, as opposed to the sporadic event that produces a solitary exostosis, the long bones may be a little shorter than normal.

The clinical features of each exostosis are similar to those described for the solitary variety. They are multiple and especially common on the limb bones. They can grow to a considerable size, 5–10 cm in diameter.

Callus

Perhaps the commonest cause of thickening of a bone is callus. Callus is the buttress of new bone formed around a fracture site to unite and strengthen it, while the cortical bone is being slowly repaired.

HISTORY

In the majority of cases the patient knows of the injury and the subsequent discomfort associated with the fracture which caused the callus, but this is not always the case. Some fractures are caused by minor stress, or stress that the patient does not connect with the breaking of bones, such as coughing causing a fracture of the ribs. Furthermore, not all fractures cause severe pain, so the absence of a history of trauma or pain does not exclude the possibility that the lump might be callus, but makes it unlikely.

EXAMINATION

Position The thickening of a bone by callus should be greatest at the site of the fracture, but it may be asymmetrical if the stresses on the bone do not run directly down the centre of the shaft.

Tenderness Mature callus is not tender. Once a fracture has united there is no local tenderness, and if an area of thickening in a bone is tender it is unlikely to be callus around a united fracture. It may be callus around non-union, but other signs of non-union will be present.

Shape Callus usually causes a fusiform enlargement of the whole bone – thickest at the site of the fracture.

Surface Young callus has an irregular surface but it becomes smooth as time passes. In young people callus is eventually completely resorbed.

Local tissues The callus may surround a deformed bone – angulated or rotated – if the fracture was not set properly.

Paget's disease of bone

(Osteitis deformans)

This condition occurs in later life. Normally, bone is continually repaired and replaced throughout life. This process follows the same pattern as the original ossification. The ossified cartilage which is reorganized into mature bone is called osteoid bone. In Paget's disease the repair process stops at the osteoid bone stage so that the healthy mature bone is gradually replaced by thick, bulky, very vascular osteoid bone. If the repair process stops a stage earlier, the old bone which has been absorbed by the osteoblasts is replaced by fibrous tissue. This makes the bone very weak. Paget's disease of bone usually affects many bones but can affect just one bone in the whole skeleton (monostosic Paget's disease). Osteogenic sarcoma complicates 5 per cent of cases.

HISTORY

Age The patient is rarely under 50 years of age, often much older.

Symptoms **Pain** is the commonest symptom. As the bones enlarge and become more vascular the patient feels a deep-seated aching, gnawing pain in the bone. He can usually tell that it is deep-seated but may have difficulty in appreciating its skeletal origin. The back is the commonest source of pain. Make a careful note of any change in the nature and severity of the pain. This may indicate malignant change.

Deformity The bone grows bigger and bends. The typical complaints are:

- **Enlargement of the skull** so that the hat no longer fits and the frontal bones become prominent.
- **Curvature of the spine**, causing a kyphosis and difficulty with fitting clothes. The patient occasionally complains that he is getting shorter.
- **Bowing of the legs.**

Headache This pain is caused by the changes in the vascularity of the skull bones but is mentioned as a separate symptom because the patient rarely associates the headache with the skull changes.

Deafness Paget's disease in the temporal bones may affect the middle ear and cause a form of otosclerosis. The patient may also have vertigo.

EXAMINATION

General appearance The patient with generalized disease has a large head, a bent back, arms that seem too long (because of the kyphosis) and bow legs.

Cardiovascular system Examine the cardiovascular system with care. The increased bone blood flow causes an increased cardiac output. The heart may be enlarged, there may be an aortic ejection murmur and the blood pressure elevated. It is claimed that Paget's disease can cause a high-output heart failure,

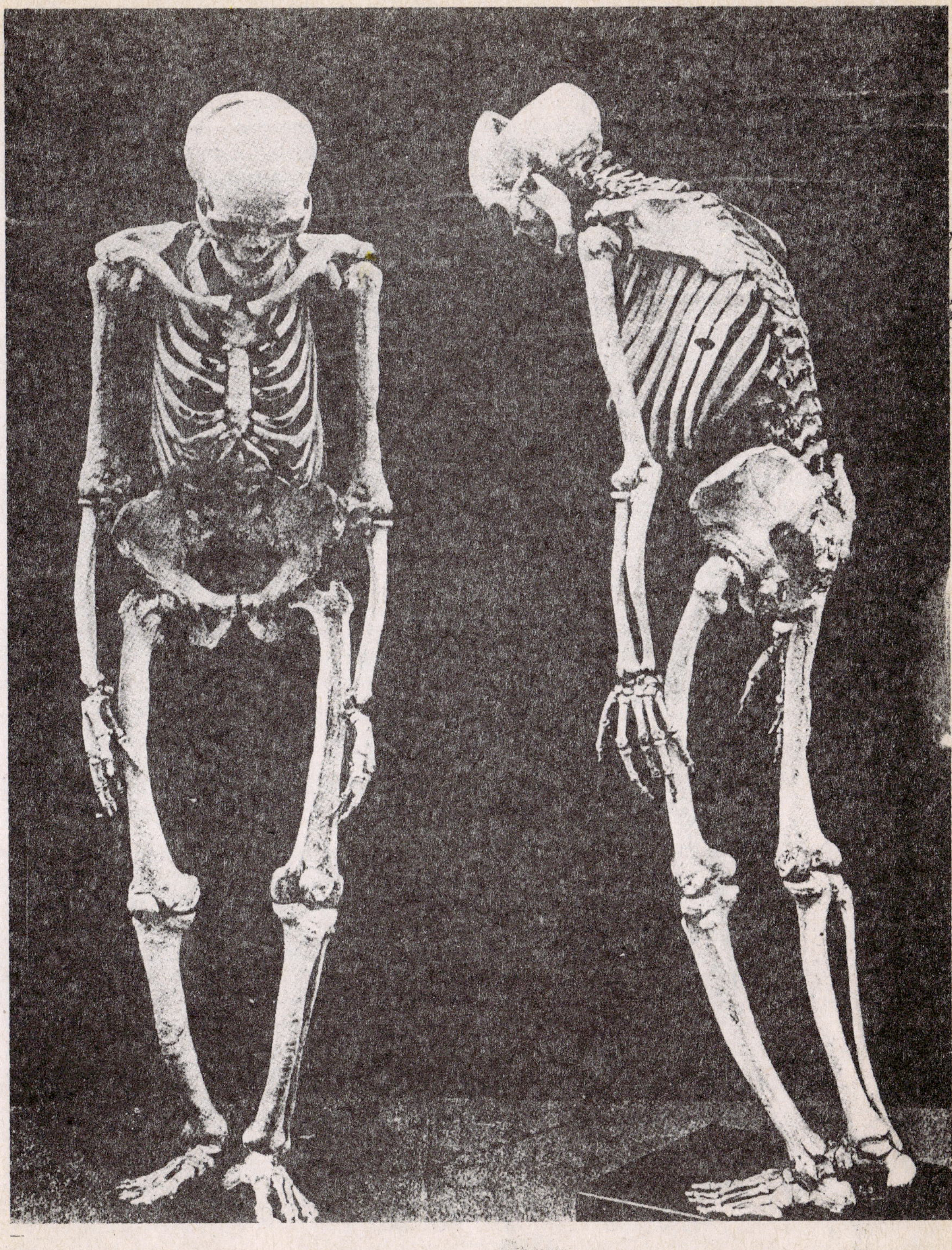

FIG. 4.9 The skeleton of a man who had extensive Paget's disease. All the bones are thick. The kyphosis makes the arms seem long. The left femur is split in the coronal plane, revealing the thickening of the cortical bone (reproduced by kind permission of the Curator of the Pathology Museum of the Royal College of Surgeons and the Medical Illustration Unit)

but this is a very uncommon occurrence. What is common is the exacerbation of any myocardial ischaemia, secondary to coronary vessel disease, by the extra demands placed upon the heart of an old person.

Respiratory system The patient may have râles and rhonchi at both lung bases if the kyphosis is severe enough to interfere with the movements of the chest wall.

Skeleton (see Fig. 4.9)

- *Skull.* The enlargement occurs in the vault. The dome looks swollen and the enlarged frontal bones make the forehead bulge forwards.
- *Spine.* The disease usually affects the whole skeleton, so producing an even kyphosis. The shoulders are rounded and the head and neck protrude anteriorly.
- *Legs.* The femur and the tibia may bow in both anteroposterior and lateral directions. The sharp anterior edge of the tibia becomes so prominent that the description 'sabre tibia' is apt, although this expression is usually reserved for bowing caused by syphilis and yaws.

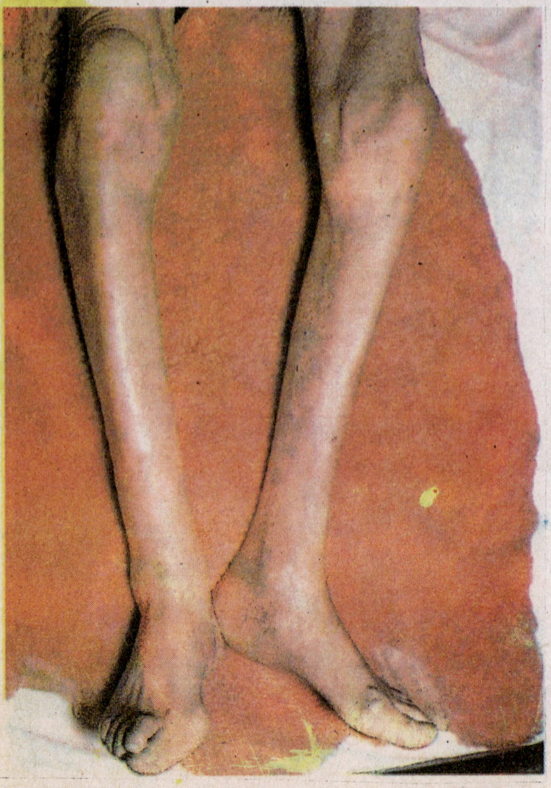

FIG. 4.10 'Sabre tibiae'. The anterior edge of the tibia is normally straight and sharp. In this patient, Paget's disease has made them thick and curved

When examining the skeleton look for any localized bony enlargement, especially in the areas where the pain is severe or has changed. A swelling of the bone which is painful, a little tender and warm to the touch suggests a sarcomatous change.

Central nervous system The patient may have a conduction deafness and difficulty when standing, caused by middle ear and vestibular apparatus damage. The function of other cranial nerves can be affected if the thickening of the bones reduces the size of the foraminae in the base of the skull. Blindness can occur if the optic nerves are compressed.

Spinal nerves may be damaged by collapse of the vertebrae.

BENIGN TUMOURS OF BONE

Benign tumours of bone fall into two categories: those arising from cortical bone (the so-called 'ivory' osteoma) and those which are primarily cartilage tumours but arise within or on the surface of long bones (enchondroma and ecchondroma). An exostosis, described earlier in this chapter, is not a benign neoplasm.

Malignant tumours are either primary or secondary. The secondary deposit is by far the most common variety of malignant tumour in bone.

Osteoma

HISTORY

The patient complains of a lump which he has felt or had drawn to his attention. It is not painful and rarely occurs in a site that interferes with joint or tendon movements.

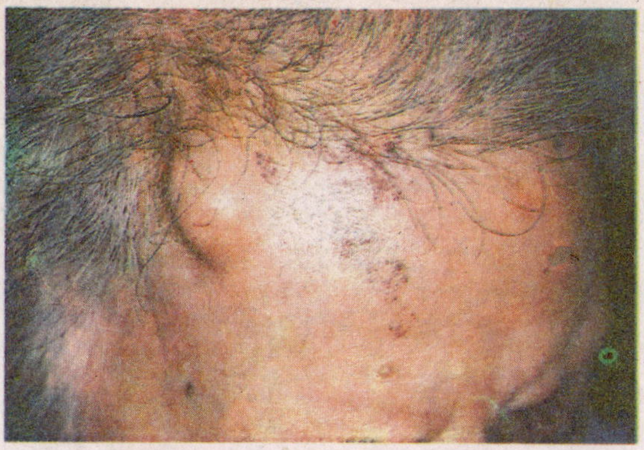

FIG. 4.11 An osteoma of cortical bone – an 'ivory' osteoma – on the forehead, which has been present for 40 years

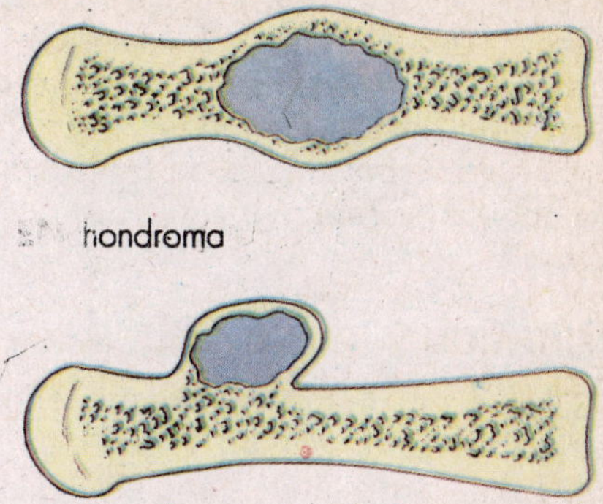

FIG. 4.12 The two varieties of chondromata that are found in long bones

EXAMINATION

Site Osteomata are common on the surface of the vault of the skull, frequently the forehead

Shape and size They are sessile, flattened mounds with a smooth surface.

Composition Osteomata are bony hard – hence the name 'ivory' osteoma.

Relations Nearby muscles and fascia move freely over the lump which is obviously fixed to and an integral part of the underlying bone.

Chondroma

A chondroma can grow in a long bone only if a piece of the cartilage from which the bone developed fails to become converted to bone.

An **enchondroma** is a chondroma growing in the centre of the bone; an **ecchondroma** is a chondroma growing on the surface of the bone. There is no pathological difference between these two varieties of chondroma.

When the chondromata are multiple and congenital (but not familial) the condition is called dyschondroplasia or **Ollier's disease.**

HISTORY

Age Chondromata usually present in teenage or early adult life.

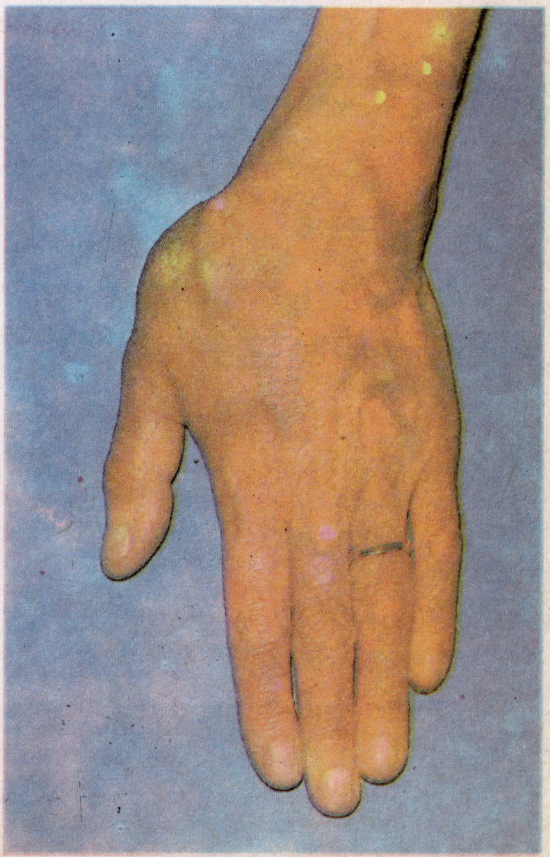

FIG. 4.13 A large ecchondroma of the metacarpal bone of the thumb

Symptoms The patient notices either that a bone is gradually expanding or that a lump is appearing on the side of a bone.

Neither symptom is painful but an ecchondroma may interfere with joint and tendon movement.

EXAMINATION

Site Chondromata are common in the bones of the hands and feet but may occur anywhere. Large, long bones are rarely affected except when the patient has congenital and multiple chondromata (Ollier's disease).

Temperature The overlying skin has a normal temperature.

Shape Enchondromata cause a fusiform enlargement of the shaft of the bone. Ecchondromata form a sessile lump on the surface of the bone.

Surface The surface of both varieties is smooth.

Composition As chondromata are usually covered by a thin layer of cortical bone they feel hard.

COMMON SOURCES OF BONE METASTASES

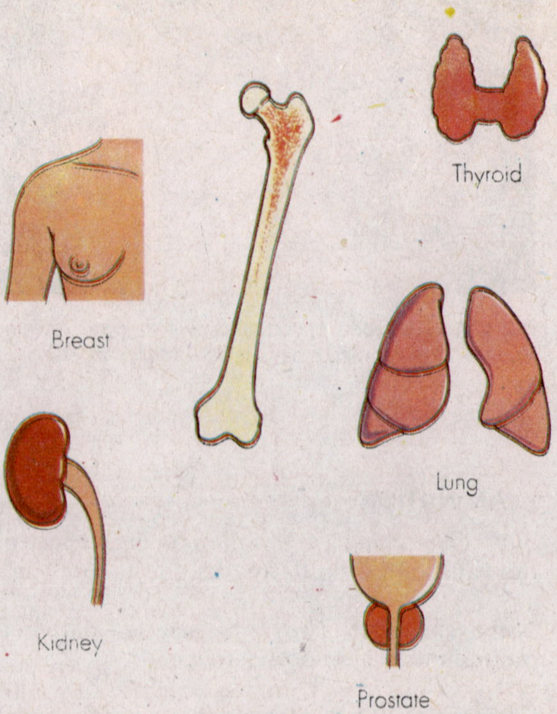

FIG. 4.14

MALIGNANT TUMOURS OF BONE

The commonest malignant tumours in bone are metastases from distant carcinomata. There are four primary tumours of bone: osteosarcoma, Ewing's tumour, multiple myeloma and the giant cell tumour (osteoclastoma). They are all relatively rare tumours.

Secondary (metastatic) tumour

The cancers that commonly metastasize to bone are to be found in the lung, breast, prostate, kidney and thyroid.

These are the five to keep uppermost in your mind, but also remember that any tumour can metastasize to bone.

The bones most often afflicted by secondary deposits are the vertebral bodies, pelvis, ribs and the upper ends of the femur and the humerus, because these bones contain red bone marrow and so have a good blood supply.

HISTORY

General features The patient often gives a history of a previous disease and its treatment (e.g. a mastectomy for a lump in the breast). If not, he is likely to be complaining of symptoms related to the primary growth, such as a cough with haemoptysis, or difficulty with micturition.

Some patients develop bony secondary deposits with no signs or symptoms to indicate the site of the primary lesion.

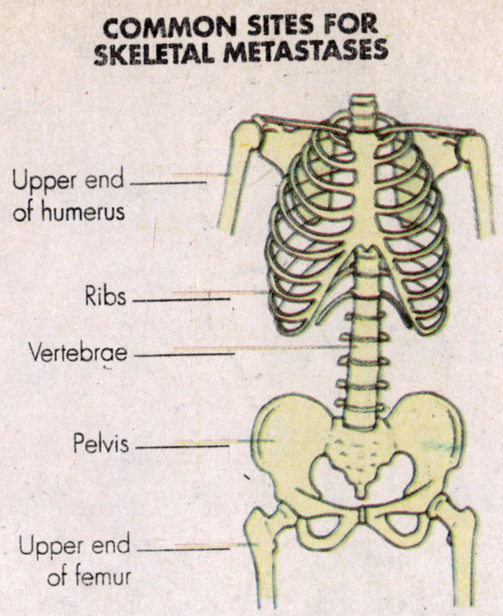

FIG. 4.15

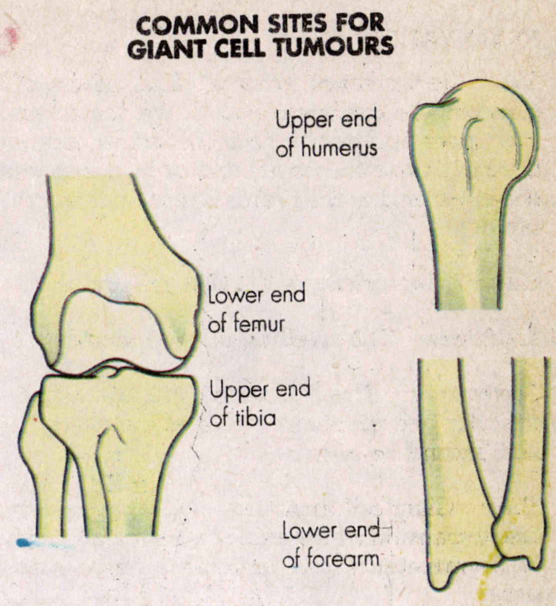

FIG. 4.16

Symptoms The commonest symptom is pain. Low back pain or pain in the pelvis and hip are often the first indication of the existence of secondary deposits.

Acute pain will occur if there is a pathological fracture, such as the collapse of a vertebral body or a fracture of the femur. The patient rarely notices any swelling at the site of a metastasis unless it is in a superficial bone such as the vault of the skull, the clavicle or a rib.

EXAMINATION

If the metastases are deep-seated they may present no physical signs except pain on movement and tenderness on percussion.

When superficial, they may cause a swelling of the bone which appears rapidly, and grows steadily.

The consistence of a secondary deposit in a bone may vary from hard and bone-like to soft, compressible and pulsatile.

Carcinoma of the kidney is a source of very vascular secondary deposits, so vascular that they may pulsate and be misdiagnosed as aneurysms.

Giant cell tumour

(Osteoclastoma)

These tumours are sometimes classified as half-way between benign and malignant because approximately one-third are entirely benign, one-third invade nearby tissues and only one-third metastasize.

HISTORY

Age The patient is usually between 20 and 40 years old.

Symptoms The usual presenting symptom is **pain**. The pain is a dull ache but may become acute if there is a pathological fracture.

The patient may also notice **swelling** of the lower end of the femur or the upper end of the tibia.

The nearby joint may get **stiff** if the swelling disturbs the tendons around it, or if the tumour invades the bone just beneath the articular cartilage.

EXAMINATION

Site The common sites to find giant cell tumours are the lower end of the femur and the upper end of the tibia (i.e. either side of the knee); and the upper end of humerus and the lower end of the radius (i.e. away from the elbow).

Colour The colour of the skin is normal.

Tenderness The swelling may be tender.

Temperature These tumours are not usually vascular and the temperature of the overlying skin should be normal.

Shape Giant cell tumours usually cause a diffuse expansion of the end of a bone but it may be asymmetrical and noticeable on one side only.

Surface Their surface is smooth.

Composition If the outer layer of bone is reasonably thick the lump feels bony hard. If it is thin it may feel firm and slightly pliable. When it is very thin it crackles and bends when touched, and feels like a broken egg shell.

It does not pulsate unless very thin walled and malignant.

Relations The surrounding structures are usually freely mobile over the swelling.

Lymph drainage The local lymph nodes should not be enlarged.

Osteosarcoma

This is the malignant sarcoma of bone. It is seen in two groups of patients: the young, and the elderly with Paget's disease. Sarcoma complicating Paget's disease has already been described (see page 106).

Osteosarcoma spreads early and rapidly by the blood stream.

HISTORY

Age Primary osteosarcoma occurs in childhood and the teenage.

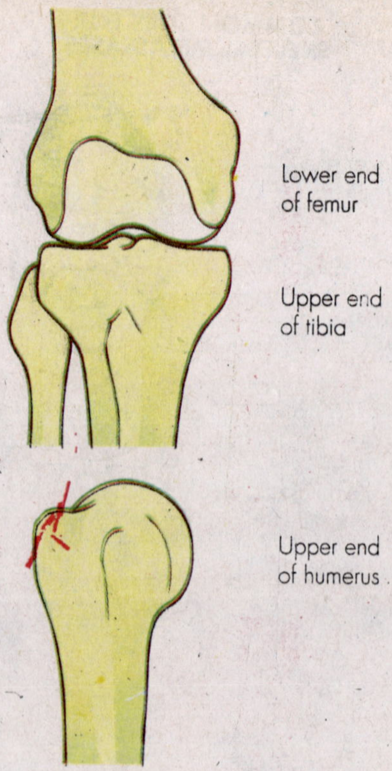

FIG. 4.17 The common sites to find osteosarcomata

Symptoms **Pain** is the predominant symptom. It usually begins before the patient notices a lump and is a persistent ache or throb.

Swelling of the bone may be noticed and in some instances this increases rapidly.

The development of **general malaise, cachexia and loss of weight** may precede or coincide with the appearance of local symptoms.

Pulmonary metastases may cause a **cough and haemoptysis.**

Abdominal discomfort and jaundice may follow the enlargement and destruction of the liver by metastases.

Cause The patient will often relate the onset of his symptoms to an injury but there is no evidence that trauma causes sarcoma. The injury simply focuses the patient's attention on symptoms which he had previously dismissed as trivial and insignificant.

EXAMINATION

Site The commonest place to find an osteosarcoma is the lower end of the femur. The upper end of the tibia is the second common site, followed by the upper end of the humerus.

Colour The overlying skin may be reddened and the subcutaneous veins visibly distended.

Tenderness The swelling may be slightly tender but not exquisitely so like osteomyelitis. Any red, warm, non-tender bony swelling should, in the first instance, be considered to be a tumour, not an infection.

Temperature The skin over the swelling is usually warm, sometimes quite hot.

Shape The swelling tends to appear on one side of the lower end of the bone, making it asymmetrical.

Surface Its surface is smooth unless it has spread into the surrounding tissues when it becomes irregular.

Composition Bony sarcomata feel **firm** but not bony hard. It is a clinical aphorism that benign tumours of bone feel hard whereas malignant tumours of bone feel soft. A very vascular tumour may pulsate.

Relations The structures overlying a small osteosarcoma are mobile but become fixed to it if it spreads locally beyond the bone.

Lymph drainage The lymph nodes will not be enlarged in the early stages of the disease, another indication that the red, warm swelling is not an infection. But when the tumour invades the soft tissues it may spread to local lymph nodes.

Local tissues The nearby **joint** often becomes stiff and develops an effusion. The adjacent artery and nerves are only involved in advanced local disease.

GENERAL EXAMINATION

Take particular care when examining the chest and the abdomen because the lungs and the liver are common sites for metastases. There may be generalized wasting, and wasting of the muscles of the affected limb.

Reticulum cell sarcoma

(Ewing's tumour)

This is a tumour which appears in the centre of long bones – a feature which helps distinguish it from osteosarcoma and osteomyelitis. The cells of this tumour have a distinct reticulate staining. In many instances this tumour is a secondary deposit from an adrenal neuroblastoma, but there is a primary variety whose cell of origin is not known.

HISTORY

Age Ewing's tumour occurs in childhood and the teenage.

Symptoms The commonest symptom is a persistent **ache** or **pain** made worse by movement.

As the femur is the bone most often affected, many children present with a **limp**.

These tumours can sometimes present as a **pyrexia of unknown origin** (PUO) and cause rigors and night sweats.

There may be **weight loss** and **malaise**, especially if the lesion is a metastasis from a neuroblastoma.

EXAMINATION

Site The mid-shaft of the femur is the commonest site to find these tumours, but the tibia and the humerus can be affected.

Colour The overlying skin may be reddened.

Tenderness The swelling is usually a little tender.

Temperature The increased vascularity makes the whole area feel warm.

Shape The tumour causes a symmetrical fusiform enlargement of the shaft of the bone, the upper and lower limits of which are indistinct.

Surface The surface of the swelling is smooth.

Composition When the bone is so expanded that the tumour mass is palpable, it feels firm and rubbery, not bony hard.

Relations The overlying structures can be moved over the mass because, although they are displaced, they are not usually infiltrated.

Lymph nodes The lymph nodes should not be palpable.

Local tissues The arteries and nerves of the limb are rarely involved.

GENERAL EXAMINATION

There may be pyrexia and generalized wasting. The lungs and liver may reveal evidence of secondary deposits and very rarely a primary neuroblastoma may be palpable in the abdomen – a lobulated mass in the upper part of the abdomen which may cross the mid-line.

RELATIONSHIP BETWEEN THE SITE OF A BONY LUMP AND ITS CAUSE

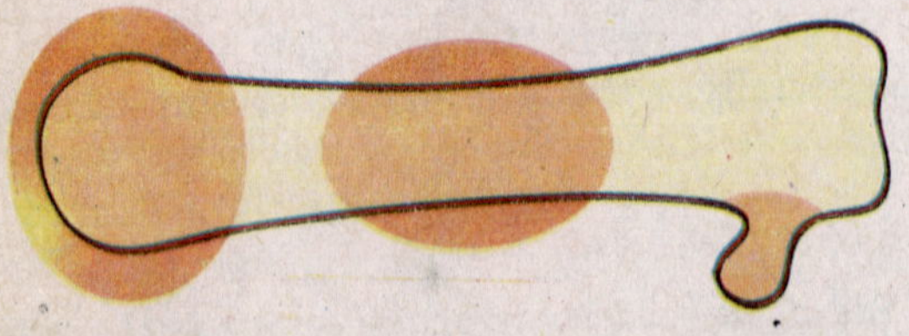

Expanding one end	**Centre**	**On surface, at end**
Osteoclastoma	Callus	Exostosis
Osteosarcoma	Secondary tumour	Ecchondroma
	Enchondroma	

FIG. 4.18

Multiple myeloma

(Plasmacytoma)

This is a disease of the blood and bone marrow in which multiple deposits of myeloma cells (plasmacytes) are found throughout the bones containing red bone marrow – the vertebral bodies, ribs, pelvis, skull and proximal ends of the femur and the humerus.

The patient presents complaining of general malaise, loss of weight and intractable pain in the skeleton – mostly the back and chest wall.

There may be signs of involvement of other parts of the blood-forming tissues – enlarged lymph glands, hepatomegaly and splenomegaly.

Occasionally a deposit in a subcutaneous bone causes a palpable lump and is the presenting symptom.

The urine contains Bence–Jones protein.

Acute osteomyelitis

Bone can become infected by organisms which reach it through the blood stream or directly through a wound. Blood-borné organisms are probably trapped in thrombi or haematomata, caused by minor trauma, in the capillary loops in the part of the shaft adjacent to the epiphyseal line known as the metaphysis.

The common infecting organisms are streptococci and staphylococci.

HISTORY

Age Patients with acute osteomyelitis are usually between 1 and 12 years old.

Symptoms The site of infection is **painful,** though in the early stages this is only a deep-seated ache. When pus forms and the intramedullary tension increases, the pain becomes intense and throbbing.

There is usually some **swelling** around the painful area, but this is not marked as it is caused by a diffuse oedema of the overlying tissues.

The patient may notice that the nearby joint is **swollen** and **stiff.**

The infection causes a loss of appetite and general debility. Most patients feel **hot and sweaty** and some have **rigors.**

EXAMINATION

Site The bones commonly infected are the tibia, femur, humerus, radius and ulna.

Colour The skin over the painful area may be red or reddish-brown.

Temperature The skin does not become palpably hot until the infection has spread through the bone into the subperiosteal layer.

Tenderness The swollen area is tender and the whole bone is sensitive. Percussion on the end of the the bone is painful.

The swelling The swelling is soft and indistinct because it is caused by oedema of the overlying structures. If there is pus near the surface there may be an area within the swelling which fluctuates.

Lymph nodes The local lymph nodes will only be enlarged if the infection has spread outside the bone.

Surrounding structures The **overlying skin may be oedematous.** The **neighbouring joint may be swollen** by an effusion and its movements limited and slightly painful. If the joint movements are very restricted and painful the infection has probably spread into the joint and caused a septic arthritis.

The **veins** of the limb are often **dilated.**

GENERAL EXAMINATION

The patient looks ill and feverish. The face is flushed and the temperature raised. If the patient has a septicaemia he may be hypotensive, sweating, possibly shaking and have a dry tongue and oliguria.

The joints

Use the same basic approach to examine a joint – inspection, palpation and movement – look at it, feel it and move it.

A PLAN FOR THE EXAMINATION OF A JOINT

Inspection

Overlying skin

Colour? Sinuses? Scars?

Shape

What is the shape of the joint? Is there any general or localized **swelling?** Are there any **deformities?**

Malalignment of a joint in the coronal plane, the plane of abduction and adduction, is known as a **valgus** or a **varus** deformity. Figure 4.19 defines these terms. When the part of the limb below the joint is angled away from the mid-line (abducted) there is a valgus deformity; when the part of the limb below the joint is angled **towards** the mid-line (adducted) there is a **varus** deformity. Students often get these deformities confused. The easiest way to remember them is to remember one deformity and work out the rules.

knock-knees – genu valgum
(the tibia is angled away from the mid-line)

Revision Panel 4.1

The causes of joint deformities

Skin	Contractures
Fascia	Contractures
Muscle	Paralysis, fibrosis, spasm
Tendon	Division, adhesion
Ligament	Rupture, stretching
Capsule	Rupture, fibrosis
Synovium	Inflammation
Bone	Changes in shape, trauma, pressure atrophy

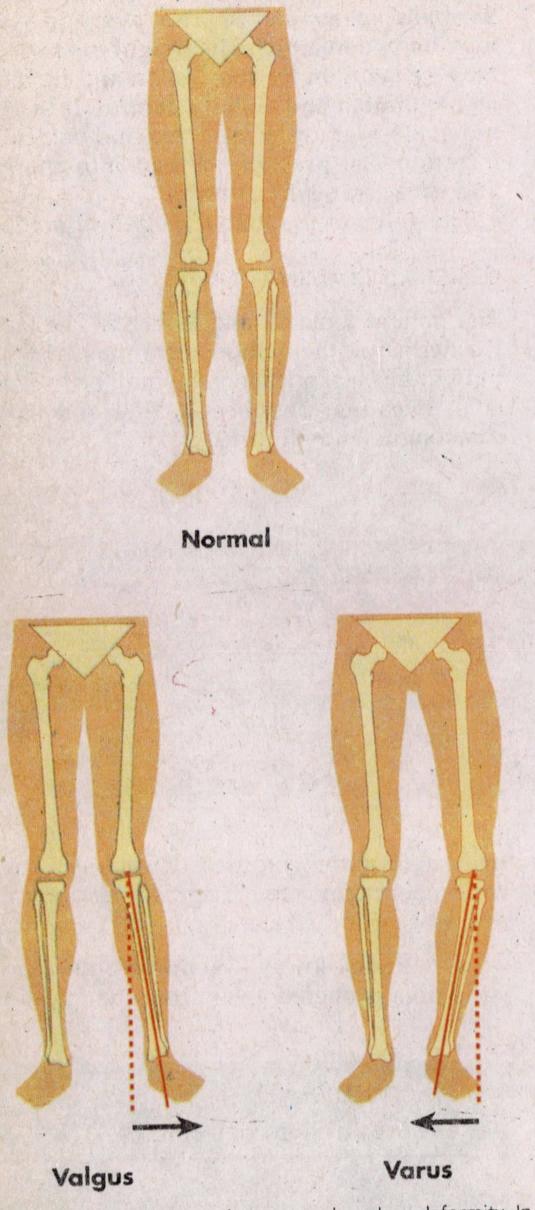

FIG. 4.19 The definition of a varus and a valgus deformity. In valgus deformity the distal bone forming the joint is abnormally abducted. In a varus deformity it is abnormally adducted. Remember, knock-knee = genu valgum

Do the **muscles** that move the joint look normal or wasted? What do the other joints in the limb look like? In what **position** does the patient hold the joint?

Palpation

Skin

Feel the temperature and texture of the skin over the joint.

Subcutaneous tissues

Are the subcutaneous tissues normal or thickened?

Muscles

Feel the texture of the local muscles for wasting and tone. The muscles may be in spasm if joint movement is painful.

Joint capsule

Is the capsule thickened? Is the thickening diffuse or localized?

Synovium

Is the synovial membrane thickened and palpable? Is there excess synovial fluid (i.e. an effusion)?

Bones

Define the contours of the bones that form the joint. Check that they are in their correct anatomical positions.

Movement

Active movement

Ask the patient to move the joint through its full range of movements. Record the degree of any limitation of movement.

Strength of movements

Make the patient move the joint against resistance so that you can assess the strength of the muscles producing each movement.

Passive movements

Move the joint through its full range of movement with the patient's muscles relaxed. Note any **crepitus** (grating sensations) felt during this passive movement.

Ligaments

Check the integrity of each ligament by stretching it. This will also reveal any **abnormal** movements.

Examine the arteries, nerves and the other joints of the limb

The majority of joints have simple movements (e.g. extension and flexion) and their examination presents no problem. The examination of the two complex joints of the lower limb, the hip and the knee, which are frequently diseased or deranged, deserves a detailed description.

EXAMINATION OF THE HIP JOINT

Position

Ask the patient to lie flat and straight on the couch, and then check that the pelvis is square to the mid-line by feeling the positions of the anterior superior iliac spines.

Inspection

Skin Remember that sinuses and scars from the hip joint are often on the buttock and posterior aspect of the upper thigh, so look at the skin over the back of the joint as well as the front.

Shape Check the contours of the thigh and buttock. **Asymmetrical skin creases** indicate joint displacement.

Position When the hip joint is painful or distended by an effusion it is held slightly flexed and abducted.

Palpation

The capsule and synovium of the hip joint cannot be felt but the muscles and the bony contours can be examined.

Relationship between pelvis and femur

The position of the greater trochanter with respect to the pelvis (i.e. acetabulum) can be checked in three ways:

1 Bilateral palpation To compare the two sides, put your thumbs on the anterior superior iliac spines and your fingers on the tops of the greater trochanters. You will appreciate any difference in the distance between these points through the position of your fingers.

2 Nelaton's line Turn the patient on his side. Imagine a line drawn from the anterior superior iliac spine to the ischial tuberosity. The top of the greater trochanter should just touch this line. If it lies above the line, there is shortening of the neck of the femur or a dislocation of the hip.

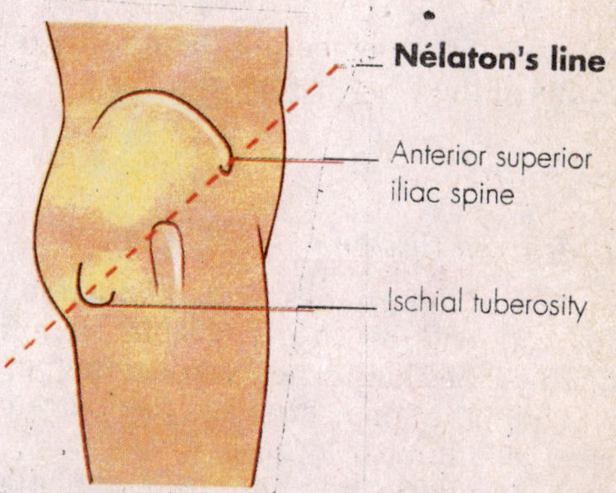

FIG. 4.20 Nélaton's line is a line drawn through the anterior superior iliac spine and the ischial tuberosity. It should just touch the top of the greater trochanter

3 Bryant's triangle This gives a measurement of the distance between the top of the greater trochanter and the coronal plane of the iliac spine. Lie the patient supine. Imagine a horizontal line passing through the anterior superior iliac spine. Measure the vertical distance between this line and the top of the greater trochanter.

Nélaton's line and Bryant's triangle are rarely used for precise measurements (radiographs are much more accurate), but they are

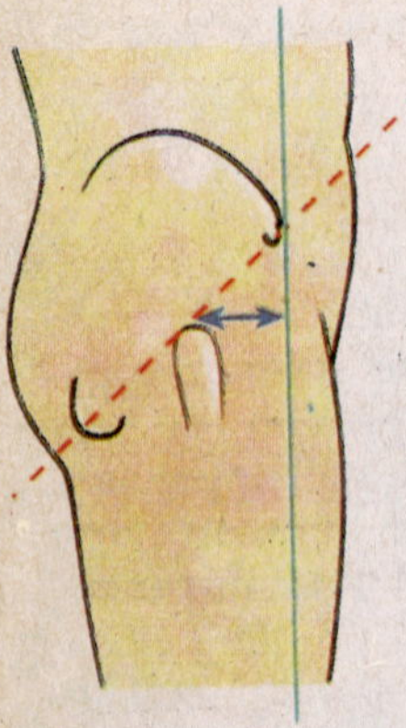

FIG. 4.21 Bryant's triangle measures the vertical distance from the anterior superior iliac spine to the greater trochanter, and the horizontal distance between the coronal planes of the iliac spine and trochanter

useful ways of remembering the normal relationships of the bony landmarks.

Movement

Test for fixed flexion

Other fixed deformities (e.g. abduction or adduction) will be clearly visible from the position of the thigh when you set the pelvis square with the spine, but fixed flexion can be masked by a lumbar lordosis.

Place your left hand underneath the hollow of the lumbar spine. Grasp one leg and flex the hip and knee until the lumbar spine straightens and presses against your left hand. If the other hip joint is normal, the thigh on that side will remain flat on the couch. If it has a fixed flexion deformity it will lift up from the couch to an angle corresponding to the degree of fixed flexion. This is called **Thomas' test for fixed flexion**.

Flex the other leg to check the opposite joint.

Passive movements

You can only test the movements of a joint by keeping one of the bones that forms the joint still, and moving the other bone.

During all passive movements of the hip you must continually check that the pelvis is not moving by keeping the thumb and little finger of one hand resting upon the two anterior superior iliac spines.

Flexion Flex the hip and knee until the thigh presses against the abdomen. Keep your left thumb on the anterior spine but spread your fingers over the iliac crest to detect when the pelvis first begins to tilt.

Abduction and adduction Keeping the left hand firmly on the pelvis, abduct or adduct each leg until the pelvis begins to move.

Rotation Check internal and external rotation either by rolling the whole limb or twisting the femur after flexing the hip and the knee to 90°.

Abnormal movements The only abnormal movement you are likely to meet, excepting those caused by acute trauma, is 'telescoping' of the joint, caused by a dislocated head of the femur sliding up and down the outer aspect of the ilium.

This abnormal movement is detected by pushing and pulling the femur along its long axis while steadying the pelvis and feeling the top of the greater trochanter. It is sometimes easier to do this by flexing the hip to 90° and pulling the thigh upwards.

Extension Do this last, as you need to turn the patient on his face. Put your hand under the knee and lift up the thigh. A normal hip extends only 10°.

Measurements

Measure the real and apparent lengths of the limb and the individual bones to determine the site of any shortening you detect (see pages 102–104).

Make the patient stand up

Look for deformities and abnormal skin creases.

Check any measurement of shortening by putting blocks under the short limb until the iliac spines are horizontal. Measure the height of your blocks.

Figure 4.22 Some important aspects of the examination of the hip joint

A

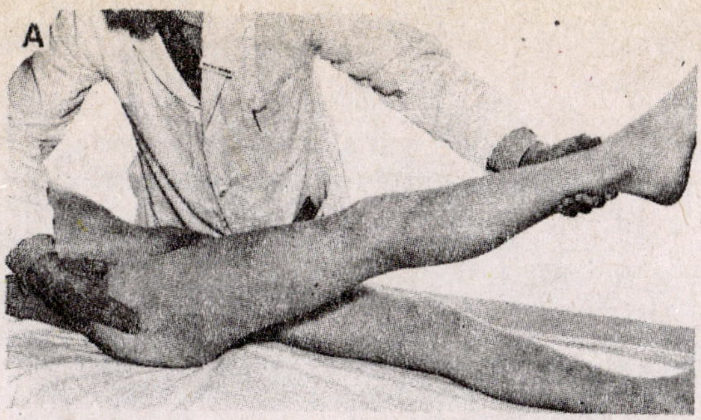

(A) When testing flexion, place your fingers on the great trochanter and your thumb on the iliac spine so that you detect any tilting of the pelvis.

B

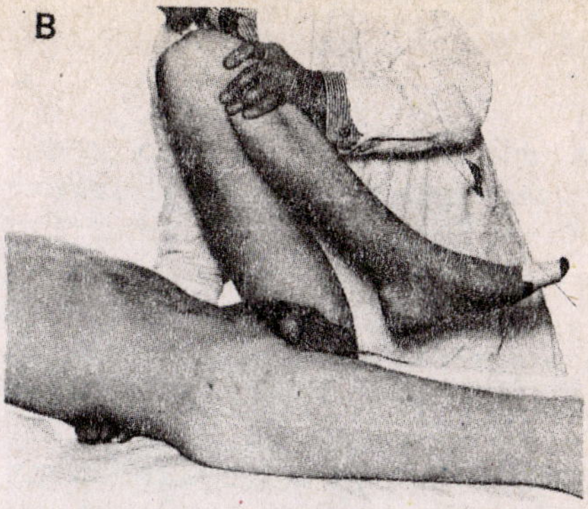

(B) Measure the degree of fixed flexion by flexing the good hip until the lumbar spine straightens and presses on your other hand placed beneath the lumbar spine. This is Thomas' test. This patient had no fixed flexion.

C

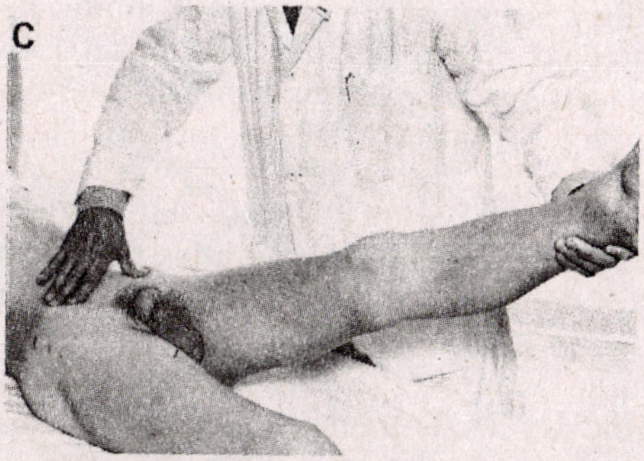

(C) Keep your fingers and thumb stretched across the iliac spines when testing ab- and adduction to detect any movement of the pelvis.

D

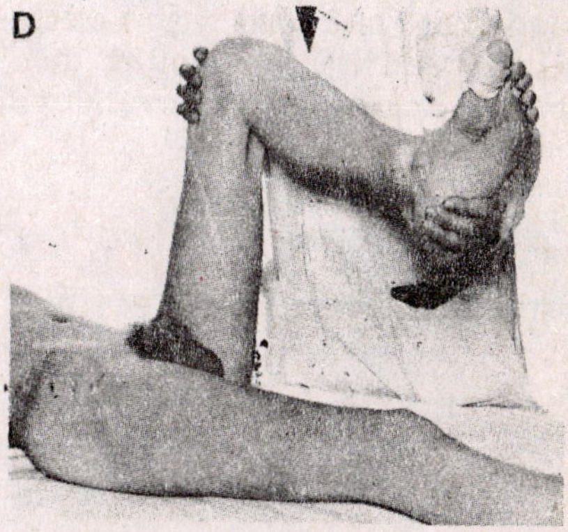

(D) Rotation is measured by flexing the hip and the knee to 90° and rotating the femur by moving the foot back and forth across the line of the limb.

E

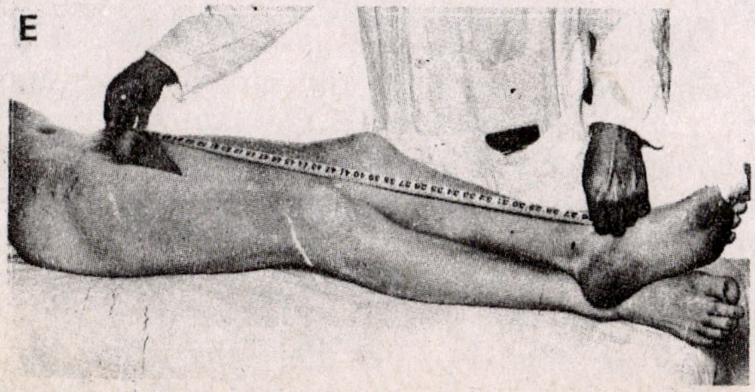

(E) This patient has fixed adduction of the right hip and fixed flexion of the right knee. The left leg must be placed in an identical position before comparing the real lengths of the limbs.

F

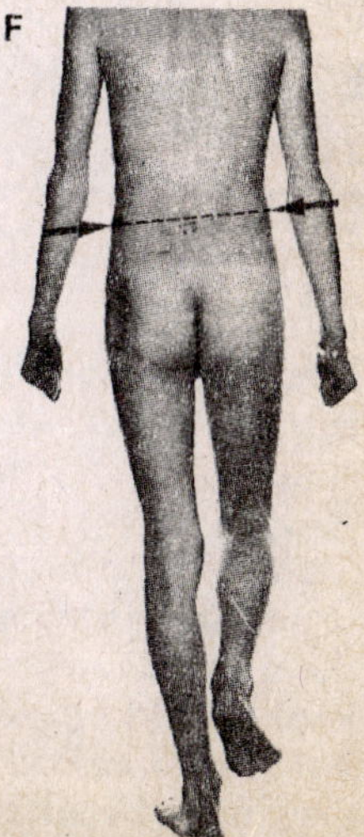

(F) Ask the patient to stand on one leg. He should raise the pelvis on the opposite side. This is Trendelenburg's test.

It is often easier to feel the relative positions of the anterior iliac spine and the greater trochanter when the patient is standing than when lying down.

Trendelenburg test Ask the patient to stand on one leg. The opposite side of the pelvis should rise to help balance the trunk on the leg. If it falls and the patient has difficulty in standing, the test is positive. A positive test means one of the following:

- Paralysed abductor muscles.
- An unstable joint (e.g. congenital dislocation of the hip or a fracture of the neck of the femur).
- Approximation of the insertion and origin of the abductor muscles preventing their proper function by a severe coxa vara or a dislocation of the hip.

Make the patient walk

Any instability of a joint becomes more noticeable during the stresses of walking.

Examine the nerves and arteries of the limb

Joint disease is often secondary to neurological abnormalities.

EXAMINATION OF THE KNEE JOINT

Inspection

Skin Look at the skin all round the joint – front and back – for discolouration, scars and sinuses.

Shape The contours of the knee joint are easy to see and any bony or joint swelling distorts them at an early stage. The size of the whole joint should be compared with the other side, but the areas in which minor degrees of swelling caused by a small effusion are first apparent are the hollows either side of, and above, the patella.

Position A knee joint that is swollen and painful is most comfortable when slightly flexed.

Palpation

Synovium

The synovium of the knee joint can be felt on either side of the patella, and in the suprapatellar pouch. In some diseases it becomes thickened and rubbery, or 'boggy'. A thickened synovium is usually hyperaemic and makes the overlying skin warm.

Bony contour

Check the position of the patella. It should be in the patellar groove of the femur, but it may be displaced laterally or superiorly if there is lengthening or rupture of the patellar ligament.

Check the position of the knee joint. When students are asked to put their index finger on the line of the knee joint, they invariably point to a spot 2.5–5 cm above it. Remember that the main bulge of the knee is formed by the lower end of the femur. The easiest way to find the joint line is to flex the knee until you can feel the anterior curved edge of the femoral condyles and can slide your finger downwards over this edge until you reach the tibial plateau.

It is important to relate areas of tenderness to the joint line and the points of attachment of the collateral ligaments.

Effusions

Effusions of the knee joint are common and easy to detect because the excess synovial fluid collects in the front of the joint where it can be seen and felt. There are three tests for detecting an effusion in the knee joint.

1 Visible fluctuation A small quantity of fluid present does not make the whole joint look swollen, but if you press gently on one side of the joint, the other side may bulge outwards.

Get the leg in a good oblique light so the hollows on either side of the patella are visible. Stroke the joint just to one side of the

Figure 4.23 Some important aspects of the examination of the knee joint

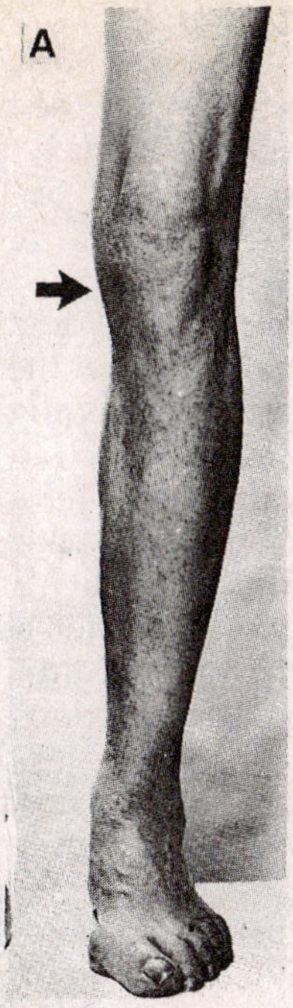

(A) Remember that the joint line is below the bulge of the knee.

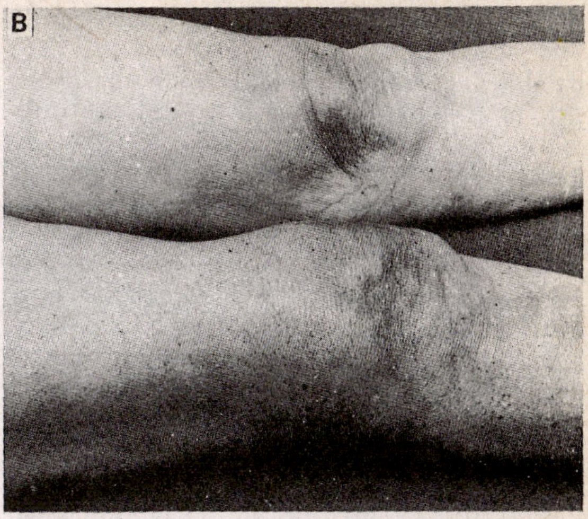

(B) Effusions fill out the hollows on either side of the patella.

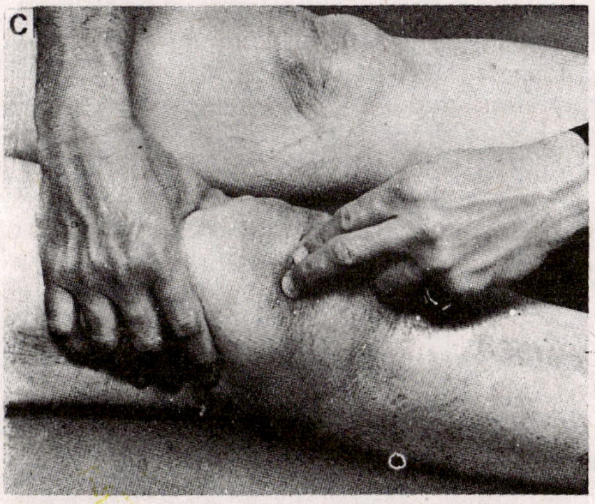

(C) Before you test for a patellar tap, compress any fluid in the suprapatellar pouch into the space beneath the patella.

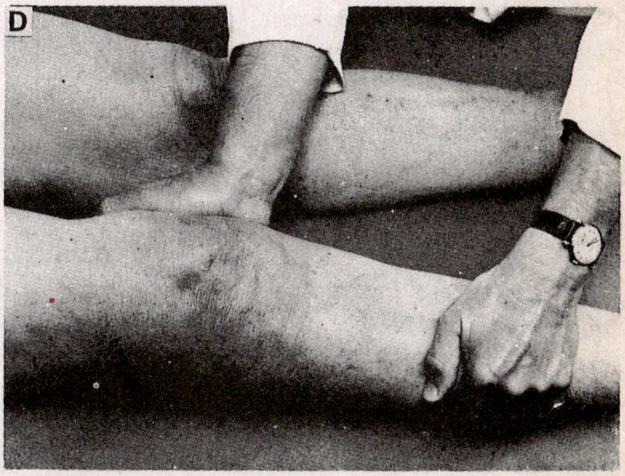

(D) Test the collateral ligaments by forcibly ab- and adducting the joint.

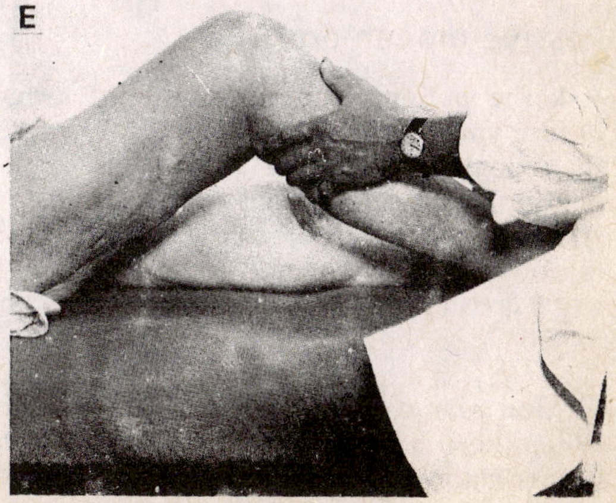

(E) Test the cruciate ligaments with the knee flexed to 90°. The anterior ligament stops anterior movement of the tibia on the femur.

patella and watch the hollow on the other side of the patella to see if it gradually fills out as the effusion is pushed into it. This is the most sensitive way of detecting a small effusion. It cannot be used if the joint is full and tense.

2 Palpable fluctuation When the knee joint is full of fluid it is possible to press on one side and feel the increase in pressure transmitted over to the other side.

Place the palm of the left hand above the patella, and the thumb and index finger either side of it. Press posteriorly and towards the toes to squeeze any fluid in the suprapatellar pouch down into the joint behind and either side of the patella. Place the thumb and index finger of the right hand either side of the patella and see if you can feel fluctuation between your thumb and finger.

3 Patellar tap This is an extension of palpable fluctuation. When the joint is full of fluid the patella is lifted off the femur. If it is pressed or tapped it can be felt to move backwards and hit the femur. This test is also helped by emptying the suprapatellar pouch into the space behind the patella with the left hand.

Surrounding tissues

Pay particular attention to the bulk and strength of the quadriceps muscle, but remember the quadriceps of the dominent leg will usually be slightly bulkier.

Passive movement

Ask the patient to move the joint himself before you check passive movement. Record the extent of the active knee movements in degrees. Remember that when the leg is straight the angle between the femur and tibia is now called 0° – zero. At full flexion the angle is usually 150–160° and full extension 0° to –10°.

Flexion Bend the knee as much as possible. When there is hip joint disease you may have to turn the patient on to his side to see the full extent of knee flexion.

Extension Lift the leg off the bed by the heel and ask the patient to relax. In women the knee joint often extends 5° or 10° past the 0° mark.

Rotation There are small degrees of rotation of the tibia on the femur but these are not easy to detect unless the knee is slightly flexed.

Abnormal movements The knee joint is a hinge joint which depends entirely on muscles and ligaments for its stability. If the ligaments are ruptured or stretched then abnormal movement can occur. Thus by testing for abnormal movements such as abduction and adduction, and anteroposterior sliding of the tibia on the femur, you are really checking the **stability** of the knee and the **integrity of its ligaments**.

1 *Lateral ligaments* Let the leg rest extended on the couch. Place the fingers of your left hand under the knee joint and the butt of your hand firmly against the lateral aspect of the joint. Keep this hand firm and use it as a fulcrum to try to abduct the knee joint by pulling the ankle towards you with your right hand. There should be only the slightest movement in the joint. If it moves easily then the medial collateral ligament is ruptured. If you stay on the same side of the patient, the same action on the other leg will adduct the joint and test the lateral collateral ligament.

To test the ligaments on the other side of the joint, change your hands around so that your left hand lies on top of the joint with the fingers resting on the side of the joint. Pull this hand towards you and push the ankle away from you with the other hand.

An alternative method is to tuck the patient's leg under your arm and then, with your hands on each side of the knee joint to detect movement, move the tibia from side to side with your body.

2 *Cruciate ligaments* Remember, the **anterior** cruciate ligament stops the **tibia** sliding **anteriorly**. The **posterior** ligament stops the **tibia** sliding **posteriorly**.

Flex the knee to 30°. Grasp the upper end of the tibia with both hands and, by pushing and pulling, see if the tibia slides back and forth over the lower end of the femur. Compare it with the other side. There should be little or no movement.

Note. It is not necessary to sit on the patient's foot and crush his toes to death to perform this procedure, but it does help if the foot is fixed by the pressure of your buttock as you sit beside the leg, facing the patient's head, so that both of your arms are in front of you and in line with the leg.

Clicks

There are some special tests which make the joint click if there is a torn cartilage. Do not try these tests. They are difficult to perform and to interpret.

Normal joints sometimes click. If the patient is complaining of clicking, find out exactly when it occurs, if it is painful, and ask the patient to reproduce it for you, but do not indulge in excessive manipulation just to hear it.

Ask the patient to stand up and walk about

Observe the gait carefully.

EXAMINATION OF THE SPINE

Many pains that are felt in the front of the trunk and down the limbs are caused by disease of the spine. The general surgeon must always bear this in mind and make the examination of the spine part of his routine examination. The routine is the same as that for examining any other joint.

Inspection

1 Skin colour.
2 Scars and sinuses.
3 Shape of the back, bony contours and deformities.
4 Muscles of the back.

Palpation

1 Temperature of the skin.
2 The bony landmarks.
3 Tenderness.

Movements

1 Flexion.
2 Extension.
3 Lateral flexion.
4 Rotation.

These movements should be performed by the patient while standing upright. It is not practicable to perform passive movements of the spine.

Nerves

1 A full neurological examination.
2 Test for irritation of the roots of the sciatic nerve with the **straight-leg raising test**.
3 Palpate the **abdomen** and do a **rectal examination** to exclude intra-abdominal and pelvic lesions which might be affecting the spine or the spinal nerves.

DISEASES OF THE JOINTS

The main object of this chapter is to ensure that you can examine the muscles and the skeleton properly. The two common joint abnormalities that you will find are swelling and deformity.

Swelling of a joint must be caused by one or more of the following:

Bony enlargement.
Synovial thickening.
An effusion.

Revision Panel 4.2
Some causes of scoliosis and kyphosis

Scoliosis
Congenital
Idiopathic (? postural)
Poliomyelitis
Muscle dystrophies
Trauma

Kyphosis
Congenital
Tuberculosis
Ankylosing spondylitis
Osteoporosis
Secondary carcinoma

Deformity of a joint must be caused by one or more of:

- Skin contractures (e.g. scar following burns).
- Fascial contracture (e.g. Dupuytren's contracture).
- Muscle spasm or weakness.
- Tendon division or fixation.
- Capsule fibrosis.
- Bone deformity.

Detailed descriptions of the diseases affecting joints are to be found in orthopaedic textbooks. The following section describes the signs and symptoms of the four common diseases of joints.

Osteoarthritis

This condition can affect any joint. It is believed to be caused by prolonged wear and tear, and exacerbated by injury and any disturbance of the normal stresses and strains associated with the transference of weight across the joint. The common causative factors are therefore:

Age.
Previous fractures involving the articular cartilage.
Previous joint diseases.
Malalignment of the skeleton following trauma or bone disease.

The articular cartilage becomes thin and ultimately wears through. The bone at the edges of the cartilage hypertrophies, but the bone beneath the cartilage degenerates.

HISTORY

Age Most patients with osteoarthritis are over 50 years old, but secondary osteoarthritis following trauma or disease may begin in early adult life.

Symptoms The principal symptom is **pain**, which comes on gradually, but steadily increases until all movements of the joint are very painful. This is a very slow process.

Associated with the pain is an **increasing stiffness.** If the arthritis is secondary to an old injury the stiffness may precede the onset of the pain.

Weakness The stiffness and pain lead to disuse atrophy so the muscles controlling the joint become weak.

Deformity As the stiffness increases, the joint becomes fixed in a flexed and often an abducted or adducted position.

Limping Pain, stiffness, weakness and deformity of the joints in the lower limb interfere with walking.

Swelling The whole joint is swollen by the bony osteophytes, and the effusion. The synovium is not usually thickened.

EXAMINATION

Inspection

Colour The skin should *not* be reddened or discoloured.

Contour The joint is usually swollen.

Deformity The joint may be fixed in an abnormal position.

Relations Other joints in the same limb, and the same joint in the other limb, may be similarly diseased. Nearby muscles are wasted.

Palpation

Skin The skin temperature is **normal,** not hot.

Tenderness Pressure on the joint, especially if it is swollen, may cause pain, but local tenderness is uncommon except during an acute exacerbation when there is an effusion.

Synovium The synovium is not usually palpable.

Muscle bulk The bulk of the muscles that control the joint is reduced.

Bony contours The bone at the edge of the articular cartilage may feel irregular and protuberant.

Movements

All movements of the joint are painful at their extremes and some movements are reduced.

(Make sure that you see the limitation of movement by asking the patient to do active movements, before you perform passive movements.)

Not all movements of the joint will be equally affected. For example, early osteoarthritis of the hip may cause limitation of abduction and medial rotation long before it affects flexion, extension, adduction and lateral rotation.

Crepitus

The joint often crackles and clicks during movement. Although the patient can feel a grating sensation associated with the crepitus, it is not usually painful.

Abnormal movements

There should be no abnormal movements because all the ligaments should be intact.

Arteries and nerves in the limb

These structures should all be normal.

Other joints

Osteoarthritis is sometimes bilateral and symmetrical. The joints most often affected are the hip, knee, spine, and fingers.

GENERAL EXAMINATION

Osteoarthritis is not associated with any other generalized disease, so the rest of the examination should be normal. As many of the patients with osteoarthritis are old and fat they frequently have unrelated diseases – especially coronary, cerebral and peripheral artery disease.

The detection of these diseases is important because their existence may alter the management of the patient.

Rheumatoid arthritis

Rheumatoid arthritis is a generalized inflammatory joint disease. Its cause is unknown. The synovial membrane becomes thickened owing to hyperaemia and lymphocyte infiltration. There may be an effusion. As the disease progresses, the cartilage becomes damaged and eroded and eventually the joint is destroyed.

Near the joints there may be nodules, which consist of necrotic collagen surrounded by fibroblasts.

HISTORY

Age Rheumatoid arthritis may appear in patients of all ages, but the common time of onset is between the ages of 30 and 40 years.

Sex Women are affected three times more often than men.

Symptoms The main symptoms are **pain** and **swelling**, which usually begin together. The commonest first complaint is of swollen, stiff fingers.

Wasting As the disease progresses the joint movements are restricted and the muscles which control the joint waste away and become **weak**. As the joints of the upper limbs are often the first to become affected the patient complains that she keeps dropping things, and cannot carry her shopping basket.

General malaise The patient may feel ill, listless and lose weight. The muscles ache, especially after exercise, and tender, painful nodules appear around the joints.

Skin rashes The patient may complain of skin irritation and rashes, especially if the joint changes are part of another generalized disease such as Reiter's syndrome or systemic lupus erythematosus.

EXAMINATION

Inspection

The disease usually starts in the small joints at the end of the limbs – fingers, wrists, toes and ankles – before it moves to the larger joints of the limb and ultimately to the joints of the trunk. The manifestations of the disease in the hands are described on page 146.

Contour The joints are evenly enlarged. The finger joints become fusiform.

Colour The skin overlying the joint may be red and, if there is much swelling, shiny and taut.

Deformity As the disease advances it affects the ligaments and tendons around the joint as well as the articular surfaces, so causing a variety of **joint deformities**. For example, there is usually ulnar deviation at the wrist joint and hyperextension of the proximal interphalangeal joints.

Wasting The muscles which control the affected joints will be wasted.

Other joints Many joints are affected and the condition is frequently symmetrical.

Palpation

Temperature The skin over the joint is warm.

Tenderness In the acute stage of the disease the joint is tender to light palpation. As the disease becomes chronic the tenderness subsides but the pain during movement persists.

Synovium Soft-tissue thickening can be felt around the joint. It is only possible to be certain that this is thickened synovium in those joints where it has a clearly palpable edge beyond the joint line.

There may be an **effusion** in the joint.

Muscle bulk The muscles which control the joint feel thin and atrophic.

Bony contours Until the joint surfaces are destroyed and pathological dislocations occur, the general bony contour of the joint remains normal, but it is often obscured by the synovial thickening.

Movements

Active movements are limited by pain and reduced in power. Passive movements are limited by pain and fibrous contractures. Abnormal movements appear when the disease has weakened the ligaments, or tendons have ruptured.

Arteries and nerves in the limb

The other structures in the limb should be normal. Patients with long-standing rheumatoid arthritis sometimes get a peripheral arteritis which causes gangrene of the tips of the toes and fingers, and ulceration of the skin of the lower third of the leg. Swelling of the joints around the wrist may cause a carpal tunnel syndrome.

GENERAL EXAMINATION

Apart from other joint involvement there may be generalized wasting and anaemia. There are three systemic diseases associated with rheumatoid joint disease:

1 **Still's disease**: a disease in which children get arthritis, splenomegaly and lymphadenopathy.
2 **Reiter's syndrome**: urethritis, conjunctivitis, skin rashes and arthritis.
3 **Systemic lupus erythematosus**: a collagen disease in which there is a scaly red rash on the face, debility and manifestations in all tissues of a small vessel arteritis.

Psoriasis and rheumatoid arthritis often coexist. The connection between these two apparently very different diseases is not understood.

Tuberculous arthritis

Any joint can become infected with the human or bovine tubercle bacillus, but the hip, knee and vertebral column are the joints most often affected. The infection reaches the joint via the blood stream and produces its typical pathological changes in the synovium – giant cells, lymphocytes, infiltration and caseation. As the disease progresses the effusion in the joint becomes purulent and the articular cartilage and the bone are destroyed.

HISTORY

Age Tuberculous arthritis occurs in young adults and children. Mild symptoms may be present for many years before the patient complains or seeks advice.

Symptoms The usual joint symptoms of **pain** and **swelling** begin simultaneously, but in the hip or the spine where the swelling is not visible, **pain** is the presenting feature.

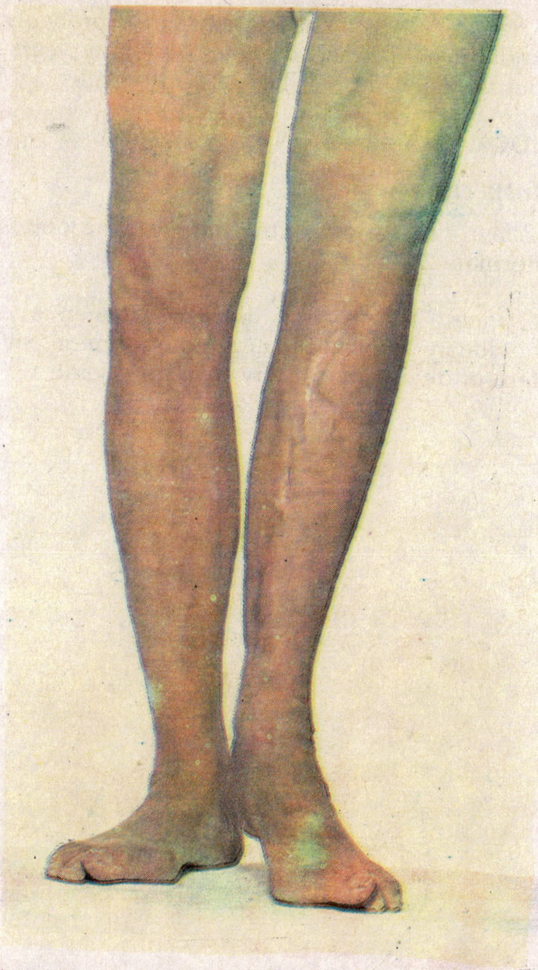

FIG. 4.24 The end-result of severe tuberculosis of the left knee joint: a fibrous ankylosis, shortening and wasting of the limb and healed sinuses

The pain **limits movement of the joint** and this usually interferes with walking, bending and stooping.

If an abscess forms in the joint it may point on the skin and then discharge. The resulting chronic sinus, with a seropurulent discharge, persists until the disease is cured or dies out.

General malaise and **loss of weight** are common symptoms.

Social history It is important to enquire about **social conditions**, such as diet and housing, and of the existence of any **family history** of tuberculosis.

LOCAL EXAMINATION

Inspection

Contour The joint (especially the knee) is diffusely swollen.

Colour The colour of the skin over the joint is normal.

Sinuses There may be a discharging sinus near the joint, or the scars of healed sinuses.

Muscle wasting There is usually **marked muscle wasting**, especially of the quadriceps femoris muscles when the knee joint is diseased.

Palpation

Skin The skin over the joint is *not* hot but the inflammatory hyperaemia in the underlying synovium may make the skin slightly warmer than normal.

Tenderness The joint is tender for a short period in the early acute phase of the disease, but, once the infection is established, the joint is not usually tender.

Synovium The swelling around the joint feels soft and pliable – something like **unbaked dough**. There is always an effusion in the joint.

Bony contour The bones are only deformed or destroyed in long-standing severe disease.

Movement

Movements are only limited if they cause pain. In these circumstances there is usually a pronounced protective muscle spasm.

There should be no abnormal movements.

When the disease has destroyed the joint it becomes fixed by a **fibrous ankylosis**.

GENERAL EXAMINATION

There may be tuberculosis elsewhere, in the lungs or the kidneys, so the general examination should be complete and thorough.

Neuropathic joints

(Charcot's joint)

The brain is unable to protect a joint which has lost its pain and position sense from harmful stresses and strains. The resulting frequent minor injuries ultimately destroy the bones and ligaments of the joint. A neuropathic joint is therefore a **painless, disorganized joint.** The possible causes of loss of joint sensation are:

- Diabetic neuropathy.
- Tabes dorsalis.
- Syringomyelia.
- Leprosy.
- Cauda equina lesions such as myelomeningocele.

Tabes dorsalis used to be the commonest cause of the Charcot joint in Great Britain, but now that untreated tertiary syphilis is rare the commonest cause is diabetes.

HISTORY

Age Neuropathic joints occur in middle and old age.

Symptoms The patient notices that the joint is becoming swollen and deformed, and gives way, but that it is **not painful**, except in the early stages of the disease when there may be a few pain fibres but no proprioceptive fibres functioning.

The mechanical weakness of the joint together with the sensory defects of the neuropathy make the patient's gait unstable.

Revision Panel 4.3

The causes of a disorganized, painless (Charcot) joint

- Diabetic neuropathy
- Tabes dorsalis
- Syringomyelia
- Leprosy
- Cauda equina lesions (e.g. myelomeningocele)

Previous illness The patient will probably know if he has had diabetes for many years, but may not know if he has had syphilis.

LOCAL EXAMINATION

Inspection

Colour The colour of the skin over the joint is normal.

Contour The joint is usually swollen and obviously deformed. There is no common pattern of deformity for any particular joint.

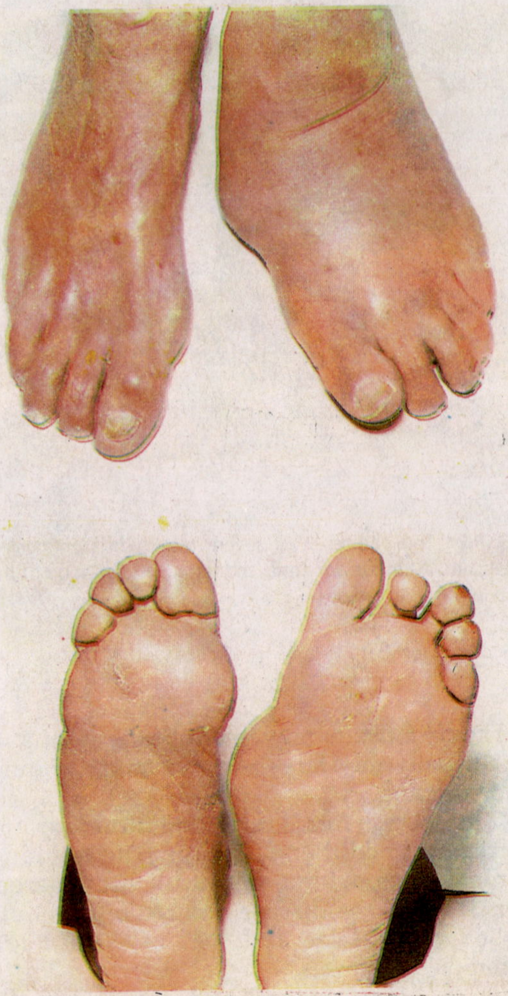

FIG. 4.25 A totally disorganized, but painless, left ankle and foot. This is a Charcot ankle and foot caused by diabetic peripheral neuropathy

Palpation

Tenderness The joint is *not* tender and movements in any direction do not usually cause pain.

Synovium The synovium is not thickened, but there is always an effusion.

Bony contours Displacement of the bony landmarks reveals that the bones are displaced or deformed. The normal shape of the bones forming the joint may completely disappear as a result of the combination of bone destruction in some areas and new bone formation and hypertrophy in others. There are two varieties of neuropathic joint: the hypertrophic and the atrophic.

The joint may be subluxed or dislocated.

Movement

The patient may be unable to perform normal movements because of the destruction of the joints and ligaments.

Some passive movements may be limited by the bony deformities, while grossly abnormal movements may be possible in other directions. It may be possible to dislocate the joint and then reduce it, and move it in a variety of abnormal ways without the patient feeling any pain or discomfort.

The knee and elbow joints may become so disorganized that the upper and lower parts of the limb flop about as if they were connected like a flail.

Nerves of the limb

Examine the nerves of the limb with great care. Vibration sense, position sense and deep pain sensitivity should all be reduced or absent. The motor innervation should be normal.

GENERAL EXAMINATION

Look for the signs of diabetes and syphilis. Take particular care to examine the whole of the nervous system and test the urine for sugar.

Ankylosis

An ankylosed joint is a fixed joint. If the bones that form the joint are fixed together by bone there is a **bony ankylosis**. If the bones are fixed by dense fibrous tissue there is a **fibrous ankylosis**.

A *bony ankylosis* is absolutely fixed and **painless** even when stressed.

A *fibrous ankylosis* moves a little and forced movement causes **pain**.

Semimembranosus bursa and Baker's cyst

The common forms of subcutaneous bursae are described in Chapter 3, pages 83–85.

The anatomically constant bursae around joints, usually between the joint and those tendons which cross it, do not enlarge very often. The one which gives most trouble is the bursa between the semimembranosus tendon and the posteromedial aspect of the femoral condyle.

This presents as a swelling behind the knee and is often confused with the other common swelling in this site, Baker's cyst.

Semimembranosus bursa

HISTORY

The common complaint is of a swelling behind the knee joint, that interferes with knee movements, particularly flexion.

The swelling grows slowly and does not usually cause pain.

EXAMINATION

The patient is usually a young or middle-aged adult.

The skin over the swelling is of normal colour and temperature.

The lump lies **above** the level of the joint line, slightly to the medial side of the popliteal fossa.

It is firm in consistence but clearly cystic because it fluctuates and often transilluminates. It may have a fluid thrill.

The swelling is in the popliteal fossa and covered only by skin.

Semimembranosus bursae often appear to empty into the knee joint with firm pressure, or during flexion of the knee joint, but this cannot occur because this bursa does not connect with the joint. The fluid is just moving

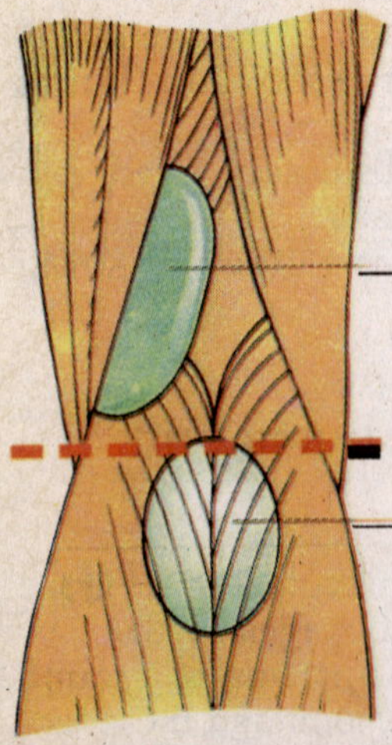

FIG. 4.26 A semimembranosus bursa appears above the joint line. A Baker's cyst appears below the joint line, deep to the gastrocnemius muscle

into the deeper recesses of the bursa between the tendons.

Lymph nodes The local lymph nodes should not be enlarged.

Adjacent structures The **knee joint** and other nearby tissues are **normal.**

Baker's cyst

Baker's cyst is a pulsion diverticulum of the knee joint, caused by chronic disease in the joint.

HISTORY

Previous illness The patient will usually give a history of chronic aches, pains and swelling of the knee joint, often known to be caused by osteoarthritis or rheumatoid arthritis.

The use of the knee is already limited when the patient notices a swelling behind the knee which further interferes with knee flexion. The swelling itself is not painful. It often fluctuates in size. The patient may have arthritis in other joints.

EXAMINATION

Baker's cyst appears in elderly patients with long-standing osteoarthritis or in younger patients with rheumatoid arthritis.

The skin over the cyst is usually a normal colour but may be a little red and warm if the arthritis in the knee joint is active.

The lump is **below** the level of the knee joint and deep to the gastrocnemius muscle. This is because the diverticulum which becomes the cyst is a blow-out through the posterior aspect of the capsule of the knee joint which is covered by the gastrocnemei as they come down from their origin on the back of the femur.

Some of the cyst may bulge out between the heads of the gastrocnemei.

The swelling is soft and fluctuant but will not usually transilluminate because of the density of the muscles which cover it. It is dull to percussion and **often reduces into the joint**. The fact that the cyst fluid is moving into the joint can sometimes be seen from the swelling which appears at each side of the patella as the cyst is compressed.

The knee joint shows evidence of arthritis – limited movements, crepitus and often an effusion.

Sometimes these cysts rupture and cause pain and swelling in the calf, this is usually misdiagnosed as a deep vein thrombosis.

Differential diagnosis It is usually easy to differentiate between Baker's cyst and semimembranosus bursa (see Fig. 4.26).

Remember the other common cause of a swelling behind the knee joint – a popliteal aneurysm. This is easy to diagnose if it has an expansile pulsation, but easy to confuse with one of the above swellings if it is thrombosed. Remember to feel the pulses at the ankle and to palpate the other leg – popliteal aneurysms are often bilateral.

Conditions peculiar to the hands

5

The hand is man's great physical asset and, anatomically, one of his most distinctive features. It has enabled him to use the tools that his brain has invented, and is indispensible to his well-being. **Everything that the doctor does to the hand should be aimed at restoring or maintaining its function.**

When you examine the hand there are four systems to assess: the muscles, bones and joints; the circulation; the nerves; and the skin and connective tissues. The general examination of these systems is described in other chapters, but the important points are repeated here and assembled into a system of examination designed to ensure that you do not miss any important abnormalities.

A PLAN FOR THE EXAMINATION OF THE HAND

Examine each system in turn.

1 The musculoskeletal system (bones, joints, muscles and tendons)

INSPECTION

Look for any abnormality of the shape, size and contour of the hand. Look for local discolouration, scars and sinuses. Look for **muscle wasting** by assessing the size of the thenar and hypothenar eminences and the bulk of the muscles between the metacarpal bones (the interossei). Look at the wrist joint.

PALPATION

Feel the bony contours, the tender areas, and any localized swellings. Feel the finger joints to assess the cause of any swelling of these joints.

MOVEMENT

Check the range and ease of movement of all the joints:

The carpometacarpal joint of the thumb (flexion, extension, abduction, adduction and opposition).
The metacarpophalangeal joints of the fingers (flexion, extension, abduction and adduction).
The interphalangeal joints (flexion and extension).

Inability to move these joints may be caused by joint disease, soft-tissue thickening, divided tendons or paralysed muscles.

2 The circulation

INSPECTION

Pallor of the fingers indicates arterial insufficiency or anaemia. During an episode of vasospasm the fingers may be white or blue. Observe the degree of filling of the veins on the back of the hands. Ischaemic atrophy of the pulps of the fingers makes the fingers thin and pointed. Ischaemic **ulcers**, small **abscesses** and even frank **gangrene** may be visible.

PALPATION

Feel the **temperature** of the skin of each finger.

Feel **both pulses** (radial and ulnar) at the wrist. Sometimes the digital arteries can be felt on either side of the base of the fingers.

Capillary return A crude indication of the arterial inflow to the fingers can be obtained from watching the rate of filling of the vessels beneath the nail, after emptying them by pressing down on the tip of the nail.

Allen's test Ask the patient to clench his fist tightly and then compress the ulnar and radial arteries at the wrist with your thumbs. After 10 seconds, ask the patient to open his hand. The palm will be white. Release the compression on the radial artery and watch the blood flow into the hand.

Slow flow into one finger caused by a digital artery occlusion will be apparent from the rate at which that finger turns pink.

Repeat the procedure but release the pressure on the ulnar artery first.

AUSCULTATION

Listen with the bell of your stethoscope over any abnormal areas. Vascular tumours and arteriovenous fistulae may produce a bruit, sometimes a palpable thrill.

Measure the blood pressure in both arms.

3 The nerves

SENSATION

When there is loss of sensation you must find out which type of sensation is lost (e.g. light touch, pain, position sense, vibration sense), as described in Chapter 1, and the distribution of the sensory loss. Does it correspond to the innervation of one nerve or to a dermatome? The areas of skin innervated by the three nerves of the hand are:

Median nerve The median nerve innervates the palmar aspect of the thumb, index and middle fingers, the dorsal aspect of the distal phalanx and half of the middle phalanx of the same fingers, and a variable amount of the radial side of the palm of the hand.

Ulnar nerve The ulnar nerve innervates the skin on the anterior and posterior surfaces of the little finger and the ulnar side of the ring finger, the skin over the hypothenar eminence, and a similar strip of skin posteriorly. The ulnar nerve sometimes innervates all of the skin of the ring finger and the ulnar side of the middle finger.

Radial nerve This innervates a small area of skin over the lateral aspect of the first metacarpal and the back of the first web space.

The dermatomes of the hand are:

C_6 – thumb
C_7 – middle finger
C_8 – little finger.

MOTOR NERVES

The muscles that control the movements of the hand lie within the hand and in the forearm (i.e. they are intrinsic and extrinsic). All the long flexors and extensors of the fingers lie in the forearm and the nerves that innervate them leave their parent nerves at or above the elbow.

The nerves that innervate the intrinsic muscles have a long course in the forearm before they reach the hand. Thus it is necessary to examine all the motor functions of the three principal nerves in the upper limb (median, ulnar and radial) if you wish to find the level at which a nerve is damaged. A rapid assessment of the motor function of these three nerves in the hand can be obtained by looking for the following physical signs.

A **median nerve palsy** causes:

- Wasting of the thenar eminence.
- Absence of flexion of the terminal interphalangeal joint of the **index** finger.
- Absent abduction of the thumb.
- Absent opposition of the thumb.

An **ulnar nerve palsy** causes:

- Wasting of the hypothenar eminence and hollows between the metacarpals.
- Absence of flexion of the **little and ring fingers.**
- Absence of adduction and abduction of the fingers.

DISTRIBUTION OF THE NERVES OF THE UPPER LIMB

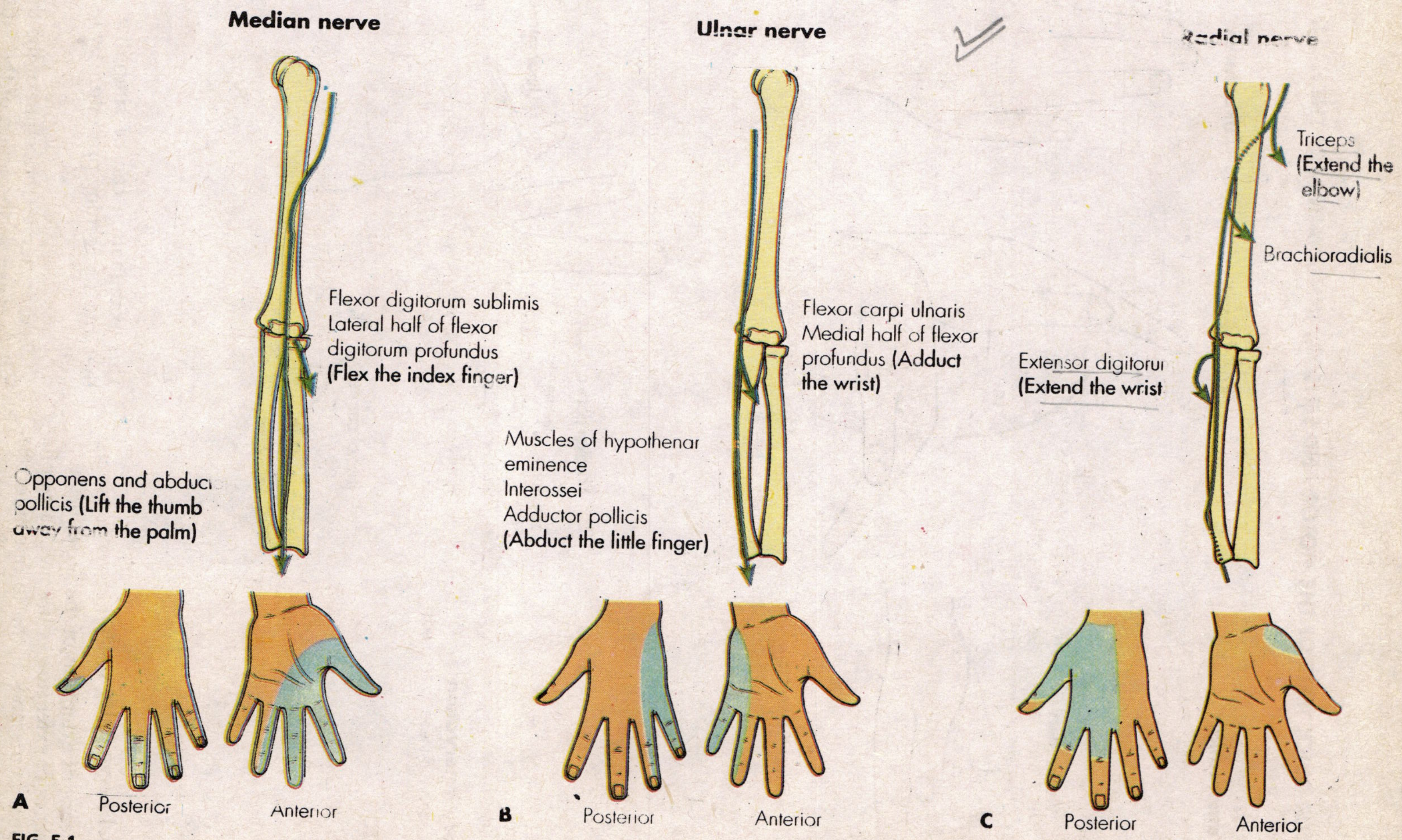

FIG. 5.1

FOUR QUICK TESTS OF THE MOTOR AND SENSORY INNERVATION OF THE HAND

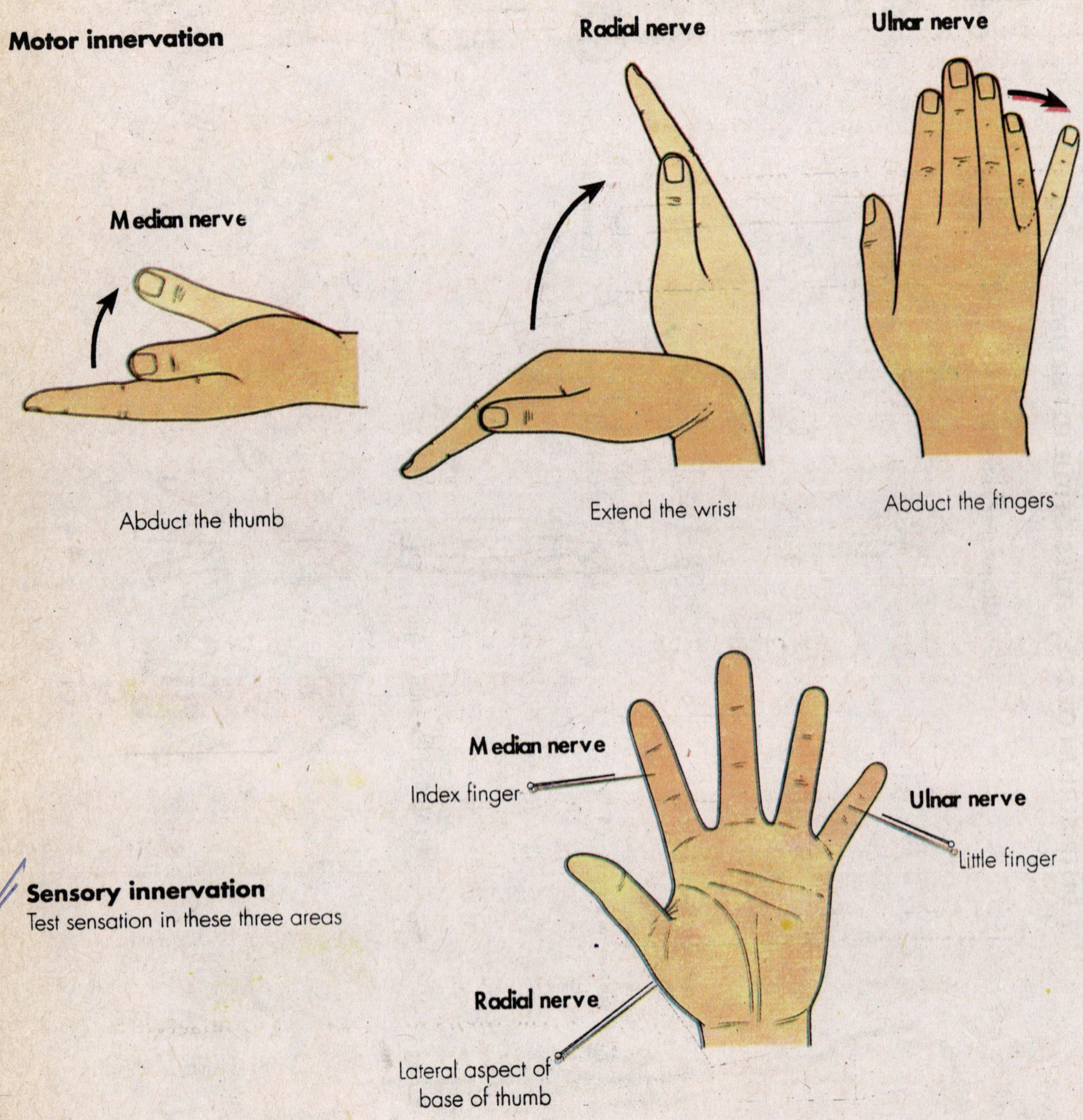

FIG. 5.2

A **radial nerve** palsy causes:

Absence of extension of the **wrist**.
Absence of extension of the metacarpophalangeal joints and of the thumb interphalangeal joint.

This examination can be simplified still further into a screening procedure by using three tests:

1 Median nerve: abduction of the thumb.
2 Ulnar nerve: abduction of the little finger.

3 Radial nerve: extension of the fingers at the metacarpophalangeal joint.

As you perform each of these tests feel the muscle you are testing to check whether or not it is contracting.

4 The skin and connective tissues

Much will have been learnt about the skin after studying its circulation and innervation. It is important to palpate the palmar fascia, as thickening and contraction of this structure is a common cause of contraction deformities (Dupuytren's contracture).

5 Wrist, elbow, shoulder, thoracic outlet, neck

Examine the wrist, elbow, shoulder, thoracic outlet and neck because abnormalities at these sites can cause symptoms in the hand.

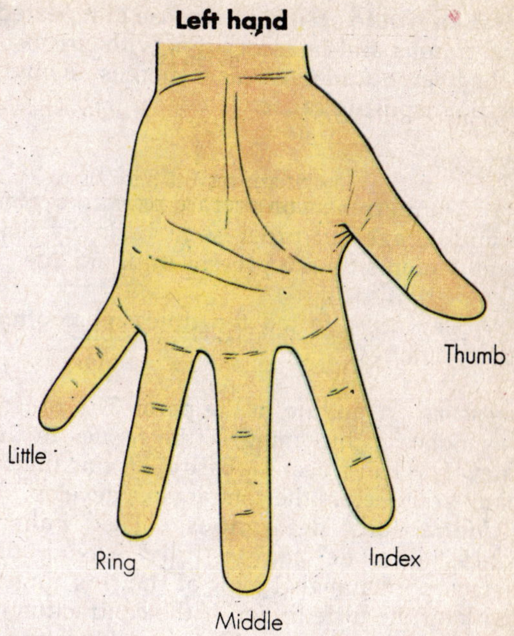

FIG. 5.3 The names of the digits of the hand

RECORDING DATA ABOUT THE HAND

Almost every issue of the Medical Insurance Societies' publications contains references to errors that have arisen because of inadequate or misleading records of lesions in the hand.

Never forget to state which hand you are describing. Write the words in full, RIGHT or LEFT; a bad R can easily be confused with an L.

Name the digits

Some people prefer to number rather than name the digits, the **first digit** being the thumb, the **second digit** the index finger and so on. But unless you remember to write the word 'digit' every time you will eventually make a mistake because the first finger, which is the index finger, is the second digit. **Do not use this system; always use names: thumb, index, middle, ring and little finger.**

It is acceptable to number the toes, as the first toe is the **great toe**.

ABNORMALITIES AND LESIONS OF THE HAND

Congenital abnormalities

There are three common skeletal abnormalities in the hand:

1 Part of the hand (usually a digit) may be absent.
2 There may be an extra digit.
3 The digits may be fused (syndactyly).

All these abnormalities are rare, but immediately recognizable.

Dupuytren's contracture

This is a thickening and shortening of the palmar fascia and the adjacent connective tissues that lie deep to the subcutaneous tissue of the hand and superficial to the flexor tendons. The cause of this change in the fascia is not known. As the thickening increases it becomes attached to the skin of the palm.

It is known to occur in response to repeated local trauma and in association with cirrhosis of the liver, but in most cases there is no obvious predisposing cause.

HISTORY

Age Dupuytren's contracture usually begins in middle age but progresses so slowly that many patients do not present until old age.

Sex Men are affected ten times more often than women.

Symptoms **A nodule in the palm.** The patient may notice a thickening in the tissues in the palm of his hand, near the base of his ring finger, many years before the contractures develop.

Contraction deformities. The patient notices that he cannot fully extend the metacarpophalangeal joint of the ring finger, and later the little finger. If the contraction of the palmar fascia becomes severe the finger can be pulled so far down into the palm of the hand that it becomes useless.

There is **no pain** associated with this condition. Very rarely, the nodule in the palm may be slightly tender.

Development The nodule gradually enlarges and the strands of contracting fascia become prominent. Deep creases form where the skin becomes tethered to the fascial thickening, and the skin in these creases may get soggy and excoriated. The deformity of the fingers slowly worsens.

Multiplicity Dupuytren's contracture is commonly bilateral and can also occur in the feet.

Revision Panel 5.1

Factors associated with Dupuytren's contracture

- Alcoholism
- Epilepsy
- Diabetes
- Repeated trauma
- Family history

Cause Dupuytren's contracture may follow repeated trauma to the palm of the hand because it used to be found in shoe repairers and other manual workers, but nowadays it is uncommon to find a convincing cause.

Systemic disease There may be symptoms of epilepsy or cirrhosis of the liver, because there is a higher incidence of the condition in patients suffering from these diseases. The reasons for these associations are unexplained.

Family history Dupuytren's contracture can be familial. If so, it is inherited in an autosomal dominant manner.

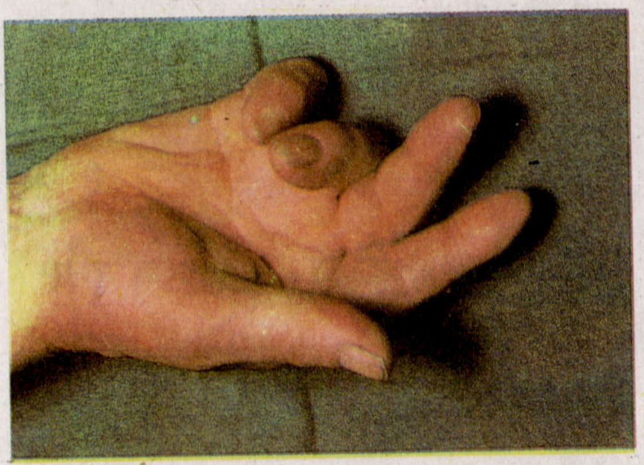

The anterior view shows the typical deformity: flexion of the metacarpophalangeal and proximal interphalangeal joints and extension of the distal interphalangeal joints.

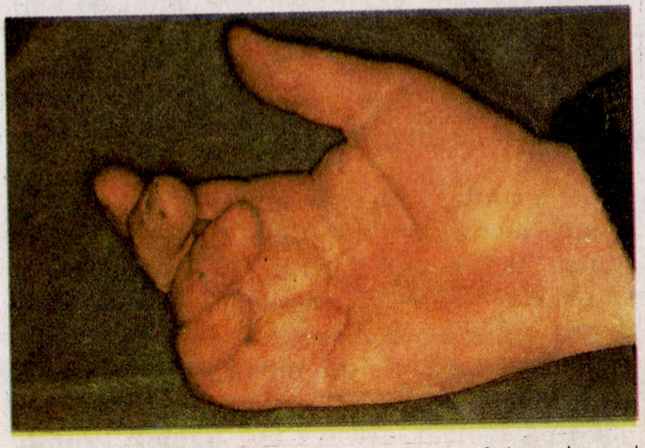

This view shows the puckering of the skin of the palm and the taut strands of palmar fascia

FIG. 5.4 DUPUYTREN'S CONTRACTURE

EXAMINATION

The palm of the hand Palpation of the palm of the hand reveals a firm, irregular-shaped nodule with indistinct edges, 1–2 cm proximal to the base of the ring finger. Taut strands can be felt running from the nodule to the sides of the base of the ring and little fingers, and proximally towards the centre of the flexor retinaculum. These bands get tighter if you try to extend the fingers.

The skin is puckered and creased, and tethered to the underlying nodule.

The deformity The metacarpophalangeal joint and the proximal interphalangeal joint are flexed because the palmar fascia is attached to both sides of the proximal and middle phalanges. The distal interphalangeal joint tends to extend. The ring finger is most affected and may be pulled down so far that its nail digs into the palm of the hand.

The flexion deformity is not lessened by flexing the wrist joint.

Local tissues The rest of the hand is normal. There may be some thickening of the subcutaneous tissue on the back of the proximal phalanges of the affected fingers, sometimes called **Garrod's pads**.

GENERAL EXAMINATION

Dupuytren's contracture is sometimes associated with epilepsy and cirrhosis of the liver. There may be systemic evidence of these diseases. These are *rare* associations.

The condition may be present in the feet.

Congenital contracture of the little finger

This is a congenital deformity of the little finger. The patient is rarely aware of the fact that he has a deformity, accepting it as the normal shape of his little finger.

It is mentioned here because, although it is the opposite deformity to a Dupuytren's contracture, the student who is unaware of its existence may misdiagnose it.

Pick up a tea cup with your thumb and index finger and hook your little finger in the manner of the affected snob at a tea party. You will find that you have extended your metacarpophalangeal joint and flexed both of the interphalangeal joints. Someone with a congenital contracture of the little finger has this deformity all the time and cannot straighten the finger.

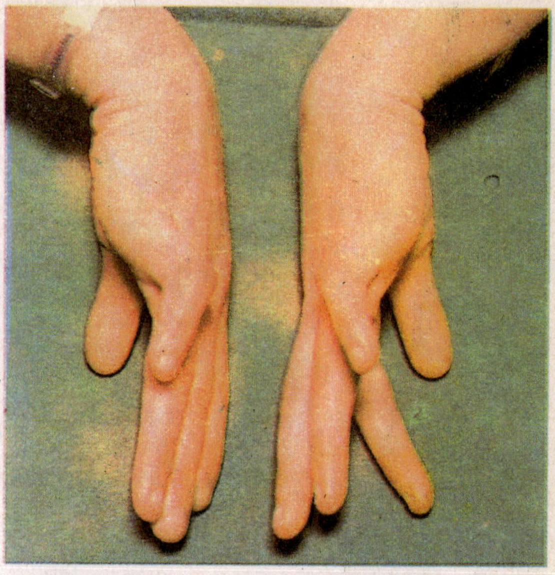

FIG. 5.5 Congenital contracture of the little finger. Extension of the metacarpophalangeal joint and flexion of the proximal interphalangeal joint

Volkmann's ischaemic contracture

Volkmann's ischaemic contracture is a shortening of the long flexor muscles of the forearm, caused by fibrosis of the muscles, secondary to ischaemia. The common causes of the ischaemia are direct arterial damage at the time of a fracture near the elbow (most often a supracondylar fracture), a tight plaster which restricts blood flow, and arterial embolism.

HISTORY

Age Supracondylar fractures are common in children and young adults, so Volkmann's contracture most often begins between the ages of 5 and 25.

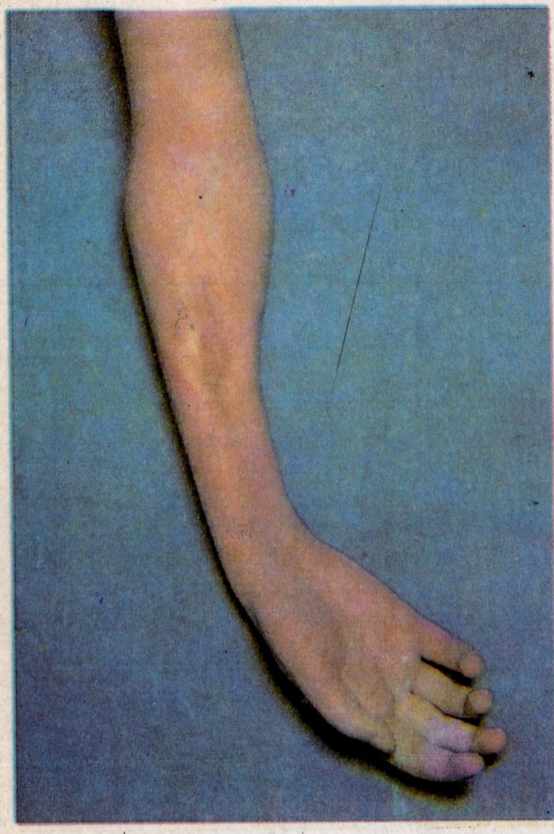

FIG. 5.6 Volkmann's ischaemic contracture. Wasting, fibrosis and contraction of the muscles of the forearm, following ischaemic damage, causing flexion and ulnar deviation of the wrist joint and flexion of all the finger joints. Further contraction will turn this into a permanently clawed hand

Cause The patient usually knows the cause of the deformity because he can clearly relate the loss of finger extension to his injury. Indeed the loss of finger movements frequently begins while the arm is immobilized for the treatment of the fracture.

Symptoms When muscles become ischaemic they are usually **painful**. If a patient complains of pain under his plaster at a point distant from the site of the fracture, remove the plaster and examine the muscles carefully.

Movements of the fingers, especially extension, become **painful and then limited**. This is more noticeable if there is no restriction of movement caused by a coexisting fracture. If the forearm is not in a plaster cast the patient soon discovers that he can extend his fingers if he flexes his wrist.

If the blood supply of the hand is also diminished, the skin of the hand will be **cold and pale**.

Ischaemia of the nerves in the anterior compartment (the median and anterior interosseous nerves) often causes 'pins and needles' (**paraesthesia**) in the distribution of the median nerve, and sometimes the severe burning pain of ischaemic neuritis.

Development As the acute phase passes, the pain slowly fades away but the restriction of finger extension increases and the hand becomes claw-like. The patient may present with a fully developed deformity.

EXAMINATION

Inspection The skin of the hand is usually **pale** and the hand looks **wasted**. All the finger joints are flexed and the anterior aspect of the forearm is thin and wasted. The deformity is called 'a claw hand'.

Palpation In the acute phase the forearm is swollen and tense, but once this has passed the forearm feels thin, the hand is cool and the pulses at the wrist may be absent. In the later stages the fibrosis and shortening make the forearm muscles hard and taut.

Movement **Extension of the fingers is limited but improves as the wrist is flexed**. This is an important sign as it differentiates Volkmann's ischaemic contracture from Dupuytren's contracture. Further flexion of the fingers (beyond the deformity) is present but the grip is weak. All other hand movements are present but may be difficult to perform with the fingers fixed in an acutely flexed position.

Passive forced extension of the fingers is painful in the acute stage and uncomfortable in the established condition. An important diagnostic feature of ischaemic contracture is that all the muscles, even the damaged ones, have some function, whereas when a claw hand is caused by a nerve lesion some of the muscles will be completely paralysed.

State of local tissues The abnormalities in the arteries and nerves of the forearm and hand have already been described. If the contracture follows a fracture, the vessels and nerves above the level of the fracture should be normal.

The heart, great vessels, subclavian and axillary arteries must be examined carefully in case they are the source of an arterial embolus.

Palpate the supraclavicular fossa for a cervical rib or subclavian artery aneurysm.

Carpal tunnel syndrome

This is a condition in which the median nerve is compressed as it passes through the carpal tunnel – the space between the carpal bones and the flexor retinaculum. The compression can be caused by skeletal abnormalities, swelling of other tissues within the tunnel, or thickening of the retinaculum. It is often associated with pregnancy, rheumatoid arthritis, diabetes, myxoedema, previous trauma and osteoarthritis.

HISTORY

Age and sex Carpal tunnel syndrome is common in middle-aged women – especially at the menopause.

Local symptoms **Pins and needles in the fingers**, principally the index and middle fingers, is the common presenting symptom. Sometimes the thumb is involved.

Theoretically the little finger should never be affected as it is innervated by the ulnar nerve, but occasionally patients complain that the whole of their hand tingles.

Pain in the forearm. For some (so far unexplained) reason the patient often complains of a pain which radiates from the wrist up along the medial side of the forearm. This is usually an aching pain, not 'pins and needles'.

Loss of function. As the compression increases, the axons in the nerve are killed and objective signs of **nerve damage** appear. Because the sensitivity of the skin supplied by the median nerve is reduced, the patient notices that she drops small articles and cannot do delicate movements. Note that this is *not* caused by a loss of muscle power, but the loss of fine discriminatory sensation. Ultimately, if the nerve damage is severe, there maybe a **loss of motor function** which presents as weakness and paralysis of the muscles of the thenar eminence and the first two lumbricals.

Exacerbations at night. Patients are often woken in the middle of the night by their symptoms. This feature is difficult to explain but is so characteristic that it is considered to be pathognomonic of the condition.

General symptoms An **increase of weight** commonly exacerbates carpal tunnel syndrome symptoms. A change in weight may be secondary to another disease such as myxoedema, diabetes or steroid therapy, or a physiological water retention as in pregnancy.

If the condition is secondary to rheumatoid arthritis or osteoarthritis the patient may have symptoms of arthritis in the wrist and other joints.

EXAMINATION

Inspection The hand usually looks quite normal except in the advanced case where there may be visible wasting of the muscles forming the thenar eminence.

Palpation Pressure on the flexor retinaculum does not produce the symptoms in the hand, but holding the wrist fully flexed for 1 or 2 minutes may induce symptoms. Light touch sensitivity and two-point discrimination may be reduced in the skin innervated by the median nerve (palm, thumb, index and middle finger). The loss of muscle bulk in the thenar eminence may be easier to feel when these muscles are contracting.

The wrist pulses and the colour and temperature of the skin should be normal.

Movement All movements of the joints of the hand, active and passive, should be present. Abduction, adduction and opposition of the thumb may be weak but the muscles that cause these movements are rarely completely paralysed.

GENERAL EXAMINATION

There are two important aspects of the general examination.

First, you must **exclude other causes of paraesthesia in the hand**, such as cervical spondylosis, cervical rib, peripheral neuritis, and rare neurological disease. This requires a detailed examination of the head, neck and arm.

Second, you must look for evidence of the cause of the carpal tunnel syndrome, such as pregnancy, rheumatoid arthritis, osteoarthritis and myxoedema.

Claw hand

Claw hand is a deformity in which all the fingers are permanently flexed. Although an ulnar nerve paralysis makes the hand claw-like, because it causes flexion of the ring and little fingers, it does not cause a true claw hand, because only part of the hand is involved.

The causes of claw hand are neurological and musculoskeletal.

NEUROLOGICAL CAUSES

Remember these causes by thinking of the course of the nerve fibres from the spinal cord through the brachial plexus into the peripheral nerves. Although the claw hand deformity caused by a neurological abnormality is caused by loss of motor function, there is often an associated sensory loss.

Revision Panel 5.2

The causes of claw hand (*main en griffe*)

Combined ulnar and median nerve palsy

Volkmann's ischaemic contracture

Advanced rheumatoid arthritis

Brachial plexus lesion (medial cord)

Spinal cord lesions
- Syringomyelia
- Poliomyelitis
- Amyotrophic lateral sclerosis

Spinal cord Poliomyelitis, syringomyelia, amyotrophic lateral sclerosis.

Brachial plexus Trauma to medial roots and cord – especially birth injuries to the lower cord as in Klumpke's paralysis. Infiltration of the brachial plexus by malignant disease.

Peripheral nerves Traumatic division of the median and ulnar nerves. Peripheral neuritis.

MUSCULOSKELETAL CAUSES

Volkmann's ischaemic contracture This only causes a claw hand at rest as the deformity can be reduced or abolished by flexion of the wrist.

Joint disease Asymmetrical muscle tension, bone and joint deformities and subluxation of the finger joints caused by rheumatoid arthritis may produce a claw-like hand.

Trigger finger

This is a condition in which a finger gets locked in full flexion and will only extend after excessive voluntary effort, or with help from the other hand. When extension begins, it does so suddenly and with a click – hence the name trigger finger. The condition is caused by a thickening of the flexor tendon, paratenon, or a narrowing of the flexor sheath, preventing movement of the tendon within the flexor sheath.

HISTORY

Age and sex There are two groups of patients affected by this condition – middle-aged women and very young children. The thumb can be affected in neonates and infants but this is a rare condition.

Symptoms The patient complains that the finger clicks and jumps as it moves, or gets stuck in a flexed position.

A trigger finger is not usually a painful condition, even when force is required to extend the finger.

The disability gradually gets more severe but a fixed, immovable flexed finger is uncommon.

Cause Occasionally the patient can recall an injury to the palm of the hand which may have caused the tendon or tendon sheath to thicken, but in most cases there is no indication of the cause.

EXAMINATION

Inspection The patient will show you how the finger gets stuck and how it snaps out into extension. The finger looks quite normal.

Palpation and movement The thickening of the tendon or tendon sheath can be felt at the level of the head of the metacarpal bone. During movement the thickening can be felt snapping in and out of the tendon sheath.

GENERAL EXAMINATION

Trigger finger is not associated with any systemic musculoskeletal disease.

Mallet finger

This is a fixed flexion deformity of the distal interphalangeal joint of a finger, caused by an interruption of the extensor mechanism: either a rupture of the extensor tendon or an avulsion fracture of its insertion. It is also known as 'baseball' finger because the commonest cause of the injury is a blow on the tip of the finger by a ball or hard object which forcibly flexes it against the pull of the extensor tendon, which then ruptures or pulls off the bone.

HISTORY

The patient usually remembers the original injury but may not come and complain immediately if the finger is not painful. He may not complain until the deformity is established and a nuisance.

Symptoms The inability to extend the tip of a finger is not a great disability, but to a person with an occupation that requires fine finger movements, including full extension of the distal interphalangeal joints, the deformity can be a serious handicap. Some patients complain that the deformity is disfiguring.

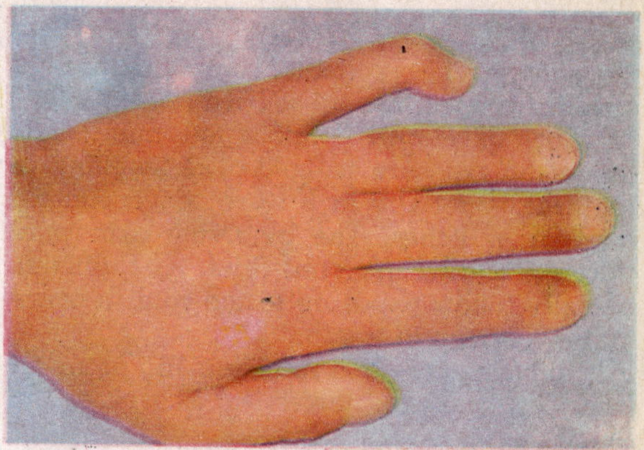

FIG. 5.7 A mallet finger. The patient's inability to extend the terminal phalanx of the little finger is only noticeable when he holds his fingers out straight

EXAMINATION

When the patient holds out his hand, with his fingers extended, the distal phalanx of the affected finger remains 15–20° flexed. If you flex the distal interphalangeal joint to 90° the patient can extend it back to the 20° position but cannot get it straight.

An x-ray is required to decide whether the tendon is ruptured or avulsed.

Chilblains

(Erythema pernio)

A chilblain is an area of oedema in the skin and subcutaneous tissues that follows a local change in capillary permeability induced by cold. Chilblains are by far the most common of that group of conditions known as **cold sensitivity states**. In addition to the oedema, there is vasospasm and interstitial infiltration with lymphocytes.

HISTORY

Age Chilblains first appear in childhood or early adult life.

Sex Woman are affected more often than men.

Occupation An outdoor occupation increases the chances of a susceptible subject getting chilblains.

Symptoms The patient complains of a **swelling** on the side or back of a finger (or toe) that has developed within a few minutes or hours of exposure to cold. The swelling is **painful**, especially in a warm environment, and often **itches**. The overlying skin may ulcerate and weep serous fluid. As chilblains usually follow exposure to the cold they are more common **in winter**.

Chilblains are often **multiple** and occur on the toes, heels and lower leg, as well as the hands.

Development Chilblains first appear in childhood and adolescence and then appear regularly every winter until the patient reaches middle age. After the susceptibility to chilblains subsides most patients continue to have some cold sensitivity problems in the hands, such as Raynaud's phenomenon (see below).

Family history The tendency to get chilblains is often familial.

EXAMINATION

Position Chilblains usually occur on the backs and sides of the fingers.

Colour At first the skin over the swelling is pale but it quickly turns a reddish-blue colour.

Temperature The temperature of the skin over the swelling is normal or slightly cooler than normal.

Shape and size The lumps on the fingers are flattened, elongated mounds, with indistinct edges that fade away into the normal finger. They vary in size. On the fingers they are usually 0.5–2 cm wide but on the legs they can be 4–5 cm across.

Surface The oedema involves the skin and subcutaneous tissues and often collects in an intradermal blister which can burst and leave a superficial ulcer. If the acute superficial ulcer fails to heal it may become deeper, destroying the full thickness of the skin and leaving a permanent scar.

Composition Although the lump is mainly oedema fluid there is often sufficient cellular infiltration to make it feel firm and sometimes hard.

Lymph nodes The axillary or inguinal lymph nodes will not be enlarged unless the chilblain is infected – a rare event.

Local tissues There may be evidence of long-standing arterial insufficiency – absent wrist pulses, a positive Allen's test (see page 132), loss of the finger pulps, recurrent paronychia and scars from previous chilblains. The nerves of the hands should be normal.

GENERAL EXAMINATION

The other extremities may be cold and show Raynaud's phenomenon or acrocyanosis.

Raynaud's phenomenon

The symptoms and signs which are commonly called Raynaud's phenomenon are a series of colour changes in the hands following exposure to cold.

To remember the order of the colour changes remember the initials WBC (the same as 'white blood count'): white, blue and crimson (red).

White The skin of one, or a number, of the fingers turns white.

Blue After a variable time, the skin turns a purple-bluish colour but is still cold and numb.

Red When the vasospasm relaxes, the skin turns red and hot and feels flushed, tingling and often painful.

One or two of these phases may be absent. The fingers may go white and then turn red, or return to normal after the blue phase, or just turn blue.

The orthodox explanation of these changes is as follows.

The **white** phase is caused by severe arteriolar spasm, making the tissues bloodless.

The **blue** phase is produced by a very slow trickle of deoxygenated blood through dilated capillaries. Venous congestion may also be caused by persistent venous spasm.

The red phase is the period of high blood flow (reactive hyperaemia) that follows relaxation of the arteriolar spasm. The increased blood flow through the dilated vessels makes the skin red, hot and painful.

There are many causes of Raynaud's phenomenon. These are described in Chapter 7, because Raynaud's phenomenon is not a condition peculiar to the hands alone, although they are invariably affected. It can also occur in the feet, ears, nose and lips.

In between attacks the tissues look quite normal. Ultimately the arteries suffer permanent structural damage which causes permanent tissue damage.

Scleroderma

Scleroderma is an uncommon disease in which the skin and subcutaneous tissues become thickened and stiff. Although it is a systemic disease affecting the bowel, especially the oesophagus and colon, as well as the skin, it often appears in the hands many years before it develops in other sites. Structural changes in the hands may be preceded for many years by Raynaud's phenomenon. The aetiology of the disease is unknown. The principal abnormality is found in the collagen fibrils which are thick and stiff.

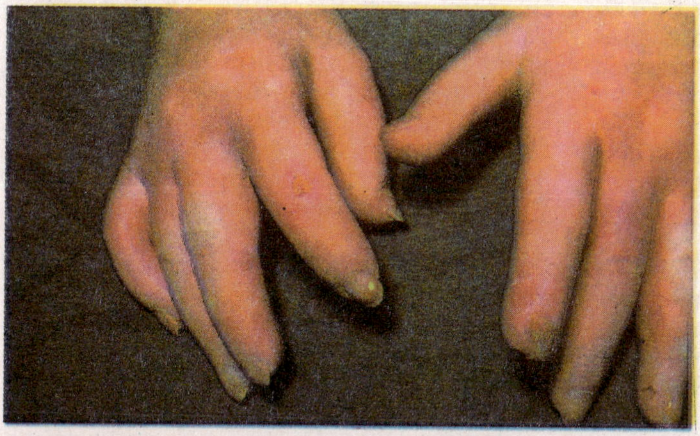

Thick stiff fingers with pale, waxy, thick skin

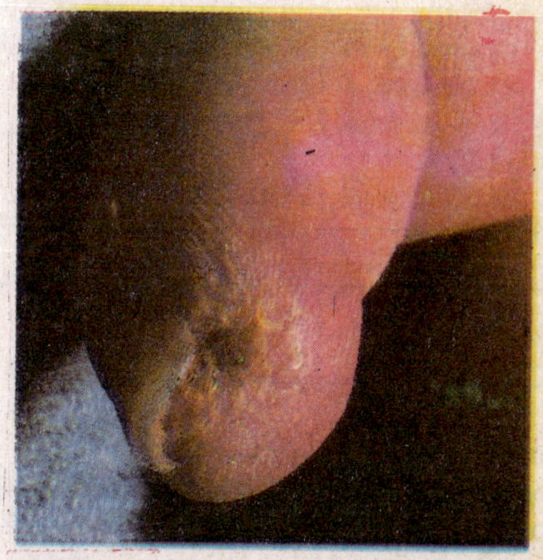

An ischaemic ulcer on the finger tip. These slowly destroy the pulp of the finger and make it pointed

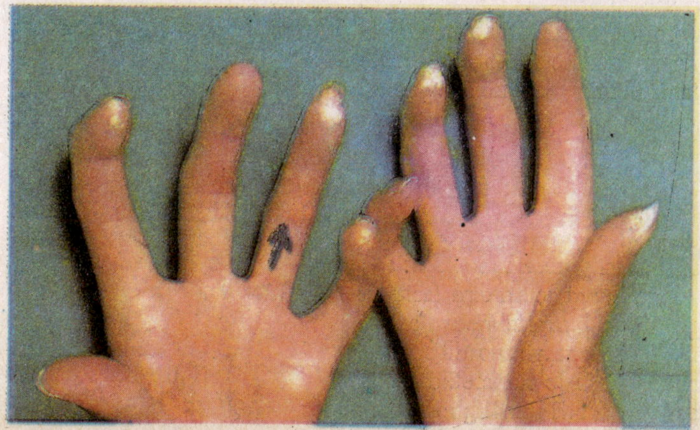

Calcinosis in the pulps of the fingers of a patient with the CREST syndrome

FIG. 5.8 THE EFFECT ON THE HANDS OF SCLERODERMA

HISTORY

Age Scleroderma commonly begins in the late 30s, but may not become severe for many years.

Sex Females are more often affected than males.

Symptoms There is **thickening of the fingers.** The patient notices that the skin of her fingers is slowly becoming pale and thick, and the movements of the interphalangeal joints are reduced.

Many patients present with the colour changes of **Raynaud's phenomenon** years before the skin changes begin.

Painful splits and ulcers appear in the skin of the finger tips.

Some patients get **multiple, recurrent small abscesses around the nails;** these abscesses throb and ache and finally discharge a small bead of pus.

Development Although the symptoms may begin in one hand or even one finger, they gradually spread to involve all the digits of both hands.

Systemic effects If the disease affects the oesophagus the patient will complain of **dysphagia**. Involvement of the colon causes **constipation** and **colicky abdominal pain.**

LOCAL EXAMINATION

Colour The skin of the hands has a white, waxy appearance caused by the combination of ischaemia and skin thickening.

Temperature The hands are cool, especially at the finger tips.

Shape and size The hands and fingers look swollen and the skin **thickened**, but the pulps of the finger tips may be **wasted**. There are often small scars on either side of the finger nails, and on the pulps, where previous abscesses have pointed and discharged.

Nodules There may be small, hard subcutaneous nodules in the finger pulps and on the dorsal aspect of the hands and fingers. These are patches of calcified fat. This abnormality is called **calcinosis**.

Pulses The pulses at the wrist are usually palpable, but Allen's test often reveals occlusions of the digital arteries.

Nerves The nerve supply of the hand is normal.

Joints The thick skin reduces the range of all movements of the finger joints. The interphalangeal joints are particularly affected, and the most noticeable abnormality is an inability to straighten the fingers.

GENERAL EXAMINATION

Other signs of scleroderma may be visible.

Face The skin of the face looks tight and shiny and the mouth is small – **microstomia**. There are often **multiple telangiectases** all over the face (and sometimes on the hands).

Wasting There may be generalized wasting if the dysphagia is causing malnutrition.

Abdominal distension Scleroderma in the large bowel inhibits peristalsis and causes chronic constipation and abdominal distension.

The combination of Calcinosis, Raynaud's phenomenon, Esophageal problems (dysphagia), Scleroderma and Telangiectases is known as the CREST syndrome.

Flexor sheath ganglion

A ganglion is an encapsulated myxomatous degeneration of fibrous tissue. When a ganglion occurs on the anterior aspect of a flexor sheath it can interfere with the grip and cause pain and disability out of proportion to its size.

HISTORY

Age and sex Flexor sheath ganglia are most common in middle-aged men.

Symptoms The patient complains of a **sharp pain** at the base of one finger whenever he grips something tightly.

He may also complain of a lump at the site of the pain.

LOCAL EXAMINATION

Colour and temperature These are normal.

Site A small tender nodule can be felt on the palmar surface of the base of a finger, superficial to the flexor sheath.

Tenderness Direct pressure on the lump is usually very painful.

Shape The nodule is spherical or hemispherical.

Size Flexor sheath ganglia are usually quite small; some cause symptoms when they are only 2–3 mm in diameter.

Surface and edge The surface of the nodule is smooth and the edge sharply defined.

Composition The nodule feels solid and hard. It is usually too small to permit the assessment of any other features such as fluctuation or translucency.

Lymph nodes The local lymph nodes should not be enlarged.

Local tissues The rest of the hand is normal.

COMMENT

Benign giant cell tumours of the flexor sheath present in an identical manner and are indistinguishable from flexor sheath ganglia.

Heberden's nodes

Heberden's nodes are bony swellings close to the distal finger joints. They are non-specific and do not indicate any particular disease.

HISTORY

The patient complains of swelling and deformity of his knuckles. There may be a history of an old injury to the finger or aching pains in both the lumps and the joints.

EXAMINATION

Heberden's nodules are commonly found on the dorsal surface of the fingers just distal to the distal interphalangeal joint. They are not mobile and can be easily recognized as part of the underlying bone.

The joint movements may be slightly restricted by osteoarthritis, and there may be radial deviation of the distal phalanx. The index finger is the finger most often affected. Small adventitious bursae may develop between the skin and the nodules. Similar nodules can appear near the proximal interphalangeal joint.

COMMENT

Heberden's nodules do not indicate any specific underlying bone or joint disease and have no clinical significance. They should not be confused with rheumatoid nodules, which are areas of necrosis surrounded by fibroblasts and chronic inflammatory cells and are found in all types of connective tissue. Patients with rheumatoid nodules invariably have other evidence of rheumatoid arthritis.

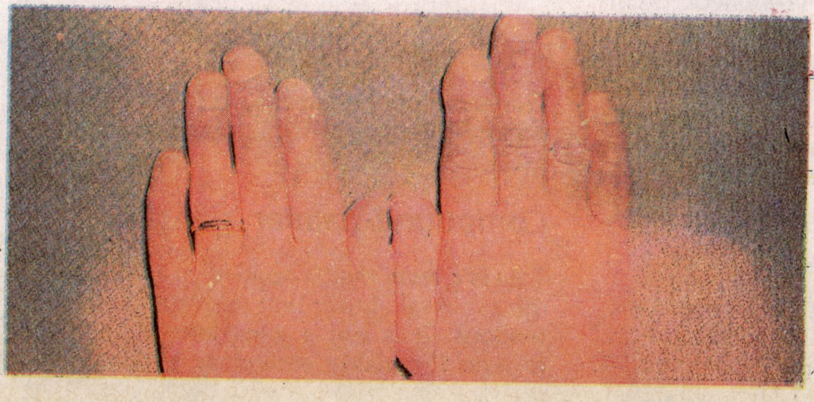

FIG. 5.9 Heberden's nodes. This patient had full painless movements of all her finger joints but large Herberden's nodes on the base of the distal phalanges of both index and middle fingers

Rheumatoid arthritis in the hand

The symptoms and signs of rheumatoid arthritis are described in Chapter 4, but, as this disease affects the hand so often, its manifestations in the hand are described here. All the deformities of rheumatoid arthritis result from the combination of uneven pull by the tendons and destruction of the joint surfaces.

Thickening of the joints

The joints most affected are the metacarpophalangeal and the proximal interphalangeal joints. Swelling of these joints gives the finger a fusiform, spindle shape.

Ulnar deviation of the fingers

The fingers are pulled towards the ulnar side of the hand, causing a varus deformity at the metacarpophalangeal joints. In advanced disease the varus deformity can be as much as 45–60°.

Flexion of the wrist

The wrist joint develops a fixed flexion deformity and usually some ulnar deviation.

'Swan neck' deformity of the fingers

This deformity is hyperextension of the proximal interphalangeal joint and flexion of the distal interphalangeal joint. It is caused by fibrotic contraction of the interosseous and lumbrical muscles.

Boutonniere deformity

The joint deformities of this abnormality are the opposite of those of the 'swan neck' deformity: flexion of the proximal interphalangeal joint and hyperextension of the distal interphalangeal joint.

It is caused by the projection and trapping of the flexed proximal interphalangeal joint through a rupture of the central portion of the extensor tendon expansion.

Tendon ruptures

In severe rheumatoid arthritis any tendon may undergo attrition (damage from friction) and rupture. This causes a variety of deformities.

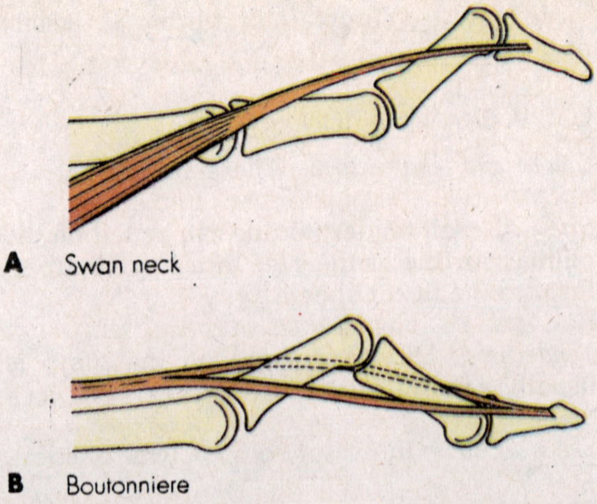

FIG. 5.10 **A**: The 'swan neck' deformity is caused by fibrotic contracture of the interosseus and lumbrical muscles. **B**: The 'boutonniere' deformity develops when the proximal interphalangeal joint pokes through the centre of the extensor expansion, following rupture of its central portion

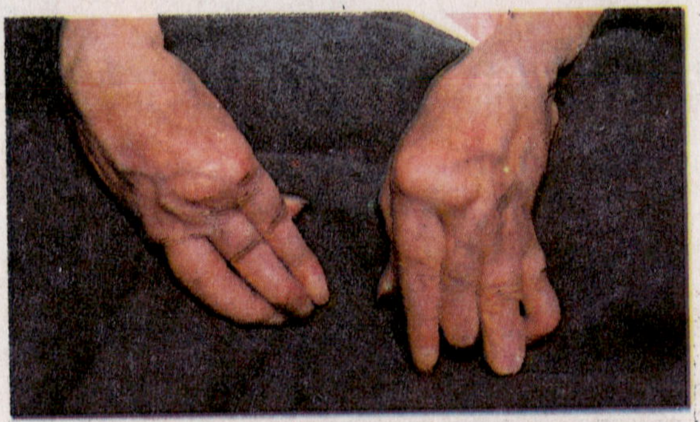

FIG. 5.11 Rheumatoid arthritis in the hands. These hands are grossly deformed. The joints are swollen, the wrists flexed and the fingers deviated. In the right hand the index finger has a 'swan neck' deformity, whereas the ring finger has a 'boutonniere' deformity

The commonest tendons to rupture are the long extensor tendons of the fingers and thumb.

Compound palmar 'ganglion'

This is a term that is applied to an effusion in the synovial sheath that surrounds the flexor tendons. It is **not** a ganglion. In the UK it is now invariably secondary to rheumatoid arthritis, but in many other parts of the world it is almost always caused by a tuberculous synovitis.

HISTORY

The commonest presenting symptom is **swelling** on the anterior aspect of the wrist and sometimes in the palm of the hand. Pain is uncommon.

The patient may notice **crepitus** during movements of the fingers.

Paraesthesia may occur in the distribution of the median nerve.

EXAMINATION

Distension of the flexor tendon synovial sheath produces a soft fluctuant swelling which can be felt on the anterior aspect of the wrist and lower forearm, and in the palm of the hand. Because the swelling passes beneath the flexor retinaculum, compression of the lump on one side of the retinaculum makes it distend on the other side.

Crepitus may be felt during palpation and when the patient moves his fingers. This is caused by the presence of fibrin bodies within the synovial sheath – commonly called 'melon seed bodies'.

There are no local signs of inflammation.

GENERAL EXAMINATION

All the joints should be examined to exclude rheumatoid arthritis, and the chest examined (and x-rayed) to exclude tuberculosis.

THE NAILS

Inspection of the nails often yields useful information about the patient's general health.

The nails are usually pale pink. The commonest cause of loss of this colour is anaemia.

Another sign of anaemia in the hands of white-skinned races is loss of skin crease colour. When the hand is relaxed the palmar skin creases are slightly darker than the rest of the skin but if the skin of the palm is stretched the creases turn a deep red. This deep red colour is not visible if the patient is anaemic.

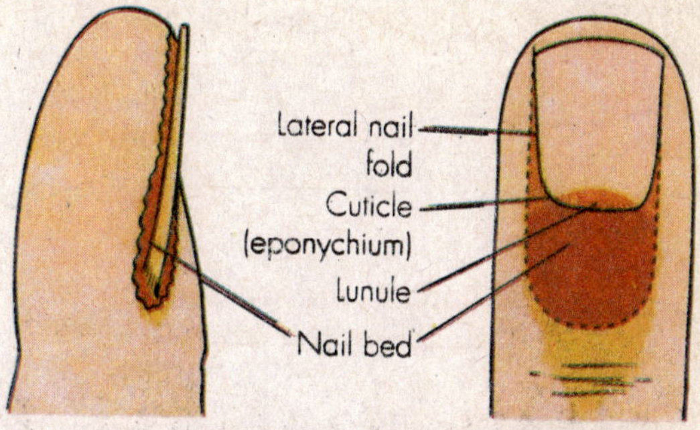

FIG. 5.12 The anatomy of the nail

Splinter haemorrhages

Splinter haemorrhages are small extravasations of blood from the vessels of the nail bed caused by minute arterial emboli. They are long, thin, red–brown streaks, their long axis running towards the end of the finger. Their colour and shape make them look like splinters of wood beneath the nail.

The presence of splinter haemorrhages is an important physical sign because they are usually caused by emboli from a bacterial endocarditis or a fulminating septicaemia. They may also occur in rheumatoid arthritis, mitral stenosis and severe hypertension.

Clubbing

Clubbing of the nails is a term used to describe the loss of the normal angle between the surface of the nail and the skin covering the nail bed.

If you look at your finger from the side you will see that the plane of the nail and the plane of the skin covering the base of the nail bed form an angle of 130–170°.

In clubbed nails there is hypertrophy of the tissue beneath the nail bed which makes the base of the nail bulge upwards and distorts nail growth so that the nail becomes curved. The planes of the nail and the skin covering the nail bed then meet at an angle greater than 180°.

It is possible to have a very curved nail but still have a normal nail/nail-fold angle, so do

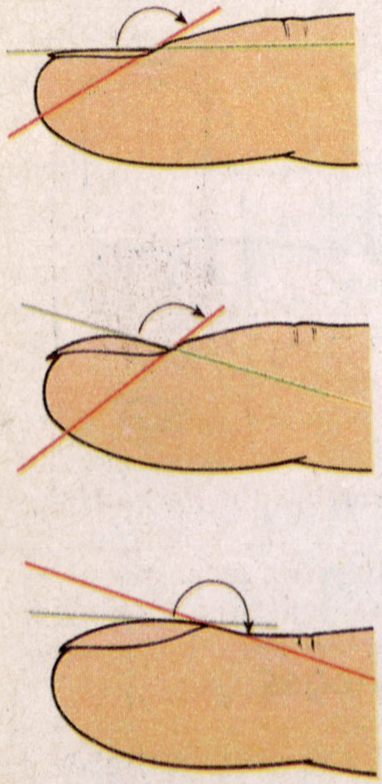

Normal and abnormal nail/nail-fold angles

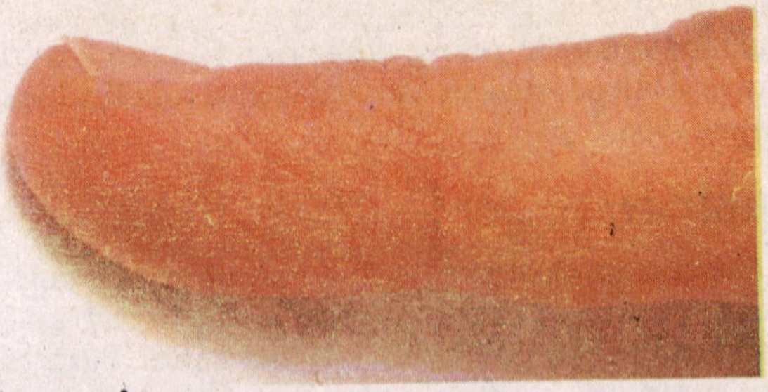

A normal finger

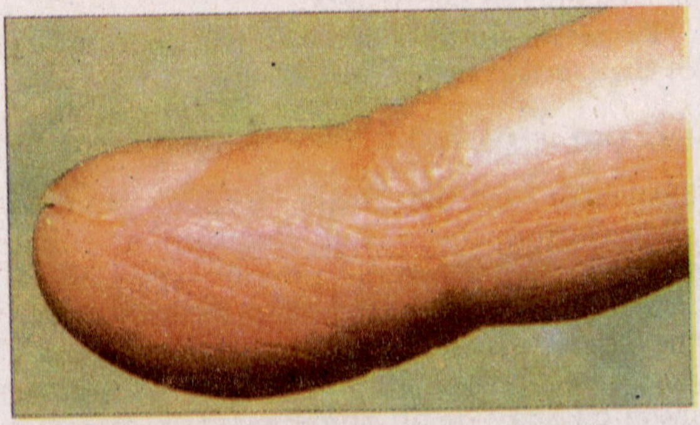

A nail/nail-fold angle greater than 180° = clubbing

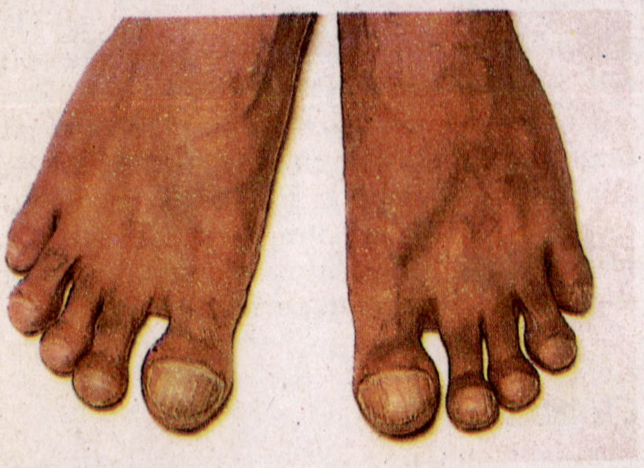

Clubbing of the toes

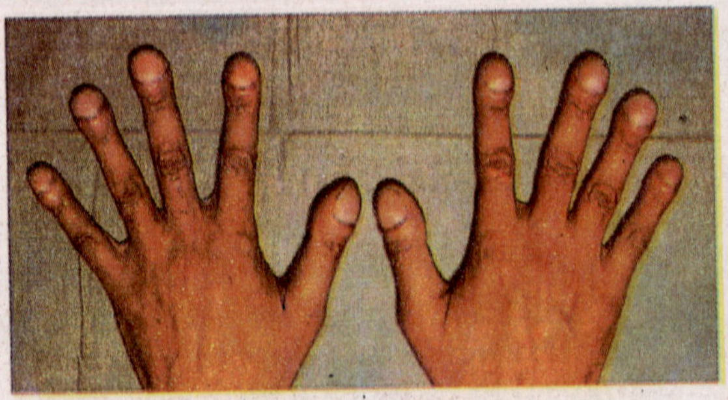

Clubbing of all the fingers. Note the swelling of the terminal phalanges

FIG. 5.13 Clubbing

Revision Panel 5.3
The signs of clubbing

Increased nail/nail-fold angle

Increased longitudinal and transverse nail curvature

Bulbous terminal phalanges

Spongy nail bed

Revision Panel 5.4
Some causes of clubbing

Congenital

Carcinoma of the bronchus

Chronic lung disease — Alveolitis, Bronchiectasis, Cystic fibrosis

Congenital cyanotic heart disease

Ulcerative colitis/Crohn's disease

not look at the shape of the nail when assessing clubbing; look at the whole finger.

The terminal phalanx may enlarge to make the end of the finger bulbous.

Spoon-shaped nails

(Koilonychia)

A normal nail is convex transversely and longitudinally, the degree of curvature varying considerably from person to person. Loss of both these curves produces a hollowed-out spoon-shaped nail (koilonychia).

When a patient complains that her nails have changed from a normal to a spoon shape, it is very likely that she has developed an anaemia following chronic loss of blood, usually from menorrhagia or haemorrhoids.

Subungual haematoma and melanoma

A blow on a nail can cause bleeding beneath it. A collection of blood beneath the nail is called a subungual haematoma. If it appears at the time of the injury the patient usually makes his own diagnosis and only comes for treatment if it is painful.

Sometimes the patient does not notice the injury and comes complaining of a brown spot beneath the nail. The clinical problem in this case is to decide whether the brown spot is haemosiderin or melanin – a haematoma or a mole.

The features of the spot sometimes help. A haematoma is usually reddish-brown, with sharp edges. A melanoma is brown with a greyish tinge, and has indistinct edges.

Inspection with a small hand-lens may solve the problem by revealing small blood vessels in the lesion, which means it is cellular.

If the patient has watched the lesion for a few weeks he will be able to tell you if it has moved down the nail with nail growth, or stayed still. Haematomata move down the nail, melanomata do not move.

If it is not possible to make a definite clinical diagnosis, the patient should be managed as if he had a melanoma until you prove otherwise.

Glomus tumour

This is a very rare tumour but is mentioned because it can cause a great deal of pain, and often occurs beneath the nail. It is an angioneuromyoma.

The patient complains of severe pain every time she touches the nail. Examination usually reveals a small purple–red spot beneath the nail. The colour is due to the angiomatous nature of the tumour; the pain comes from its abnormally rich nerve supply. Glomus tumours can occur in any part of the skin but are most often found in the hands.

Changes associated with generalized diseases

Psoriasis: pitting, ridges, poor growth.
Cirrhosis of the liver: white nails.
General debilitating illnesses: transverse furrows (Bean's lines).
Anaemia: koilonychia.

Revision Panel 5.5
Common nail abnormalities

Loosening	Psoriasis Fungal infections
Pitting	Psoriasis
Transverse ridges	Systematic illness Local damage (paronychia)
Longitudinal ridges	Old age
Thickening and twisting (Onychogryphosis)	Trauma Age
Clubbing	See Revision Panel 5.4

INFECTIONS IN THE HAND

Infections in the hand cause severe pain and swelling. They are more likely to present in a casualty department than in a routine surgical outpatient clinic, but two varieties are so common that they deserve a description in this chapter.

Paronychia

This is an infection beneath the skin at the side or base of the nail, and which develops into a small abscess.

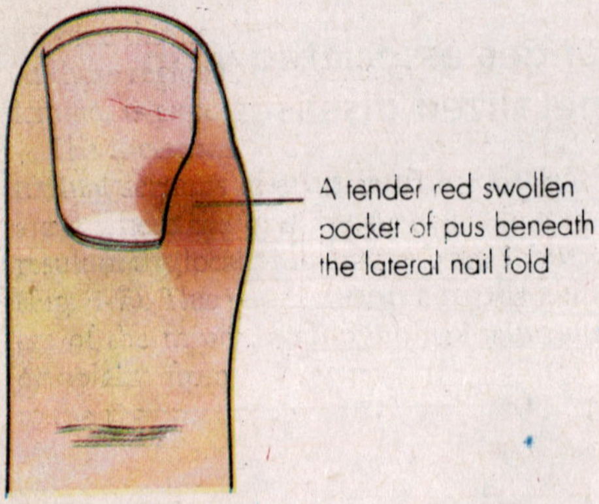

FIG. 5.14 A paronychia

The patient complains of a painful, tender spot close to the nail that may have throbbed all night and kept him awake. He may remember picking or cutting a piece of cuticle or split skin (hang nail) a few days before the pain began.

The skin at the base and side of the nail is red, shiny and bulging and the whole area is exquisitely tender.

In the early stages the pus collects between the nail and the overlying skin but later it spreads deep to the nail so that movement of the nail is painful and pus is visible through it.

Paronychia are more common in fingers with a poor circulation.

Chronic paronychia

Normally a paronychia subsides after the pus has drained out, but if there is a foreign body present or the infecting organism is an unusual bacterium or a fungus the wound may fail to heal and continue to discharge. The patient may then present with a discharging sinus in a discoloured area close to the nail, with unhealthy bluish granulation tissue protruding from it. Biopsy is an essential part of the management of such a case to exclude other conditions such as malignant melanoma and squamous cell carcinoma.

Pulp space infections

This is an infection, usually followed by abscess formation, in the subcutaneous tissue which forms the pulp of the finger tip.

It presents with throbbing pain, swelling and redness. Sometimes there is a history of a penetrating injury such as a prick with a needle. On examination there is swelling and tenderness and sometimes a pus-filled blister. If the blister is opened you will see a hole in the skin leading to the subcutaneous abscess.

If neglected or poorly treated the skin of the pulp, and the distal phalanx, may necrose.

The only lesion likely to be mistaken for a pulp space infection is a rapidly growing, vascular, secondary tumour deposit in the distal phalanx. Although this will be red, hot and tender it will progress much slower than an infection and not suppurate. There may also be clinical evidence of the primary lesion.

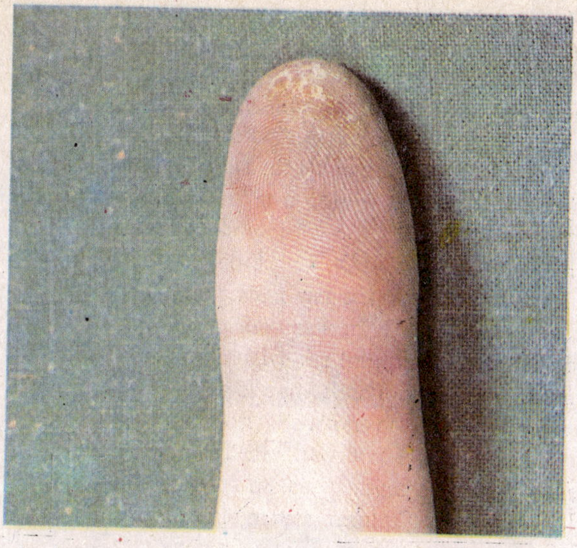

Patchy areas of discolouration and coldness, which are sometimes painful, sometimes hypoaesthetic, caused by digital artery embolism

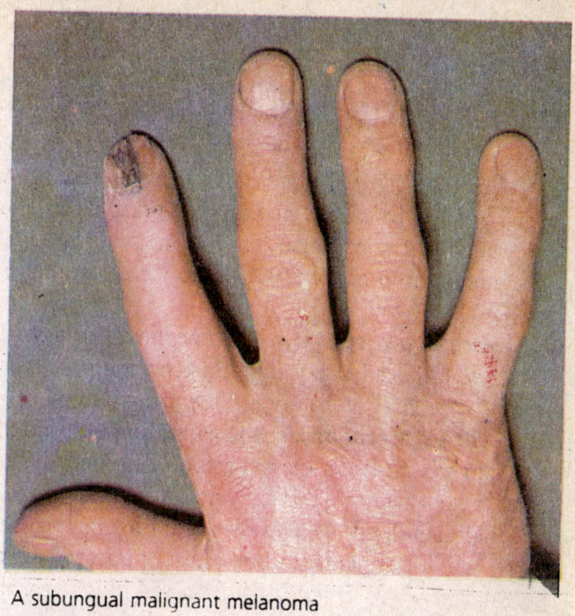

A subungual malignant melanoma

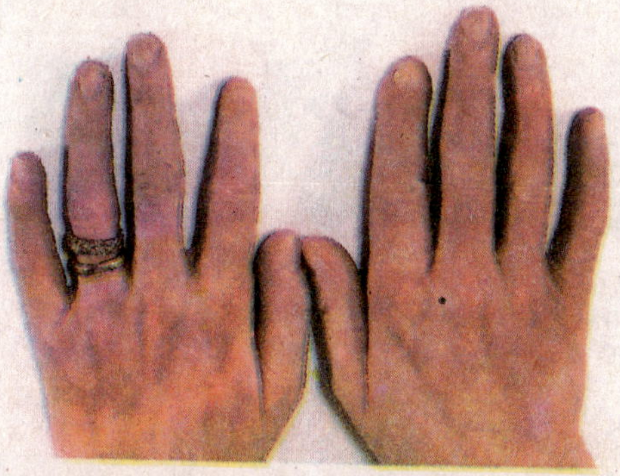

Acrocyanosis. A persistent blue discolouration of the skin of the hands caused by mild vasospasm, usually induced by a drop of ambient temperature

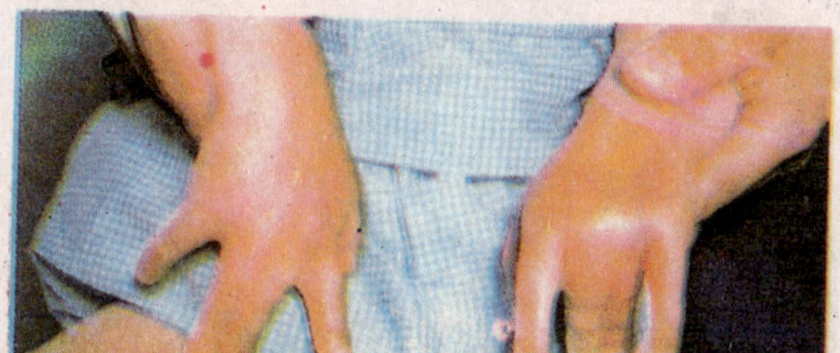

Syndactyly. Fusion of the middle and ring fingers of both hands

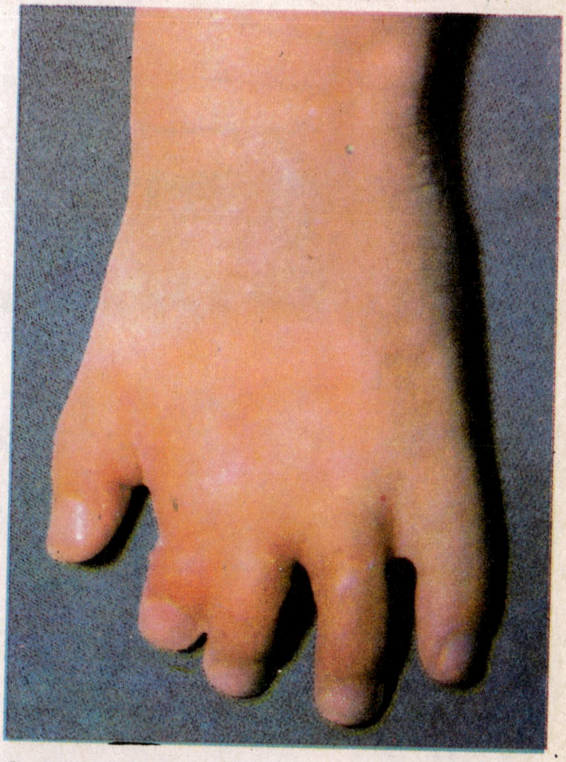

Syndactyly. Fusion of the middle and ring fingers, in this case associated with a marked failure of finger growth and other bony abnormalities

FIG. 5.15 SOME MORE CONDITIONS FOUND IN THE HANDS

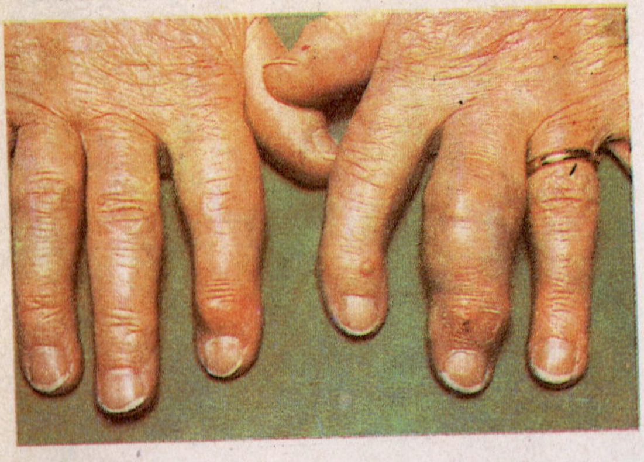

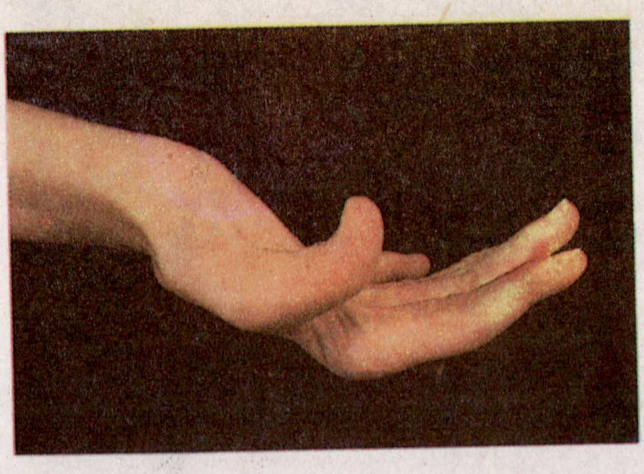

Gouty tophi

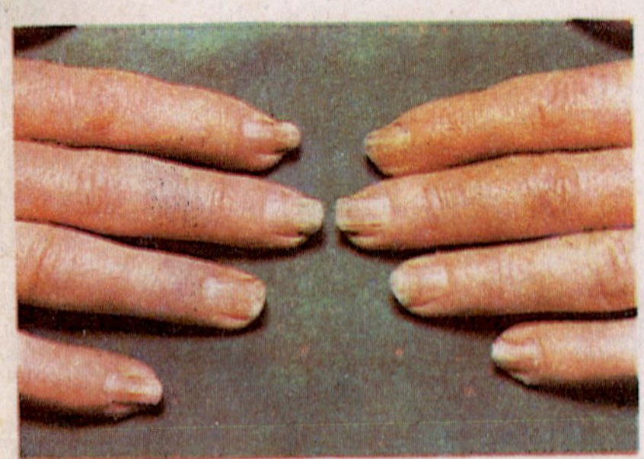

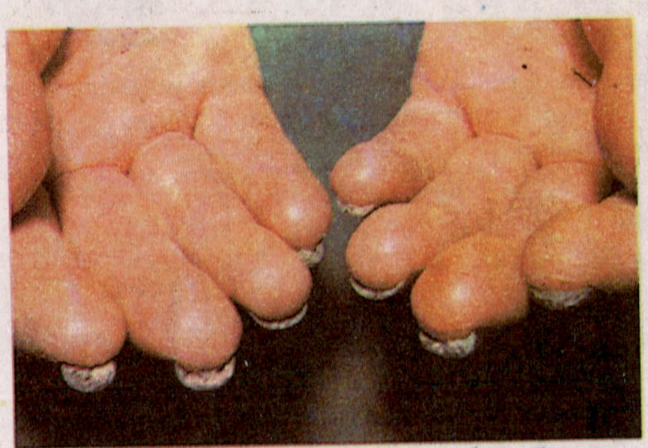

Pits, furrows and thickening of the nails caused by psoriasis

The hyperextendibility of the thumb and metacarpophalangeal joints of the Ehlers–Danlos syndrome

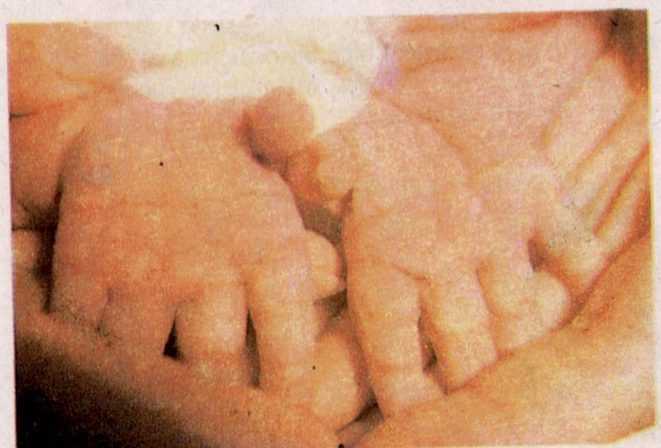

The abnormal palmar creases associated with Down's syndrome

FIG. 5.15 *Continued*

Conditions peculiar to the feet

6

CONGENITAL AND ACQUIRED DEFORMITIES OF THE FOOT AND ANKLE

Club foot

(Talipes)

There are many deformities of the ankle and foot that can develop *in utero* and be present at birth. They are classified according to the skeletal deformity but are collectively known as **talipes** or **club foot**. However, these are bad terms when used in such a broad, non-specific manner. Similar deformities can also develop in adult life after injury, paralysis and other musculoskeletal disorders.

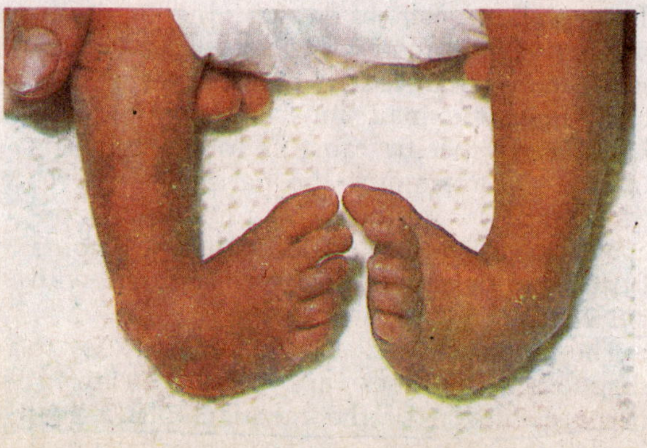

FIG. 6.1 Severe bilateral clubbed feet. The varus deformity is so gross that the feet are pulled upwards as well as inwards, making this a talipes calcaneovarus

There are two main types of deformity:

1 The ankle may be abnormally extended so that weight-bearing is on the toes – **an equinus deformity**; or abnormally dorsiflexed so that weight-bearing is on the heel – **a calcaneous** deformity.
2 The foot may be deviated into a **varus** or **valgus** position, which usually means that there is also some associated inversion and eversion, respectively. These terms are defined on page 116.

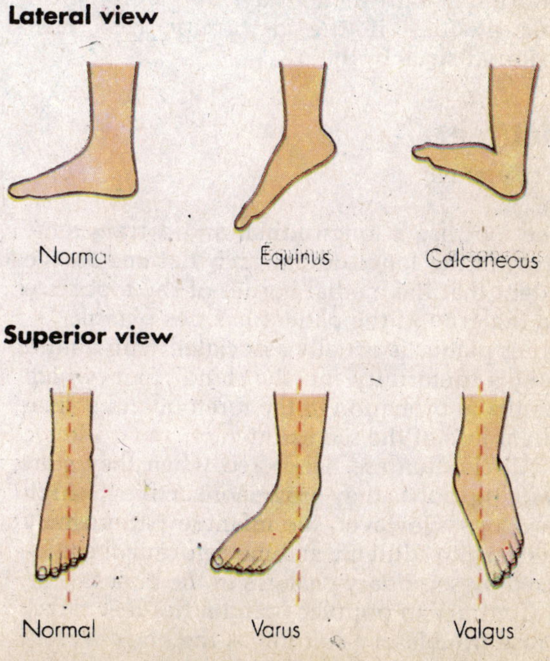

FIG. 6.2 The deformities of the foot

There are, therefore, eight types of deformity – four simple and four mixed. Each is prefixed with the term 'talipes' to indicate that the site of the abnormality is the ankle–foot (*tali–pes*):

1 *Simple:* talipes varus
talipes valgus
talipes equinus
talipes calcaneous
2 *Mixed:* talipes equinovarus
talipes equinovalgus
talipes calcaneovarus
talipes calcaneovalgus

Of these eight variations only two are common: talipes equinus caused by a short Achilles tendon, and talipes equinovarus – the true 'club foot'.

The clinical examination of the foot should follow the pattern described for bones and joints in Chapter 4: *look, feel* and *move*. The obvious deformities of the true club foot will be the equinus at the ankle, the varus of the heel with supination of the subtalar joint, and the adduction of the forefoot. The joint movements may be limited and the muscles that effect the joint movements wasted.

The nerves and arteries are usually normal when the abnormality is a congenital skeletal deformity, but there may be neurological abnormalities if the deformity has been acquired since birth.

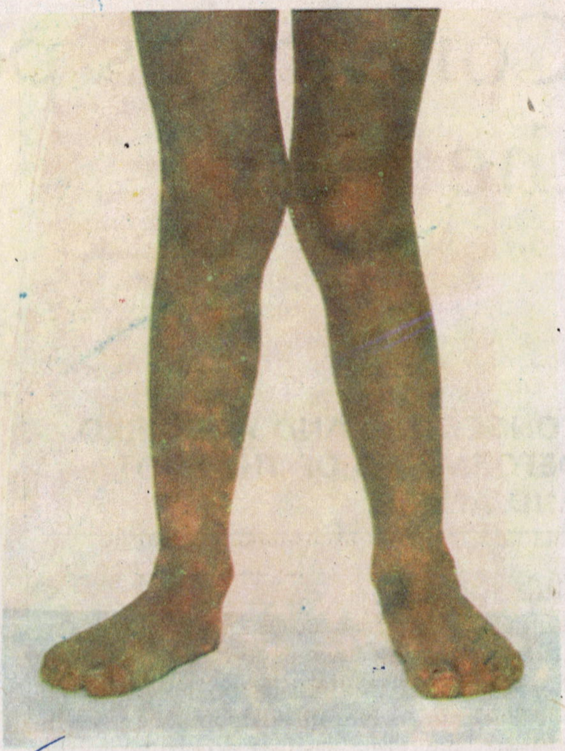

FIG. 6.3 Flat feet (pes planus). The medial border of the foot rests on the ground. There is also mild genu valgum (knock-knees)

Flat feet

(Pes planus)

The foot has a longitudinal and a transverse arch. If the longitudinal arch flattens to the extent that the medial border of the foot rests on the ground the patient has pes planus.

Pes planus is usually associated with a mild valgus deformity of the hind foot which results in pronation of the forefoot and subsequent loss of the medial arch.

All children are flat-footed when they start walking, but as they grow more active the arch develops. However, the infantile pattern may persist into adult life and the deformity become fixed by secondary changes in the bones.

Contrary to popular opinion flat feet rarely cause trouble in adult life as the body weight is spread over a large flat area.

Hollow or high-arch foot

(Pes cavus)

This is the opposite to flat foot; the longitudinal arch is accentuated. Pes cavus is secondary to muscle imbalance with relative weakness of the intrinsic (small muscles) of the foot. Usually no specific cause is found, but it is important to examine the peripheral nerves thoroughly. Peripheral neuropathies, especially Charcot–Marie–Tooth disease, **spina bifida** and **poliomyelitis**, can all present with pes cavus.

The high arch is clearly visible and easy to diagnose. The toes are always 'clawed' (hyperextension of the metatarsophalangeal joints and flexion of the interphalangeal joints) and the patient cannot straighten his toes. Extension of the metatarsophalangeal

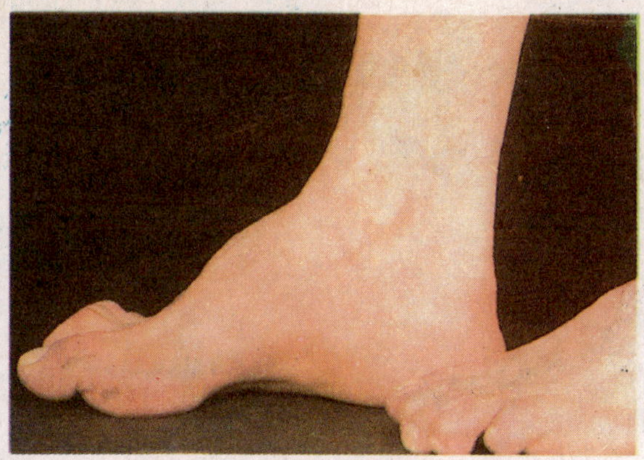

FIG. 6.4 A high-arched foot (pes cavus)

joints and the high arch make the ball of the foot more prominent and lift the tips of the toes off the ground so that they do not participate in weight-bearing. Consequently **callosities** develop on the ball of the foot beneath the heads of the metatarsal bones, and on the dorsal aspect of the toes where they rub against shoes.

Unlike the flat foot, the high-arched foot frequently causes pain and discomfort.

Hallux valgus and bunion

A valgus deformity at the metatarsophalangeal joint of the great toe is a common abnormality. It can be congenital or acquired. The acquired variety is more common in women than men and is often attributed to poorly fitting footwear.

The valgus deformity is obvious to the patient and the doctor. In itself it causes little trouble, but two secondary effects are the source of much discomfort.

Bunion

This is the name given to the bursa which forms over the medial aspect of the prominent head of the first metatarsal. It often swells up and sometimes becomes infected. The patient has difficulty in finding a comfortable pair of shoes because the bunion is painful when rubbed or touched.

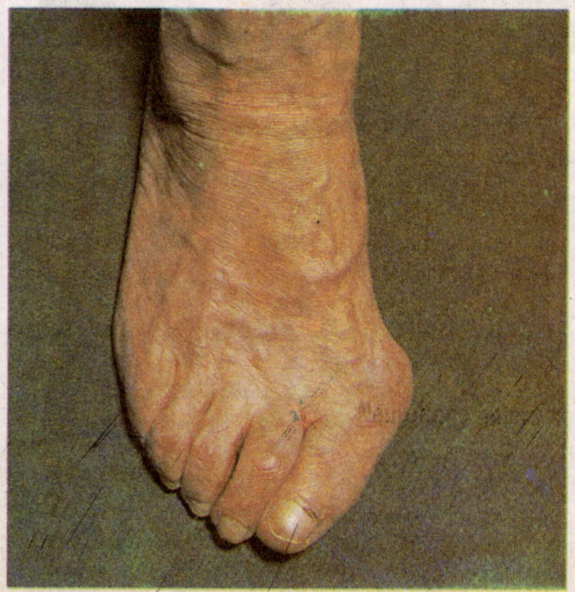

FIG. 6.5 Severe hallux valgus. The second toe is rising up over the great toe and the remaining toes are deviated towards the lateral side of the foot

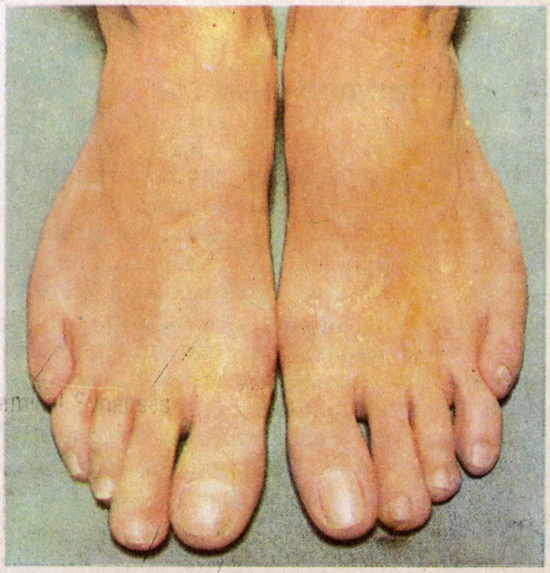

FIG. 6.6 Digiti quinti varus. This is the opposite deformity to hallux valgus and affects the fifth toe. It is a common congenital abnormality and rarely causes symptoms

The fluctuant subcutaneous swelling is easy to feel and distinguish from the underlying bony prominence.

Osteoarthritis

As a result of prolonged abnormal stresses across the deformed metatarsophalangeal joint, the joint surfaces degenerate and osteoarthritis develops. This causes pain in the joint during movement and weight-bearing, and hypertrophy of the bone which makes the deformity more obvious.

Clinical examination reveals the deformity, the adventitious bursa (the bunion), pain on moving the joint, limited movements and, sometimes, crepitus.

Hallux rigidus

The first metatarsophalangeal joint is often afflicted by osteoarthritis even when it is in normal alignment. This causes pain and a progressive reduction of joint movement.

A stiff, painful metatarsophalangeal joint secondary to osteoarthritis is known as hallux rigidus.

The pain may become less severe when the joint becomes fixed by a fibrous ankylosis.

Hammer toe and claw toe

A hammer toe is caused by a fixed flexion of the proximal interphalangeal joint. The middle phalanx points downwards so much that the distal interphalangeal joint has to hyperextend to enable the pulp of the toe to rest on the ground. There is also hyperextension of the metatarsophalangeal joint (see Fig. 6.7).

The cause of hammer toe is not understood, except that it must ultimately result from an imbalance of muscle tone.

A hammer toe causes pain and discomfort when the skin over the proximal interphalangeal joint rubs on the sole or top of the shoe, respectively.

A claw toe is caused by a contracture of its long flexor tendon. This causes flexion of both interphalangeal joints and a secondary extension of the metatarsophalangeal joint. The tip of the toe rests upon the ground and may develop a painful callosity. As the M–P joint extension develops, the tip of the toe may be lifted off the ground and a callosity develop over the proximal interphalangeal joint.

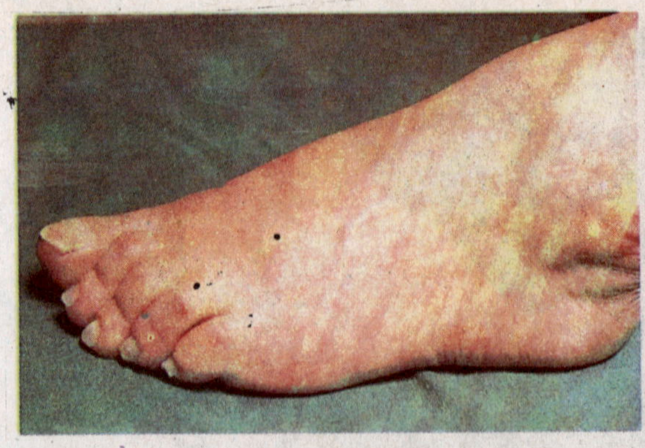

A row of hammer toes. The tips of some of the toes are off the ground and there are callosities over the flexed proximal interphalangeal joints. The distal interphalangeal joints of the fourth and fifth toes are only slightly hyperextended

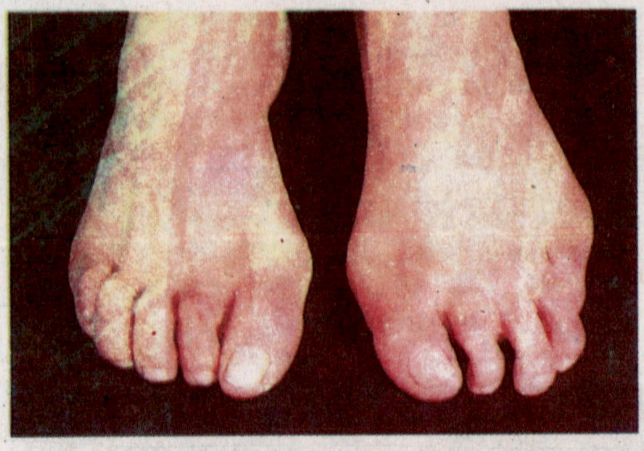

Bilateral claw toes. Claw toes are caused by hyperextension of the metatarsophalangeal joint and the flexion of ***both*** interphalangeal joints. The tip of the toe points directly downwards and may not reach the ground

FIG. 6.7 HAMMER TOES AND CLAW TOES

Callosities and corns

Continual pressure and friction on small areas of the skin of the foot caused by poor-fitting shoes or skeletal deformities stimulate

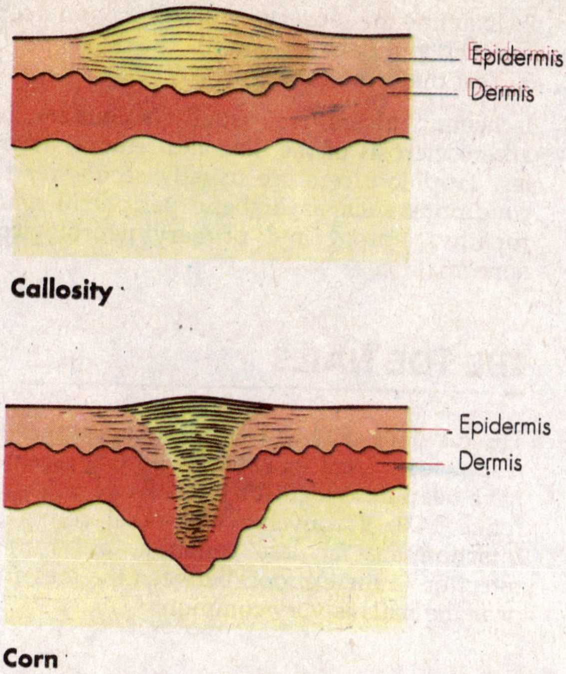

FIG. 6.8 Callosities and corns are patches of thickened, hard epidermis. A callosity protrudes above the surface of the skin; a corn is pushed into the skin

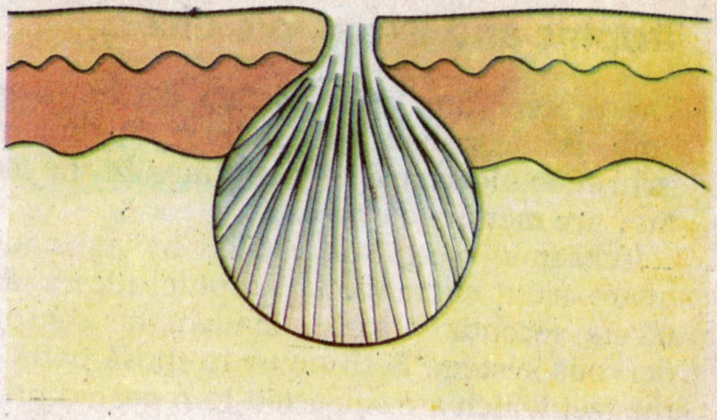

FIG. 6.9 A plantar wart (verruca). The fine fronds get pushed down into the sole of the foot

thickening of the skin. A patch of thickened hyperkeratotic skin is called a **callosity**. If it is pushed into the skin so that it appears to have a deep central core it is often called a **corn** but there is no real difference between a corn and a callosity (see Fig. 6.8 and page 59).

Plantar wart

(Verruca plantaris)

This is a wart on the sole of the foot. It is caused by a virus similar to that which causes warts on the hands, but because it gets pushed into the sole of the foot it has different physical characteristics.

HISTORY

The patient is usually a child or young adult and the main complaint is of pain in the sole of the foot during walking.

EXAMINATION

Site Plantar warts are usually found on the ball and the heel of the foot.

Colour The painful spot is pearly white in colour, with occasional brown flecks caused by haemorrhage.

Tenderness Pressure on the wart is **very painful**, in contrast to corns and callosities which are not very tender when pressed.

Size The area of tenderness may be a few millimetres, or 1 cm, in diameter.

Surface When the wart is small it is covered by apparently normal skin, but as it enlarges the skin breaks down to reveal a circular pit and the ends of the grey–white filiform strands which are the substance of the wart.

Edge A plantar wart has clearly demarcated edges, as it is really a pit containing a wart. This gives it a 'punched-out' appearance in contrast to the indistinct edge of a corn or callosity.

Consistence Because the wart is pushed into the hard, thick skin of the foot it is rarely possible to feel a well-defined lump. The fine strands in the centre of the wart are soft.

Multiplicity There may be more than one plantar wart.

Local structures The local lymph nodes, arteries and nerves should be normal.

Trophic and ischaemic ulcers

The presentation of ischaemia in the lower limb is described in Chapter 7, but as ischaemic ulcers are very common in the feet they are mentioned here.

Ischaemic ulcers are caused by an inadequate skin circulation. Trophic ulcers are ulcers secondary to an inadequate sensory nervous system. Both occur in those parts of the feet which are subjected to repeated pressure and trauma, the prime cause of both types of ulcer.

Prolonged pressure on one part of the foot causes ischaemic damage of the tissues, and pain. If the circulation is inadequate, then the tissues cannot repair themselves and an ischaemic ulcer develops. If the nerves are inadequate the patient does not feel the pain and continues to damage the area until it is beyond repair.

These ulcers occur on the heel, the ball of the foot, over the head of the fifth metatarsal and over the tips and knuckles of the toes.

When a patient is **ambulant** the main pressure areas are on the **sole of the foot** (i.e. the heel and ball of the foot and the tips of the toes). When a patient is lying **in bed** the main pressure areas are on the **back of the heel** and lateral side of the foot.

Whenever you examine a patient with an ulcer on his foot:

1 Examine the circulation (pulses, etc.).
2 Examine the sensory nerves (light and deep touch and pain sensation).
3 Test the urine for sugar.

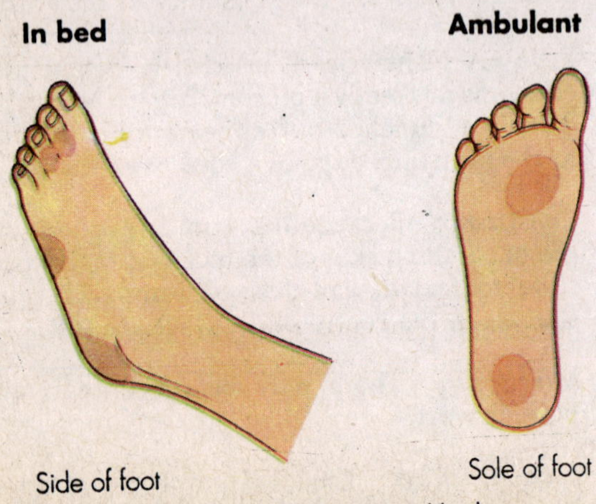

FIG. 6.10 The sites of ischaemic and trophic ulcers

Ischaemic ulcers are usually secondary to atherosclerosis of the iliac and femoral arteries. Trophic ulcers are usually secondary to conditions such as diabetic peripheral neuropathy, leprosy and primary neurological abnormalities.

THE TOE NAILS

The toe nails may show the same changes in response to local or generalized disease that have been described for the nails of the hand (page 147). Paronychia and other forms of infection are far less common, but fungal infection (athlete's foot) between the toes and near the nails is very common.

Onychogryphosis

The normal nail is a thin plate which slides along the nail bed. When the sliding mechanism goes wrong the nail begins to thicken and heap up until it appears to be growing vertically out of the nail bed. It then curves over the end of the toe and looks like an animal's claw. This deformity of the nail is called onychogryphosis. It can occur in young people after an injury to the nail bed, but is most common in elderly people where it is presumed to be a failure of the sliding mechanism caused by old age.

Ingrowing toe nail

This is a common condition in which the side of the nail, usually the lateral side of the great toenail, appears to be growing or digging into the substance of the toe.

It is a misnomer because, although the nail may be excessively curved in its transverse plane, it is growing normally as a thin plate sliding forwards on the nail bed.

If you remove an ingrowing toenail you invariably find that it has an irregular edge which is damaging the skin. The damage is

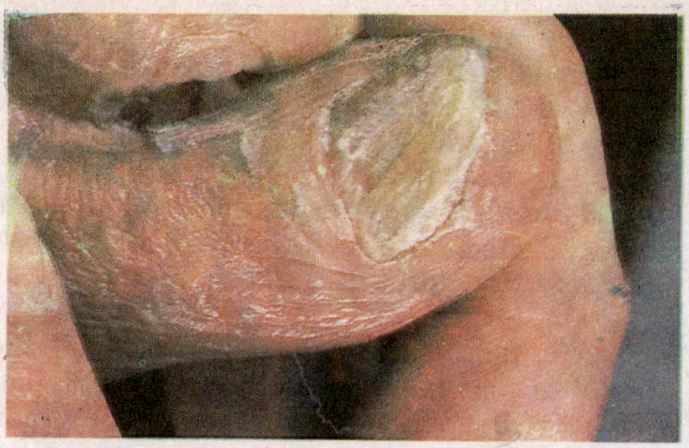

The nail is thick, growing upwards and beginning to curl around the end of the toe like a claw

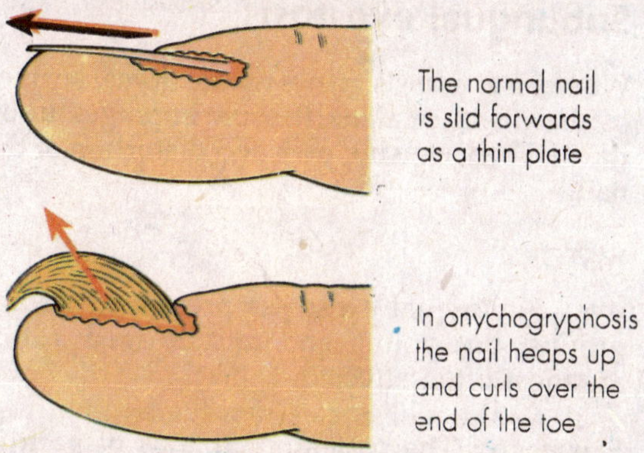

A diagrammatic representation of the disorder of nail growth that causes onychogryphosis

FIG. 6.11 Onychogryphosis

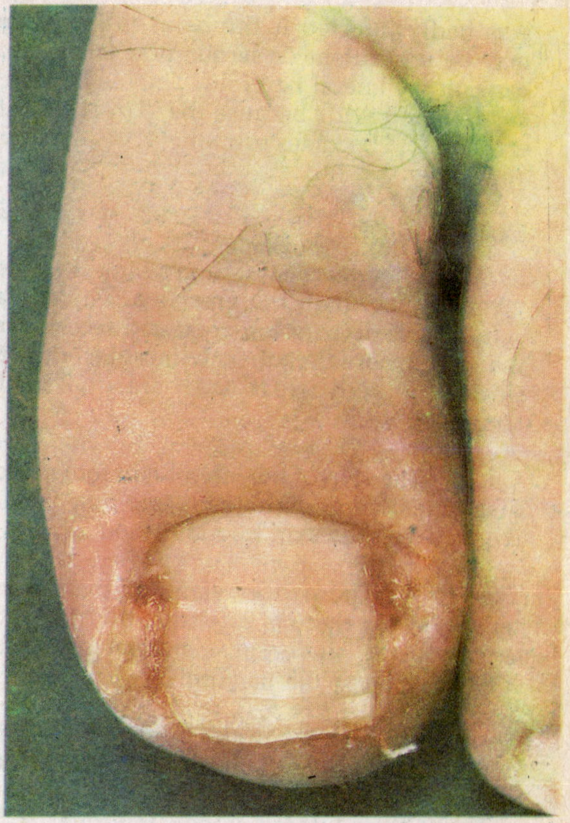

FIG. 6.13 An ingrowing toe nail. Both sides of the nail are pushing into the soft tissues which are infected and producing exuberant granulation tissue

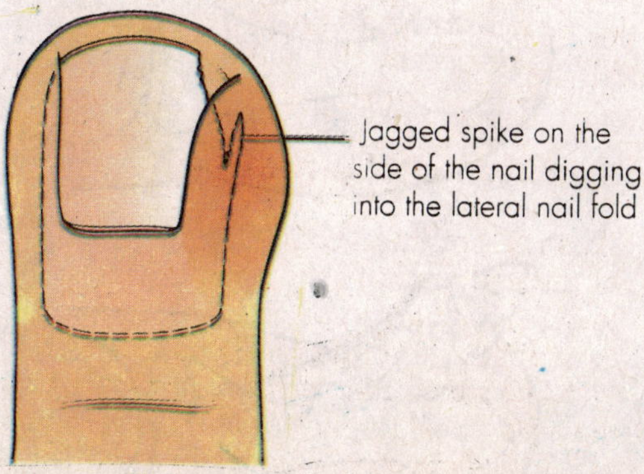

FIG. 6.12 The jagged, irregular edge of the nail beneath the lateral nail fold is the real cause of the pain and infection known as 'ingrowing toe nail'. The nail is damaged by misguided efforts to cut off the corner of the nail

exacerbated when the skin at the side of the toe is forced upwards during walking.

The usual cause of the irregularity of the nail is an attempt by the patient to cut off the corner, which has ended with the nail being torn off, leaving a jagged spike at the edge.

HISTORY

Age and sex Ingrowing toenails are commonly found in **adolescent** and young adult males. The excessive use of the feet in games such as football, and less stringent hygiene in young boys and men, may contribute to the sex incidence.

Symptoms The principal symptom is **pain**. The toe is sore and painful when walking. If it gets badly infected it throbs at night. There may be a purulent or serous **discharge** from beneath the lateral nail fold. The toe becomes **swollen and wide** because the skin at the lateral nail fold becomes prominent, oedematous and soggy.

EXAMINATION

Site The symptoms of ingrowing toe nail invariably occur in the great toe. The lateral side of the nail (between great and second toe) is affected more than the medial side, but both sides and both great toes are commonly abnormal.

Colour The skin of the lateral nail fold is reddish-blue. Red granulation tissue may be visible between the skin fold and the nail.

Tenderness The swollen skin and the nail are tender. When there is extensive infection, the whole toe is tender and movement of the interphalangeal joint is painful.

Shape The increase in the bulk of the lateral nail fold makes the great toe wide and spatulate.

The nail itself does not look abnormal. If the nail fold can be pulled away from the nail without causing too much pain, it may be possible to see the extent to which the nail is digging into the tissues and the jagged spikes on the edge of the nail.

Local lymph nodes The inguinal lymph nodes may be enlarged if there has been long-standing infection, but this is uncommon.

Complications Inadequate excision of the nail bed may result in the regrowth of spikes of nail from the residual corners of the nail bed.

Subungual exostosis

When an exostosis grows on the dorsal surface of the distal phalanx it soon impinges upon the nail bed, causing pain and distortion of the nail.

HISTORY

Age Subungual exostoses present in all age groups, but young and middle-aged adults are most often affected.

Symptoms The patient complains of **pain in the toe**, especially when it is pressed. The toe

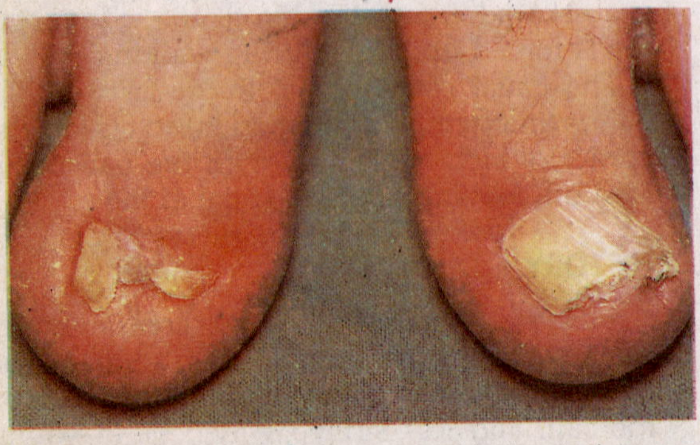

FIG. 6.14 This patient had the right nail bed excised 4 years before this photograph was taken. It shows two spikes of nail growing up the corners of the nail bed that were not excised. The left nail shows the thickening that precedes the appearance of an onychogryphosis. A fungus infection can cause a similar thickening

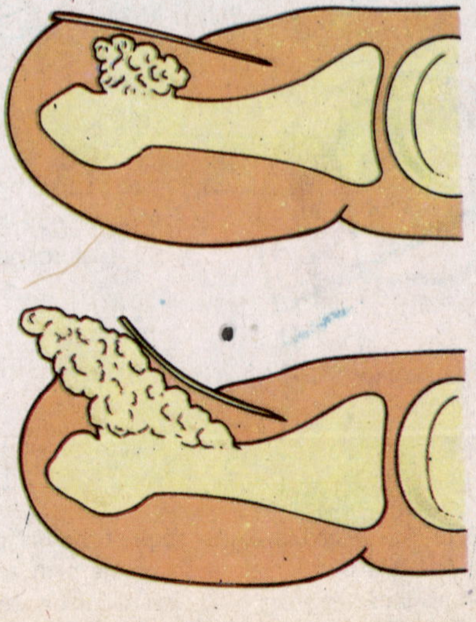

FIG. 6.15 A small and a large subungual exostosis

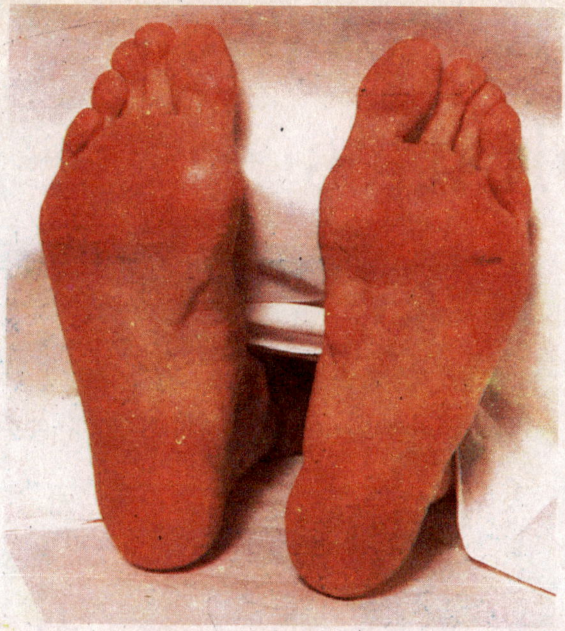

FIG. 6.16 Dupuytren's contracture of the feet. There are bilateral thick nodules in the plantar fascia but no flexion deformities of the toes

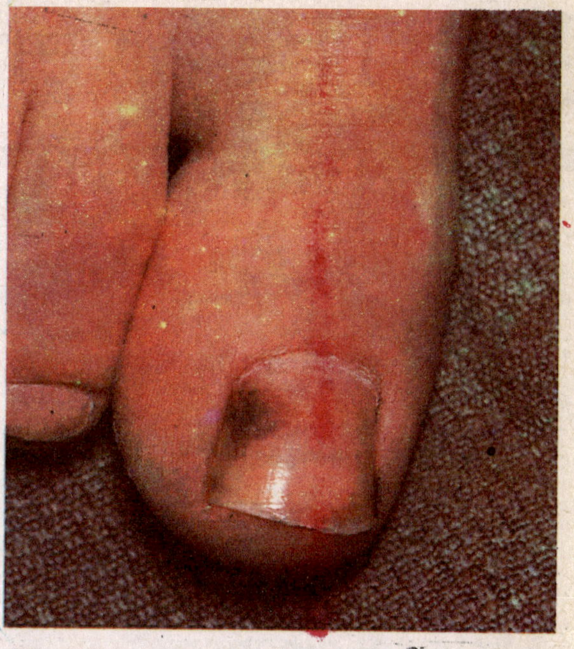

FIG. 6.17 A brown patch beneath the great toe nail. Subungual melanoma or haematoma? The latter will migrate down the toe with nail growth, but do not wait too long to detect this sign – remove the nail and biopsy the lesion

may swell slightly and the nail become pushed up and **deformed**.

EXAMINATION

In the early stages the toe looks normal but pressure on the nail causes severe pain. At this stage, when there are no visible changes in the nail, the diagnosis can only be made from a radiograph. As the exostosis grows the nail bulges upwards and then a swelling appears between the toe and the end of the nail. The skin overlying this swelling (which is the exostosis) is hard, rough and fissured.

If the exostosis is not removed it will continue to grow and form a prominent mass on the dorsal surface of the toe, with the nail tipped up and displaced posteriorly.

The cracks and fissures on the skin covering the exostosis may become infected.

Dupuytren's and ischaemic contractures

Do not forget that both these conditions may occur in the feet. Their presentation and signs are similar to those in the hands (see page 135), except that Dupuytren's contracture in the foot usually involves the whole of the plantar fascia and all of the toes.

Subungual melanoma

The features of malignant melanoma are described in Chapter 2.

Beware of the **brown spot** beneath the nail, shown in Fig. 6.17. It may be a subungual haematoma or a melanoma. Assume it is the latter unless there is a definite history of injury and clear evidence that the brown area is moving down the nail with nail growth.

7 The arteries, veins and lymphatics

The examination of the arteries, veins and lymphatics requires special examination techniques which will be described before the detailed descriptions of the history and clinical features of individual conditions.

Arterial disease

CLINICAL ASSESSMENT OF THE ARTERIAL CIRCULATION OF A LIMB

Always examine the patient's limbs in a **warm** room.

Inspection

Colour

The first, and, in white races, most noticeable feature of an ischaemic limb is its colour. Unfortunately a black skin masks these subtle colour changes, making the diagnosis of mild and moderate arterial insufficiency in the black races extremely difficult.

The skin may be as white as marble, or show varying degrees of pallor which become more obvious in the lower parts of the leg and the toes. Sometimes excessive deoxygenation of the blood in the skin capillaries gives the foot a purple–blue cyanosed appearance, but the blue fades to white within a few seconds when the patient lies down.

The vascular angle

This is also called Buerger's angle and is the angle to which the leg must be raised before it becomes white. In a normal person the straightened leg can be raised by 90° and the toes will stay pink. In an ischaemic leg, elevation to 15° or 30° may cause pallor. This angle is directly comparable to the pressure in the small vessels in the foot. The height, in centimetres, between the sternum and the heel at the elevation when the foot becomes pale is approximately equal to the pressure in the foot vessels in millimetres of mercury. A vascular angle of less than 20° indicates severe ischaemia.

Capillary filling time

After elevating the legs and estimating the vascular angle, ask the patient to sit up and hang his legs down over the side of the couch. A normal leg will remain a healthy pink colour. An ischaemic leg will **slowly** turn from white to pink, and then become a flushed purple–red colour. This is caused by blood filling the dilated skin capillaries. The time taken for the foot to become pink is the **capillary filling time** and depends upon the degree of arterial obstruction. In severe ischaemia it may be as long as 15–30 seconds. The appearance of a red–purple foot is just another indication of the severity of the ischaemia.

Venous filling

In a warm room the veins of the foot are relaxed and full of blood, even when the patient is lying horizontal. If the foot is ischaemic the veins will be collapsed, and look like pale blue gutters in the subcutaneous tissue. This appearance is often called **guttering of the veins.**

The veins collapse when the legs are raised above the level of the heart, but if the circulation is normal they do not empty completely. The veins become guttered at 10–15° of elevation only when there is considerable ischaemia.

Pressure areas

Look carefully at all those areas subjected to pressure or trauma during walking or bed-rest. These are the first sites to show evidence of trophic changes, ulceration or gangrene.

Look at the **heel**, its bottom, back and lateral side. Look at the **malleoli**. Look at the skin over the **head of the fifth metatarsal**. Look at the **tips of the toes** and **between the toes**, where one toe nail rubs against the side of the next toe, and look at the **ball of the foot**. Pressure necrosis is manifest by: thickening of the skin, a purple or blue discolouration, blistering, ulceration, or patches of black, dead (gangrenous) skin.

Palpation

Temperature

The skin temperature can only be assessed reliably if both limbs have been exposed to the same ambient temperature for a full 5 minutes. Do not pull back the sheets, or uncross the patient's legs, and feel the skin straight away. Uncover the limbs and then perform some other part of the physical examination so that by the time you are ready to feel the skin temperature it has adjusted to the temperature of the surrounding air. Some clinicians find they can appreciate temperature best with the palmar surface of the hand, but most prefer to use the backs of their fingers. The sensitivity of the back of the fingers is not a neurological phenomenon but is related to the temperature of the skin of the hand. The palmar surface of the hand is usually warm and moist and, in this state, not as good a temperature sensor as the cool, dry backs of the fingers.

Move your hand over the whole limb and assess which parts are warm or cold and the level at which the changes occur. Do not assume that a blue or even a red foot will be warm; it might be very cold.

Capillary refilling

Press the tip of a nail, or the pulp of a toe or finger, for 2 seconds and then observe the time taken for the blanched area to turn pink after you have stopped pressing. This gives a crude indication of the rate of blood flow in the capillaries and the pressure within them.

Feel all the pulses

Pulses are most easily felt where an artery is superficial and crossing a bone.

In the neck, shoulder and upper limbs the carotid, subclavian, brachial and both wrist arteries are close to the skin and easy to palpate, so with the minimum of anatomical knowledge you should have no difficulty in feeling them.

The **femoral pulse** at the groin lies mid-way between the symphysis pubis (the mid-line) and the anterior superior iliac spine. The artery is so superficial that it can usually be felt even when it is pulseless.

The **foot pulses** are also easy to feel. The dorsalis pedis artery runs from a point mid-way between the malleoli to the cleft between the first and second metatarsal bones.

The **posterior tibial artery** lies one-third of the way along a line between the tip of the medial malleolus and the point of the heel, but is easier to feel 2.5 cm higher up where it runs just behind the medial malleolus.

The **popliteal pulse** is difficult to feel because it does not cross a prominent bone and is not superficial.

There are three ways to feel the popliteal pulse, and you may have to try all three before deciding if the pulse is present.

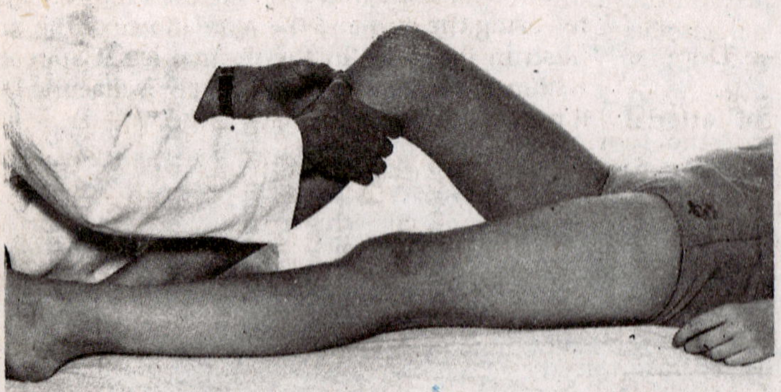

FIG. 7.1 The popliteal pulse can be felt in three ways. The method depicted here (described below) is the most convenient technique. The most reliable method, but the most inconvenient, is to turn the patient prone so that you can put the fingers of both your hands along the line of the artery

1 Flex the knee to 135°, with the heel resting on the couch. Place your thumbs on the tibial tuberosity and your fingers over the lower part of the popliteal fossa (see Fig. 7.1). Move your fingers from side to side until you catch the neurovascular bundle between them. It feels like a taut rubbery cord. Then press the bundle against the lower surface of the tibia to feel the pulse.

> **Revision Panel 7.1**
>
> **Routine for assessing the arterial circulation**
>
> *Inspection*
> - Colour:
>   - Horizontal
>   - Elevated (vascular angle)
>   - Dependent
> - Venous filling
> - Look at the pressure areas and between the digits
>
> *Palpation*
> - Skin temperature
> - Capillary refilling time
> - Palpate the pulses
>
> *Auscultation*
> - Listen for bruits
> - Measure the blood pressure
> - Reactive hyperaemia time

You cannot feel the popliteal artery above the level of the knee joint in this way because it is deep between the condyles of the femur in a large pad of fat.

2 With the leg straight, place one hand behind the knee with the finger tips along the mid-line of the popliteal fossa, and hyperextend the knee against this hand and the couch with your other hand.

3 Turn the patient into the prone position and feel along the line of the artery with the finger tips of both hands. This is the most reliable method. Whenever you are doubtful about the presence of a pulse, check its rate against your own superficial temporal pulse to make sure that you are not feeling your own finger-pulp pulses. In general if you are doubtful about a pulse, excepting the popliteal, it is probably absent.

Test the muscles and nerves

Severe ischaemia, acute or chronic, will cause loss of muscle and nerve function, producing ultimately an immobile, numb limb.

Auscultation

Listen along the course of all the major arteries. It is an important part of the routine examination to listen to the arteries in the neck, the abdomen, the groin and the thigh. If you have

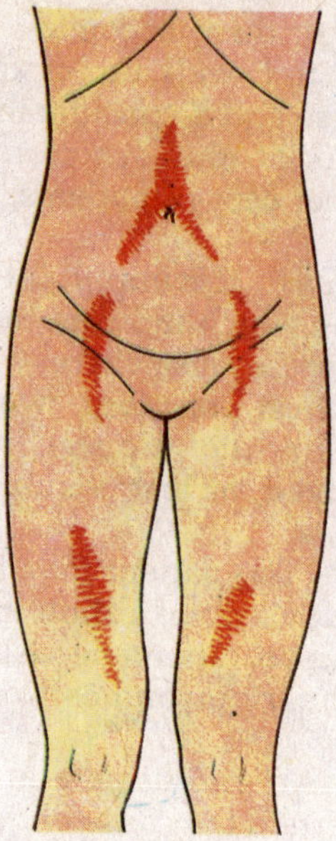

FIG. 7.2 The common sites to hear bruits over the arteries of the lower limbs

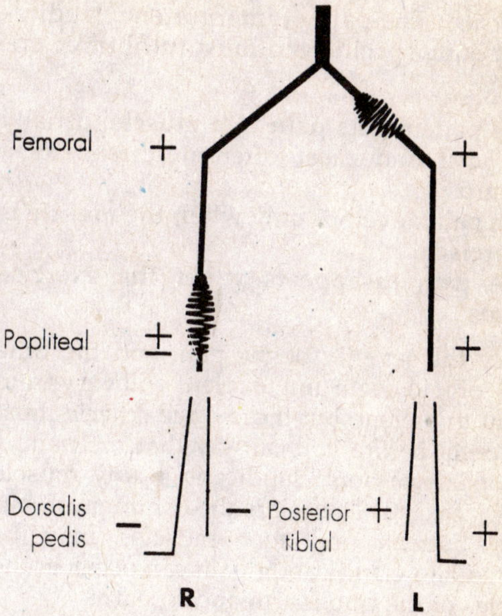

FIG. 7.3 Record the pulses and bruits on a simple diagram

any suspicion of a stenosis in an artery after feeling the pulses – listen to it.

You need a small bell on your stethoscope to listen along the line of an artery with ease. Do not press too hard over a superficial artery. Pressure can distort the artery and cause a bruit.

Bruits are caused by the vibration of the arterial wall, induced by the turbulent flow beyond a stenosis. They may change in volume and character if the blood flow through the stenosis changes.

Measure the **blood pressure in both** arms to exclude subclavian or innominate artery disease.

It is possible to measure the thigh blood pressure with a stethoscope and a sphygmomanometer, but auscultation has now been replaced by the Doppler flow detector.

An indication of the severity of arterial ischaemia can be obtained from the **reactive hyperaemia test**. Inflate a sphygmomanometer cuff around the limb to 250 mmHg for 5 minutes, and then measure the interval between releasing the cuff and the appearance of the red flush in the skin. In the normal leg it appears within 1–2 seconds. In a severely ischaemic leg it may never appear.

DISTURBANCES OF ARTERIAL BLOOD SUPPLY

Intermittent claudication

Strictly speaking 'intermittent claudication' means intermittent limping (*claudicatio* = to limp); but by common usage, albeit illogical, the term is now used to describe the muscle pain which appears during exercise when there is an inadequate arterial blood flow.

HISTORY

Age The age distribution of patients with intermittent claudication is related to the age distribution of obliterative arterial disease. Thus, although the majority of these patients are over 50 years old, some are young adults afflicted by arterial embolism, Buerger's disease or traumatic occlusion of the arteries.

Sex This complaint is ten times more common in men than women, and when caused by aortic bifurcation stenosis may be associated with impotence.

Symptoms The **pain** of intermittent claudication is quite specific and must fulfil three criteria:

1 The patient gets **pain in a muscle**, usually the calf and most often described as a cramp.
2 The pain develops only **when the muscle is exercised.**
3 The pain **disappears when the exercise stops.**

Clearly the severity of the pain and the time taken for it to begin and to relent will vary from patient to patient, but these three criteria must be present before you can say that the pain is that of intermittent claudication. Any muscle can be affected. The calf is the commonest, but thigh, buttock and foot muscles may be affected and claudication pain can occur in the muscles of the upper arm and forearm.

Pains that appear at rest, or as soon as the patient stands up, or in tissues other than muscles, and which do not abate with rest, are not claudication pains – however much they may also be related to exercise.

The patient often notices **numbness, pins and needles** and other paraesthesiae in the **skin of the foot** at the time that the muscle pain begins. This is caused by the shunting of blood from the skin to the muscle.

Limitation of walking is the principal complaint. The patient finds that he can walk a certain distance normally but then starts to develop an ache, which becomes a cramp in the muscles of his leg, that prevents him walking further.

The distance he can walk is called the **claudication distance**. Record this as accurately as possible.

Also ask how long the patient must stand still before the pain goes away and whether he can walk the same distance again.

Some patients complain of an ache which does not stop them walking and which fades away if they force themselves to continue; others find that they can prevent the pain appearing by walking slowly.

Onset and progression The pain of claudication may begin suddenly or insidiously. The latter onset is the most common, with the walking distance gradually shortening over a few months and then becoming static. In many patients the walking distance then begins to **increase** and a considerable spontaneous remission of the symptoms can be expected in 30 per cent of patients.

Systematic questions It is important to enquire about symptoms which indicate the presence of vascular disease elsewhere. Ask about **pains in the chest, fainting, weakness** or **paraesthesiae** in the upper limbs, and episodes of **blurred, or lost, vision.**

Previous history The patient may have had a previous episode of claudication in either leg which has regressed spontaneously. He may have had a **coronary thrombosis** or a **stroke**.

Family history Arterial disease is sometimes familial, so ascertain the cause of death of parents and siblings or the presence of any vascular disease symptoms. It is surprising how often you will find that all the other members of the family have arterial disease.

EXAMINATION

General appearance

Arterial disease appears in all types of patient; some are fat, some are thin. Although there is a preponderance of obese persons in those suffering from angina, there are also many thin men with severe arterial disease.

An arcus senilis, a white ring around the iris, is not diagnostic of vascular disease.

General examination

Although the main complaint is probably of pain in the legs you must examine the whole cardiovascular system with care – blood pressure, the heart, listen to the carotid arteries in the neck and feel the abdominal aorta in case it is aneurysmal.

Examination of the legs

The legs usually look remarkably normal.

Inspection The skin of the foot of the affected leg may be **pale and blanch on elevation** – but the vascular angle is usually greater than 30°. The skin colour is often normal.

Venous filling is normal except in severe cases.

The skin over the **pressure areas** should be healthy.

Palpation The foot and leg will be cooler than the normal side.

The **pulse** immediately above the affected group of muscles is likely to be weak or absent. Thus if the claudication is in the calf you will find no popliteal pulse but the femoral pulse is likely to be present. If the pain is felt in the thigh muscles the femoral pulse is likely to be absent.

Thus the level of the symptoms gives an indication of the level of the disease, but beware; it is possible to have claudication in the lower limb and normal pulses, but careful examination often reveals a bruit, and if you examine the legs after exercise the ankle pulses may have disappeared.

Auscultation The common sites to find bruits in association with intermittent claudication are at the aortic bifurcation, over the iliac and common femoral arteries and over the superficial femoral artery at the adductor hiatus.

The **musculoskeletal system** of the leg should be normal. There may be slight wasting of the affected muscles, but movement and power are normal. Remember that many of these patients are old and likely to have arthritis of the hip or knee.

The **nervous system** of the limb – motor, sensory and reflex – should be normal. This is a very important part of the examination because nerve root pains such as sciatica can mimic the pain of claudication.

Rest pain

This is a term used to describe the continuous pain caused by severe ischaemia. In contrast to the pain of intermittent claudication, which only appears during exercise, this pain is present at rest throughout the day and the night.

HISTORY

Age Most patients with arterial disease bad enough to cause rest pain are 60 or more years old, but Buerger's disease and trauma can cause rest pain in young men.

Sex The majority of patients with rest pain are men.

Symptoms The patient complains of a **continuous, severe pain, aching in nature** but bad enough to stop him sleeping and using the limb.

Rest pain usually occurs in the most distal part of the limb – **the toes and the forefoot**. If there is associated gangrene the patient feels the pain at the junction of the living and the dead tissues.

Rest pain is often relieved by putting the leg below the level of the heart. The patient **hangs his leg over the side of the bed**, and prefers to sleep sitting in a chair.

The painful part is very sensitive, and movement or pressure cause an acute exacerbation. When in bed the patient often sits with the knee bent, holding the foot still to try to relieve the pain, but strong analgesic drugs are the only substances that will give any relief.

Rest pain is usually unremitting and if not relieved gets steadily worse until the patient asks for an amputation.

Systematic questions The patient may have suffered from intermittent claudication in the affected limb for many years before the onset of rest pain.

There may be symptoms of arterial disease elsewhere, such as angina, muscle weakness, and transient loss of vision.

There may be symptoms of diabetes – polyuria, thirst, loss of weight, weakness and fatigue.

Previous history Many of these elderly patients have had strokes and myocardial infarctions in the past. Some have had rest pain or claudication in one or both legs which has been treated successfully or perhaps necessitated amputation.

The patient may have diabetes.

Family history There may be a family history of vascular disease.

EXAMINATION

General appearance

The patient looks drawn and haggard – the effect of continuous pain and sleepless nights. Most have lost some weight and less than half are obese and overweight.

The patient will be unwilling to lie flat on a couch with the leg horizontal for more than a short period because it makes the pain worse.

General examination

Examine the whole of the cardiovascular system with care. Hypertension and vascular bruits are common findings.

Local examination

Inspection **When dependent** the painful foot will be a deep **reddish-purple** colour. The tips of the toes may be **grey** or white if they are completely bloodless. There may be black patches of gangrene on the toes or the heel.

When horizontal the foot will be pale or marble white, and the veins will be empty and guttered. Elevation of the leg increases the pallor. If the foot is not white when horizontal it will certainly become so when elevated to 20°.

It is possible to have severely ischaemic **toes** and a good circulation in the rest of the foot. In these circumstances the description above applies to the toes only.

If the whole foot is painful but stays pink above an angle of 20°, the pain is unlikely to be an ischaemic pain. The 20° angle corresponds to a pressure in the small ankle vessels of approximately 30 mmHg. If the ankle pressure is above this level the tissues are not usually painful, although there may be severe claudication.

If the patient has been sitting with the leg dependent (to ease the pain), the foot may be swollen, but if he has been resting in bed it will be thin and look atrophic.

Look at the **pressure areas**. Pay particular attention to the heel and the skin between the toes. These areas may be gangrenous, ulcerated, or infected. There may be infection under the nails.

Palpation The skin temperature from the midcalf downwards is usually reduced even when the foot is dependent and congested. **Capillary refilling** is retarded.

There is no fixed pattern of pulselessness with rest pain. It is possible for a patient to have no palpable pulses in a leg and have no symptoms, or all the pulses present down to the ankle and have rest pain in all his toes.

In general, rest pain is caused by a combination of large- and small-vessel disease, so it is common to find that the popliteal or the femoral pulse is absent. If they are present you must suspect small vessel disease, and the most likely causes are diabetes or Buerger's disease.

Auscultation Bruits are commonly heard over the iliac and femoral pulses. It is often the appearance of disease in these large vessels in the presence of a blockage lower down the limb which precipitates the rest pain.

The **musculoskeletal system** should be normal; but there may be muscle wasting caused by disuse, and if the patient has been sitting holding his foot for many weeks there may be a **fixed flexion deformity** of the knee or hip joint.

The **nervous system** of the limb will be normal except when the arterial disease is secondary to long-standing diabetes. In these cases there may be loss of deep and superficial sensation caused by diabetic peripheral neuropathy. Patients with severe diabetic neuropathy do not get pain from their ischaemic tissues because they have lost all pain sensation.

Pregangrene and gangrene

The term **pregangrene** is used by clinicians to describe the changes in a tissue which indicate that its blood supply is so precarious that it will soon be inadequate to keep the tissue alive.

The principal symptom of pregangrene is **rest pain**, which is described in detail above.

The principal signs are: pallor of the tissue when elevated, congestion when dependent, guttering of the veins, atrophic changes manifest in thickening and scaling of the skin and wasting of the pulps of the toes or fingers, coldness and poor capillary refilling. Ischaemic tissues are tender.

Many textbooks state that loss of hair on the skin of the lower legs and toes is a sign of ischaemia. It is a useless and unreliable sign, so forget about it.

Those symptoms and signs already described in association with rest pain indicate that the tissue is balanced on a knife-edge between life and death. Any further reduction of the blood supply will result in tissue death – gangrene. Hence these symptoms must be treated with the utmost urgency and energy.

Gangrene is the term used to describe dead tissue (see Figs 7.4 and 7.5).

Dead tissue is **brown or black** and gradually contracts into a **crinkled, withered, hard mass.** These changes can happen to a patch of skin, a toe, or the whole of the lower limb.

The dead part is **senseless** and **not painful.**

The junction between dead and living tissues gradually becomes distinct and is known as the **line of demarcation**. If left alone the dead tissue may eventually fall off. The living tissue on the proximal side of the line of demarcation is likely to be ischaemic and so it is often painful and tender. It may give rise to rest pain. This does not happen when the gangrene is due to local trauma and the surrounding tissues are normal.

The areas of skin most likely to become gangrenous, secondary to vascular disease, are the extremities of the limbs (the tips of the toes and fingers) and areas subjected to pressure.

If the dead tissue becomes infected then it does not become shrivelled and hard but **soft and boggy. Pus** appears at the line of demarcation.

A hard, non-infected patch of gangrene is sometimes called **dry gangrene**. A soft infected patch of gangrene is sometimes called **wet gangrene**. These are not very useful names. It is better to talk about gangrene which is infected or non-infected. This difference is important because in some instances (particularly in diabetes) the gangrene is actually secondary to the infection.

Ischaemic ulceration

An ischaemic ulcer is the aftermath of gangrene because an ulcer – whether superficial or deep – can only occur if part of the skin is removed or dies. By definition, an ischaemic ulcer is an ulcer caused by an inadequate blood supply.

HISTORY

Ischaemic ulcers are common in the elderly, but can occur in the young following trauma. The elderly often have symptoms of coronary or cerebral vascular disease.

Symptoms Ischaemic ulcers – except those associated with a neurological abnormality – are very **painful**. They cause **rest pain**.

They do not bleed much, but discharge a thin serous exudate which is sometimes purulent.

The patient sometimes remembers a minor precipitating injury.

They show no sign of healing and, despite the patient's care and attention, often get slowly deeper and larger. Ischaemic ulcers near joints may penetrate into the joint, making joint movements very painful.

The causes of ischaemic ulcers are:

1 **Large-artery obliteration**: atherosclerosis, embolism.
2 **Small-artery obliteration**: Raynaud's disease, scleroderma, Buerger's disease, embolism, diabetes and physical agents such as pressure necrosis, radiation, trauma and electric burns.

Systematic questions and past history These often indicate the presence of long-standing generalized vascular disease.

Revision Panel 7.2

The symptoms and signs of acute ischaemia

Pain, becoming

Painless (numb)

Pallor

Paralysis

Pulseless

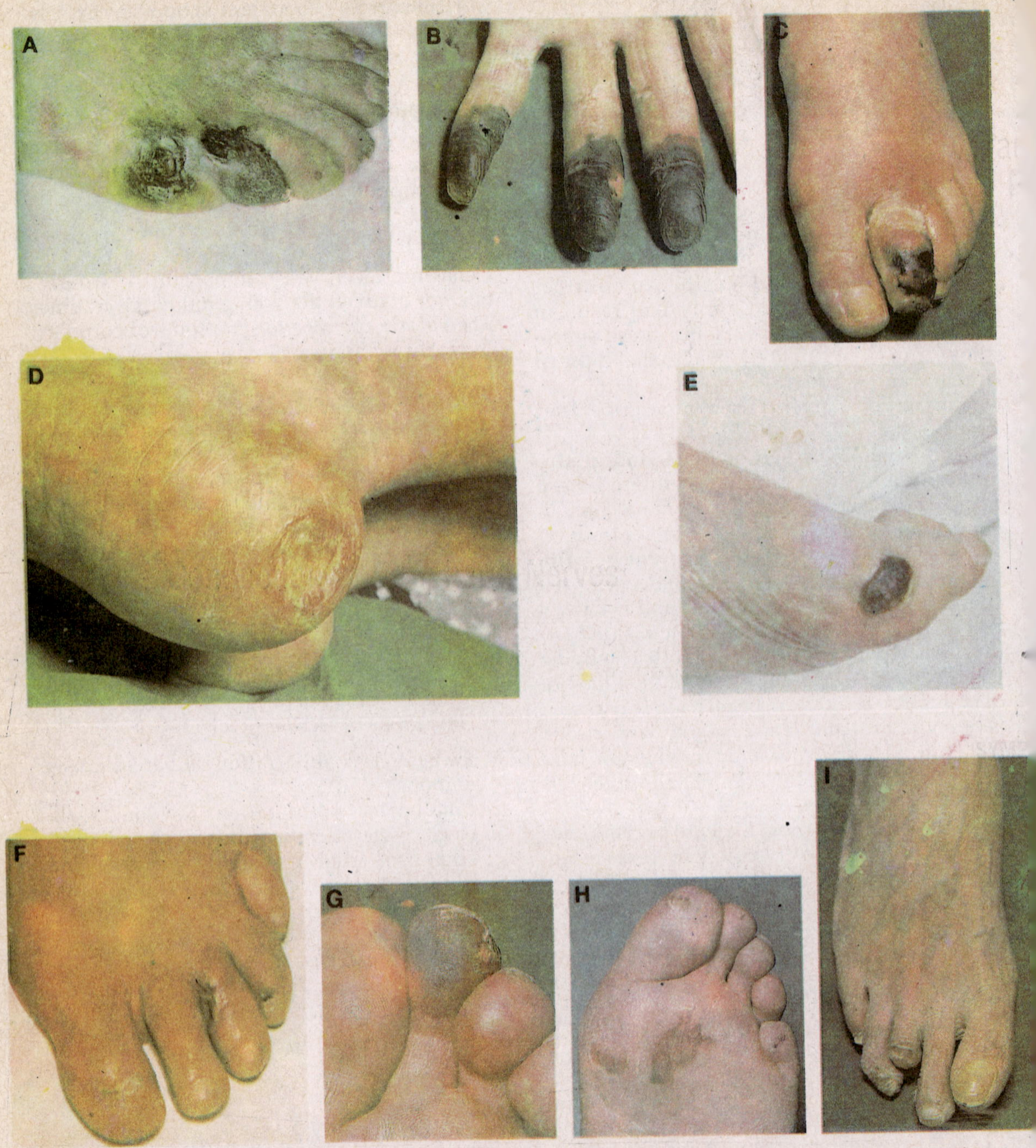

FIG. 7.4 The common sites and causes of gangrene. **A**: Gangrene of the fifth toe caused by atherosclerotic obstruction of the iliac and femoral arteries. **B**: Gangrene of the finger tips caused by emboli from a subclavian aneurysm. **C**: Infected (wet) gangrene caused by a mixture of infection and mild ischaemia in a diabetic. **D**: Pressure necrosis on the heel following a prolonged period of unconsciousness (normal circulation). **E**: Pressure necrosis over a slight bunion caused by a tight bandage and mild occlusive vascular disease. **F**: Infected gangrene between the second and third left toes in a diabetic. **G**: A blue ischaemic toe caused by emboli from a femoral artery stenosis. **H**: Multiple ischaemic areas on the sole of the foot caused by emboli from the left side of the heart. **I**: Long-standing ischaemia of the toes with gangrene of the third toe that has proceeded to autoamputation

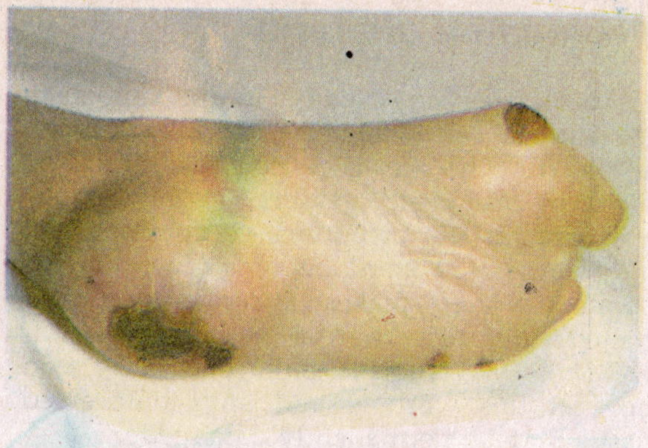

FIG. 7.5 An ischaemic foot with patches of gangrene on all the pressure areas: the heel, the head of the first metatarsal and the base of the fifth metatarsal

LOCAL EXAMINATION

Position Ischaemic ulcers secondary to vascular disease are found at the tips of the toes (or fingers) and over the pressure areas.

Tenderness The ulcer and the surrounding tissues are very tender. Removing a dressing can cause an exacerbation of the pain that lasts 2–3 hours.

Temperature The surrounding tissues are usually cold because they, too, are ischaemic. Warm, healthy tissues suggest that the ulcer is due to local factors.

Size Ischaemic ulcers can be any size from small, deep lesions 1–2 mm across to large, flat ulcers on the lower leg, 10 cm in diameter.

Edge The edge of an ischaemic ulcer is punched-out (square-cut) because there is no attempt at healing by the surrounding tissues. If healing does begin, the edge becomes sloping. The skin at the edge of the ulcer is usually a blue–grey colour.

Base The base may contain grey–yellow sloughing tissue and is often infected. If all the slough has separated, the base has a flat, pale pink colour. The tissue forming the base has a blood supply but it is not sufficient to support the growth of healthy red granulation tissue.

Revision Panel 7.3
The causes of ischaemic ulceration

Large-artery obliteration
- Atherosclerosis
- Embolism

Small-artery obliteration
- Raynaud's disease
- Scleroderma
- Buerger's disease
- Embolism
- Diabetes
- Physical agents:
  - Pressure necrosis
  - Radiation
  - Trauma
  - Electric burns

Revision Panel 7.4
The clinical features of an ulcer

The ulcer

Position	Shape
Number	Size
Tenderness	Edge
Temperature	Base
	Depth
	Discharge

The surrounding tissues
- Relations
- State of adjacent glands
- Local circulation
- Local innervation

Revision Panel 7.5
The causes of chronic ulceration

Infection

Repeated trauma

Ischaemia

Oedema

Denervation

Localized destructive disease (tuberculosis, carcinoma)

Depth Ischaemic ulcers are often very deep, penetrating down to bone and into the underlying joints.

They may ramify beneath the skin because subcutaneous tissue is more susceptible to ischaemia plus infection than skin.

Discharge The discharge is either clear fluid (serum) or pus. It is unlikely to be heavily blood-stained.

Relations The base may be stuck to, or be part of, any underlying structure. It is not uncommon to see **bare bone, ligaments and tendons** exposed in the base of an ischaemic ulcer.

Lymph drainage Any infection in the ulcer is usually localized to the ulcer, so the local lymph glands (groin or axilla) are not normally enlarged.

State of the local tissues The surrounding tissues may show signs of ischaemia – pallor, coldness and atrophy.

The **pulses** may be absent. There may be loss of **superficial and deep sensation**, weakness of movement and loss of reflexes.

It is **essential to examine the nerves of the limb** of any patient presenting with an ischaemic ulcer.

GENERAL EXAMINATION

Look for signs of vascular disease elsewhere. Look for evidence of neurological abnormalities. **Test the urine** for sugar.

Revision Panel 7.6

The causes of neuropathic ulceration

(Ulcers secondary to a loss of sensation)

Peripheral nerve lesions
- Diabetes
- Nerve injuries
- Leprosy

Spinal cord lesions
- Spina bifida
- Tabes dorsalis
- Syringomyelia

Neuropathic ulceration

Tissue ischaemia is usually painful. Pain is the mechanism by which the body knows when any part of the skin is becoming deprived of blood by prolonged pressure.

When our feet or buttocks become painful after prolonged standing or sitting the discomfort we feel makes us move about and remove the pressure from the painful part. If we do not have normal pain sensation we do not get this warning and any compressed tissue may be permanently damaged.

Neuropathic ulcers are, therefore, only indirectly caused by local ischaemia; the main cause is the lack of sensation in the tissue.

Neuropathic ulcers are deep penetrating ulcers, similar to ischaemic ulcers. They occur over pressure areas (see Fig. 7.6), but the surrounding tissues are **healthy** and have a good circulation.

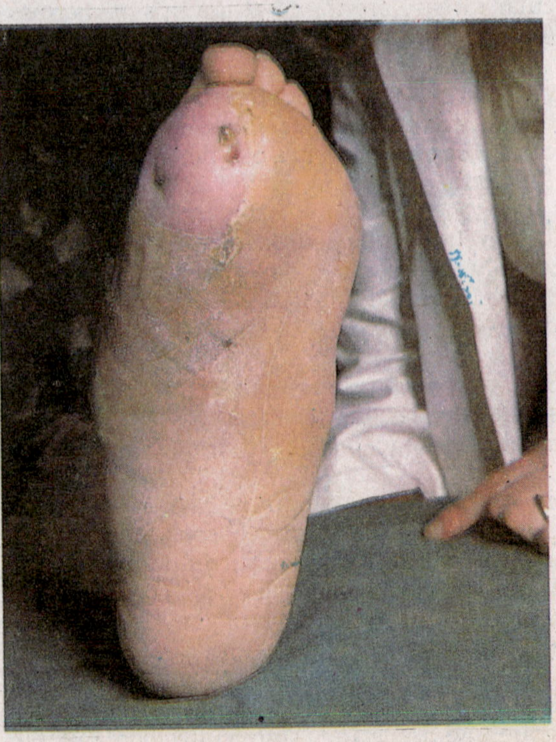

FIG. 7.6 Trophic ulcers on the sole of the foot in a patient with diabetic peripheral neuritis. The circulation was good and all the pulses were present, but there was a total loss of pain sensation. The great toe had been amputated 2 years earlier for similar ulceration

Their three diagnostic features are:

1 They are **painless.**
2 The surrounding tissues are unable to appreciate pain.
3 The surrounding tissues have a normal blood supply.

These ulcers can easily be mistaken for ischaemic ulcers, hence the importance of a full neurological examination.

The causes of neuropathic ulceration are:

1 **Peripheral nerve lesions:** diabetes, nerve injuries, leprosy.
2 **Spinal cord lesions:** spina bifida, tabes dorsalis, syringomyelia.

Diabetes can be associated with both true ischaemic ulcers (because of large-vessel atherosclerosis) and neuropathic ulcers (because of peripheral neuritis). It is sometimes difficult to decide the prime cause of an ulcer in such cases.

Aneurysms

An aneurysm is a dilatation of the whole or part of an artery. The majority of aneurysms are associated with, and probably caused by, atherosclerosis.

The causes of aneurysms are as follows:

1 **True aneurysms.**
Congenital: **Weak areas** (berry aneurysm).
Weak walls (Marfan's syndrome, Ehlers–Danlos syndrome).
Arterial dilatation associated with a congenital arteriovenous fistula.
Acquired: **Trauma:** direct injuries, irradiation.
Infection: non-specific bacterial arteritis (often called mycotic), syphilis.
Degeneration: atherosclerosis, arteriomegaly, cystic medionecrosis.
2 **False aneurysms.**
Following trauma.

Although an aneurysm can occur in any artery there are a few common sites.

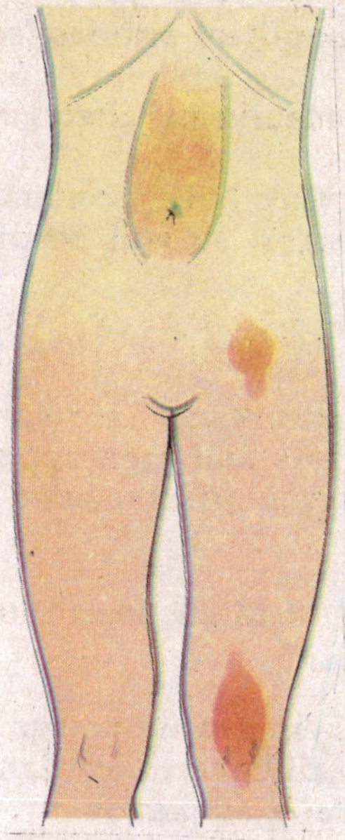

The common sites to find aneurysms

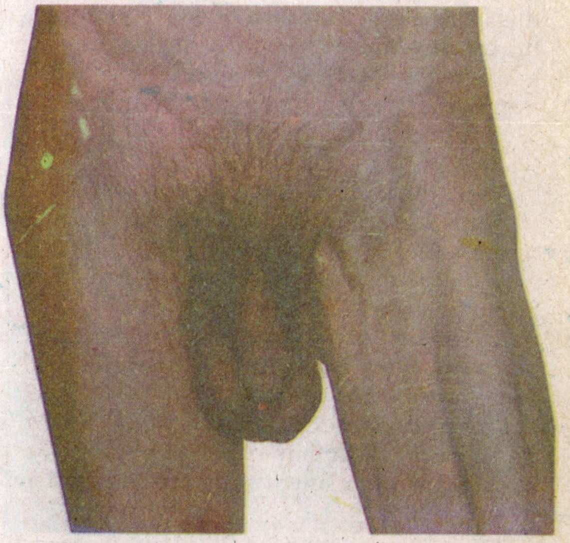
An aneurysm of the left common femoral artery compressing the femoral vein and causing distention of the long saphenous vein

FIG. 7.7 ANEURYSMS

Congenital aneurysms occur within the skull on the circle of Willis. They cause subarachnoid haemorrhages and sudden death.

Acquired atherosclerotic aneurysms are usually found in the **abdominal aorta** and the

common femoral and popliteal arteries (see Fig. 7.7).

Acquired syphilitic aneurysms affect the thoracic aorta.

Atherosclerotic aneurysms have a common set of symptoms and signs, so will be discussed collectively.

HISTORY

Age Atherosclerotic aneurysms are rare before the age of 50 years and then appear with increasing frequency in direct relation to age.

Sex Men are affected 10 to 20 times more often than women.

Symptoms Many aneurysms cause no symptoms during life and are discovered by chance during a routine physical examination.

The commonest presenting symptom is a **dull aching pain**. With abdominal aneurysms, this is usually a dull ache over the swelling in the centre of the abdomen. It does not radiate, is not relieved or exacerbated by any natural event, and is often thought to be indigestion. This pain is caused by stretching of the artery wall.

Aneurysms may also cause pain in the back if they press upon and erode the bodies of the vertebrae.

Acute pain can occur if the vessel suddenly stretches or begins to tear.

A severe pain, bursting in nature, is common when an aneurysm ruptures and a large haematoma forms.

Referred pain caused by pressure on a nerve is not uncommon. Some patients with abdominal aortic aneurysms present with **sciatica**.

Some patients notice a **pulsatile mass**. This is a common presentation for femoral and popliteal aneurysms, but not so common for the abdominal aortic aneurysm.

Severe ischaemia of the lower limb will follow thrombosis of an aneurysm. This is a rare event in aortic and femoral aneurysms but a common occurrence with popliteal aneurysms. Less severe ischaemia is often caused by **emboli** originating in the aneurysm. One of the best examples of this complication is the multiple small emboli which block the digital arteries from a subclavian aneurysm. In the lower limb the patient may complain of intermittent claudication or rest pain.

Venous thrombosis and obstruction may occur. The aorta, femoral and popliteal arteries are closely related to the vena cava, femoral and popliteal veins. Enlargement of the artery can block the vein by direct pressure or cause it to **thrombose**. The patient presents with a **swollen, blue, painful limb or calf**.

Systematic questions and past history These often reveal evidence of coronary or cerebral vascular disease or previous aneurysms. Femoral and popliteal aneurysms are often bilateral but do not necessarily appear at the same time.

EXAMINATION

Abdominal aneurysms

The abdominal aorta divides into the iliac arteries at the level of the umbilicus, and so abdominal aortic aneurysms are found in the umbilical and epigastric regions. Their distinctive feature is that they have an **expansile pulsation**. It is essential to put your hands on either side of the mass to confirm that the

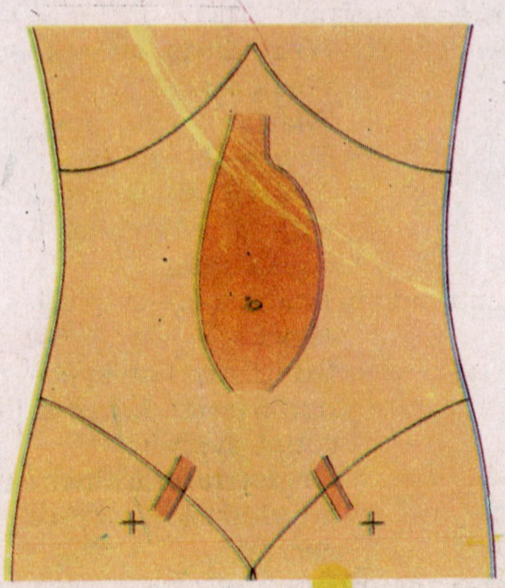

FIG. 7.8 The abdominal aortic aneurysm. If there is a gap between the top of the aneurysm and the costal margin, the aneurysm probably begins below the origin of the renal arteries. The femoral pulses are usually palpable

swelling is expanding. Many lumps in the upper abdomen – particularly carcinoma of the pancreas and stomach – have a transmitted pulsation and are misdiagnosed as aneurysms.

Aneurysms are often tender; they are usually firm, not compressible and immobile. Sometimes an elongated and dilated aorta will move from side to side.

The **pulses** at the groins and in the legs are usually **present**; in fact these arteries are often slightly dilated.

Most students expect to find blocked peripheral arteries when they discover an aneurysm. This is *not* a common combination of abnormalities.

When an aneurysm **ruptures** it becomes tender and the patient may show the signs of hypovolaemia – pallor, tachycardia and hypotension. If the blood leaking from the aneurysm spreads laterally or downwards it may be palpable as a soft mass in the loin or iliac fossa.

Femoral aneurysms

These are usually in the common femoral artery and bulge forwards just below the inguinal ligament. They are so superficial that it is difficult to miss their pulsatility, but it is still important to confirm that the pulsation is **expansile**. A mass of enlarged lymph nodes may have a marked transmitted pulsation and be misdiagnosed as an aneurysm.

The other pulses in the leg may be absent or there may be a popliteal aneurysm.

Examine the limb carefully for any evidence of arterial insufficiency or venous obstruction.

Popliteal aneurysms

Aneurysms of the popliteal artery are noticed once they are large enough to bulge out of the popliteal fossa. They have usually been present for some time and may have caused many of the symptoms described above.

Once again the diagnosis is obvious provided you make sure that the pulsation is **expansile**.

Thrombosed popliteal aneurysms are more difficult to diagnose and may be confused with a Baker's cyst or a semimembranosus bursa.

The lump is solid, dull to percussion and does not fluctuate. It may move slightly from side to side but not up and down and its size does not change when the knee is flexed.

The ankle pulses will not be palpable if the aneurysm is thrombosed, and are often not palpable when it is pulsating because of stenotic disease or emboli blocking the popliteal trifurcation.

Examine the leg carefully for evidence of venous obstruction. Popliteal vein thrombo-sis is a common complication of popliteal aneurysms.

False aneurysms

A false aneurysm is a large haematoma whose centre contains fluid blood which is in direct connection with the lumen of a blood vessel (see Fig. 7.9).

The common cause is a stab wound. A haematoma forms outside the artery and thrombus plugs the hole in the artery, but the pulsatile blood pressure gradually forces the haemostatic plug outwards into the haematoma to form a cavity connected to the lumen of the vessel.

Revision Panel 7.7

The causes of aneurysms

True

Congenital

- Weak area (berry aneurysm)
- Arterial dilatation associated with an arteriovenous fistula

Acquired

- Trauma:
  - Direct injuries
  - Irradiation
- Infection:
  - Non-specific bacterial (often called mycotic)
  - Syphilis
- Degeneration:
  - Atherosclerosis
  - Arteriomegaly
  - Cystic medionecrosis

False

Following trauma

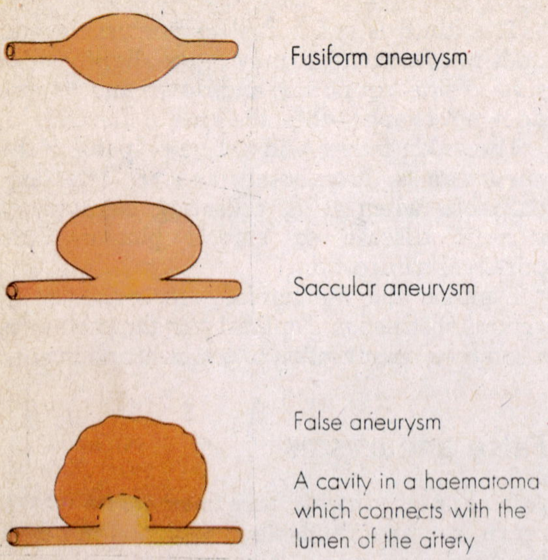

FIG. 7.9 The types of aneurysm

The symptoms, signs and complications of a false aneurysm are exactly the same as those of true aneurysms, except for:

1 A history of trauma. (This is not always remembered.)
2 Sudden appearance of the swelling after the trauma.
3 An aneurysm at an unusual site, e.g. wrist or ankle.

Coarctation of the aorta

This is not a common condition, but it is important to know its physical signs because if it can be discovered when it is symptomless it can be corrected surgically and so prolong the patient's life.

Coarctation is a narrowing of the aorta just beyond the origin of the left subclavian artery close to the site of the ligamentum arteriosum, the remnant of the ductus arteriosus.

Provided the ductus arteriosus closes normally a coarctation often causes no symptoms until adult life (hence the need to be aware of its physical signs); but if the ductus arteriosus is patent the patient will have symptoms and often has other cardiac abnormalities.

The common symptoms which usually begin in adult life are **dyspnoea on exertion**, and **cerebrovascular accidents**, both caused by hypertension in the upper half of the body in the vessels proximal to the coarctation.

Examination reveals hypertension in the brachial arteries; visible and palpable collateral arteries in the shoulders and around the scapulae; weak and delayed femoral pulses; a strong cardiac impulse and a systolic murmur, loudest posteriorly to the left of the vertebral column at the level of T4 and T5.

The detection of the unexpected coarctation is another reason for always feeling the femoral pulses during a routine examination.

Congenital vascular deformities

The vascular deformities seen in the skin (e.g. strawberry naevi) are discussed in Chapter 2. Congenital abnormalities of major vessels are rare. They present in two main forms: multiple arteriovenous fistulae, and abnormalities of the venous system.

Multiple arteriovenous fistulae

(Robertson's giant limb)

The effect of the abnormal fistulae is to increase the blood flow through the leg and to increase the cardiac output and blood volume.

These changes cause overgrowth of the leg and heart failure.

The principal local symptom is **overgrowth of the whole** of the lower limb, in length and volume. The skin of the leg is **warmer** than the normal side and **pinker**.

Small ulcers may develop around the ankle.

The heart enlarges and left ventricular failure may develop.

Occluding the circulation of the limb with a sphygmomanometer cuff causes a bradycardia because it increases the peripheral resistance (**Branham's bradycardic response**).

Venous abnormalities

(Klippel–Trénaunay syndrome)

These abnormalities take a variety of forms but the principal signs are:

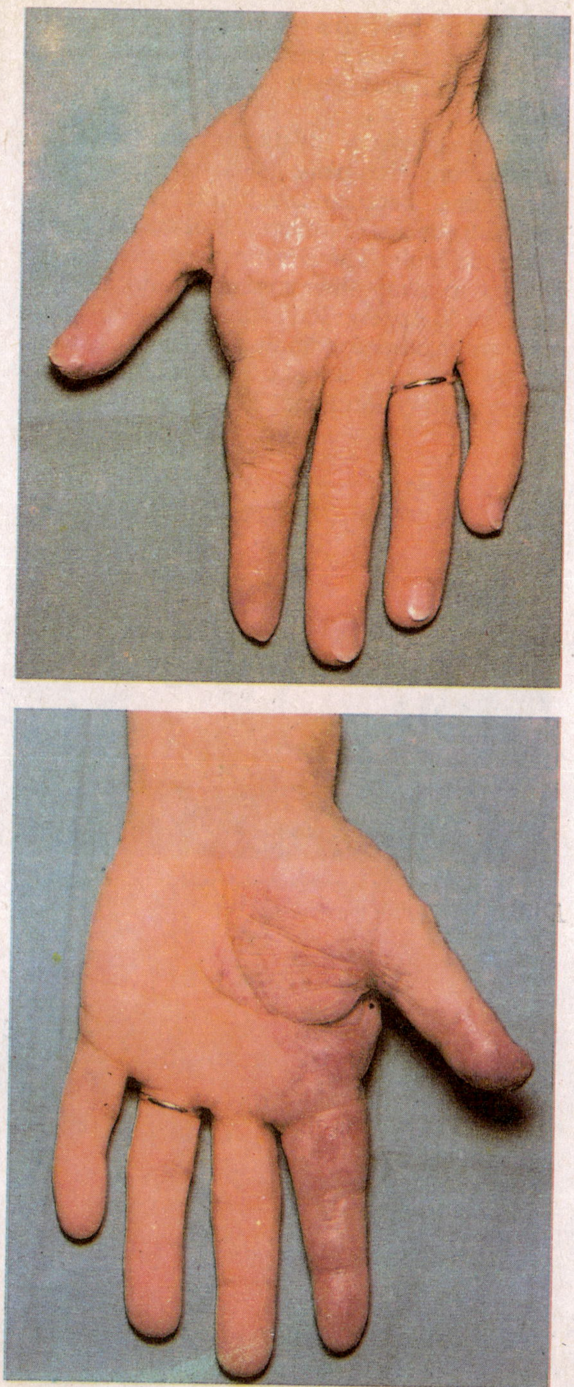

FIG. 7.10 A congenital arteriovenous fistula of the hand. The index finger and thenar eminence are enlarged, the veins are distended and the thenar eminence is pulsatile. There is ischaemic ulceration on the tip of the thumb. A bruit could be heard, on auscultation, all over the hand

1 Dilated, varicose veins (often large vessels running down the lateral side of the leg).
2 Cutaneous angiomata, port-wine stains.
3 Overgrowth of the limb.

In these cases there is no arteriovenous shunt so the heart is normal and the bradycardia test negative.

Transient cerebral and retinal ischaemia

The sudden reduction of cerebral or retinal blood flow can cause a mild stroke, paraesthesiae and fainting, or a transient loss of vision.

These attacks are often called transient ischaemic attacks (TIAs). The disadvantage of this term is that it does not indicate which tissue is being made ischaemic.

Do not forget that the right side of the brain controls the left side of the body, and vice versa. Disease in the right carotid artery may therefore cause symptoms in the right eye and left arm and leg.

Transient cerebral ischaemia is caused by small emboli from the heart or great vessels or transient hypotension, as in Stokes–Adams attacks.

Small emboli most often come from an atheromatous stenosis or ulcer at the origin of the carotid bifurcation. If such a lesion is left untreated it may cause a major stroke, so it is important to be aware of the significance of the early symptoms.

When anyone presents with brief episodes of weakness, tingling or pins and needles, or loss of sensation on one side of the body, which last for a few minutes and then fully recover, remember the possibility of carotid artery disease and **listen over the carotid artery**. There is likely to be a **bruit** which is maximal at the level of the hyoid bone.

Transient monocular blindness (amaurosis fugax) is also often caused by emboli from the carotid artery. The patient suddenly sees a grey veil cutting out the whole or part of the vision of one eye. This lasts a minute or so and then returns to normal.

Again, examine the carotid artery and listen for **bruits**.

Also examine the visual fields – there may be some permanent defects. Look at the fundi with an ophthalmoscope – if there have been previous emboli you may see an artery which suddenly gets narrow, and at the narrowing some yellow–white exudate.

Transient blindness can also be caused by migraine, multiple sclerosis, temporal arteritis and hysteria.

Raynaud's phenomenon

Raynaud's phenomenon is a series of colour changes in the skin of the hands or feet following exposure to the cold (see also page 142).

The skin first turns **white**, and becomes cold and numb. It next turns **blue**, but remains cold and numb; and lastly turns **red, hot and painful.**

The diagnosis of the phenomenon is usually made from the patient's description of her symptoms, because the hands look normal between attacks. The diagnosis of the cause is far more difficult. These symptoms can be secondary to many other conditions and the diagnosis of idiopathic Raynaud's disease is made only when other conditions have been excluded.

The causes of Raynaud's phenomenon are given in Revision Panel 7.8.

Revision Panel 7.8

The causes of Raynaud's phenomenon

Irritation of nerves
- * Cervical spondylosis and cervical disc protrusion
- * Cervical rib
- Thoracic outlet syndrome
- Spinal cord diseases
- Old poliomyelitis

Platelet emboli from:
- Subclavian aneurysm (secondary to cervical rib)
- Atherosclerotic stenosis of subclavian artery
- Damaged subclavian artery crossing a cervical rib

Collagen diseases
- * Scleroderma

Vibrating tools

Repeated immersion in cold water

Blood abnormalities
- Cold agglutinins
- Cryoglobulins

Cold sensitivity
- * Primary Raynaud's disease

Drugs
- Ergot

General diseases
- Hypothyroidism
- Diabetes
- Malnutrition

* Common causes

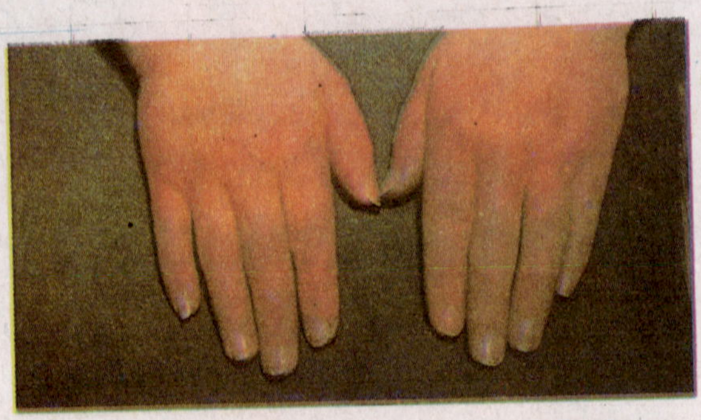

Hands showing the transition from the blue to the red phase. Ten minutes earlier the fingers of both hands had been white and numb

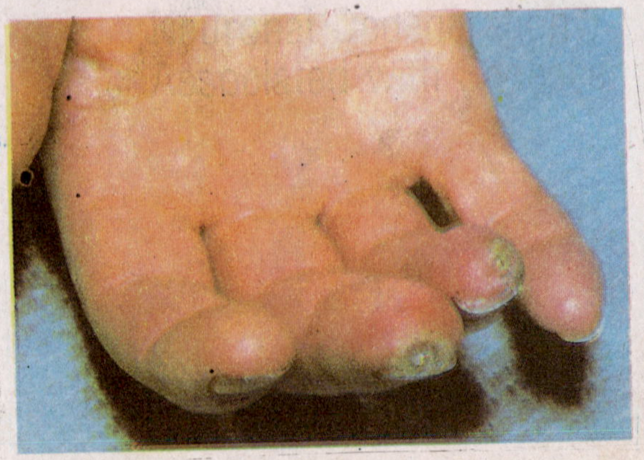

Ischaemic ulceration of the finger tips. This usually indicates permanent, rather than spastic, occlusion of the digital vessels

FIG. 7.11 RAYNAUD'S PHENOMENON

The common causes of Raynaud's phenomenon are cervical spondylosis, scleroderma, cervical rib and idiopathic Raynaud's disease.

Patients with **cervical spondylosis** are likely to have pain and discomfort on moving the neck, limitation of neck movements and, sometimes, neurological abnormalities in the arm or hand.

Patients with **scleroderma** may have visible changes in their skin and face, and dysphagia (see Fig. 8.10 on page 207).

Cervical ribs are rarely detectable on clinical examination, though they may be suspected if there is a fullness in the supraclavicular fossa.

The effect of long-standing Raynaud's phenomenon

Repeated episodes of digital artery spasm or temporary blockage by emboli damage the tissues of the fingers. Ultimately the digital artery stays blocked with embolus or thrombus.

The fingers waste, especially the pulps, to become thin and pointed. The hand is cold and the joints stiff.

Small scars appear following necrosis of small areas of skin. Sometimes there are small, very painful **ischaemic ulcers** on the finger tips.

Repeated infections around the nails (paronychia) are common. They are very painful and slow to heal.

The patient may eventually get **rest pain** and **gangrene** of the finger tips.

In long-standing disease it is not uncommon to see the gradual appearance of signs of scleroderma – evidence that the symptoms, though present for many years, have been a secondary not a primary phenomenon (see Fig. 5.8 on page 143).

Primary Raynaud's disease is quite common in teenage girls. It is mild, familial, often associated with chilblains and often disappears in the late twenties. A few women have symptoms all their life and very rarely the disease becomes severe.

When the phenomenon starts in adult women, often around the menopause, it is unlikely to be the primary disease, but likely to herald the appearance of scleroderma.

Acrocyanosis

This is a condition in which the hands and feet are persistently blue and cold. The colour of the skin does not vary with the environmental temperature as it does in Raynaud's phenomenon, but the blueness may come and go, leaving the hands pink and normal between attacks.

The hands are not painful but are susceptible to chilblains.

The diagnosis is based solely on the temperature and colour of the skin.

Erythrocyanosis crurum puellarum frigida

This condition occurs in young girls 15–25 years old, in response to cold. The lower **posterior and medial aspect of the lower leg becomes red–blue** (erythrocyanosis) and **swollen**. The swollen area is tender and susceptible to **chilblains** and **superficial ulceration**. Often the swelling is more noticeable than the discolouration, and if it spreads around the ankle it can be mistaken for lymphoedema. This is a form of cold sensitivity on a part of the leg frequently exposed to the wind, rain and cold.

Venous and lymphatic disease

CLINICAL ASSESSMENT OF THE VENOUS CIRCULATION OF THE LOWER LIMB

The history and examination of the venous circulation of the lower limb gives you information on two features of this circulation – whether it is adequate in cross-sectional area to allow a normal outflow of blood from the limb, and whether the valves ensure one-way flow. With these objects in mind, perform the examination in the routine way.

The common symptoms of venous disease are pain, swelling and changes of the skin of the lower leg. These are discussed fully in the description of individual diseases.

Inspection

Ask the patient to stand up (veins are collapsed when lying down).

The majority of patients with venous disease have abnormal **visible subcutaneous** veins. If these veins are dilated and tortuous they are called varicose veins.

It is important to note their size and course, and record this on a drawing of the leg. The site often gives a good indication of their cause.

Some veins are very large and prominent, others may be minute and intradermal so that they cause a blue patch. If these patches are carefully inspected you will see that they consist of minute veins radiating from a single feeding vein. They are often called **venous stars.**

Compare the size of the legs, especially at ankle level, for evidence of **oedema.**

Inspect the skin of the whole leg but particularly the lower medial one-third of the lower leg. Venous disease affects this area first, causing pigmentation, **eczema and ulceration.**

Palpation

Feel along the course of the veins and feel the tension in the veins. The veins in the lower leg often lie in a gutter of indurated subcutaneous tissue.

Feel at the sapheno-femoral and the sapheno-popliteal junctions, and ask the patient to cough. A strong **cough impulse** indicates that the valves in the subcutaneous veins that protect these junctions are incompetent.

Feel along the medial side of the lower leg, with the patient standing, and then lying flat, for tender defects in the deep fascia. Such areas are often the site of incompetent superficial to deep communicating veins.

The important sites at which the superficial and deep systems are connected are shown in Fig. 7.12.

Palpate the skin of the lower leg. Look for pitting **oedema**, and thickening and tenderness of the subcutaneous tissues.

Brown pigmentation caused by the loss of red blood cells into the tissues, **eczema** and **ulceration** will be obvious.

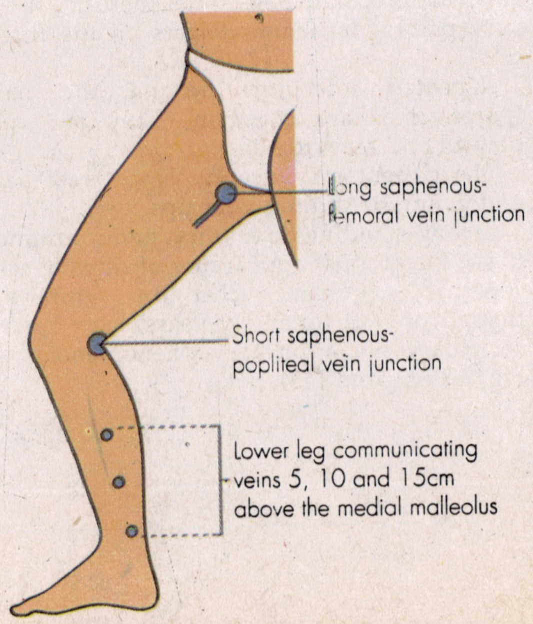

FIG. 7.12 The common sites where the superficial veins connect with the deep veins

Tourniquet tests

These are designed to reveal the presence and site of incompetent valves, in particular the valves in the veins that connect the deep to the superficial veins.

Lie the patient flat. Elevate one leg until all the blood has drained from the superficial veins.

Place a rubber tourniquet around the upper third of the thigh, tight enough to occlude the superficial veins.

Ask the patient to stand up.

If the veins above the tourniquet fill up but those below it stay collapsed, there must be an incompetent communicating vein above the tourniquet. If the veins below the tourniquet fill rapidly there must be an incompetent communicating vein below it.

Figures 7.13 and 7.14 explain how this test works. It is possible to use a number of tourniquets at once or move one tourniquet progressively down the leg and so define the segment of the limb which contains the incompetent communicating vein.

When the anatomical site of the communication between superficial and deep veins is known (e.g. the long saphenous–femoral vein junction), it is possible to compress it with direct digital pressure to see if this prevents retrograde filling, instead of using a tourniquet. When this is done for the long saphenous vein it is called the **Trendelenburg test**.

When you raise the limb, check that the veins collapse when they are above the level of the heart. If they do not collapse, the outflow from the limb must be obstructed or the pressure abnormally high because of increased blood flow.

Percussion

When the veins are full they transmit a percussion wave along them. The larger the vein and the fewer the valves, the better this wave is transmitted. It is more significant if a percussion wave is transmitted from above downwards, as this implies absent or incompetent valves.

Place the fingers of one hand on the lower limit of the visible veins and tap them at their upper limit. A palpable percussion impulse indicates a dilated incompetent vein between the sites of palpation and percussion.

Auscultation

Listen over clusters of veins, particularly if they remain distended when the patient lies down, as they may indicate the site of an arteriovenous fistula.

Revision Panel 7.9

Routine for assessing the venous circulation

Ask the patient to stand up

Inspection
- Site and size of visible veins
- Effect of elevation and dependency
- Swelling of the ankle
- Colour of skin

Palpation
- Sites of fascial defects
- State of skin and subcutaneous tissues
- Trendelenburg test
- Tourniquet tests

Percussion
- Percussion wave conduction

Auscultation
- Listen for bruits

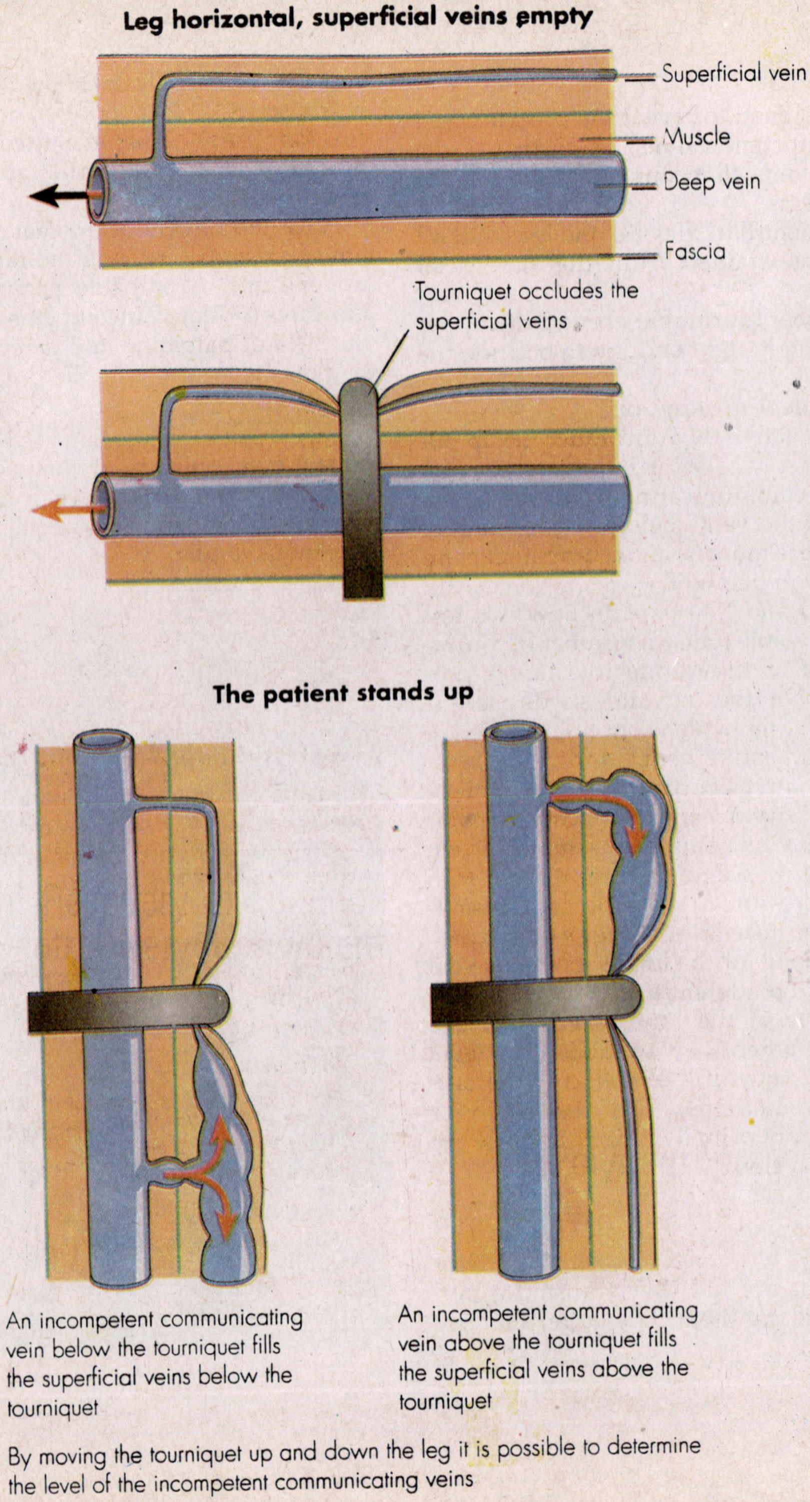

FIG. 7.13 THE PRINCIPLES OF THE TOURNIQUET TEST

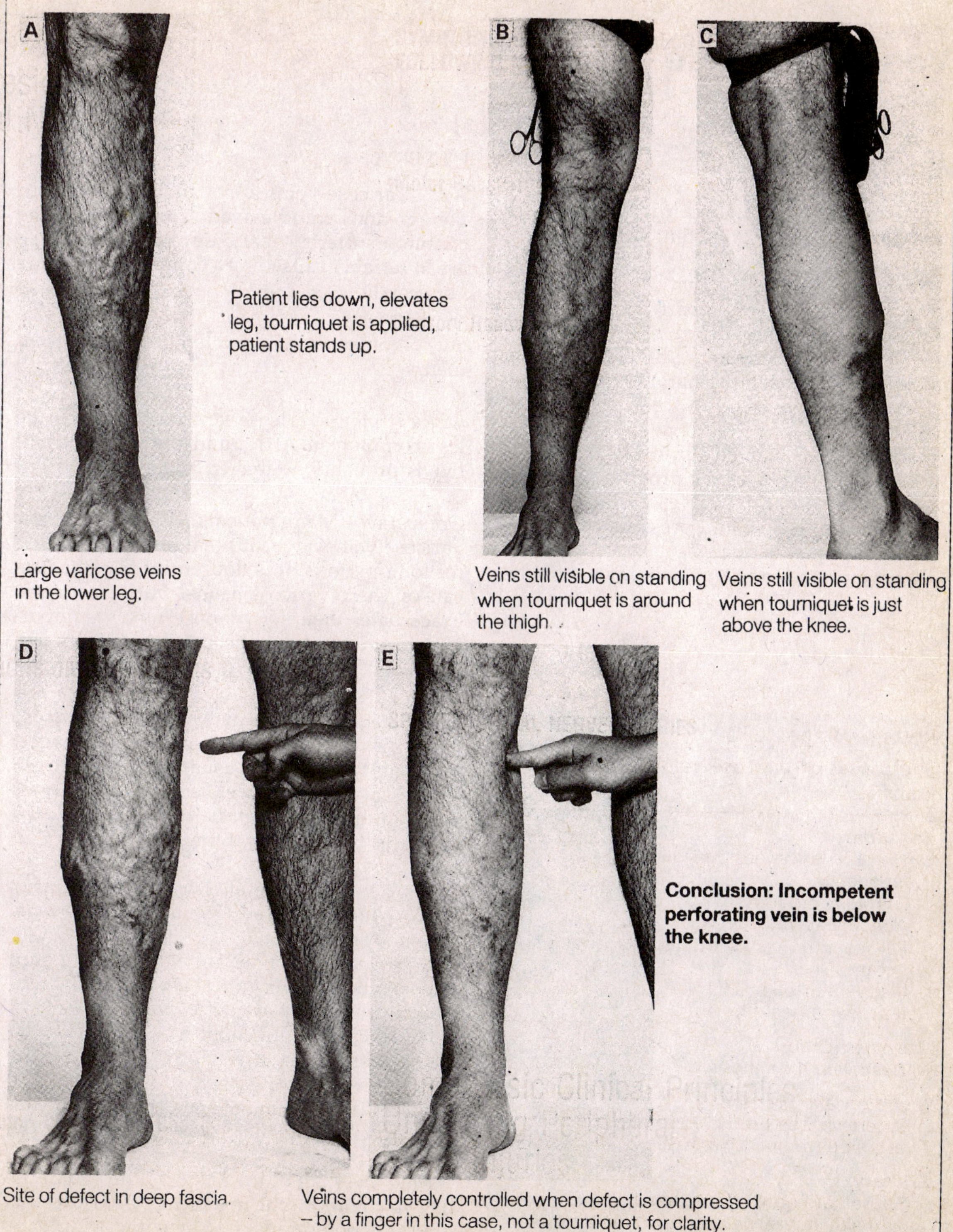

FIG. 7.14 THE TOURNIQUET TEST FOR INCOMPETENT COMMUNICATING VEINS

Venous disease

Varicose veins

A varicose vein is a dilated tortuous vein. Its valves are usually incompetent but not always (see Fig. 7.15).

It is not the varicosities that cause the symptoms of varicose veins, apart from cosmetic complaints, but the disordered physiology caused by the incompetent valves. Thus it is possible to have asymptomatic varicose veins or severe symptoms with very few visible varicose veins.

Varicose veins may be a primary abnormality, or secondary to either proximal obstruction, destruction of the valves by thrombosis, or an increase in flow and pressure caused by an arteriovenous fistula.

The symptoms and signs will depend on the cause.

Revision Panel 7.10

The causes of varicose veins in the lower limbs

Secondary

Obstruction to venous outflow

- Pregnancy
- Fibroids/ovarian cyst
- Abdominal lymphadenopathy
- Pelvic cancer (cervix, uterus, ovary, rectum)
- Ascites
- Iliac vein thrombosis
- Retroperitoneal fibrosis

Valve destruction

- Deep vein thrombosis

High flow and pressure

- Arteriovenous fistula (especially the acquired traumatic variety)

Primary

- Cause not known; often familial
- Probably a weakness of vein wall that permits valve ring dilatation
- Very rarely, congenital absence of valves

HISTORY

Age Varicose veins affect all age groups but young and middle-aged women are the common sufferers. Varicose veins in children are invariably caused by a congenital vascular abnormality.

Sex Women are affected ten times more than men.

Ethnic group Varicose veins were said to be less common in Africa and the Far East, but this is probably no longer true.

Occupation Many patients with symptomatic varicose veins have jobs that involve standing for long periods. It is doubtful if the standing causes their varicose veins, but it certainly exacerbates their symptoms. Thus it is important to know about the patient's occupation when considering treatment.

Symptoms Many patients with varicose veins have no symptoms. The commonest complaint is **pain**. It is usually a **dull ache** felt in the calves and lower leg that gets worse through the day, especially when standing up. It is **relieved by lying down** for 15–30 minutes.

Some patients present with a red, painful, tender lump caused by acute superficial thrombophlebitis.

A few patients complain of a **bursting pain** when walking. This indicates a deep vein deficiency. It is rarely caused by varicose veins.

Night cramps are common.

The disfiguring effects of the veins on the skin are often the principal complaint. The dilated visible veins, venous stars, pigmentation, eczema and ulceration all disfigure the legs.

Mild swelling of the ankle by the end of the day is common but marked ankle oedema is not, and other causes of swelling should be eliminated before accepting that it is caused by the varicose veins.

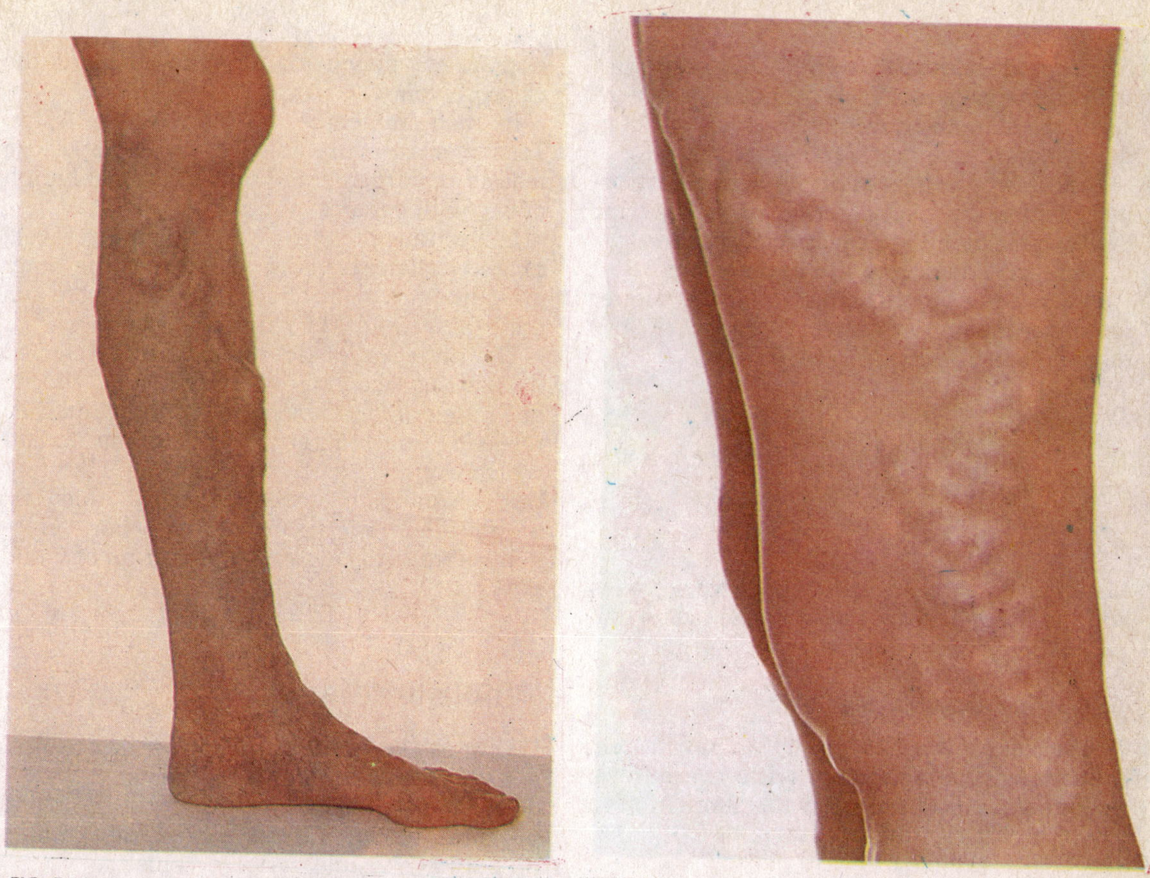

FIG. 7.15 Varicose veins are, by definition, dilated and tortuous, and usually have incompetent valves. They occur on both the medial and lateral sides of the leg

Ask carefully about symptoms that would indicate a cause of the varicose veins, especially **pregnancy** and abdominal symptoms from pelvic tumours. These may become apparent in the answers to the systematic questions.

Previous history Most patients with varicose veins have had them for years and have had various forms of treatment such as operations and injections.

Ask about any episodes of deep vein thrombosis that may have accompanied previous illnesses, operations, accidents or pregnancies.

Ask women if they had swelling of their legs, thrombosis or a 'white leg' during their pregnancies.

Family history It is common to find that the patient's mother and sisters also have varicose veins.

LOCAL EXAMINATION

Inspection

Look for large visible veins. Record their **site, extent and size**. You need a large drawing of the front and back of the limb to do this properly.

Look at the skin of the leg, especially the lower third of the medial side of the lower leg, for signs of chronic venous hypertension – brown pigmentation, eczema and ulceration.

Palpation

Palpate the texture of the skin and subcutaneous tissues of the lower leg.

There may be pitting oedema or thickening, redness and tenderness. These changes are caused by chronic venous hypertension and are called by various names, the best being

lipodermatosclerosis, which indicates that the change is caused by a progressive sclerosis of the skin and subcutaneous fat by fibrin deposition, tissue death and scarring.

Feel along the course of the veins, particularly behind the medial border of the tibia, for tender defects in the deep fascia.

Feel for a cough impulse in the groin.

Perform the Trendelenburg and tourniquet tests (see above) to detect the site of any incompetent communicating veins.

Percussion

Test for the conduction of a percussion impulse up and down the vein.

Auscultation

Listen over any large bunch of varicosities and, if the veins do not collapse when the patient lies down, along the whole leg.

GENERAL EXAMINATION

This is the most important part of the examination.

Examine the abdomen with great care, including a rectal and vaginal examination to exclude any pelvic or abdominal cause for the varicose veins.

In men, remember to palpate the testes. Testicular tumours can be small but cause massive enlargement of the abdominal lymph nodes with vena caval obstruction.

Inspection of the abdomen may reveal dilated collateral veins crossing to the other groin or up over the abdomen and chest to join the tributaries of the superior vena cava.

The direction of flow in a vein is detected by placing two fingers on the vein, sliding one finger along the vein to empty it and then releasing one finger and watching to see which way the empty segment fills (**Harvey's test**). You may have to repeat this test moving the fingers in either direction before being able to decide on the direction of blood flow.

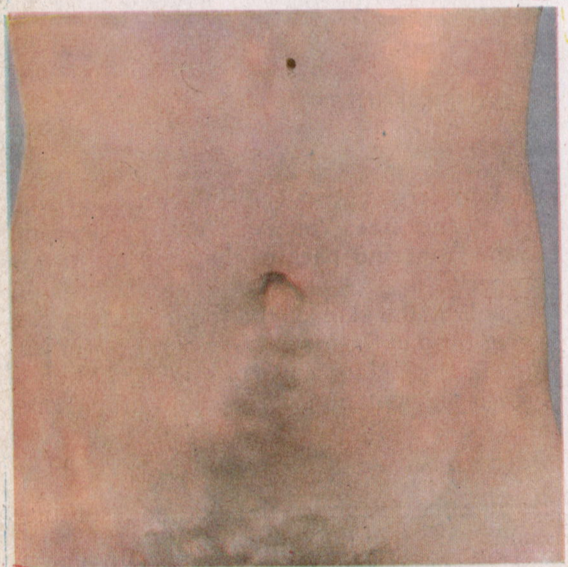

FIG. 7.16 Dilated tortuous collateral veins crossing the abdomen in a patient with an inferior vena cava thrombosis. The common cause of inferior vena caval obstruction is intra-abdominal malignant disease

Venous ulceration

Do not use the term 'varicose ulcer'. The ulcer is not caused by the varicose veins but by the disordered pattern of venous blood flow and pressure. Many patients with venous ulcers do not have visible varicose veins.

HISTORY

Age Venous ulcers usually follow many years of venous disease, so most are seen in patients 40–60 years old, many of whom have had recurrent ulceration for some years before seeking medical help. Severe disease can cause ulceration in young adults, and ulcers can appear in children and teenagers with congenital venous malformations.

Sex Women are affected far more often than men.

Symptoms The patient has usually suffered from aching pain, discomfort and tenderness of the skin, pigmentation and eczema for months or years before an ulcer appears.

The ulcer is painful at first but as it settles down and becomes chronic it is rarely very painful. The main symptoms are **discomfort when dressing it, discharge and unsightliness.**

Previous history The majority of venous ulcers follow deep and communicating vein damage, so there is often a history of deep vein thrombosis during an illness or pregnancy. The patient may have had previous episodes of ulceration.

Cause The ulcer invariably begins after the skin of the leg has been knocked and damaged. Sometimes the patient remembers the initial incident; usually she does not.

EXAMINATION

The leg

Examine the whole limb for the presence of varicose veins and especially try to detect the presence of incompetent communicating veins, as described in the previous sections.

The majority of patients with venous ulcers have incompetent communicating veins.

Examine the arteries and the nerves of the leg to exclude other causes of ulceration.

The ulcer

Site Venous ulcers are commonly found around the 'gaiter' area of the lower leg (the lower third) and usually on the medial side, but they can occur lower down, even on the foot.

They are 'never' found above the junction of the middle and upper thirds of the lower leg.

Shape and size Venous ulcers can be of any shape and size (see Fig. 7.17).

Edge The edge is sloping and pale purple–blue in colour.

Base The base is usually covered with pink granulation tissue, but areas of white fibrous tissue can be seen between the granulations. In the chronic ulcer there may be more white fibrous tissue than granulation tissue.

There may be sloughing skin and fat covering the granulation.

The deep structures rarely die but tendons and bone may be exposed.

Depth Venous ulcers are usually shallow and flat.

Discharge The discharge is seropurulent with an occasional trace of blood. Heavy infection and thick pus are *not* common.

Surrounding tissues The base of the ulcer is fixed to the deep tissues. The surrounding tissues show signs of chronic venous hypertension – induration and pigmentation, warmth, redness and tenderness.

There may be scars from previous ulcers and many dilated veins.

The movements of the ankle joint may be limited by the scar tissue and there may be an equinus deformity of the joint.

Local lymph nodes The infection in an ulcer rarely spreads to the inguinal lymph nodes, so these glands should not be enlarged or tender.

Remember that squamous carcinoma can arise in a chronic benign ulcer. If a patient presents with a long history suggestive of venous ulceration but with an ulcer whose edge is raised or thickened, or in any way different from the typical ulcer described above, be suspicious of malignant change, especially if the inguinal lymph glands are enlarged. Malignant change in a chronic ulcer is known as a **Marjolin's ulcer**.

GENERAL EXAMINATION

A patient with a venous ulcer has probably had venous disease for many years and so is unlikely to have any malignant intra-abdominal disease. Nevertheless, examine the abdomen, and the other leg, with care.

Deep vein thrombosis

Deep vein thrombosis is usually thought of as a complication of an operation or an illness. Remember that it can occur spontaneously, especially in women taking oral contraceptives.

Only one-quarter of deep vein thromboses cause symptoms and signs.

HISTORY

The patient complains of pain and swelling in the calf or whole leg. The onset of symptoms is sudden and they are usually severe enough to make walking difficult.

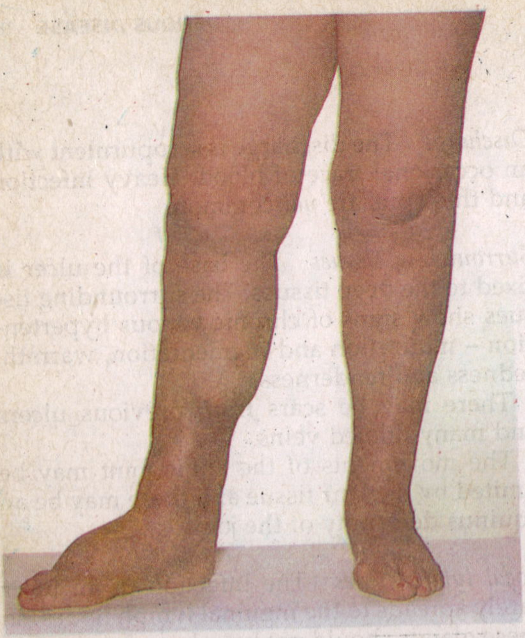

The 'gaiter area'. This photograph shows the medial aspect of the lower third of the leg, narrowed and hardened by venous lipodermatosclerosis. This is the area in which most venous ulcers develop

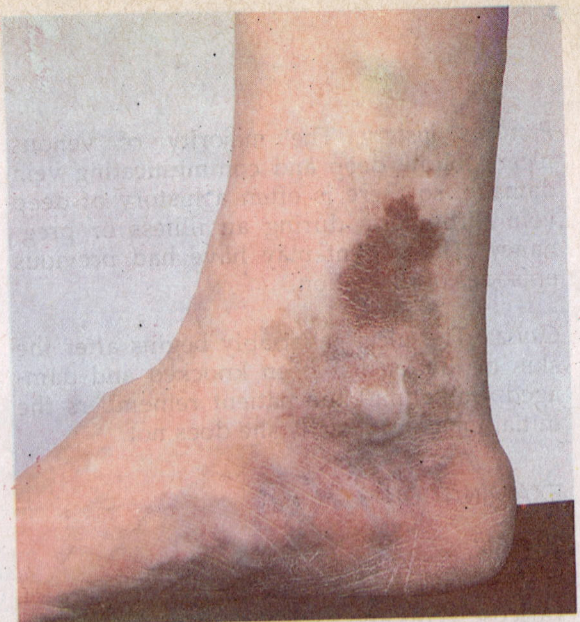

Chronic venous insufficiency causes '*pigmentation*' of the skin and dilated '*intradermal venules*'. The venules first appear in a triangular area over and below the medial malleolus, with the apex of the triangle over the first or second lower leg communicating vein (see Fig. 7.12). This is known as the 'ankle-flare' or 'corona phlebectatica'

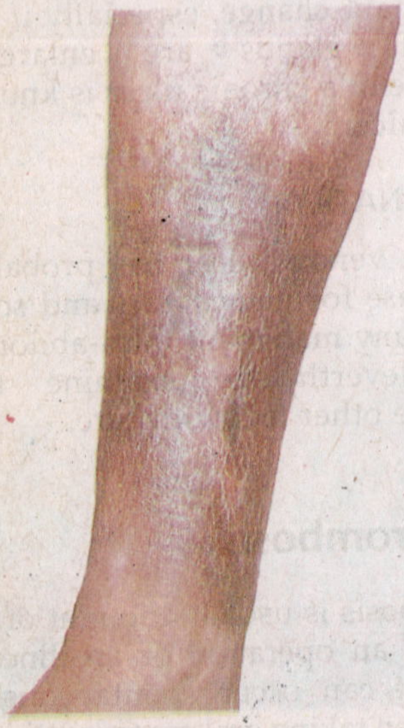

The pigmentation of chronic venous disease may cover the whole of the lower limb

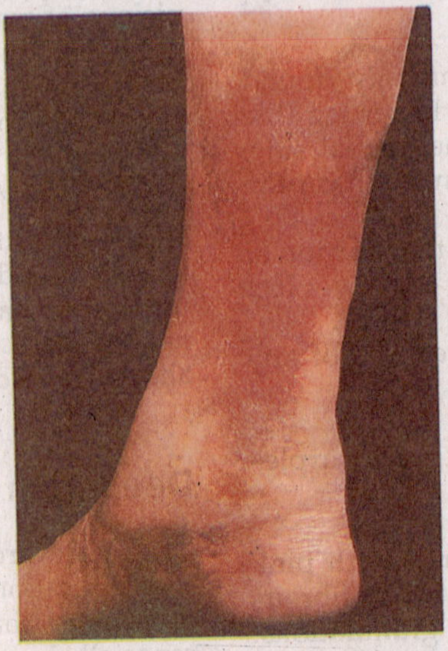

Acute lipodermatosclerosis usually begins on the medial side of the gaiter area and is painful, hot, red and tender. It is often misdiagnosed as cellulitis or acute thrombophlebitis

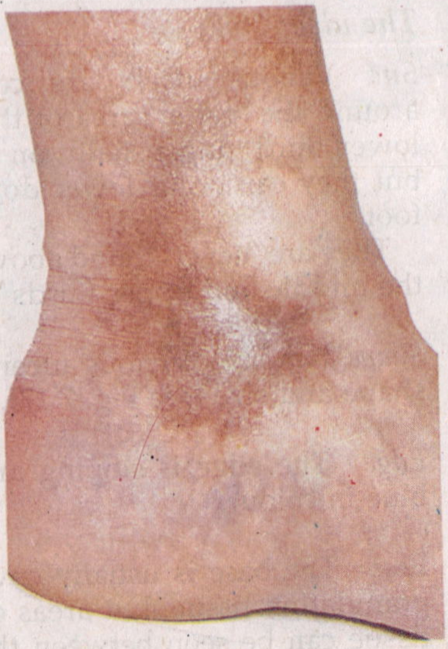

Atrophie blanche is the name given to white scars in the skin that appear without the skin ever having broken down or ulcerated

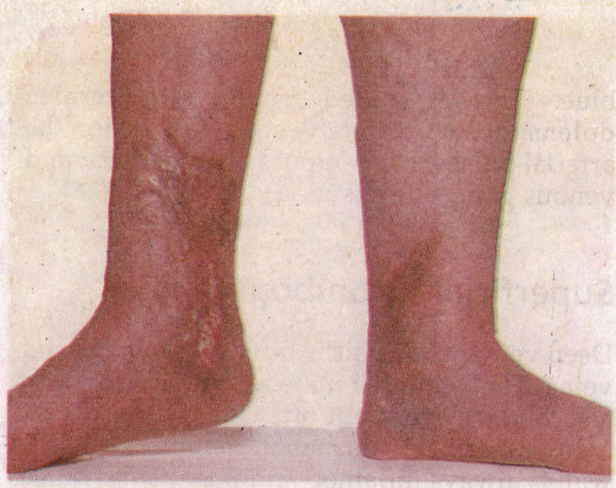

Subcutaneous fibrosis, following chronic lipodermatosclerosis, and/or painful ulceration may cause a 'fixed flexion' of the ankle joint

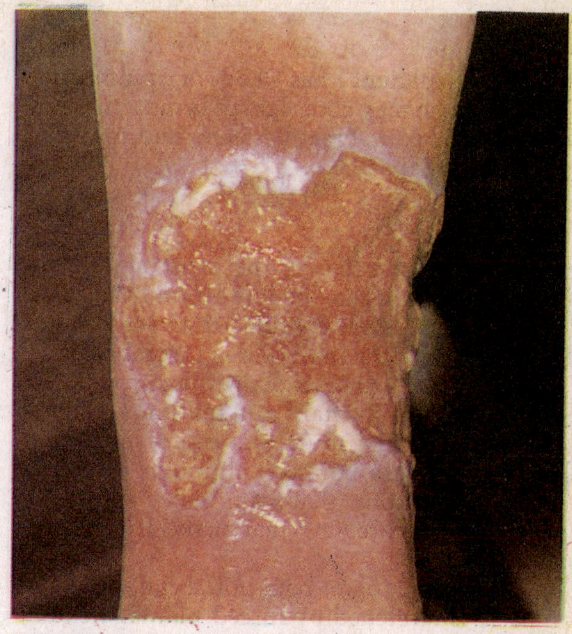

A chronic recurrent, infected, enlarging venous ulcer. The base contains little healthy granulation tissue and many areas of avascular fibrous tissue

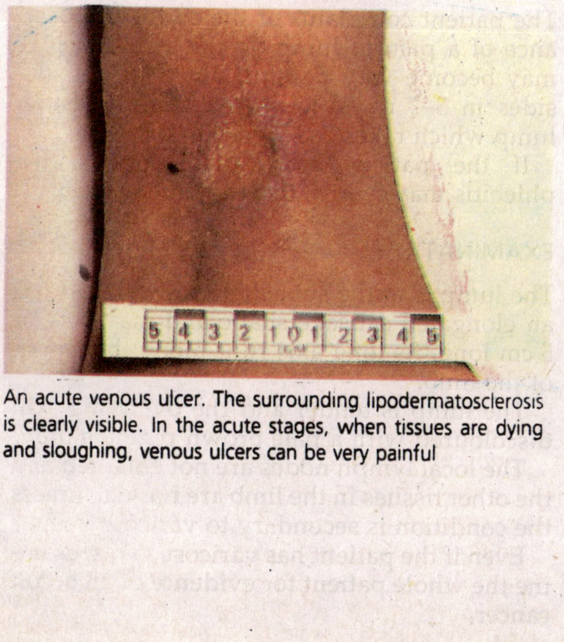

An acute venous ulcer. The surrounding lipodermatosclerosis is clearly visible. In the acute stages, when tissues are dying and sloughing, venous ulcers can be very painful

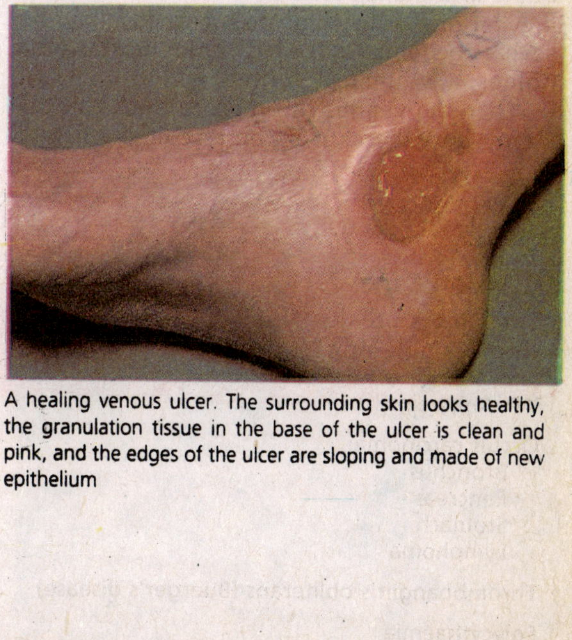

A healing venous ulcer. The surrounding skin looks healthy, the granulation tissue in the base of the ulcer is clean and pink, and the edges of the ulcer are sloping and made of new epithelium

FIG. 7.17 THE CUTANEOUS MANIFESTATIONS OF CHRONIC VENOUS INSUFFICIENCY

If the patient has had a pulmonary embolism he may complain of symptoms such as pleuritic pain, breathlessness and haemoptysis, or collapse.

EXAMINATION

Swelling of the leg is the most significant physical sign. It may be just around the ankle if the thrombosis is confined to the calf, or up to the groin if the iliac vein is thrombosed.

The muscles that contain the thrombosed veins may become **hard and tender**. A change in texture of the muscle is more significant than tenderness because, although there are many conditions that can make a muscle tender, there are few that make it stiff and hard.

The production of pain in the calf when the muscle is stretched by forced plantar flexion, known as **Homan's sign**, is another (but inaccurate) way of detecting muscle tenderness.

If the thrombosis obstructs the outflow of blood from the limbs the superficial veins dilate and the leg feels hot.

A large swollen limb that is made pale by severe oedema is called **phlegmasia alba dolens**, a 'white leg' or 'milk leg'.

When the venous thrombosis blocks all the main veins the skin becomes congested and blue. This is called **phlegmasia cerulea dolens**. In such severe venous obstruction the arterial pulses may temporarily disappear and venous gangrene ensue.

> **Revision Panel 7.11**
>
> **The causes of superficial thrombophlebitis**
>
> Varicose veins
>
> Occult carcinoma:
> - Bronchus
> - Pancreas
> - Stomach
> - Lymphoma
>
> Thromboangiitis obliterans (Buerger's disease)
>
> Polycythaemia
>
> Polyarteritis
>
> Idiopathic
>
> Iatrogenic
> - Intravenous injection and injuries

Superficial thrombophlebitis

Deep vein thrombosis is thrombosis in normal veins. The vein wall may become inflamed as a secondary event but often stays normal.

In superficial thrombophlebitis the vein wall is always inflamed and may be the cause of the thrombosis.

The causes of superficial thrombophlebitis are given in Revision Panel 7.11.

When the episodes occur in the **arms** of patients over the age of 45 years, and when they are **transient** and **migrate**, they frequently indicate an occult carcinoma.

Idiopathic thrombophlebitis migrans is a rare disease.

HISTORY

The patient complains of the sudden appearance of a painful lump on the arm or leg. It may become very painful, but the pain subsides in 3–7 days, leaving a slightly tender lump which takes 2–3 weeks to disperse.

If the patient has varicose veins, the phlebitis may follow an injury to the vein.

EXAMINATION

The lump is in the subcutaneous tissue. It has an elongated sausage shape and may be 4 or 5 cm long. Its long axis runs along the length of the limb.

The lump is tender and the overlying skin discoloured with a pale brown pigmentation.

The local lymph nodes are not enlarged and the other tissues in the limb are normal, unless the condition is secondary to varicose veins.

Even if the patient has varicose veins, examine the whole patient for evidence of an occult cancer.

Axillary vein thrombosis

Thrombosis of the axillary–subclavian vein may follow excessive use of the limb, especially above the head, or compression of the vein by musculoskeletal abnormalities or enlarged lymph nodes.

HISTORY

The patient complains of a sudden discomfort and swelling of the arm. The arm, forearm and hand swell up, in that order, and there is discomfort on the medial side of the upper arm and in the axilla.

The arm may feel hot and, if it becomes very swollen, movements become restricted.

The patient may give a history of an unusual activity in the preceding 24 hours. Clearing a shelf high above head level is not an uncommon precipitating cause.

EXAMINATION

The whole arm is swollen, sometimes slightly congested and blue, and the veins are distended. When the hand is raised above the level of the heart the veins on the back of the hand will *not* collapse.

The axillary vein in the axilla is tender.

There may be distended subcutaneous veins crossing the shoulder.

Make sure that you examine the head and neck, breast and abdomen for possible sources of enlarged deep cervical, axillary, supraclavicular and mediastinal lymph glands.

Congenital vein abnormalities

These are rare vascular malformations but are mentioned because they are often misdiagnosed as simple varicose veins. The typical appearance is shown in Fig. 7.18.

There are dilated veins, which have been present since birth or early childhood, often on the outer side of the leg, not the inner side where most varicose veins appear. The leg is often longer than the normal leg and there are cutaneous angiomata (port-wine stains).

This clinical syndrome is often given the eponym Klippel–Trénaunay syndrome. There is **no** arterial abnormality and no arteriovenous fistulae (see also page 176).

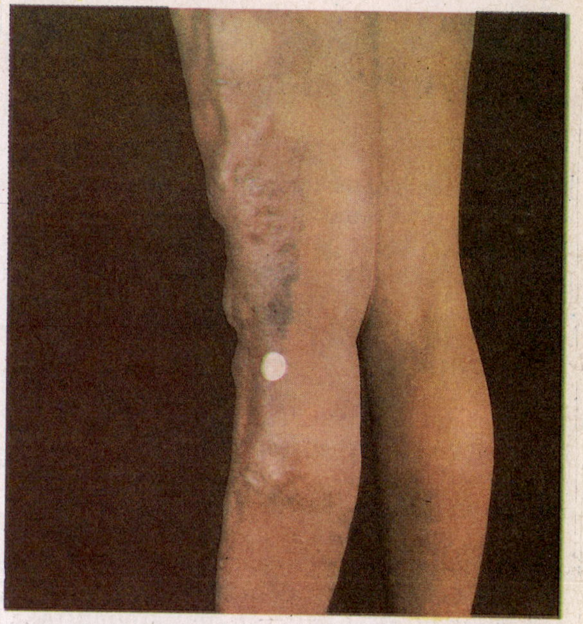

The dilated, anatomically abnormal varicose veins of a congenital venous deformity. There are also patches of port-wine staining

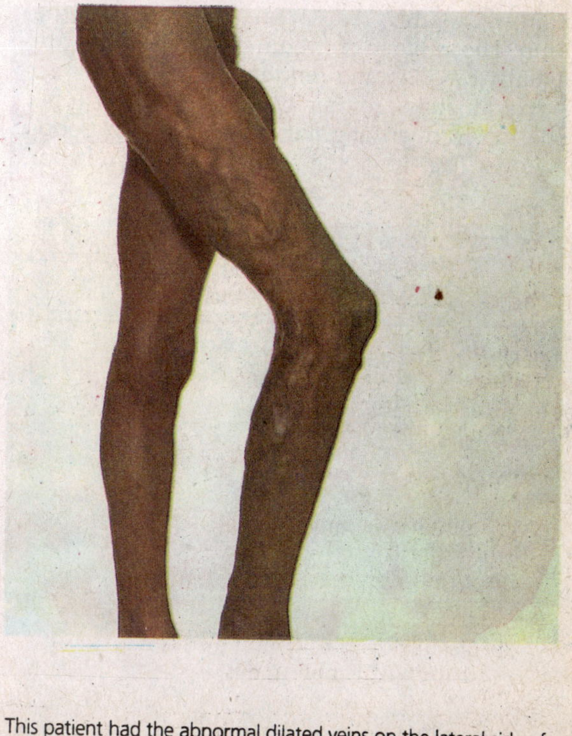

This patient had the abnormal dilated veins on the lateral side of the leg typical of the Klippel–Trénaunay syndrome, with marked overgrowth of the length and circumference of the leg

FIG. 7.18 CONGENITAL VARICOSE VEINS

The lymphatics

Primary disease of the lymph vessels is rare, but secondary involvement of the lymph nodes which lie on the pathways of lymph flow is common, so secondary lymphoedema is not rare.

Lymphangitis

When bacterial infection spreads through the tissues it gets into the lymphatics and the bacteria then pass along in the lymph to the nearby lymph nodes.

If the lymphatics become inflamed they become visible as a thin, tender red streak on the skin. Lymphangitis is most often seen as a complication of infection in and around the hands and feet.

The patient complains of a throbbing pain at the site of the primary infection and the painful, tender red streak running up the limb. The axillary or inguinal lymph nodes are usually swollen and tender.

Examination reveals the red tender lymphatic. The overlying skin may be slightly oedematous. The site of the primary infection is not always obvious – it may be just a small crack between the toes or alongside a finger nail.

Lymphangitis occurs in the normal lymphatics of normal tissues. When infection gets into oedema – whatever the cause of the oedema – it spreads diffusely to cause a cellulitis.

Revision Panel 7.12

The causes of lymphoedema

Secondary

Neoplastic infiltration of lymph nodes
- Secondary carcinoma
- Primary reticuloses

Infection
- Filariasis
- Lymphogranuloma inguinale
- Tuberculosis
- Recurrent non-specific infection

Iatrogenic
- Surgical excision of lymph nodes
- Irradiation of lymph nodes

Primary
- Congenital or acquired deficiency of the lymphatics
- Dilatation and incompetence of the lymphatics

Lymphoedema

Lymphoedema is interstitial oedema of lymphatic origin. This means that it is rich in protein. The oedema of heart and kidney failure has a low protein content.

The causes of lymphoedema are given in Revision Panel 7.12.

The most important and commonest cause of lymphoedema is secondary lymph node disease. Primary lymphoedema is diagnosed only when all the causes of secondary lymphoedema have been eliminated.

HISTORY

Age Primary lymphoedema may present at birth, in young adults, or, less often, in middle age.

Secondary lymphoedema presents in middle and old age.

Sex Females are affected more than males. Even secondary lymphoedema is more common in women because tumours of the uterus, ovary and vagina can metastasize to the iliac and inguinal nodes, and carcinoma of the breast spreads to the axillary nodes.

Geography Filariasis (infestation with the parasite *Wuchereria bancrofti*), which is found in tropical and subtropical countries, is a common cause of severe lymphoedema (elephantiasis).

Symptoms The patient complains of a **slowly progressive swelling** of the limb or genitalia.

The lower limb is most often affected by primary lymphoedema and there is frequently a history of an injury, such as a sprained ankle, starting the swelling. The swelling takes years to develop.

In secondary lymphoedema the swelling may appear in a few weeks and progress rapidly.

The swelling is **not painful** and there is no discomfort in the swollen limb apart from that caused by the increased weight and any mechanical disability.

Lymphoedema of the lower limb is commonly complicated by **athlete's foot** (tinea pedis) between the toes and by episodes of acute **cellulitis**, sometimes accompanied by septicaemia. The patient complains of pain and tenderness, sweats, rigors and malaise.

Vesicles may appear on the skin and leak clear-coloured fluid.

There may be symptoms of the cause of the oedema.

Family history Some forms of primary lymphoedema are familial.

EXAMINATION

The lymphoedema (see Fig. 7.19)

Lymphoedema has no special characteristics. It is often stated in textbooks that it does not pit. This is not so. **All oedema pits**. The longer it has been present, the denser the accompanying fibrosis and the **harder** the oedema, but if you press hard enough and long enough it will pit.

Lymphoedema of the lower limb affects the toes much more than other forms of oedema, and if it has been present for years the toes get squashed together and become **squared-off**. This hardly ever occurs with venous, cardiac or renal oedema.

The skin of a lymphoedematous leg gets thick and **hyperkeratotic**. The thick scales grow outwards and look like warts.

Lymphoedema is usually diagnosed, when other general causes (cardiac and renal) and local causes (venous obstruction, venous thrombosis) have been *excluded*. It is, therefore, essential to examine the whole patient, particularly the heart, abdomen and veins of the limb.

The lymph nodes

The lymph nodes draining the lymphoedematous area will not be enlarged in primary lymphoedema but may be big and hard if they are infiltrated with tumour.

Examine all the areas which drain to any palpable nodes.

GENERAL EXAMINATION

Search widely for a cause for the lymphoedema.

Postmastectomy oedema

Swelling of the arm is a common complication of any form of mastectomy, or combination of mastectomy and radiotherapy, that disturbs the axillary lymph nodes.

When the oedema occurs in the first few days or weeks after the initial treatment it is usually caused by an **axillary vein thrombosis**.

If it begins 1–2 months after operation and progresses rapidly, it may be caused by scar tissue **constricting the axillary vein** or **lymphatic obstruction**.

If the oedema starts months or years after the initial treatment in an arm that otherwise has been normal, then it is most likely to be caused by **recurrent carcinoma** in the lymph nodes.

Lymphangioma

Lymphangioma is a rare condition but sufficiently distinct to make it easy to diagnose and worthy of a short description (see page 53).

HISTORY

The patient, or the patient's mother, complains of a soft subcutaneous swelling, or sometimes small vesicles containing clear or red–brown fluid on the skin. These abnormalities may be present at birth or appear later. As the years pass the lumps often get bigger and the vesicles increase in number.

The lesions are not painful.

EXAMINATION

The skin

The skin over the lesions, which are commonly found at the junction of leg, arm or neck with the trunk, contains multiple small vesicles. The contents of the vesicles are a clear yellow, red or dark brown fluid.

They cannot be compressed or emptied.

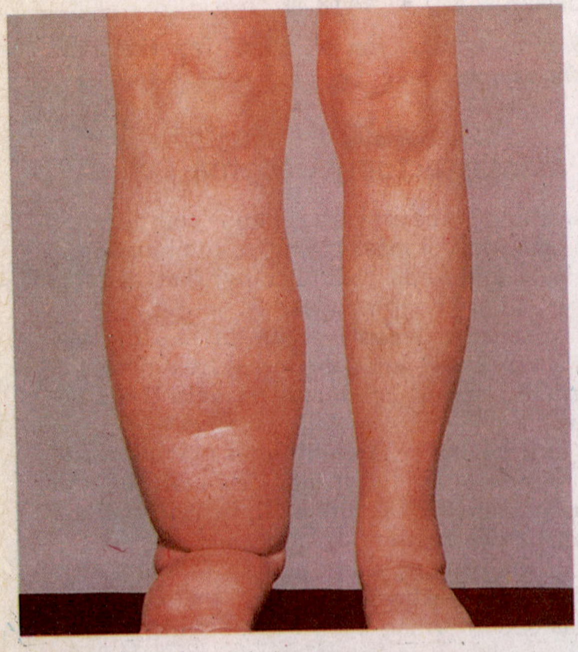

Lymphoedema of the right leg

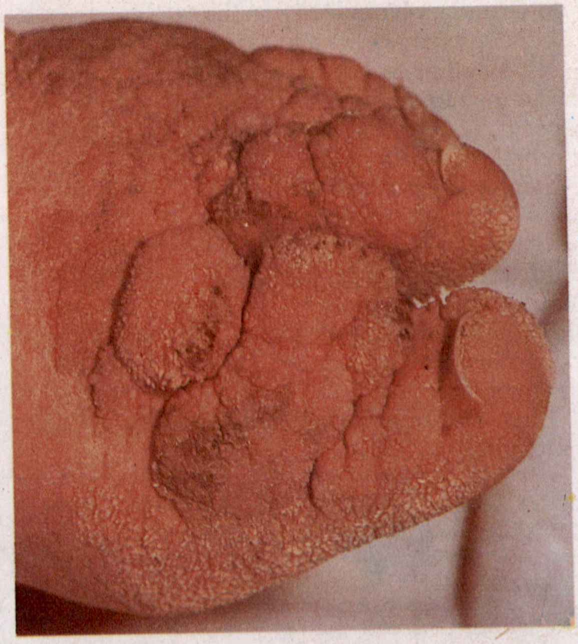

The complications of chronic lymphoedema. The skin becomes covered with nodules and filiform hyperkeratoses. The fissures become infected and attacks of cellulitis affecting the whole limb may cause fevers and rigors

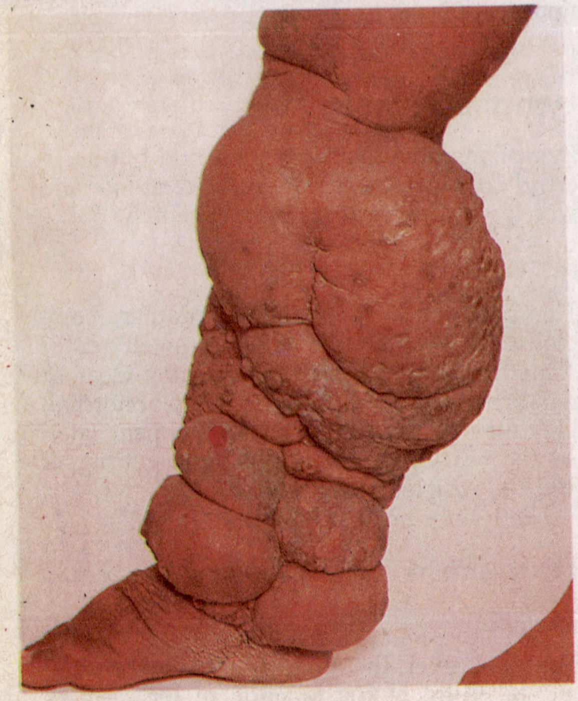

Severe long-standing lymphoedema. The skin is thickened and hyperkeratotic

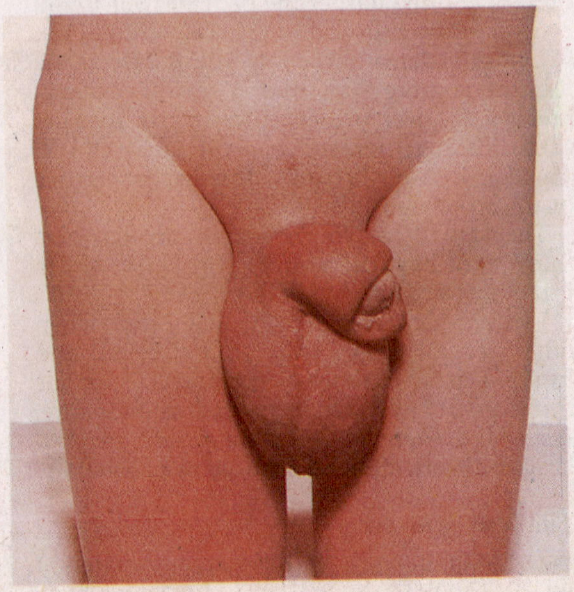

Genital lymphoedema. This usually affects the penis and scrotum but may be confined to the scrotum. In about 50 per cent of patients there is also mild lymphoedema of the legs

FIG. 7.19 LYMPHOEDEMA

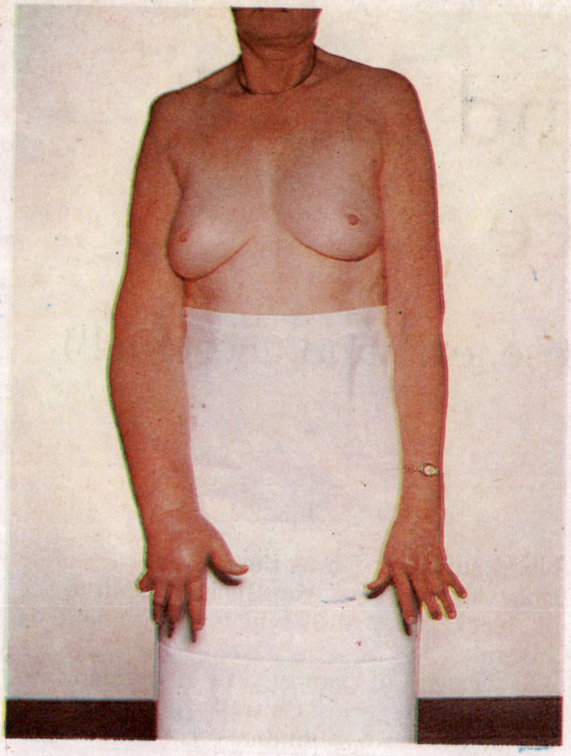

Secondary lymphoedema. This patient's right arm lymphoedema was caused by infiltration of the axillary lymph glands by metastases from a carcinoma in the right breast. Some carcinomata of the breast present in this way

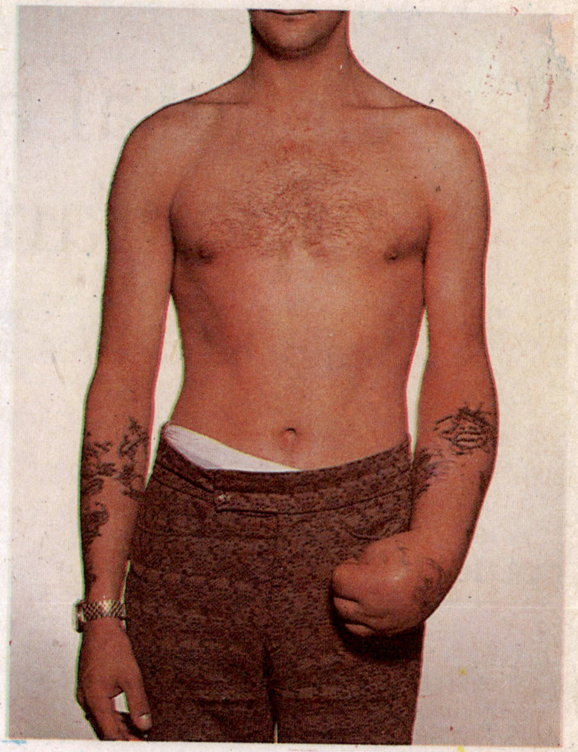

'Hysterical' oedema. Immobility and dependency, in this case caused by a 'hysterical' paralysis, can cause severe oedema. This is not a true lymphoedema but a gravitational oedema. The limb is often bluish in colour because of the concomitant venous congestion – hence the name 'hysterical oedeme blue'

FIG. 7.19 *Continued*

The lump

Deep to the skin are a series of soft indistinct cysts. If they are large enough they fluctuate and transilluminate. They have the same signs as a cystic hygroma (see page 266). Indeed, the skin over some cystic hygromata eventually develops vesicles.

Lymphadenopathy

Enlargement of lymph nodes is commonplace. The causes are partly related to the site of the nodes involved, and some are discussed elsewhere in this book; but they are so important that they are presented here again for further revision (Revision Panel 7.13).

Revision Panel 7.13

The causes of lymphadenopathy

Infection
- Non-specific
- Glandular fever
- Tuberculosis
- Toxoplasmosis
- Syphilis
- Cat-scratch fever (*Rochalimaea henselae*)
- Filariasis
- Lymphogranuloma (inguinale)

Metastatic tumour

Primary reticuloses

Sarcoidosis

8 General and facial appearance

(scalp, head, eyes, nose, ears and chest wall)

COLOUR

One of the first things that one notices about a patient is the colour of his skin: not his racial colour, though it is important to record his racial origin, but changes from his normal colour. Although minor colour variations are easier to appreciate in white-skinned people, they are also visible in dark-skinned races.

The skin may be pale or tinged blue, yellow or brown.

Pallor

Normal skin colour varies according to the thickness of the skin, the state of the skin circulation and the degree and type of pigmentation. If the skin thickness and the circulation appear to be normal, then pallor of the skin usually indicates **anaemia**. Anaemia is best detected by looking at the colour of the mucous membranes.

1 Look at the colour of the conjunctiva on the inner side of the lower eyelid.
2 Look at the colour of the **buccal** mucous membrane.
3 Stretch the skin of the palm and look at the colour of the **palmar creases**.

Cyanosis

Cyanosis is the purple–blue colour given to the skin by deoxygenated blood. It is most apparent in areas with thin skin but a rich blood supply, such as the *lips, tongue, finger nails* and *ear lobes*. Cyanosis is difficult to see in black skin and when the patient is anaemic.

The causes of cyanosis can be divided into two large categories: **central**, when the defect lies in the cardiopulmonary circulation and **peripheral**, when there is excessive deoxygenation in the tissues, usually because of inadequate tissue perfusion.

If the cyanosis is caused by a central abnormality it will be generalized and the patient's extremities will usually be warm.

If the cyanosis is caused by a peripheral abnormality the extremities will be **blue and cold**, but central organs such as the tongue will be pink.

Polycythaemia

An excess of circulating red blood cells gives the patient a purple–red, florid appearance. This may be mistaken for cyanosis. It differs from cyanosis in that it heightens the colour of all the skin, especially the *cheeks, neck, backs of hands* and *feet*. The discolouration of cyanosis is usually limited to the tips of the hands, feet and nose.

Jaundice

Jaundice is a yellow discolouration of the skin, caused by an excess of bile pigments in the plasma.

The yellow colour is first visible against the white background of the **sclera** but as the jaundice increases the whole skin turns yellow.

The colour changes with the depth of the jaundice. White skin first turns a pale lemon yellow. As it deepens it becomes yellow–orange, sometimes almost brown, and in those rare conditions where severe jaundice may exist for many years, such as biliary cirrhosis, the skin eventually turns a yellowy grey–green colour.

It is not possible to diagnose the cause of jaundice from its presence. The most useful diagnostic features are the sequence of events preceding its onset and the presence or absence of pain.

Jaundice can be caused by excessive haemolysis – prehepatic jaundice; by liver malfunction – hepatic jaundice; or by obstruction of the bile ducts – posthepatic jaundice.

The common causes of these three types of jaundice are:

1 Prehepatic jaundice – haemolytic anaemia.
2 Hepatic jaundice – infectious hepatitis.
3 Posthepatic jaundice – gallstones and carcinoma of the pancreas.

Figure 8.1 describes the principal premonitory symptoms, pain and fluctuations of jaundice that accompany the four main causes of jaundice.

Brown pigmentation

An increase in the natural brown pigmentation of the skin can be generalized or localized.

Causes of generalized pigmentation

- **Addison's disease** is the important cause of increased pigmentation to remember, because if it is not diagnosed and treated it can cause sudden death. The brown pigmentation of Addison's disease is visible in the buccal mucous membrane.
- **Arsenic and silver poisoning.**
- **Haemochromatosis.**
- **Gaucher's disease.**

Causes of localized pigmentation

- **Pregnancy** Around the areolae and along the mid-line of the abdomen.
- **Chronic venous hypertension** Lower medial third of the lower leg.
- **Erythema ab igne** Frequently seen on parts of the legs exposed to heat.
- **Ultraviolet and high-voltage irradiation.**
- **'Café au lait' patch** Associated with neurofibromatosis.
- **Various forms of melanoma.**
- **Pellagra** Nicotinic acid deficiency.
- **Rheumatoid arthritis.**
- **Acanthosis nigricans.**

Vitiligo

Vitiligo is the name given to white depigmented areas of skin. It commonly occurs without a generalized cause, but it can be secondary to leprosy, scleroderma, syphilis, and some organ-specific autoimmune diseases such as Hashimoto's thyroiditis, Addison's disease, pernicious anaemia and diabetes.

Excoriation/pruritus

This is itching of the skin caused by a local or general abnormality. The presence of multiple scratches on the skin is usually very obvious and noticed during your initial inspection. Itching of the skin is caused by:

1 **Skin diseases**:
Urticaria.
Eczema.
(Psoriasis does not usually cause itching.)
2 **Local irritation**:
Clothing/washing powder.
Parasites – fleas, scabies.
Discharges – vaginal and rectal.

Revision Panel 8.1

Causes of a generalized increased skin pigmentation

Sunlight
Pregnancy
Addison's disease
Renal failure
Haemochromatosis
Drugs (e.g. busulphan)

THE DISTINGUISHING FEATURES OF THE FOUR COMMON CAUSES OF JAUNDICE

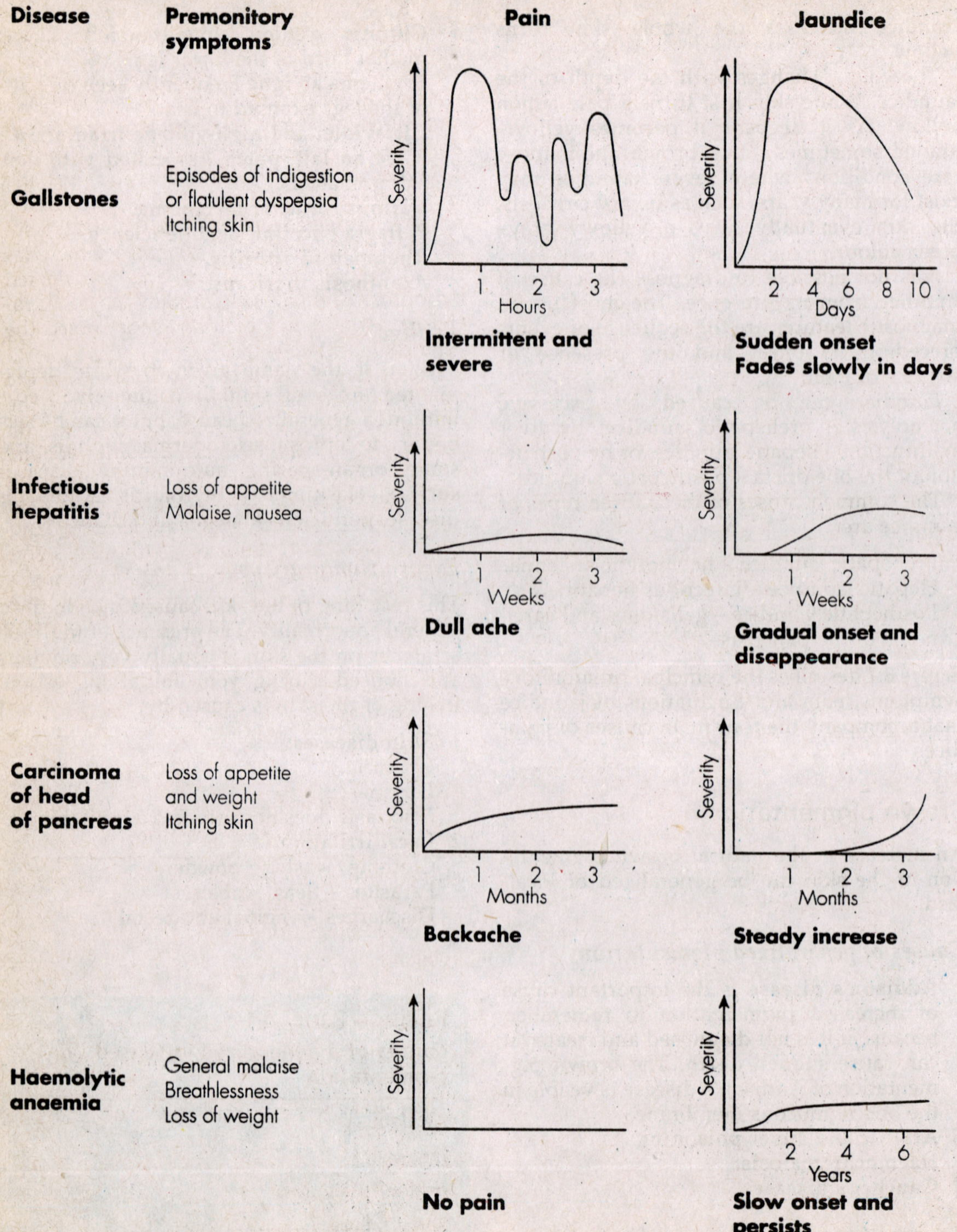

FIG. 8.1

3 **Occult disease:**
Subclinical jaundice with bile salt retention.
Hodgkin's disease.
Leukaemia.
Uraemia.
Food sensitivity.
Polycythaemia.
Thyrotoxicosis.

If a skin disease or local irritation is the initiating stimulus, the cause of the pruritis and excoriation is usually obvious on inspection, so the causes to remember are the occult diseases. Any patient presenting with an itching, but otherwise normal skin, should be suspected of having subclinical jaundice, Hodgkin's disease or uraemia until you prove otherwise.

GENERAL APPEARANCE

When you look at the patient's size, shape and physical characteristics you will subconsciously put him into one of four categories. His body will look normal, wasted, overweight, or have some skeletal or sexual characteristics which look out of proportion.

The following sections describe the principal conditions that cause these three changes in body build.

Wasting

There are many causes of wasting. Almost all serious diseases cause some loss of appetite and weight so only the common conditions are listed in Revision Panel 8.3.

Severe wasting of the upper half of the body and oedema of the lower half is a common physical appearance in the elderly and is usually caused by advanced carcinoma which has either destroyed the liver and so caused hypoproteinaemia, or formed large intra-abdominal masses which have obstructed the vena cava or iliac veins.

The degree of wasting is apparent from the way in which the skeleton, particularly the shoulder girdle, and the folds of loose skin on the arms, trunk and buttocks becomes visible.

This clinical picture can also be caused by the combination of two diseases: a disease which causes wasting, such as carcinoma, and congestive heart failure. Although you should always try to make one diagnosis, many elderly people have more than one disease.

Revision Panel 8.2

The common causes of itching

General
Cholestasis (subclinical jaundice)
Hodgkin's disease
Lymphoma
Renal failure (uraemia)
Food sensitivities
Iron deficiency
Polycythaemia

Skin disease
Infestations (e.g. scabies)
Insect bites
Eczema
Urticaria
Prickly heat
Clothing/washing powder sensitivities

Revision Panel 8.3

The common causes of wasting

In children
Severe gastroenteritis
Malabsorption syndromes

In young adults
Tuberculosis
Reticuloses
Anorexia nervosa

In middle age
Diabetes
Thyrotoxicosis
Carcinoma

In old age
Carcinoma
Senility
Gross cardiorespiratory disease

All age groups
Starvation

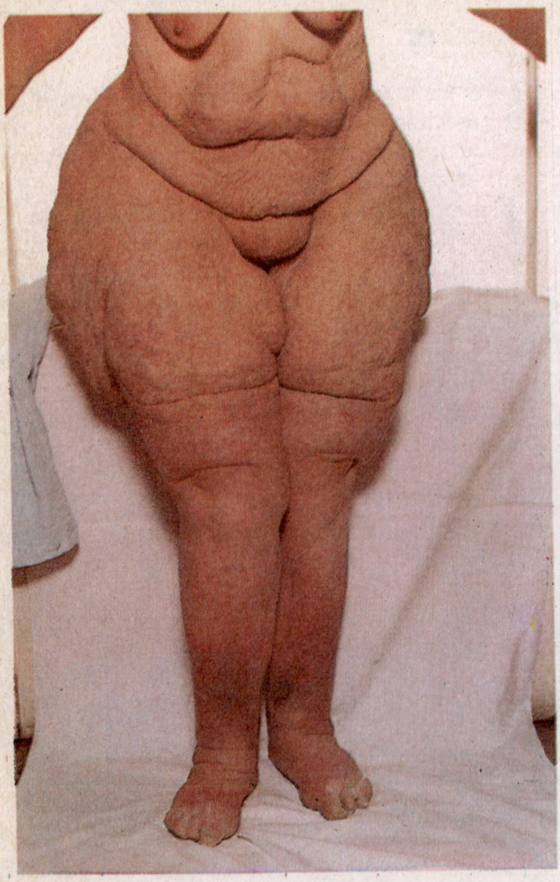

FIG. 8.2 Gross obesity usually affects the whole body, but may, as in this patient, be predominantly confined to the buttocks and thighs

Overweight

Patients with normal skeletal and sexual proportions but whose bodies are bigger than they should be are most likely to be obese from overeating, but three serious pathological conditions cause an increase in weight that can easily be mistaken for obesity: water retention, myxoedema and Cushing's syndrome.

Water retention

Nephrosis and other causes of water retention (renal, cardiac or hepatic) cause an increase in weight. The whole body swells but the

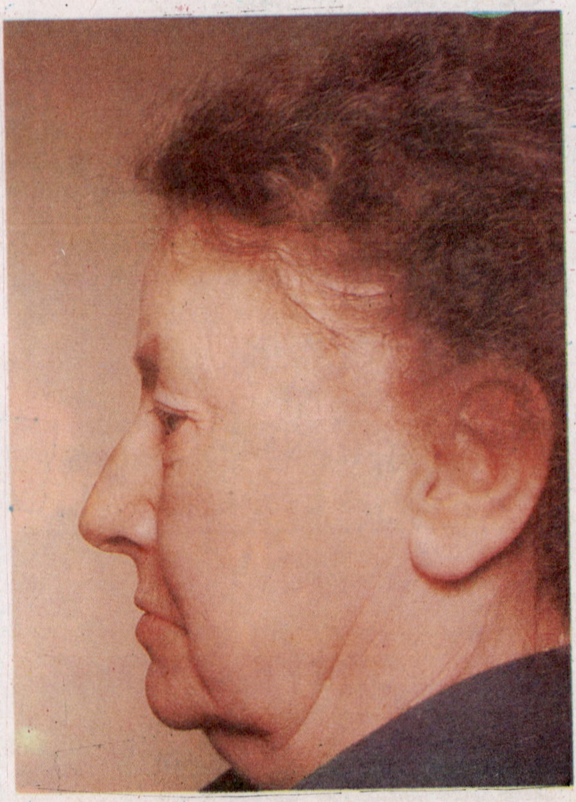

FIG. 8.3 This woman has myxoedema. There is some loss of hair, especially the outer third of the eyebrows, heaviness of the face and creamy skin, but none of these features is diagnostic. This photograph is included to emphasize that early myxoedema is extremely difficult to recognize (see also Fig. 11.26, page 285)

Revision Panel 8.4

The common causes of an increase in weight

- Obesity
- Pregnancy
- Interstitial fluid retention (renal, cardiac or hepatic failure)
- Localized fluid retention (massive ovarian cysts, ascites)
- Myxoedema
- Cushing's syndrome

swelling is most noticeable in the dependent parts. The patient has oedema of the legs, or the sacral region if he is confined to bed, but also in the loose tissues of the face, especially in the skin below the eyes. The swelling around the eyes is often the first symptom and is present when the patient wakes up. Cardiac oedema is also most apparent in the dependent parts and similarly tends to disperse to other areas (not resolve) at night in response to the change of body position.

Myxoedema

Myxoedema, which is caused by a deficiency of thyroid hormone, causes a puffy face, a generalized non-pitting increase in the subcutaneous tissues of the trunk and limbs, a 'peaches and cream' complexion and a dulling of thought, speech and action (see pages 286–287).

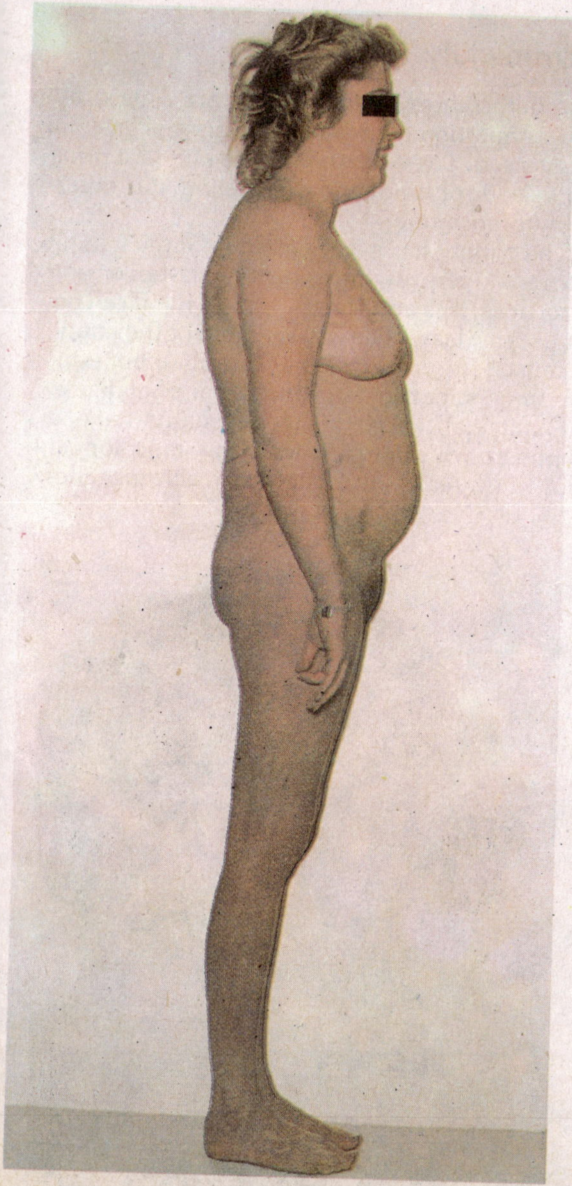

An increase of fat on the trunk and shoulders but thin arms and legs. Red striae on the abdomen and breasts

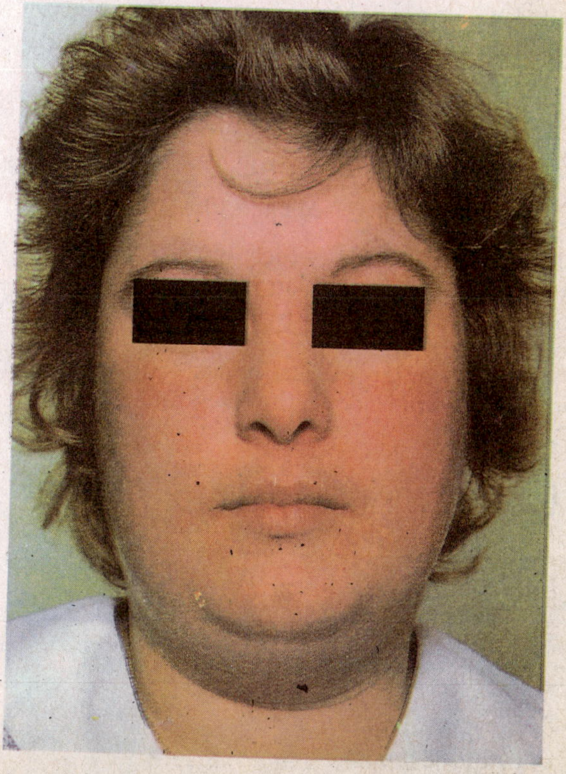

A round 'moon' face, some early hypertrichosis and an unusually florid acniform rash

FIG. 8.4 CUSHING'S SYNDROME

Cushing's syndrome

(Fig. 8.4)

Cushing's syndrome is produced by an excess of adrenal glucocorticoids. One in four patients with Cushing's syndrome has an adrenal adenoma; the remainder have a pituitary abnormality, either an adenoma or excess hypothalamic stimulation.

The patient puts on weight, particularly on the face, neck and trunk. The arms and legs stay thin. The face becomes 'moon-shaped' and the rounded thickened shoulders are often described as a 'buffalo hump'.

There is excess of lanugo hair, an increase in skin pigmentation and red (fresh) striae in the skin that has been stretched, particularly the skin of the abdomen. Hypertension is common.

Skeletal or sexual disproportion

There are a variety of skeletal abnormalities and a few rare disorders of general body development usually associated with chromosomal abnormalities that will be apparent from your initial general inspection.

Paget's disease of bone

(Osteitis deformans) (see page 106)

This is a disease in which normal bone is absorbed and replaced by primitive vascular (osteoid) bone. This makes the bones thick but soft.

The skull enlarges. The bones of the vault bulge outwards above the eyes and ears so much that the patient may complain that he has had to buy larger hats.

The spine bends into a marked kyphosis which reduces the patient's height and may make respiration difficult. The bending of the spine makes the arms look longer.

The long bones of the limbs become thicker and curve forwards and outwards.

Acromegaly

The deformities of acromegaly are caused by the stimulation of growth after normal growth has ceased. The primary abnormality is a pituitary acidophil adenoma secreting too much growth hormone.

The patient has a large face and large hands. There is overgrowth of the soft tissues of the face, nose, lips and tongue and of the facial air sinuses and jaw. The enlargement of the hands is caused by overgrowth of the small bones of the fingers, particularly the distal phalanges.

Giant (tall) acromegalics usually have a kyphosis which makes the arms look longer than they really are, but many acromegalics

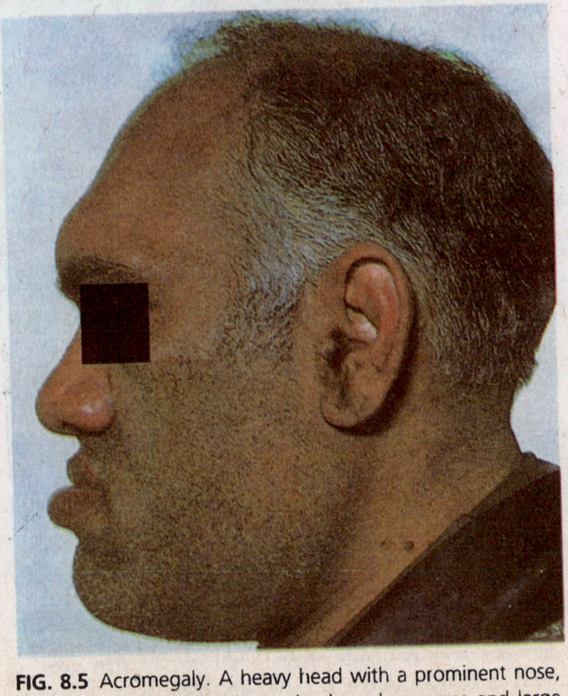

FIG. 8.5 Acromegaly. A heavy head with a prominent nose, chin and lips. These patients also have long arms and large hands and feet

Revision Panel 8.5

The common causes of hair loss

Local
- Male balding
- Alopecia areata
- Skin infections

General
- Hypothyroidism
- Cytotoxic drugs
- Hypopituitarism
- Iron deficiency
- Severe illness

are not tall or kyphotic. Their joints are often enlarged by exuberant osteoarthritis.

The big nose, protuberant jaw and large hands have been compared to the facies of Punch of 'Punch and Judy'.

The skin is greasy, not dry, and there is no loss of mental faculties. These two features help distinguish early acromegaly from myxoedema.

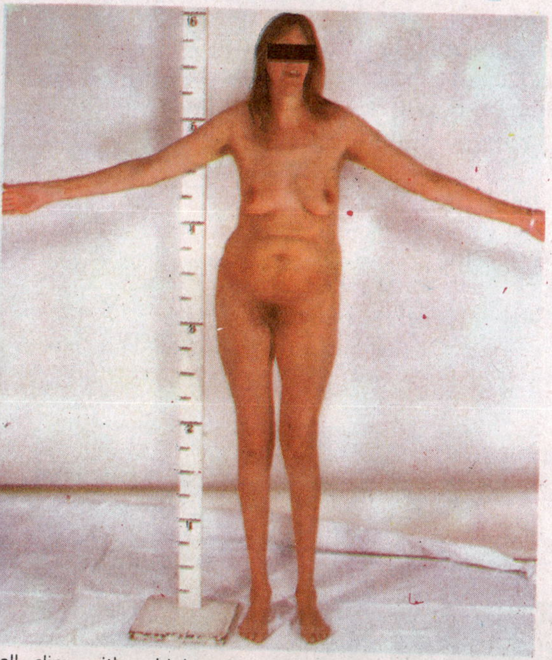

Tall, slim, with a high-arched palate, long arms, and long spindly fingers

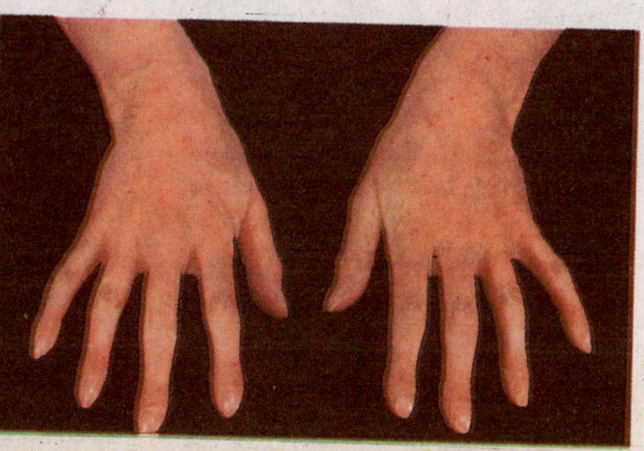

ne long spindly fingers of a patient with Marfan's syndrome

IG. 8.6 MARFAN'S SYNDROME

Marfan's syndrome

Although this is a rare syndrome, you must know of its existence because of the blindness, caused by lens dislocation, and the vascular catastrophes, such as dissecting aneurysm and aortic incompetence, that often accompany it. It is caused by an abnormality of the mucopolysaccharides that form the ground substance of intercellular cement.

Patients with Marfan's syndrome are tall and thin, with very long fingers and toes (arachnodactyly) and a high arched palate.

When this syndrome causes only minor skeletal changes it is difficult to recognize.

Klinefelter's syndrome

(Fig. 8.7)

Klinefelter's syndrome is a congenital abnormality in which a male has an extra female (X) chromosome. Thus instead of being a normal XY male, he is XXY, and testosterone production is subnormal.

The patients are tall, with a female distribution of fat around the breast and pelvis, but normal male hair growth on the face and pubis.

The testes are very small and soft and do not produce spermatozoa, so the patients are sterile.

Turner's syndrome

(Fig. 8.8)

Turner's syndrome is a congenital abnormality in which a female has only one female (X) chromosome. Thus instead of being a normal XX female, she is XO.

There are no skeletal abnormalities but the patient has a masculine shape – wide shoulders and narrow pelvis – and is invariably shorter than the average woman.

The most distinctive feature, when present, is 'webbing' of the shoulders. This is a thickening of the neck and a prominence of the skin folds that run from the neck to the shoulders.

The breasts and pubic hair are usually underdeveloped.

Dwarfism

(Fig. 8.9)

There is a multitude of causes of dwarfism, many of which are obscure endocrine abnormalities. The common causes are as follows.

Rickets Bowed long bones. Scoliosis. Prominent costochondral junctions ('rickety rosary'). Transverse groove across rib cage at attachment of diaphragm (Harrison's sulcus).

Achondroplasia (the circus dwarf). Large head. Flattened bridge of nose. Stunted trunk, hands and fingers. Waddling gait. Umbilicus is below the mid-point of vertical height.

Renal dwarfism

Cretinism

Pituitary deficiency

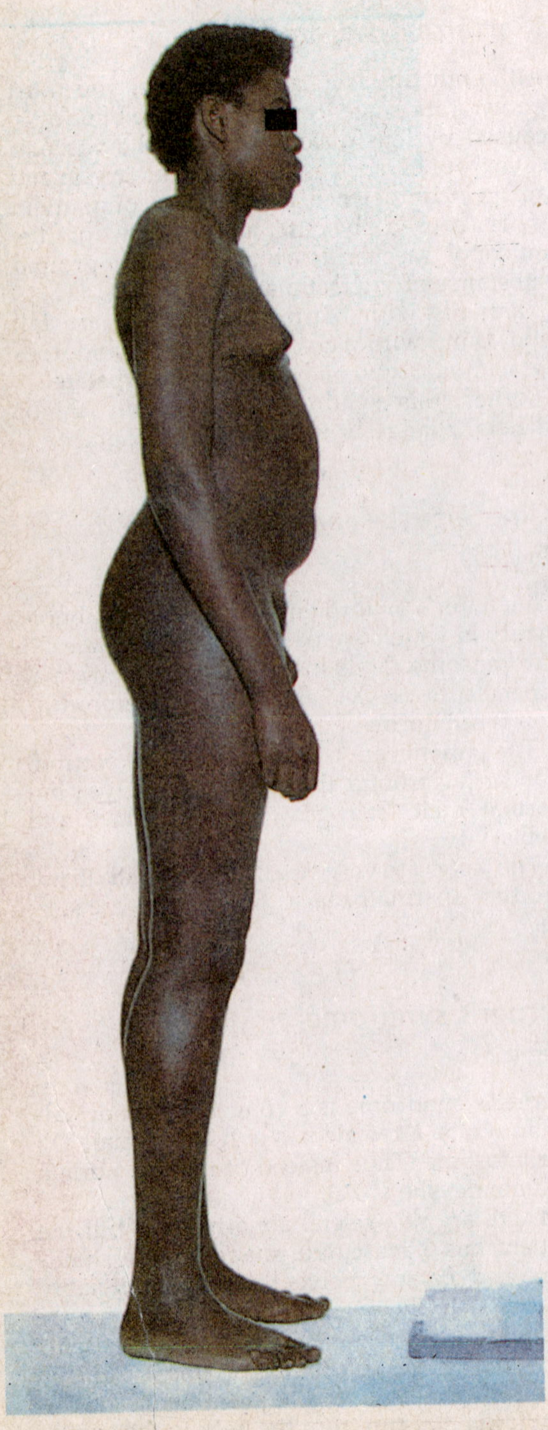

A tall male with a female body shape, a female distribution of body fat and hair, and atrophic testes

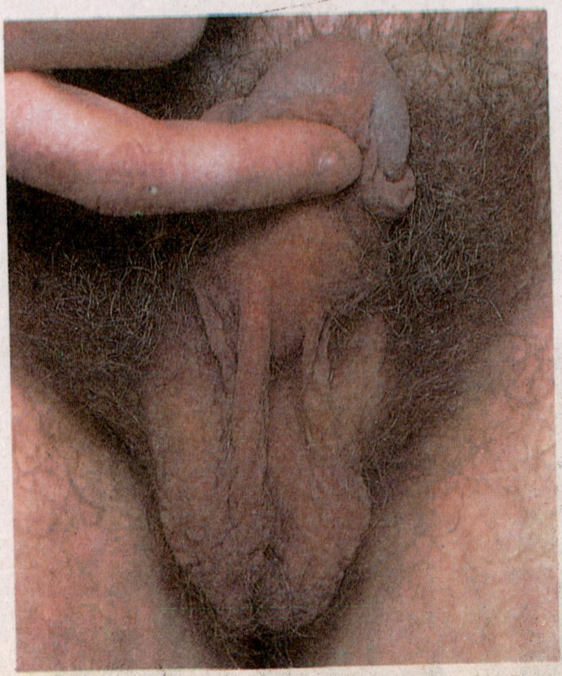

The small underdeveloped scrotum, containing atrophic testes, of a patient with Klinefelter's syndrome

FIG. 8.7 KLINEFELTER'S SYNDROME

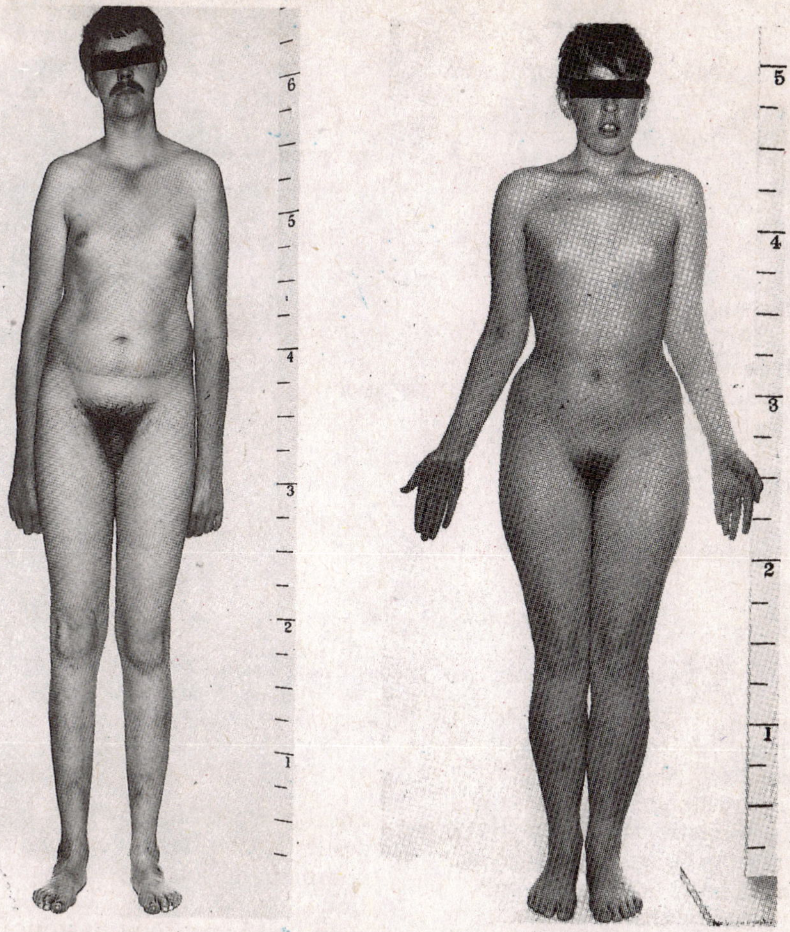

FIG. 8.8 A comparison between the bodybuild of **A**: a young man with **Klinefelter's syndrome** – a tall male with a female distribution of body fat and **B**: a young woman with **Turner's syndrome**, – a short female with a masculine shape and amenorrhoea. The 'webbing' of the shoulders is not very pronounced in this patient

Signs and stigmata of congenital syphilis

This is now a rare condition.

In infants Signs of congenital syphilis rarely appear before 7 years of age. Any symptoms that do occur are usually similar to the symptoms of the secondary stage of acquired syphilis: snuffles, condylomata around the mouth and anus and a ham-coloured, symmetrical, transient rash.

In children and young adults Congenital syphilis causes:

- Interstitial keratitis.
- Deafness.
- Periostitis (sabre tibia).
- Synovitis (Clutton's joints).

These conditions leave permanent defects, aptly described as making the patient blind, deaf and lame.

The *stigmata* of the infection remain with the patient for the rest of his life. They are:

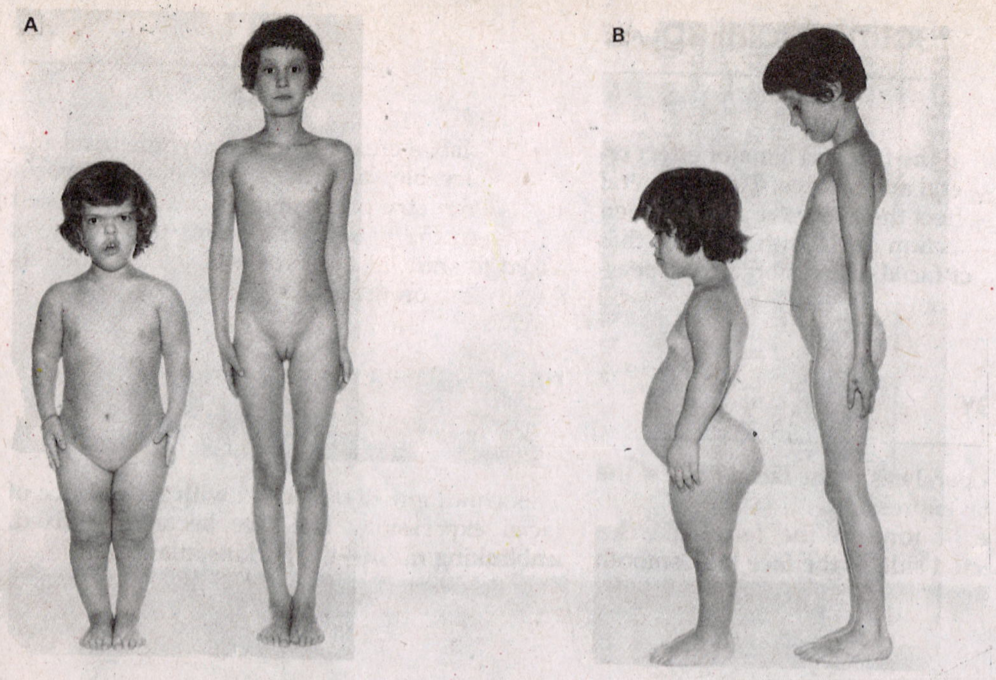

FIG. 8.9 An achondroplastic child standing beside a normal child of the same age. The facial and skeletal abnormalities are all obvious. Note that the umbilicus of the achondroplastic is below the mid-point of the vertical height

Remnants of interstitial keratitis (loss of vision).
Nerve deafness.
Depressed bridge of nose (saddle nose).
Perforated palate or nasal septum.
Radiating scars and creases around the mouth (rhagades).
Hutchinson's teeth (small permanent incisors with a notched border).
Sabre tibiae.
Painless joint effusions (Clutton's joints).
Retardation of growth.

Interstitial keratitis, nerve deafness and Hutchinson's teeth are known as **Hutchinson's triad**.

Hysteria

Beware of the patient whose mental attitude to his symptoms seems out of proportion, either over-responding to them or ignoring them. The patient whose symptoms do not fit any known pattern who tells you with a big smile that he has severe pain, or who, while complaining of severe symptoms, appears quite unconcerned ('la belle indifference') may well be neurotic, hysterical, or fabricating the symptoms and the signs.

A diagnosis of hysteria should only be made when all possible organic causes for the symptoms have been excluded.

In this situation your clinical experience is your greatest help.

DISEASES AFFECTING FACIAL APPEARANCE

The appearance of the face has a major effect on the patient's general appearance. Those general conditions that affect the face have already been described. This section deals with diseases that particularly affect facial expression and appearance.

Bell's palsy

Bell's palsy is a paralysis of the facial nerve affecting the muscles of facial expression.

The absence of tone in the facial muscles makes the affected side of the face look smooth and sloppy. The corner of the mouth droops, the nasolabial creases become asymmetrical and less noticeable, and the lower eyelid droops. The asymmetry of the mouth can be increased by asking the patient to bare his teeth. If he is asked to shut his eyes you will see that the lids fail to close on the affected side.

Parkinson's disease

(Paralysis agitans)

This condition is associated with an absence of facial expression. The face becomes a fixed, unblinking mask – the Parkinsonian mask.

In addition to the facial changes, all movements become stiff and restricted. The patient walks with short shuffling steps, back bent, and head poked forwards.

The hands, limbs and head develop a **tremor**. The repetitive shaking of the thumb and index finger give the appearance of 'pill-rolling'

In its florid state Parkinson's disease presents an unmistakable clinical picture, but it can be detected long before this if you look out for the loss of facial expression.

Scleroderma

The progressive thickening of the skin of the face that occurs with scleroderma can also reduce the patient's ability to use her muscles of facial expression. The skin thickens and has a pale, waxy appearance.

The mouth gets small **(microstomia)** and jaw movements may be restricted.

Telangiectases appear on the cheeks, around the mouth and across the nose.

Fine white horizontal scars appear on the neck in the lines of the transverse skin creases.

When the patient smiles and laughs the face does not respond fully. This is different from

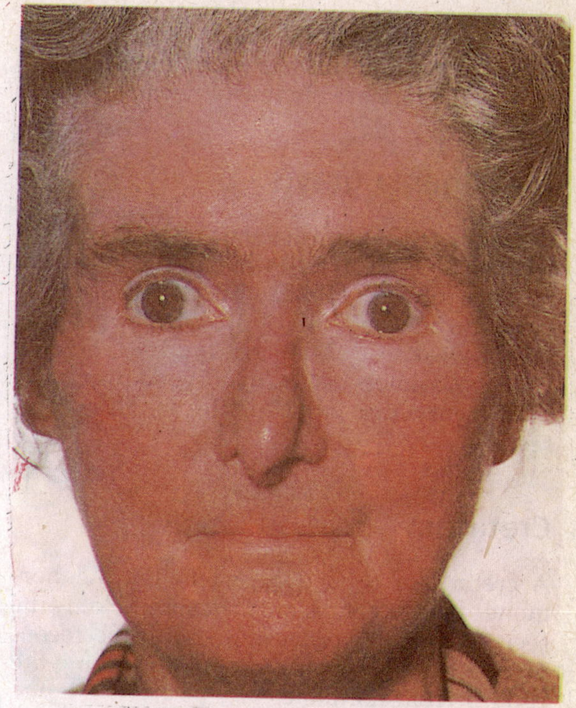

Note the tight skin, small mouth, fine wrinkles around the mouth and small telangiectases

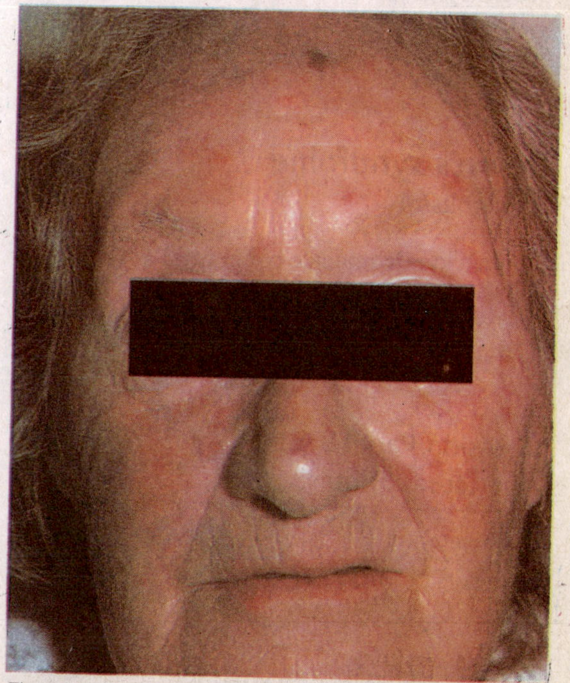

The telangiectases of scleroderma

FIG. 8.10 SCLERODERMA

Parkinson's disease in which there is not a flicker of facial expression even though the tissues of the face are obviously normal.

Myasthenia gravis

Remember that myasthenia gravis causes weakness of all muscles but particularly the muscles of the eyelids. Suspect it in any patient who complains of tired, drooping eyelids or weakness of the face and jaw.

The weakness is transitory; power and movement return if the muscles are allowed to rest.

Cretinism

A cretin is a child deficient in thyroid hormone. It is a condition that should only be seen in neonates because it should be recognized soon after birth and cured by giving the child thyroid hormone.

In an advanced case the face is broad and flat, the eyes are wide apart and the tongue protrudes from the mouth.

If the condition is not treated, growth is slowed so that the child is short, fat and mentally retarded.

Down's syndrome

(Mongolism)

Down's syndrome is a congenital abnormality usually associated with an extra chromosome 21.

Revision Panel 8.6
The causes of ptosis

- Inflammation
- Tumours
- Excess eyelid skin
- Muscle weakness (myopathies, myasthenia)
- Third nerve palsy

Males and females, and all races are equally affected. The prime abnormalities are mental retardation, floppiness and a short stature. The old name describes the dominant facial features; the outer ends of the palpebral fissures slant upwards and there are prominent epicanthic folds. The face is flattened, and the

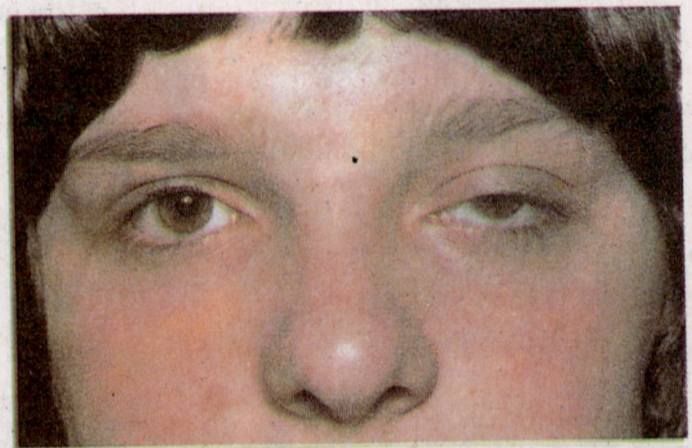

FIG. 8.11 Myasthenia gravis. Heavy, drooping eyelids, much worse on the left. The eye signs of generalized diseases are often asymmetrical, even unilateral

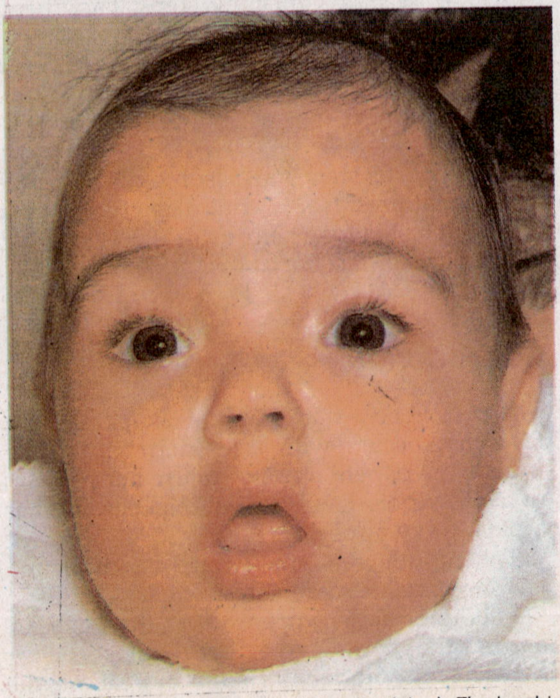

FIG. 8.12 Congenital hypothyroidism (cretinism). The head is broad, the eyes wide apart, the tongue protrudes from the mouth and all movements and responses are slow and sluggish

tongue protrudes. The child often has a squint and one-third have congenital heart disease.

The Down's baby is distinguishable from the cretin because its skin and hair are smooth and fine, not coarse and thick, and though it is more floppy than a normal baby it is not slow and sluggish like a cretin.

THE EYES

The condition of the eyes profoundly affects the facial appearance. This book cannot discuss the many diseases of the eye, some of which are part of generalized conditions, but a few easily recognizable and surgically relevant conditions are presented.

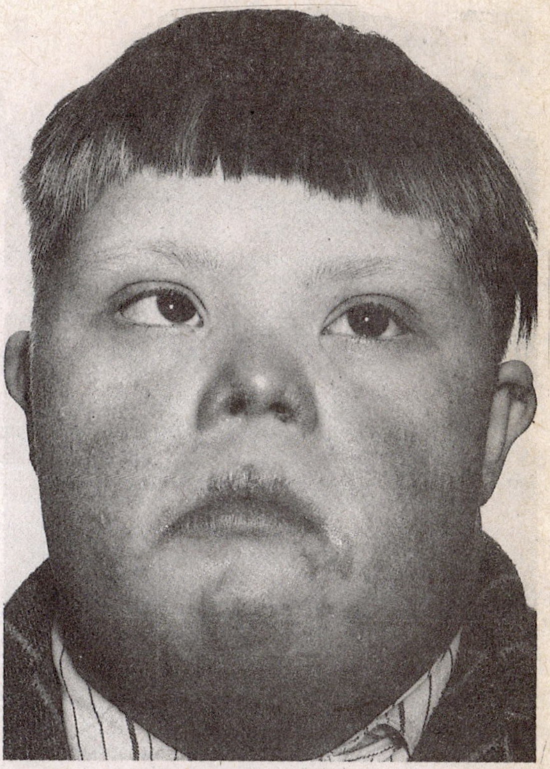

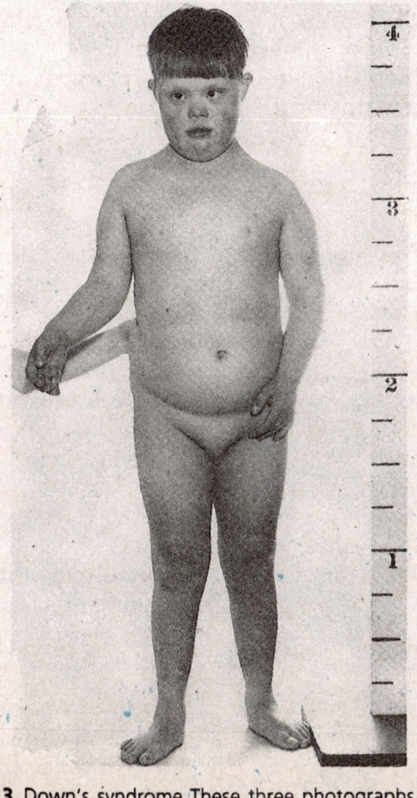

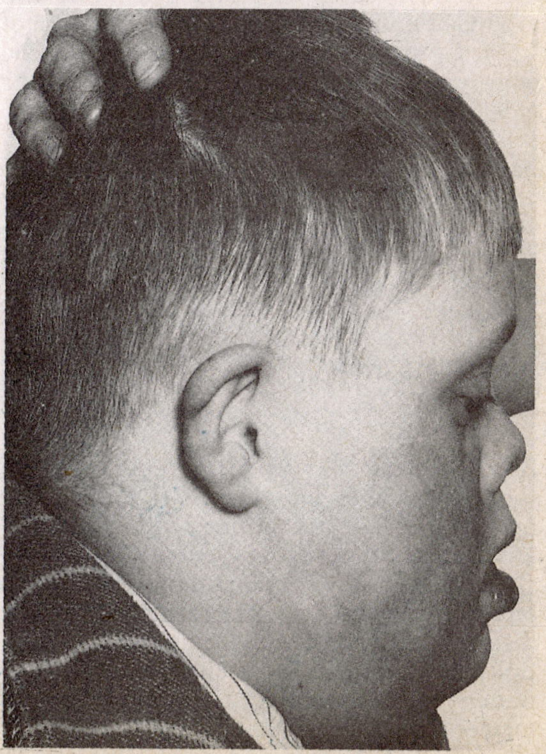

FIG. 8.13 Down's syndrome These three photographs show the short stature, floppiness and typical facial features of Down's syndrome

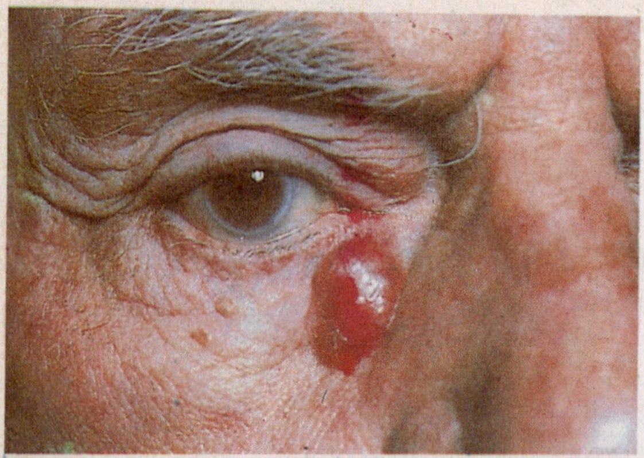

FIG. 8.14 Arcus senilis This is a thin white rim around the iris. It is a common abnormality and does not indicate advanced arterial disease. Note that the patient also has a basal cell carcinoma

Arcus senilis

This term is used to describe a white rim around the outer edge of the iris. It is a rim of sclerosis and cholesterol deposition in the edge of the cornea and is common in the elderly.

It has no great clinical significance, except in patients below the age of 40 when it may be associated with hyperlipoproteinaemia. It is *not* associated with generalized degenerative arterial disease, although both conditions often coexist.

Xanthelasma

(Xanthoma)

Xanthelasmata are fatty plaques in the skin of the eyelids. They look like masses of yellow opaque fat. They are confined to the skin and are not painful or tender.

Xanthomata are very common. One or two on the eyelids do not indicate any underlying disease, but if the patient has extensive, multiple, growing lesions, you should exclude any underlying abnormality of cholesterol metabolism, diabetes, or arterial disease.

Exophthalmos

(Proptosis)

Exophthalmos is the forward protrusion of the eye from its normal position in the orbit.

Figure 8.15 shows the relationship of the eyelids to the iris in the normal and the protruding eye.

In the normal eye the lower eyelid just touches the lower edge of the iris (the inferior limbus), provided the lower lid is normal, while the upper lid crosses the eye mid-way between the pupil and the superior limbus.

The first sign of exophthalmos is the appearance of sclera *below* the inferior limbus. The proptosis has to be considerable before sclera is visible above the superior limbus.

The position of the upper eyelid is also altered by the tone of the levator palpebrae superioris muscle. Retraction of the upper eyelid will reveal sclera above the superior limbus, but you will not mistake this for exophthalmos if you remember to check the position of the lower eyelid.

When the eye is pushed forwards four secondary physical signs appear:

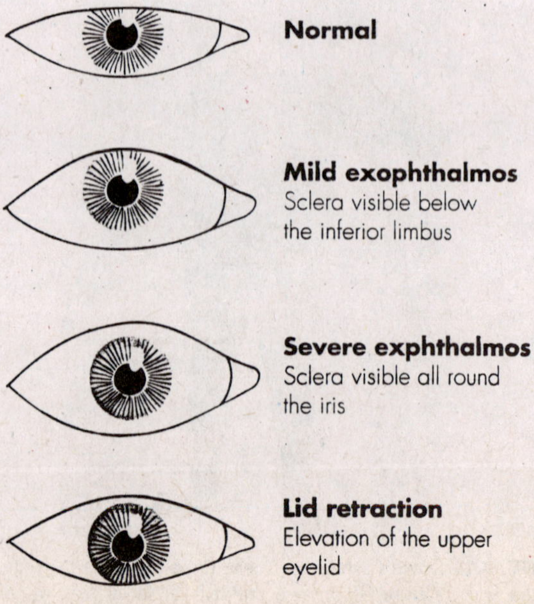

FIG. 8.15 The relations of the eyelids to the iris

1 The patient can look up without wrinkling the forehead.
2 Convergence for very close vision is restricted.
3 The patient blinks less often.
4 The patient may not be able to close his eyes and **corneal ulceration** may develop.

If the protrusion of the eye interferes with the venous and lymphatic drainage of the conjunctiva, it becomes oedematous and wrinkled. This is called **chemosis**.

The causes of exophthalmos are listed in Revision Panel 8.7.

The commonest cause of both bilateral and unilateral exophthalmos is thyrotoxicosis.

Revision Panel 8.8 lists the causes of a pulsating exophthalmos. This is a rare condition but easy to recognize. It is usually associated with severe chemosis.

Revision Panel 8.7

The causes of exophthalmos

* *Endocrine*
Thyrotoxicosis (before, during and after its onset)
Cushing's syndrome (rare)

Non-endocrine
* *Congenital deformities of the skull*
(Craniostenosis, oxycephaly, hypertelorism)

Orbital or periorbital tumours
Periorbital meningioma
Optic nerve glioma
Orbital haemangioma
Lymphoma
Osteoma
Pseudotumour (granuloma)
Carcinoma of antrum
Neuroblastoma

Inflammation
Orbital cellulitis
Ethmoid or frontal sinusitis

Vascular causes
Cavernous sinus arteriovenous fistula
Cavernous artery aneurysm

Eye disease
* Severe myopia
* Severe glaucoma (buphthalmos)

* Likely to be bilateral

Ectropion

Deformities of the lower eyelid often cause the lid to evert. This reveals sclera below the inferior limbus and so mimics exophthalmos, but should not lead to a misdiagnosis because the eyelid looks deformed. When the eyelid becomes everted its inner surface of shiny conjunctiva may become scarred, dull and immobile.

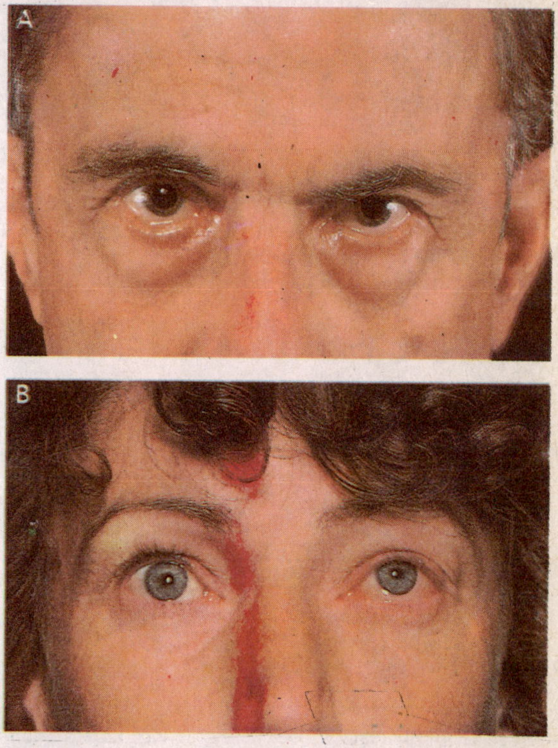

FIG. 8.16 A: Ectropion: Eversion of the lower eyelid. **B**: Proptosis: the sclera is visible between the inferior limbus and the left lower eyelid but the lower eyelid is normal. Thus this is not ectropion but proptosis caused, in this patient, by a retro-orbital tumour

Revision Panel 8.8

The causes of pulsating exophthalmos

Carotid artery–cavernous sinus arteriovenous fistula

Aneurysm of the ophthalmic artery

Vascular neoplasm in the orbit

Cavernous sinus thrombosis

Subconjunctival haemorrhage

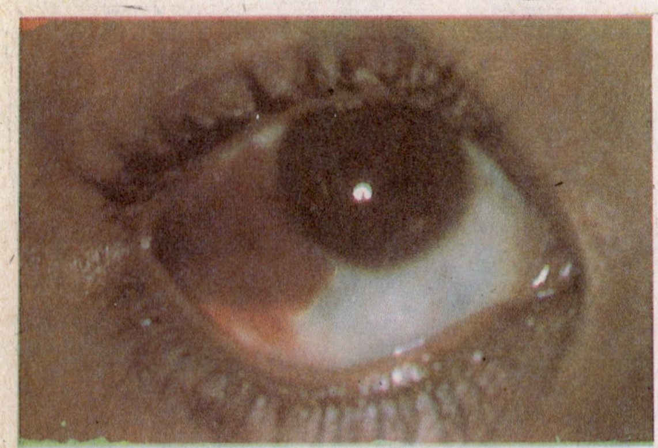

A subconjunctival haemorrhage may arise from a subconjunctival vessel or be blood which has tracked forwards from behind the eye – usually from a fracture of the base of the skull. When this patient looked to the left, white sclera could be seen to the right of the haemorrhage, confirming that the bleeding was solely from subconjunctival blood vessels

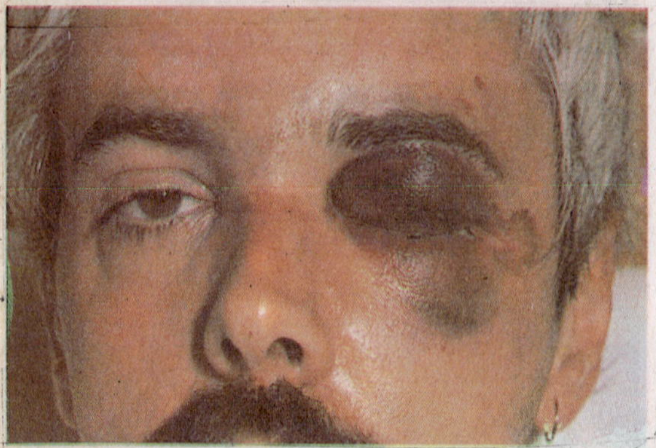

Extensive bleeding from a fracture of the base of the skull may cause a large periorbital haematoma as well as a subconjunctival haemorrhage

FIG. 8.17 SUBCONJUNCTIVAL HAEMORRHAGE

Horner's syndrome

Horner's syndrome comprises the physical signs that follow interruption of the sympathetic nerve supply to the head and neck.

The preganglionic sympathetic fibres of the head and neck arise in the first and sometimes second thoracic segments of the spinal cord. They synapse with the cells in the three cervical sympathetic ganglia whose fibres (postganglionic) are distributed to the structures of the head and neck along the nerves and blood vessels.

The sympathetic pathway to the face and eye can, therefore, be interrupted by trauma or disease anywhere between the appearance of the preganglionic fibres from the spinal cord and their termination.

Absence of sympathetic tone causes myosis, ptosis, vasodilatation and anhidrosis.

The causes of Horner's syndrome are as follows (the common causes are in bold type):

- Brain lesions – **posterior inferior cerebellar artery thrombosis.**
- Spinal cord lesions – syringomyelia, tumours.
- Injuries to the lower roots of the brachial plexus.
- Surgical excision of the inferior cervical ganglion (**cervical sympathectomy**).
- Tumours in the apex of the lung (**Pancoast's tumour**).
- Tumours in the neck.
- Aneurysm and dissection of the carotid artery.

Revision Panel 8.9
Horner's syndrome

- A small pupil (myosis)
- Drooping of the upper eyelid (ptosis)
- A warm pink cheek (vasodilatation)
- Absence of sweating (anhidrosis)
- Nasal congestion (nasal vasodilatation)
- (Apparent enophthalmos)

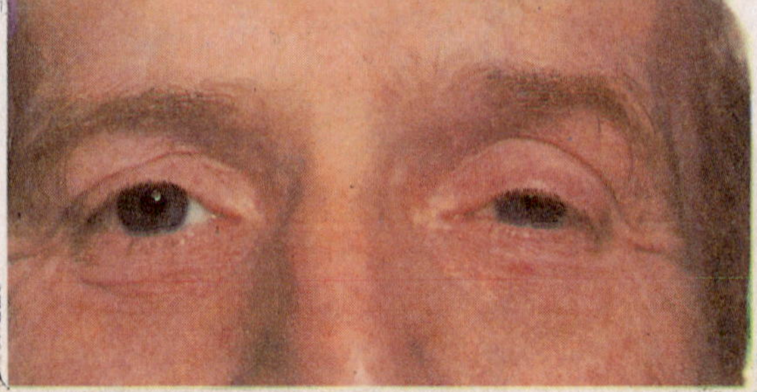

FIG. 8.18 Horner's syndrome of the left eye. See Revision Panel 8.9

When these nerve fibres are interrupted by disease there may be a period before the paralysis when the sympathetic activity is increased. Stimulation of the sympathetic nerves makes the pupil dilate, the upper eyelid retract and the skin of the face pale, cold and sweaty. The causes of sympathetic nerve irritation are the same as the causes of paralysis.

THE NOSE

The appearance of the face is altered by the shape of the nose. In addition to the infinite variability of the shape of the normal nose, there are two pathological conditions which alter its shape.

Saddle nose

A nose whose bridge is depressed and widened is called a saddle nose. This deformity is caused by congenital abnormalities such as achondroplasia and hypertelorism, or destruction of the nasal cartilages, commonly caused by leprosy, cutaneous leishmaniasis and congenital syphilis.

Rhinophyma

Rhinophyma is a thickening of the skin over the tip of the nose caused by hypertrophy and adenomatous changes in its sebaceous glands. It is not caused by an excessive intake of alcohol.

SHAPE OF THE SKULL

There are a number of congenital deformities of the skull, all with long names that describe the skull's shape, but they are all very rare.

The abnormality of shape that you should look out for in neonates and young children is the progressive and disproportionate enlargement of the skull caused by **hydrocephalus**.

The normal scalp consists of hairy skin, subcutaneous fat and a fascial aponeurosis. All

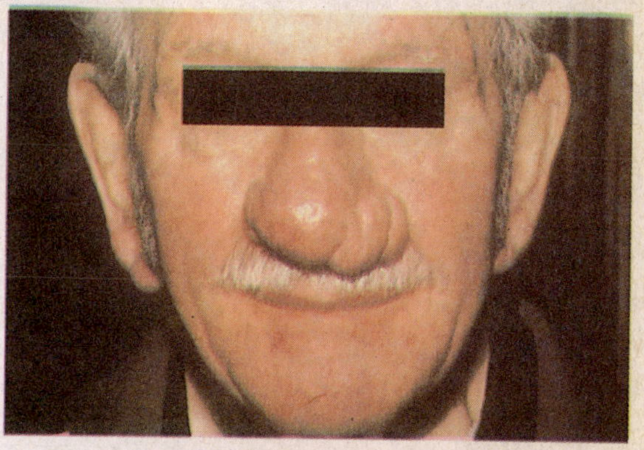

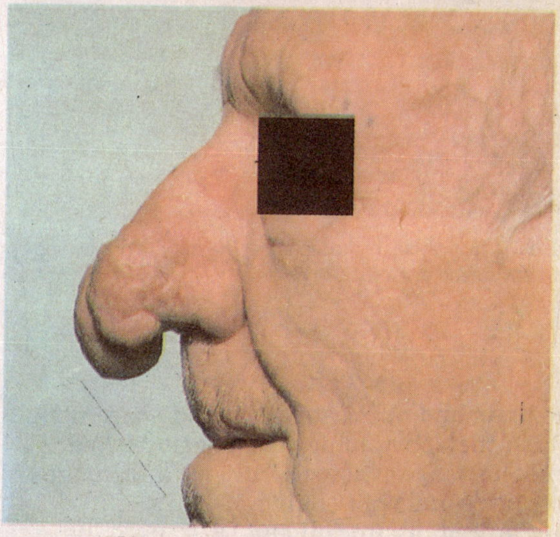

FIG. 8.19 Two examples of rhinophyma: hypertrophy of the sebaceous glands in the skin of the nose

these structures can give rise to the common lesions of the skin and subcutaneous tissues described in Chapters 2 and 3, but some are so common on the scalp that they deserve special mention.

Hydrocephalus

Hydrocephalus is a pathological accumulation of cerebrospinal fluid within or around the brain – internal or external hydrocephalus.

Congenital hydrocephalus is caused by a failure of cerebrospinal fluid absorption, so that there is distension of the ventricles within

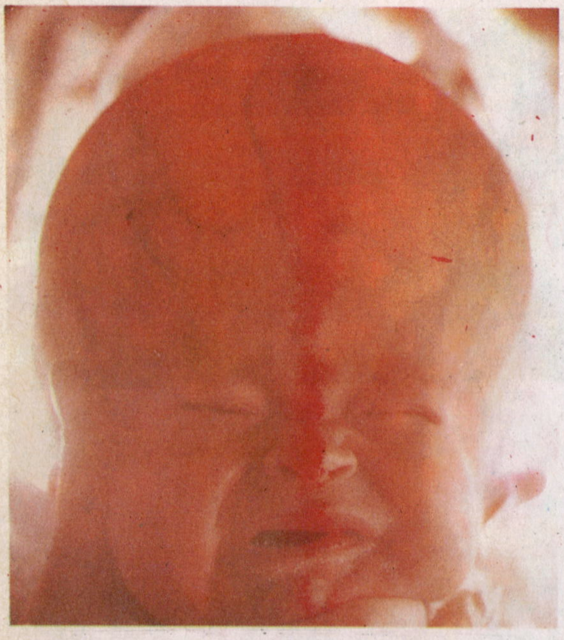

FIG. 8.20 Congenital hydrocephalus. The bright light behind the baby's head reveals the thinness of the bones of the skull

the brain and of the subarachnoid space with which they communicate. Congenital hydrocephalus is often associated with a meningomyelocele and spina bifida.

Acquired hydrocephalus is caused by a block of the aqueduct of Sylvius or the foramina over the fourth ventricle, by tumour or infection. In this type of hydrocephalus the distended ventricles do not communicate with the subarachnoid space.

Multiple sebaceous cysts

The scalp may be covered with sebaceous cysts of all sizes. They are diagnosed by their spherical shape and hard, tense composition (see also page 78). They are by far the commonest cause of a lump on the scalp. They rarely have a visible punctum.

A suppurating sebaceous cyst with granulation tissue bulging out of it is sometimes called **Cock's peculiar tumour** (see page 80). It is easily mistaken for a squamous cell carcinoma.

Turban tumour

There are four pathological conditions that can cause multiple lumps on the scalp which grow steadily, coalesce and eventually produce an irregular mass that covers the whole scalp and looks like a turban. All are **rare**.

As the term 'turban tumour' is purely descriptive, it can be applied to all four conditions. However, it is most often used to describe **multiple cylindromata**, which present as firm pink nodules in the skin.

Multiple nodular basal cell carcinomata may also cover the scalp, but they are firm, retain their pearly-white appearance and covering of fine blood vessels, do not really look like a turban and can usually be diagnosed by examining one of the smaller lesions.

Multiple sweat gland tumours, **hidradenomata**, form soft, boggy swellings in the scalp. Although very soft (they feel like lumps of oedematous skin), they are not fluctuant and cannot be compressed or indented.

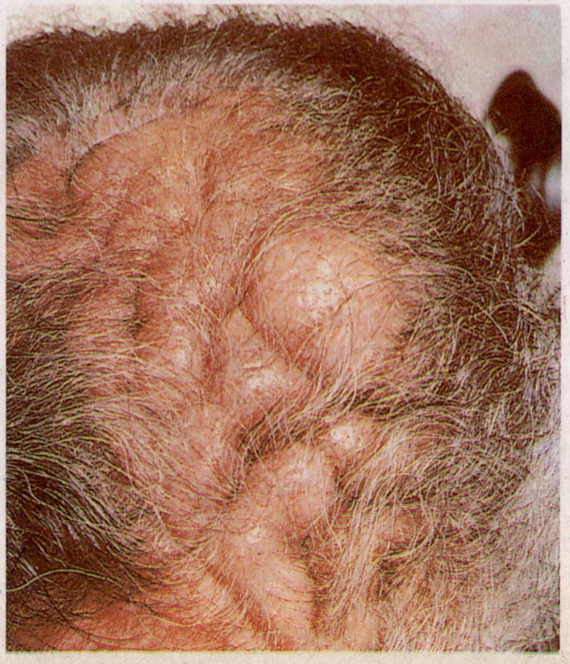

FIG. 8.21 A 'turban tumour'. This one was a cylindroma

Finally, and rarest of all, is subcutaneous **plexiform neurofibromatosis** of the scalp. This is usually associated with neurofibromata in other sites and café au lait patches.

Pott's puffy tumour

Pott's puffy tumour is a diffuse oedematous swelling of the scalp over a patch of osteomyelitis in the skull. It is most often seen in the frontal region overlying frontal bone osteomyelitis caused by frontal sinusitis.

Cephalhaematoma

This is a subperiosteal haematoma. It occurs in neonates following a traumatic delivery, and in infants following direct trauma. The haematoma spreads beneath the pericranium (periosteum) to the fissures between the skull bones.

For a few days it forms a soft, fluctuant swelling covering one of the bones of the vault of the skull but, when the blood begins to resorb, the residual blood clot forms a ridge around the edge of the swelling. Ultimately all that is left of the swelling is a **hard, raised edge**, which is often compared to a dinner plate, and is easily mistaken for a depressed fracture if you do not observe that the lip is above the level of the rest of the skull.

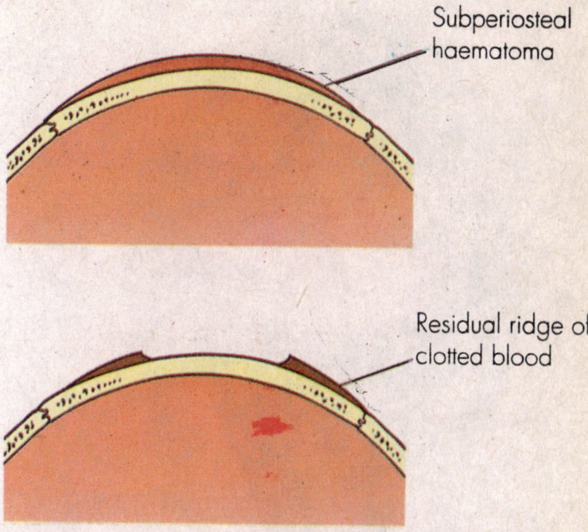

FIG. 8.22 A cephalhaematoma is a subperiosteal haematoma limited by the fissures between the bones. When the blood is absorbed, a ridge of clotted blood forms a rim around the edge of the haematoma

Ivory osteoma

This is an osteoma of the cortical bone that forms the outer table of the skull. Ivory osteomata appear during adolescence and young adult life but cause no symptoms and need no treatment.

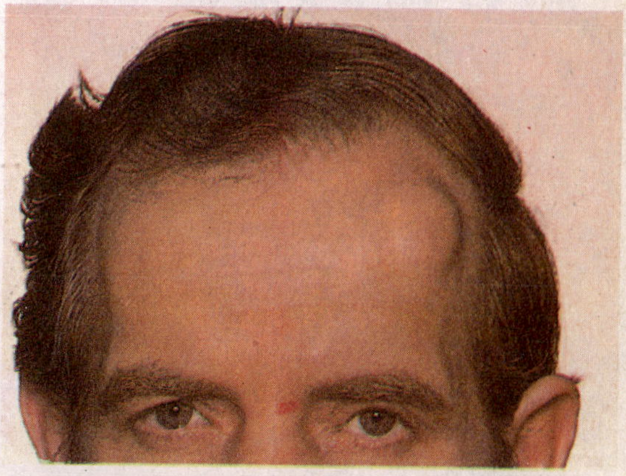

FIG. 8.23 An ivory (cortical) osteoma on the forehead

THE EARS

Bat ears

Congenital bat ears are ears which jut out from the side of the head rather than lying flat against it. Bat ears are *not* associated with any mental abnormalities. Cup-shaped ears that protrude from the side of the skull are a feature of Down's syndrome but these are not true bat ears.

If the patient complains that his ears have become prominent, look behind them for swellings in the subcutaneous tissue or bone that may be pushing the ear outwards. For example, a mastoid abscess makes the ear more prominent.

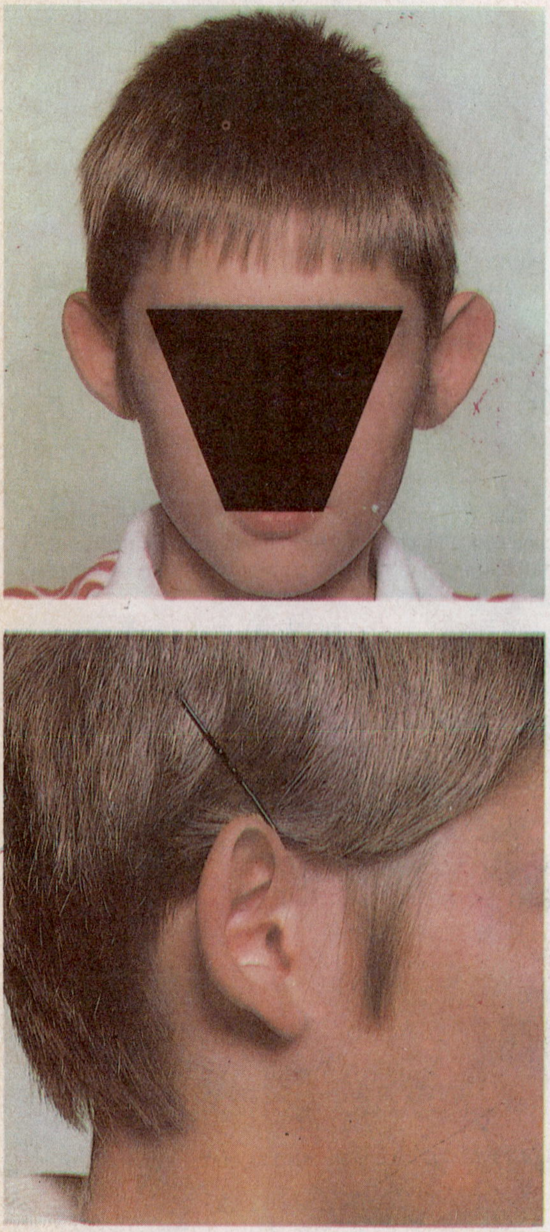

FIG. 8.24 Bat ears

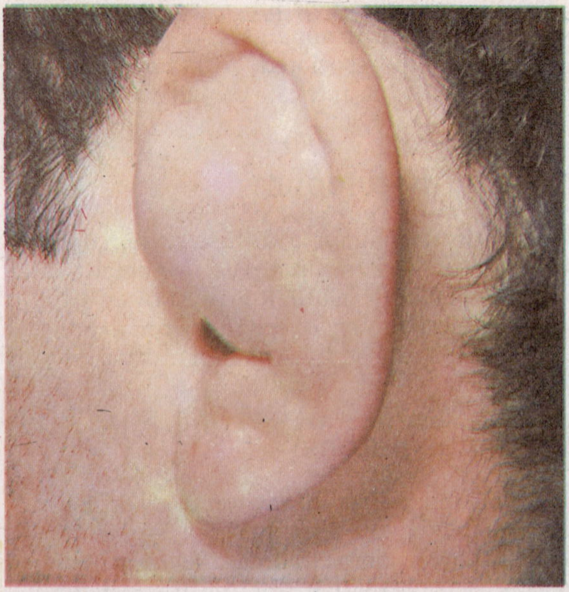

FIG. 8.25 A 'cauliflower ear'. The swelling is a subperichondral haematoma and is almost blocking the external auditory meatus

Cauliflower ears

Cauliflower ears are ears distorted by multiple subperichondral haematomata. Unlike most other haematomata, those beneath the perichondrium of the ear are slow to resorb. Some actually absorb fluid and swell. The patient complains of a flattened, sometimes fluctuant, sometimes firm, swelling fixed to the cartilage of the ear, which fills the hollows of the ear and distorts its shape.

Cauliflower ears are common in boxers and wrestlers.

Keloid nodules

Many women have their ears pierced. If the hole becomes infected, or if the patient has an inherent tendency towards keloid scarring, the scar tissue may overgrow and produce a large nodule behind the lobe of the ear. The nodule is soft, spherical and sometimes pedunculated. It is often misdiagnosed as an inclusion dermoid cyst but is usually a solid mass of keloid scar.

Accessory auricle

Accessory auricles are small pieces of cartilage separate from the pinna. They are found

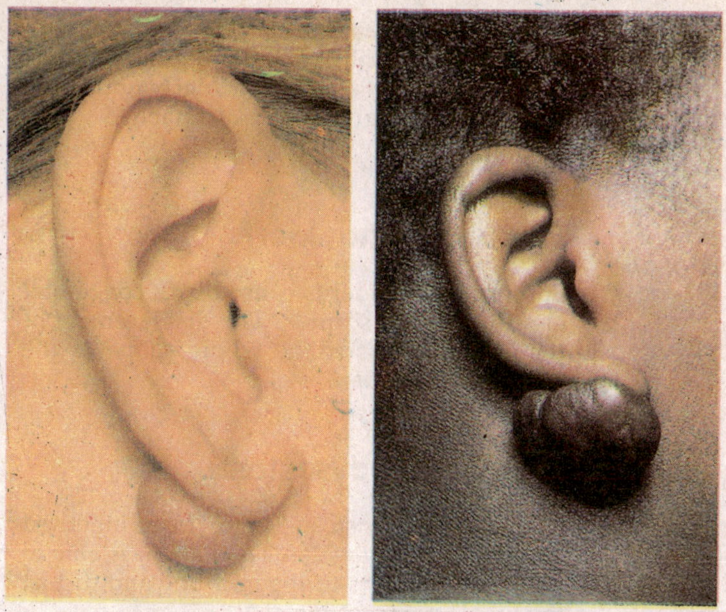

FIG. 8.26 Keloid scars at the site of ear piercing. The mass of scar tissue usually protrudes from the posterior aspect of the ear lobe. Keloid scars are more common in black-skinned races

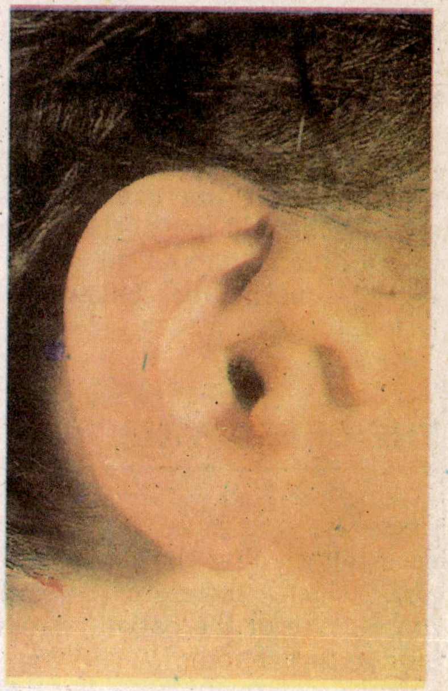

FIG. 8.27 An accessory auricle

on the side of the face just in front of the tragus. They cause no symptoms and can be differentiated from the other two lumps that develop in front of the ear, an enlarged pre-auricular lymph gland or a parotid gland tumour, by the fact that they have been present from birth.

MENINGOCELE

A **meningocele** is a protrusion of the meninges through a defect in the spinal canal or skull. It contains cerebrospinal fluid. A meningocele is covered by skin.

A **meningomyelocele** is a protrusion of the meninges plus part of the spinal cord or cauda equina through a defect in the spinal canal. A meningomyelocele is *not* completely covered by skin and the thin meninges rupture a few days after birth.

There are two other uncommon congenital abnormalities of spinal cord and canal development. A **myelocele** is an open, exposed spinal cord. The infant is stillborn or dies

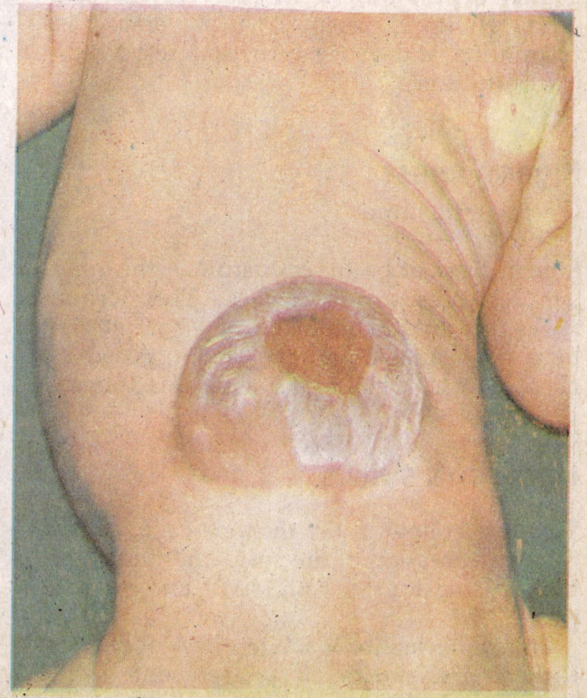

FIG. 8.28 A meningomyelocele of the spine

within a few days of birth. A **syringomyelocele** is the bulge of a dilated spinal cord (hydromyelia) through the spinal canal.

The diagnosis of a meningocele, or meningomyelocele, is made on the basis of its composition – soft, fluctuant and translucent; its site – in the mid-line of the lower back, or the back of the skull; and the presence of neurological abnormalities below the level of the lesion.

THE CHEST WALL

There are a number of deformities and diseases which alter the shape of the chest wall and which, therefore, affect the general appearance of the patient; hence their inclusion in this chapter.

Funnel chest

(Pectus excavatum)

Funnel chest, or pectus excavatum, is a congenital depression of the body of the sternum. If it is deep it may embarrass respiration and cause recurrent respiratory tract infection.

Pigeon chest

(Pectus carinatum)

Pigeon chest, or pectus carinatum, is the opposite deformity to funnel chest. The sternum sticks forwards like the keel of a boat. It may be a congenital deformity or be caused by chest disease in childhood, such as asthma.

Harrison's sulcus

This is a hollow in the thoracic cage, caused by the depression of the costo-chondral junctions of the fourth, fifth, sixth and seventh ribs.

This abnormality is a late effect of **rickets.** Rickets first causes an enlargement of the costo-chondral junctions – **the rickety rosary** – but later the costo-chondral junctions and the ends of the ribs soften and sink inwards. The resulting hollow is particularly noticeable over the lower group of ribs attached to the sternum.

Sprengel's shoulder

Sprengel's shoulder is caused by a congenital elevation of the scapula. The displacement of the scapula distorts the whole shape of the chest and shoulder.

Craniocleidodysostosis

Craniocleidodysostosis is a rare inherited absence of the clavicles. The patient is able to pull the shoulders to the mid-line and distort the whole shape of the chest.

Winging of the scapulae

The scapula is normally held against the chest wall by the serratus anterior muscle. This muscle also rotates and moves the scapula forwards around the chest during those movements which involve holding the arm out forwards.

The nerve to the serratus anterior (the long thoracic nerve of Bell) may be divided or stretched by direct trauma, carrying heavy weights or wearing a knapsack, or be affected by a viral neuritis. When the serratus anterior muscle is paralysed the scapula pokes out from the chest wall – a deformity called 'winging'. If the patient complains of weakness of the arms or deformity of his back, remember to ask him to put his hands and arms out forwards and press against a wall. If the serratus anterior muscles are paralysed the scapulae will protrude backwards.

Myopathy affecting the serratus anterior muscle will also cause 'winging'.

Tietze's syndrome

This is a condition which occurs in young women. It is a painful swelling of the second, third and fourth costal cartilages. The cause is

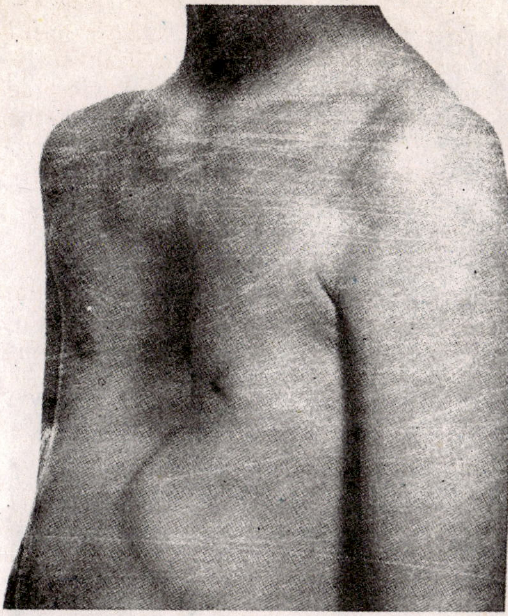

Funnel chest

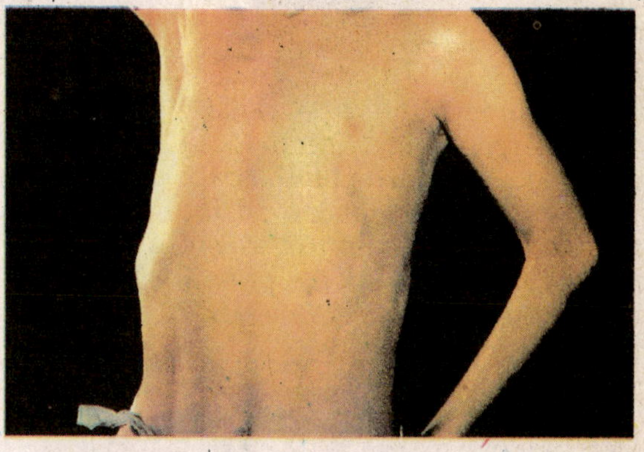

A rickety rosary

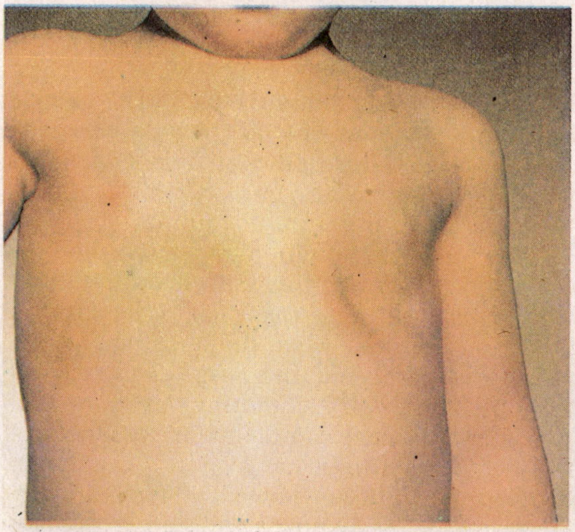

Pigeon chest

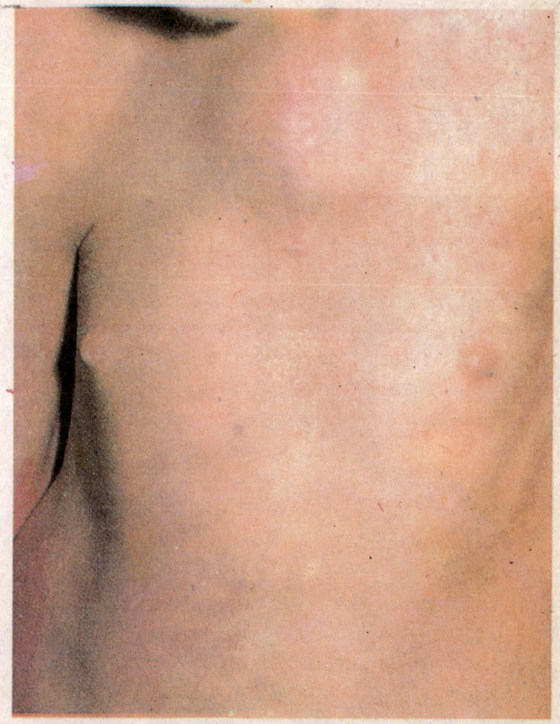

An aortic aneurysm eroding through the sternum

FIG. 8.29 DEFORMITIES OF THE CHEST WALL

unknown but the symptoms, pain and swelling in or near the breast cause the patient great concern because she thinks she has a carcinoma of the breast.

The diagnosis is based solely upon the clinical detection of hard, immobile, tender swellings of the costo-chondral junctions. It is a self-limiting condition.

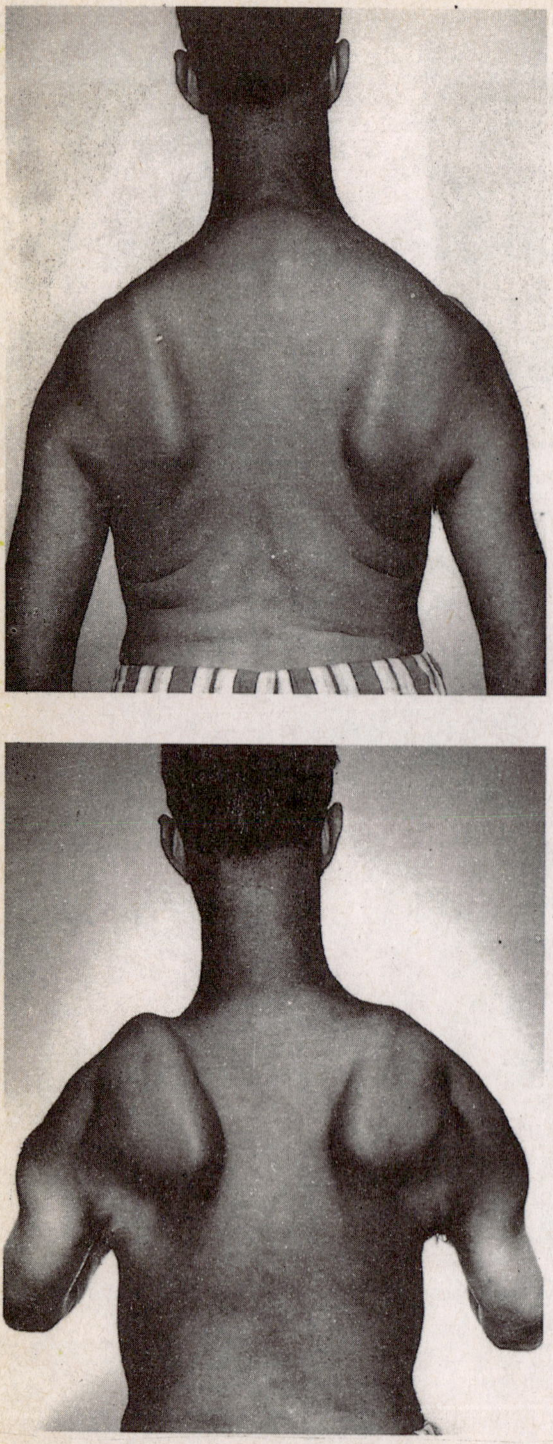

Winging of the scapulae, accentuated by asking the patient to hold out their arms in front of their trunk, and press against a wall

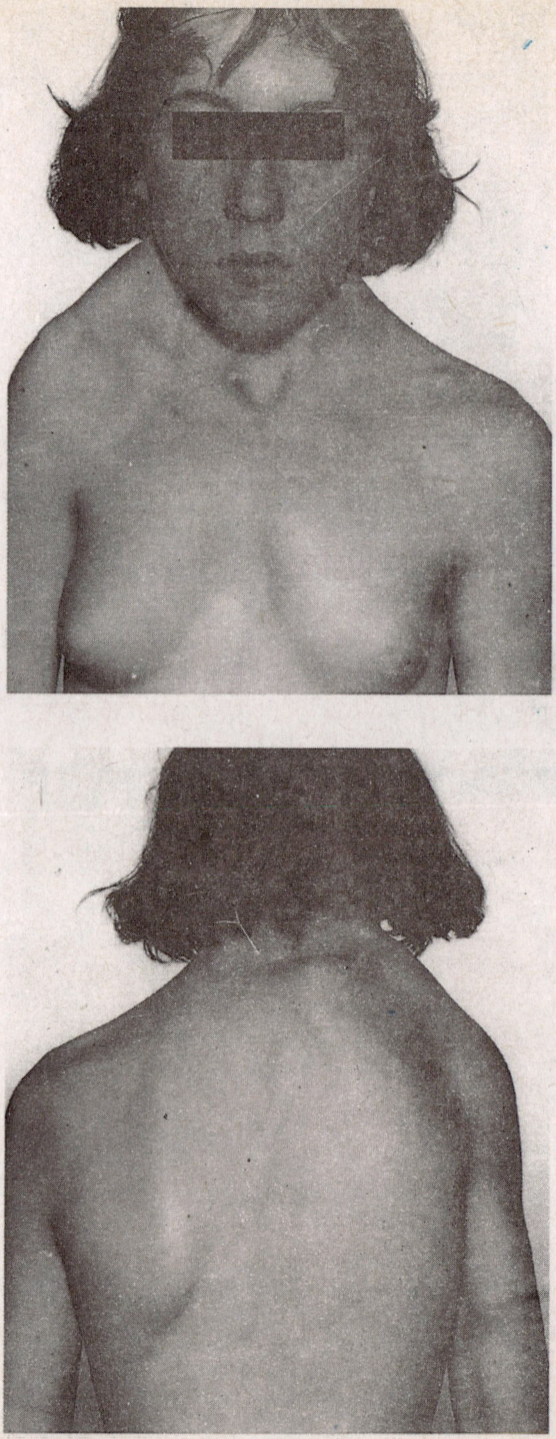

Sprengel's shoulder. A congenitally high scapula

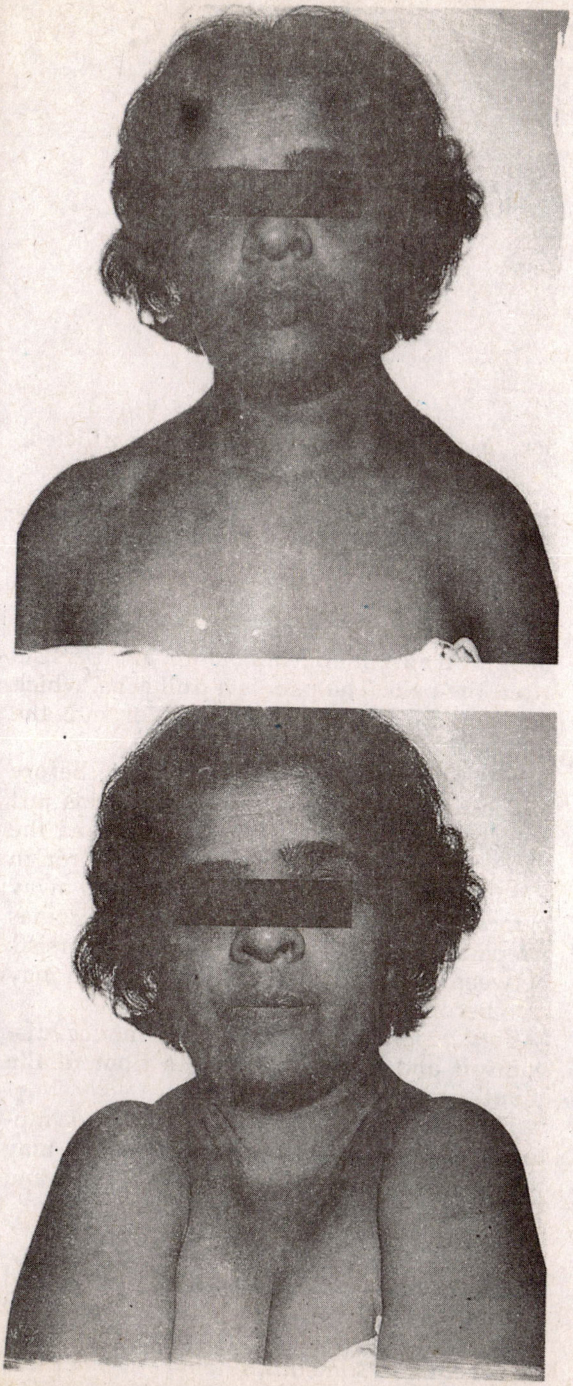

Craniocleidodysostosis. Congenital absence of the clavicles

FIG. 8.30 SOME ABNORMALITIES AFFECTING THE APPEARANCE OF THE CHEST WALL

Lumps on the chest wall

The tissues that form the chest wall can give rise to all the benign and malignant swellings that have been described in Chapters 2, 3 and 4.

Chondromata and secondary tumours in the ribs are quite common.

Aneurysms of the arch of the aorta eroding through the sternum and causing sudden death by rupturing are now extremely rare.

Revision Panel 8.10

The causes of swellings of the chest wall

Bony hard
- Secondary carcinoma
- Chondroma
- Osteoma
- Exostosis (diaphyseal aclasis)
- Myeloma

Fluctuant
- Tuberculosis abscess of rib or lymph node
- Empyema necessitas
- Infected haematoma

Pulsatile
- An eroding aortic aneurysm

9 The salivary glands

Saliva is produced by the paired parotid, submandibular and sublingual glands and many other small, unnamed glands scattered beneath the buccal mucous membrane.

The commonest surgical diseases of the salivary glands are infection and calculus formation in the submandibular gland, and tumours of the parotid gland. Mumps is the commonest medical disease; all other diseases of the salivary glands are uncommon.

THE SUBMANDIBULAR SALIVARY GLAND

Submandibular calculi

Submandibular calculi are common because the submandibular gland lies below the opening of its duct on the floor of the mouth, and because the secretions of the submandibular gland contain a considerable quantity of mucus, two factors which encourage stasis in the duct. Calculi in the parotid gland are less common.

A salivary gland calculus is composed of cellular debris, bacteria, mucus, and calcium and magnesium phosphates – a mixture similar to the 'scale' (tartar) that the dentist scrapes off our teeth.

HISTORY

Age Most submandibular salivary calculi occur in young to middle-aged adults. They are rare in children.

Sex Males and females are equally afflicted.

Symptoms The main symptoms are **pain and swelling** beneath the jaw, caused by obstruction of Wharton's duct.

These two symptoms vary in predominance. Swelling is usually the principal complaint, because it appears before, and persists after, the pain. The pain is a dull ache, which occasionally radiates to the ear or into the tongue.

Both symptoms appear, or worsen, **before and during eating**. The swelling begins just before eating and the pain develops as the gland enlarges. Both symptoms last through the meal, but afterwards the pain goes away before the swelling. If the gland becomes irreparably damaged the swelling persists between meals and the dull aching pain may also become constant.

Very rarely, the patient may notice **discomfort** and a **swelling in the floor of the mouth**.

The patient may be able to relieve his symptoms by pressing on the gland, and he may notice that this action produces a foul-tasting fluid in the mouth (purulent saliva).

Development The symptoms may recur and remit for periods of a few days or weeks if the stone moves about in the duct, sometimes obstructing it, sometimes not.

If the stone passes through the orifice of the duct the symptoms disappear.

Persistent obstruction damages the gland, making it harder and more tender.

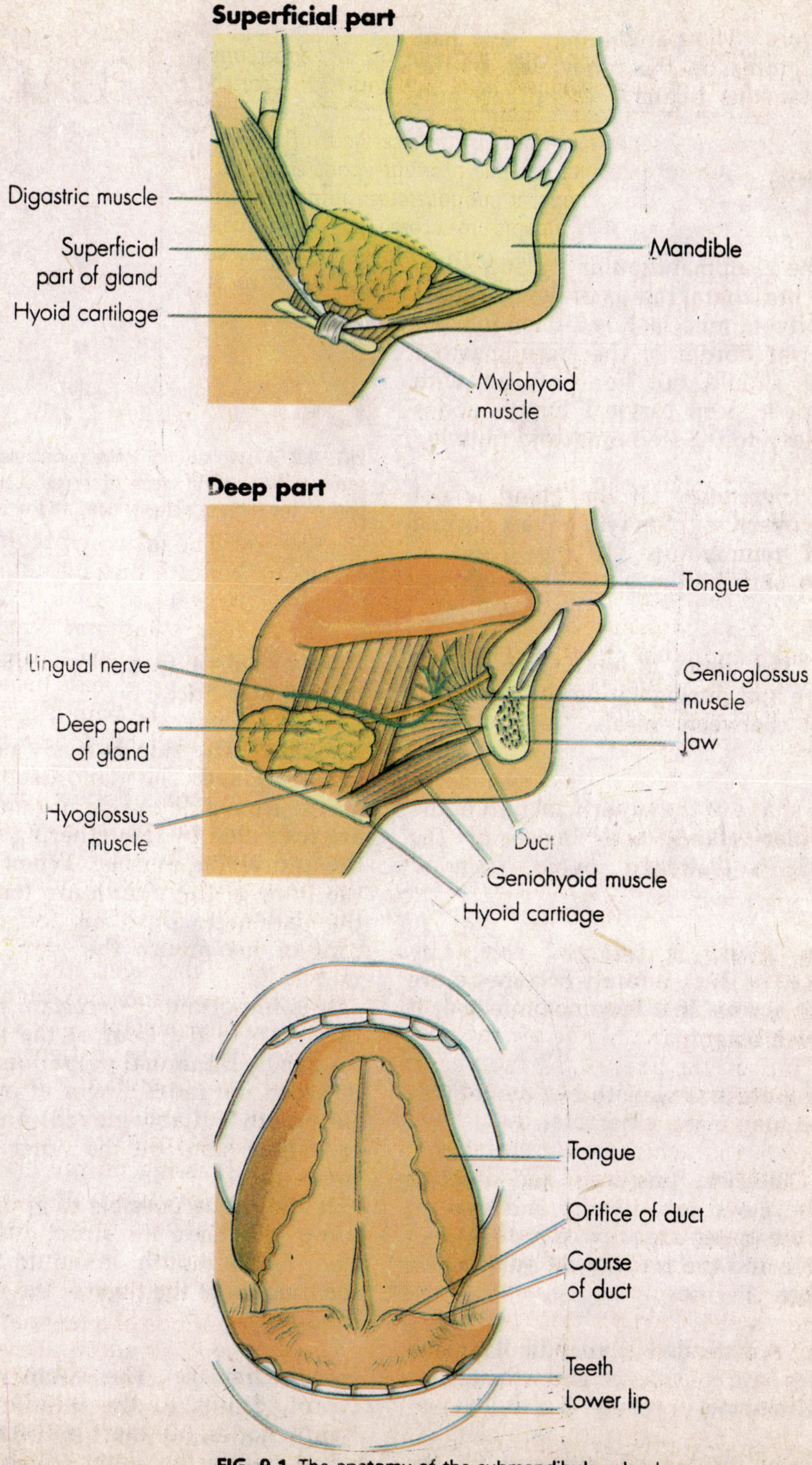

FIG. 9.1 The anatomy of the submandibular gland

Previous history The patient may have had similar symptoms on the other side of the face. Simultaneous bilateral calculi are uncommon.

EXAMINATION

The lump

Position The submandibular gland lies beneath the horizontal ramus of the mandible on the mylohyoid muscle. It is 2–3 cm in front of the anterior border of the sternomastoid muscle and should not be confused with enlarged upper deep cervical lymph nodes which are deep to the sternomastoid muscle.

Colour and temperature If the gland is not infected the overlying skin will have a normal colour and temperature. If the gland is infected the skin becomes red, oedematous and hot.

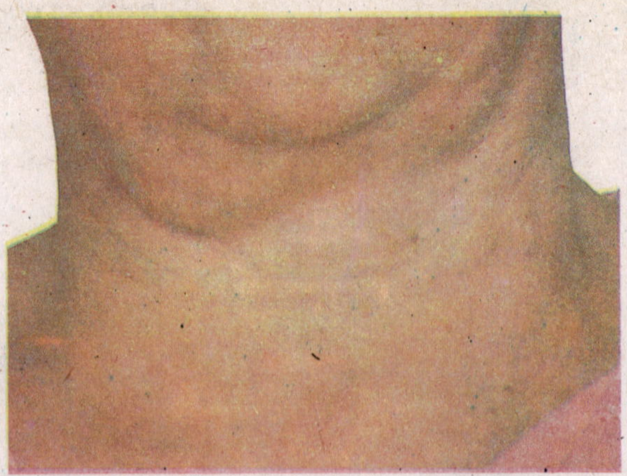

FIG. 9.2 A swollen right submandibular gland. Although some of the swelling seems to spread over the jaw, the upper part of the lump is actually deep to the mandible

Tenderness The gland is tender when it is tense (before and during eating) but not usually tender between meals, unless it is infected.

Shape The shape of the superficial part of the submandibular gland, and hence of the swelling, is a flattened ovoid (almond shaped).

Size If the gland is enlarged solely by obstruction of its duct, it rarely becomes more than 3–5 cm across. If it becomes infected, it may get much bigger.

Surface Its surface is smooth but the lobules of the gland may make it bosselated.

Edge The anterior, posterior and inferior edges of the gland are distinct and easy to define, but the upper edge is wedged between the mandible and the mylohyoid muscle and is impalpable.

Composition A distended submandibular gland has a **rubbery** hard consistence, and will not fluctuate, transilluminate or reduce. It is dull to percussion.

Occasionally, prolonged pressure on the gland may make it a little smaller and produce a jet of saliva from the orifice of the submandibular duct.

Relations The skin is freely mobile over the swollen gland. The gland itself can be moved a little from side to side but most movements are restricted by the tethering of the gland to the underlying muscles. When the muscles of the floor of the mouth are tensed by asking the patient to push his tongue against the roof of his mouth the gland becomes less mobile.

It is important to ascertain the relations of the lump to the floor of the mouth and the tongue by **bimanual palpation**. Feel the lump between the index finger of one hand inside the mouth (suitably gloved), and the fingers of the other hand on the outer surface of the lump.

It should be possible to appreciate that the lump is outside the structures that form the floor of the mouth. It should not be fixed to the mucosa of the floor of the mouth or to the tongue.

Lymph drainage The submandibular gland lymph drains to the middle deep cervical lymph nodes, but there is also some lymphoid tissue within the gland which can contribute to its enlargement.

The local lymph glands will not be enlarged if the gland is not infected.

Local tissues The nearby tissues, except the submandibular duct in the floor of the mouth, should be normal.

The floor of the mouth

Inspection Ask the patient to open his mouth and lift his tongue up to the roof of the mouth.

This displays the orifices of the submandibular ducts on their small papillae on either side of the frenulum of the tongue (Fig. 9.1).

If a stone is impacted at the end of the duct, its grey–yellow colour may be visible through the open orifice of the duct.

The presence of a stone in the duct makes that side of the floor of the mouth bulge upwards and look pink.

Press the gland gently and watch for any discharge from the orifice of the duct.

Palpation Feel along the course of the duct in the floor of the mouth for lumps and tenderness.

A stone in the duct will not feel stony hard if it is small and surrounded by inflammatory oedema. The lump caused by such a stone will feel soft with a hard centre.

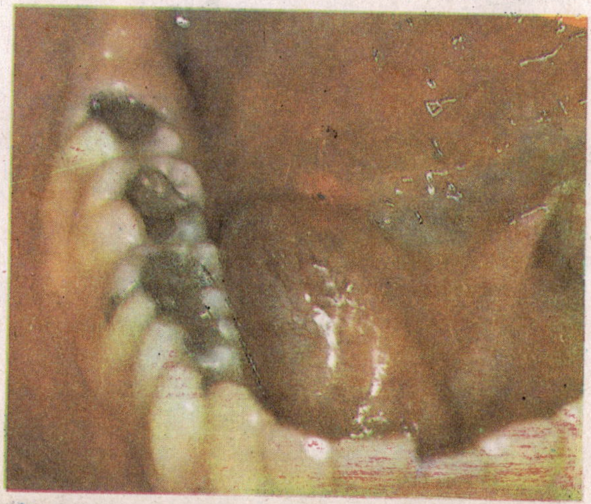

FIG. 9.3 When a stone impacts at the end of the submandibular duct, the floor of the mouth looks asymmetrical. In this photograph there is a bulge over the patient's right duct. Palpation revealed a firm lump

General examination

Examine all the salivary glands in case the symptoms are due to a systemic disease such as Sjögren's syndrome (see page 232), not a stone.

Submandibular sialitis

Infection of a submandibular gland is invariably secondary to the presence of a stone in its duct or the damage done by a stone which has passed through the duct. The infecting organism is usually a staphylococcus.

The symptoms are identical to those caused by a stone except that when the gland is infected the **pain is severe, throbbing, continuous**, and exacerbated by eating.

The physical signs of the lump in the neck are similar to those of the obstructed gland described above, with the addition of **heat** and **tenderness**. An infected gland may become quite big (5 × 10 cm). If the duct system becomes dilated (**sialectasis**) the pus may pool in the gland and the whole structure turn into a multilocular abscess, which may then point onto the skin.

Submandibular salivary gland tumours

The tumours that often occur in the parotid gland – pleomorphic adenoma, cylindroma and carcinoma – may occur in the submandibular gland, but they are rare.

The physical features of pleomorphic adenoma and carcinoma in the submandibular gland are identical to the physical features of these tumours when they occur in the parotid gland, apart from the site.

The pleomorphic adenoma forms a painless, slow-growing, non-tender, hard, well-defined spherical mass within the gland. Carcinoma causes an indistinct, hot, slightly tender, rapidly growing, painful mass. Numbness of the anterior two-thirds of the tongue indicates infiltration of the lingual nerve, and is diagnostic of carcinoma.

It may be difficult to distinguish a pleomorphic adenoma from enlargement of the lymph tissue within the gland. A long history of slow, gradual growth is the most useful distinguishing feature.

THE PAROTID GLAND

Acute bacterial parotitis

The commonest infection of the parotid gland is mumps. This is an **epidemic viral parotitis;** when it occurs in an epidemic with bilateral painful swollen glands and excessive oedema, which spreads down into the neck giving the child a double chin, it is easy to diagnose.

When it causes unilateral gland enlargement, little pain, no oedema, and there are no obvious contacts with the infection, it can be much more difficult to diagnose.

Remember, **mumps is the commonest cause of parotitis.**

Non-specific parotitis, usually a staphylococcal infection, is caused by:

1 Poor oral hygiene.
2 Dehydration.
3 Obstruction of Stensen's duct by stone or scar tissue.

In the days before the fluid balance of sick patients was properly controlled, fulminating parotitis with a subsequent septicaemia was a common cause of death.

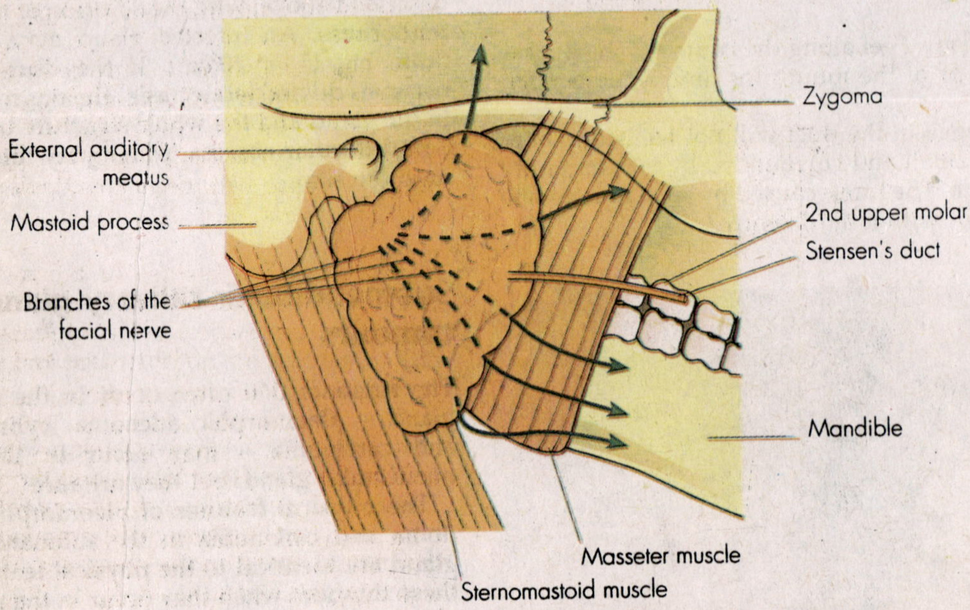

N.B. The parotid gland extends below and behind the angle of the mandible. Lumps in this part of the gland are easily mistaken for enlarged upper deep cervical lymph glands.

FIG. 9.4 The anatomy of the parotid gland

HISTORY

Age Acute parotitis is more common in the elderly and the debilitated.

Symptoms The patient complains of the sudden onset of **pain and swelling** in the side of his face.

The pain is continuous and throbbing, and radiates to the ear and over the side of the head.

Speaking and eating cause pain because any movement of the temporomandibular joint is painful.

The patient feels hot, sweaty and ill. He may complain of shivering attacks (rigors).

Systematic questions The answers to these questions may reveal symptoms of another illness, such as a bronchial carcinoma, which has caused the debility and dehydration.

Previous history The patient may have recently undergone a major operation or suffered a severe medical illness.

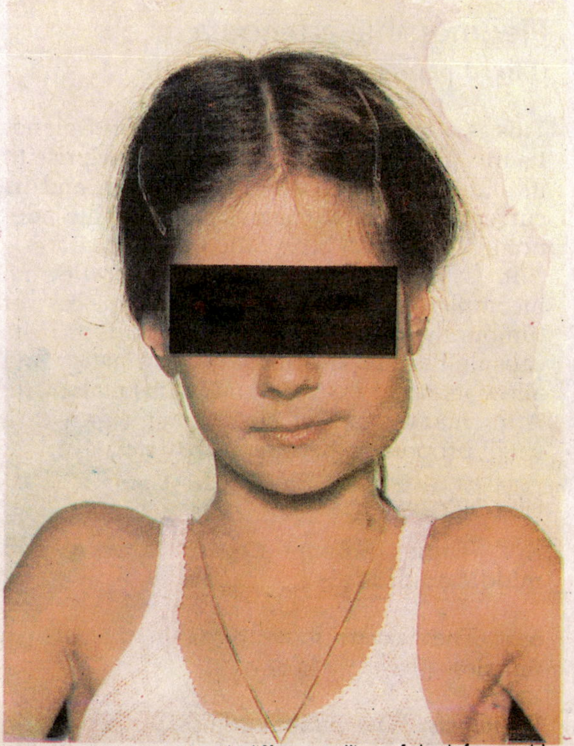

FIG. 9.5 A young girl with diffuse swelling of the left parotid gland caused by mumps. Much of the swelling is caused by oedema

EXAMINATION

The lump

Position The parotid gland lies in front of and below the lower half of the ear. It is wrapped around the vertical ramus of the mandible, with its deep portion in between this bone and the mastoid process.

In acute parotitis the whole gland is swollen, so the whole of the face in front of the lower half of the ear bulges outwards.

Colour and temperature The skin over the swelling is discoloured a reddish-brown, feels hot, and is smooth and shiny.

Tenderness The swelling is very tender.

Shape The mass has the shape of the normal parotid gland: a semicircular anterior edge, a vertical edge just in front of the ear, and a bulge running into the gap between the mandible and the mastoid process.

Size The swollen gland may be three or four times larger than a normal gland.

Surface Its surface is smooth but difficult to define because of the oedema, inflammation and tenderness.

Composition The texture of the swelling is often described as **brawny**. This means that it has a firm consistence but is indentable. It is dull to percussion, not fluctuant and not compressible.

Relations If the overlying skin is red and oedematous it will be tethered to the swelling. The swelling cannot be moved over the deep structures and becomes more prominent when the patient contracts the masseter muscles by clenching his teeth.

Lymph drainage The upper deep cervical lymph nodes are usually enlarged and tender.

Local tissues Apart from the changes in the skin, and the restricted movements of the temporomandibular joint, the surrounding tissues are normal. The function of the facial nerve is *not* impaired.

The mouth

Inspection Remember that the orifice of Stensen's duct is opposite the *second upper molar tooth*. The mouth of the duct may be patulous and the mucous membrane over the course of the duct slightly oedematous.

Palpation Feel the mouth of the duct for any thickening or lumps.

The parotid gland cannot be palpated bimanually because it lies behind the anterior edge of the masseter muscle and the vertical ramus of the mandible.

Gentle pressure on the gland may produce a purulent discharge from the mouth of the duct.

Chronic parotitis

Chronic parotitis is usually caused by a small calculus or a fibrous stenosis blocking the mouth of Stensen's duct.

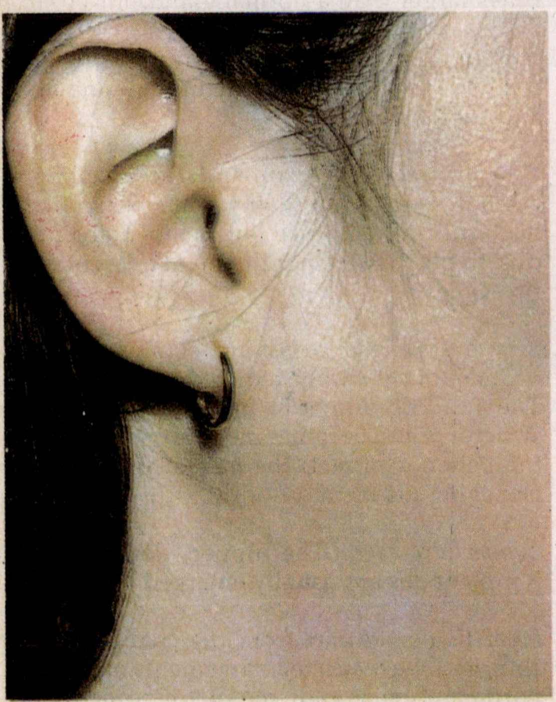

FIG. 9.6 Chronic parotitis. A firm, slightly tender enlargement of the whole of the parotid gland caused by recurrent infection secondary to a stone in Stensen's duct

HISTORY

The patient complains of **recurrent swelling** of the parotid gland. The swelling is particularly noticeable before eating and is associated with an aching pain.

In severe cases the gland becomes permanently swollen, but the pain does not usually become constant.

Chronic parotitis is sometimes bilateral.

EXAMINATION

The whole gland is easy to feel because it is slightly bigger and firmer than a normal gland and its edges are distinct. It is also tender and feels **rubbery hard**.

If there is partial obstruction to the flow of saliva, pressure on the gland may produce a copious squirt of fluid through the orifice of the duct.

Examine all the other salivary glands to exclude a generalized abnormality.

Pleomorphic adenoma

(Mixed parotid tumour, sialoma)

This is a **true adenoma** of the parotid gland. Its mixed histological appearance gave rise to its old name, mixed parotid tumour, and its currently favoured name, pleomorphic adenoma. It has also been called a sialoma.

It is a slow-growing adenoma with an incomplete capsule. The small pieces of tumour that protrude through the defects in its capsule limit its treatment by enucleation and allow its rapid extension if it turns malignant. After many years of slow, benign growth a small proportion become locally invasive.

HISTORY

Age These tumours appear in early and middle adult life.

Sex They occur more often in males than females.

Symptoms The patient complains of a **painless swelling** on the side of his face which has been present for months or years and which is **slowly growing**.

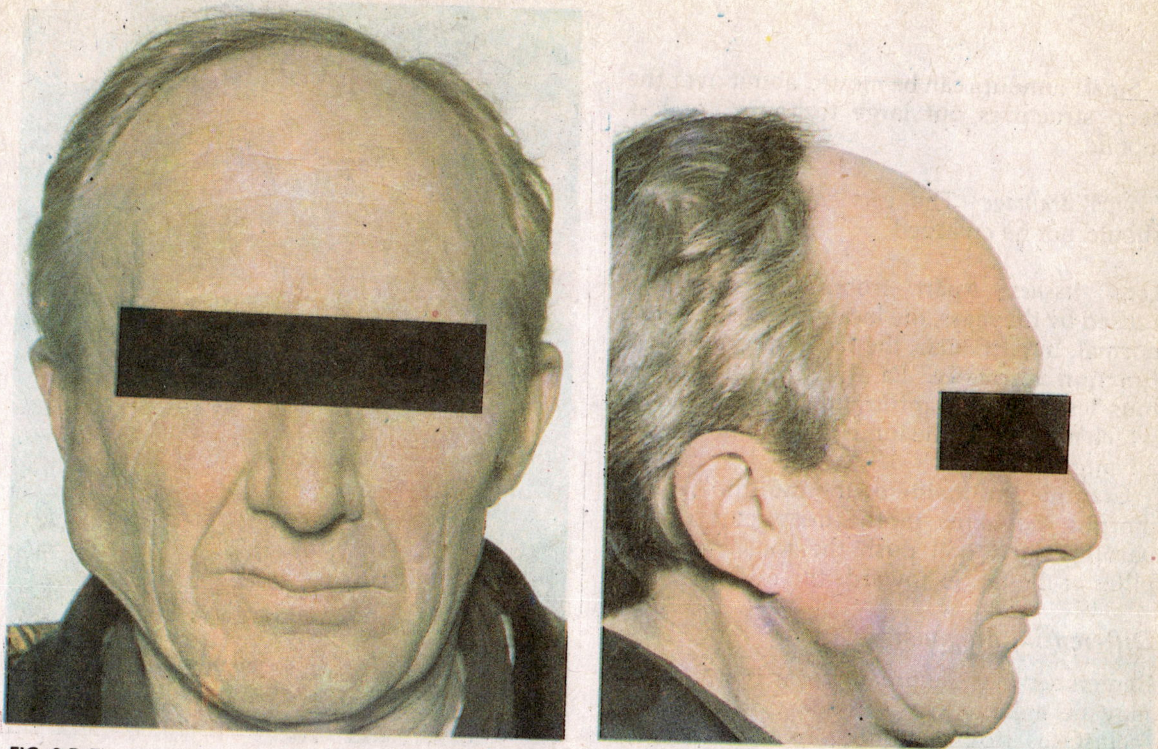

FIG. 9.7 The pleomorphic adenoma. These pictures show the typical site, the healthy overlying skin, the absence of facial nerve involvement and the lobulation that develops as the tumour grows

The lump may be more prominent when the mouth is open, or when eating. The latter symptom can cause confusion so it is important to find out whether the lump just becomes more prominent because of contraction of the masseter muscle or actually increases in size.

EXAMINATION

Position The majority of parotid adenomata begin in the portion of the gland that lies over the junction of the vertical and horizontal rami of the mandible, just anterior and superior to the angle of the jaw.

Why the majority begin here is not known, for they can occur in any part of the gland.

Colour and temperature The temperature and colour of the overlying skin are normal.

Tenderness The lump is **not tender**.

Shape Most pleomorphic adenomata are spherical when they are small, but as they grow they become flat on their deep surface and slightly pointed superficially. They may become lobulated when very large.

Size These tumours can vary from pea-sized nodules to large, almost pendulous, masses, 20 cm across.

Surface Their surface is smooth, sometimes bosselated, and occasionally crossed by deep furrows.

The surface of any deep extension between the mandible and the mastoid process is impalpable.

Edge The edge is quite distinct and easy to feel.

Composition The tumour mass has a rubbery hard consistence, is dull to percussion, not fluctuant or translucent, and not compressible.

Relations The overlying skin and the ear are freely movable, **not attached** to the lump.

Small tumours can be moved about over the deep structures but large tumours are less mobile.

Lymph drainage The cervical lymph nodes should not be enlarged.

Local tissues Apart from any distortion caused by the mass, the local tissues should be normal. In particular, the **facial nerve should function normally**. Paralysis of any facial muscles indicates infiltration of the nerve, which means that the lump is a carcinoma, not a benign adenoma.

Examine the inside of the mouth. A pleomorphic adenoma in the deep part of the parotid gland will push the tonsil and the pillar of the fauces towards the mid-line.

Differential diagnosis

Remember that the **preauricular lymph node** may be enlarged by secondary infection or metastases from a tumour in the forehead, scalp, eyelids, cheek or external auditory meatus. The resulting firm, smooth swelling just in front of the tragus can be indistinguishable from a pleomorphic adenoma if it is not tender and there are no obvious abnormalities in its drainage area.

The most distinctive physical sign of an enlarged preauricular lymph node is its mobility. Most tumours in the parotid can only be moved a short distance because they are tethered to the gland; the preauricular lymph node is outside the capsule of the parotid gland and usually very mobile.

Adenolymphoma

(Warthin's tumour)

This is a cystic tumour which contains epithelial and lymphoid tissues. The epithelial element is believed to originate from embryonic parotid ducts which have become separated from the main duct system of the gland. The lymphoid element comes from normal lymph tissue that happened to be close to the developing gland.

The tumour arises on the surface of, or just beneath, the capsule of the parotid gland.

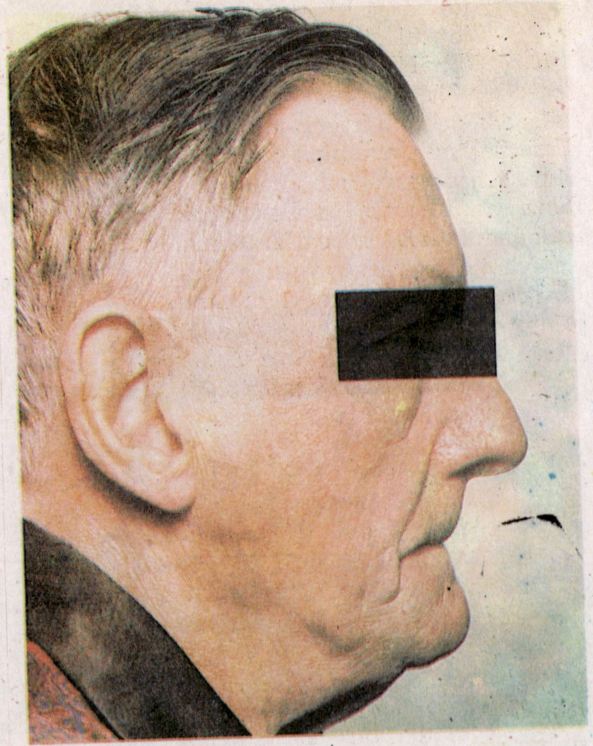

FIG. 9.8 Warthin's tumour. An adenolymphoma of the parotid gland. This photograph has been chosen because it shows so well the typical site of the adenolymphoma – just over the angle of the jaw. Although it looks similar to the pleomorphic adenoma shown in Fig. 9.7, it had a soft consistence

HISTORY

Age Adenolymphomata appear in middle and old age.

Sex They are more common in men than women.

Ethnic group They do not occur in Negroes.

Symptoms The patient complains of a **slow-growing, painless swelling** over the angle of the jaw. The swelling may be bilateral.

EXAMINATION

Position The adenolymphoma usually develops in the lower part of the parotid gland, level with the lower border of the mandible. This is slightly lower than the common site of origin of the pleomorphic adenoma.

Temperature and colour The overlying skin looks and feels normal.

Tenderness The lump is not tender.

Shape and size It is spherical or hemispherical, and usually 1–3 cm in diameter.

Surface The surface is smooth and well defined.

Edge Its edge is distinct and sometimes makes the lump seem separate from the parotid gland.

Composition Adenolymphomata have a **soft** consistence, are dull to percussion and not translucent, but they often **fluctuate**. The fluctuation is sometimes a true sign of the fluid content of the cysts but more often is a reflection of the soft solid consistence and strong capsule.

Relations The lump can usually be moved a little in all directions and is not attached to the skin.

Lymph drainage The cervical lymph nodes should not be enlarged.

Local tissues The adjacent tissues are all normal.

The site and consistence are the features which make one suspect that a parotid swelling is an adenolymphoma.

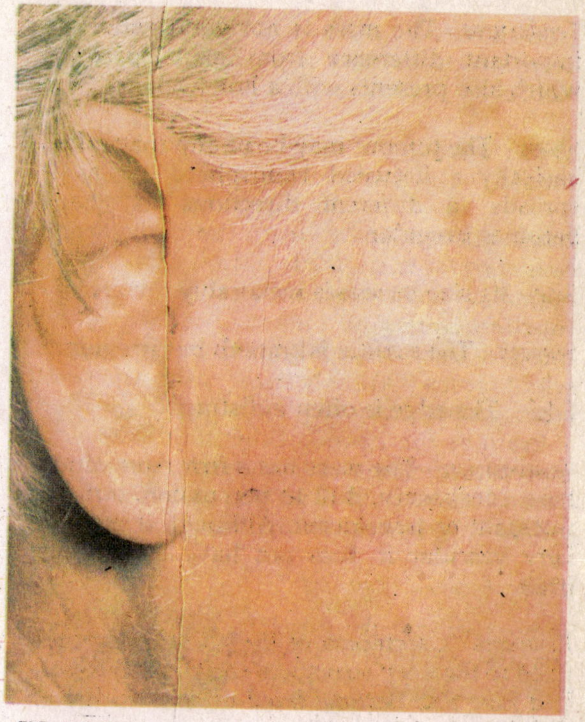

FIG. 9.9 Carcinoma of the parotid gland. This patient complained of a painful swelling in front of his ear. The swelling was hot and the overlying skin reddened. Although the swelling was not very large, there was some weakness of the muscles of facial expression

Carcinoma of the parotid gland

Carcinoma of the parotid gland is uncommon, but not very rare. It can arise *de novo*, or in a long-standing pleomorphic adenoma.

HISTORY

Age The patient is usually over the age of 50 years.

Sex Males and females are equally affected.

Symptoms The common complaint is of a **rapidly enlarging swelling** on the side of the face. The swelling is persistently **painful**, especially during movements of the jaw. The pain may radiate to the ear and over the side of the face. The patient may give a history of a preceding painless lump which has been present for many years.

The patient may also complain of asymmetry of the mouth and difficulty in closing the eyes.

EXAMINATION

Position The swelling is in the site of the parotid gland.

Colour If the overlying skin is being infiltrated by the tumour it may be reddish-blue.

Temperature The skin and the mass are hyperaemic and hot.

Tenderness The mass is not very tender, an important difference from acute parotitis which also presents with a hot swelling.

Shape The tumour may be of any shape. It is basically a flattened hemisphere but as it spreads in different directions its shape becomes irregular.

Size Its size increases inexorably.

Surface The surface is smooth but irregular.

Edge The edge is often indistinct.

Composition The mass has a firm, sometimes hard consistence, dull to percussion, but not fluctuant or translucent. Although it may be very vascular it does not have an audible bruit.

Relations Carcinoma of the parotid becomes fixed to the deep structures early in its growth and may also become fixed to, and infiltrate, the skin.

The thickening of the tissues around the temporomandibular joint may restrict jaw movements.

Lymph drainage The cervical lymph nodes are likely to be enlarged and hard.

Revision Panel 9.1

Causes of swelling of a salivary gland

Acute infection
- Viral (e.g. mumps)
- Bacterial (e.g. staphylococcus)

Duct obstruction

Sialectasis (chronic infection)

Tumour
- Benign
- Malignant

Sarcoidosis

Sjögren's syndrome

Local tissues If the **facial nerve** is infiltrated by tumour, the patient will be unable to use the muscles of facial expression. The signs may vary from mild weakness of the lower lip when baring the teeth, to a complete seventh nerve palsy.

If the tumour has infiltrated into the mandible, the jaw may be swollen and tender.

GENERAL EXAMINATION

There may be evidence of disseminated blood-borne metastases.

AUTOIMMUNE DISEASE

There are two syndromes of slow, progressive, but relatively painless enlargement of the salivary glands, in which biopsy reveals that the swelling is caused by replacement of the glandular tissue by lymphoid tissue. Both conditions are believed to be autoimmune diseases.

Mikulicz's syndrome

Mikulicz's syndrome is:

1 Enlargement of the salivary glands. Usually both parotid and both submandibular glands enlarge, but the syndrome can begin and remain in one gland for quite a long time.
2 Enlargement of the lachrymal glands. This causes a bulge at the upper outer end of the eyelid and narrowing of the palpebral fissures.
3 A dry mouth, which may be the presenting symptom. The patient is **not** thirsty.

Sjögren's syndrome

Sjögren's syndrome is all the above conditions although the degree of salivary gland enlargement is often not so gross, *plus*:

1 Dry eyes.
2 Generalized arthritis.

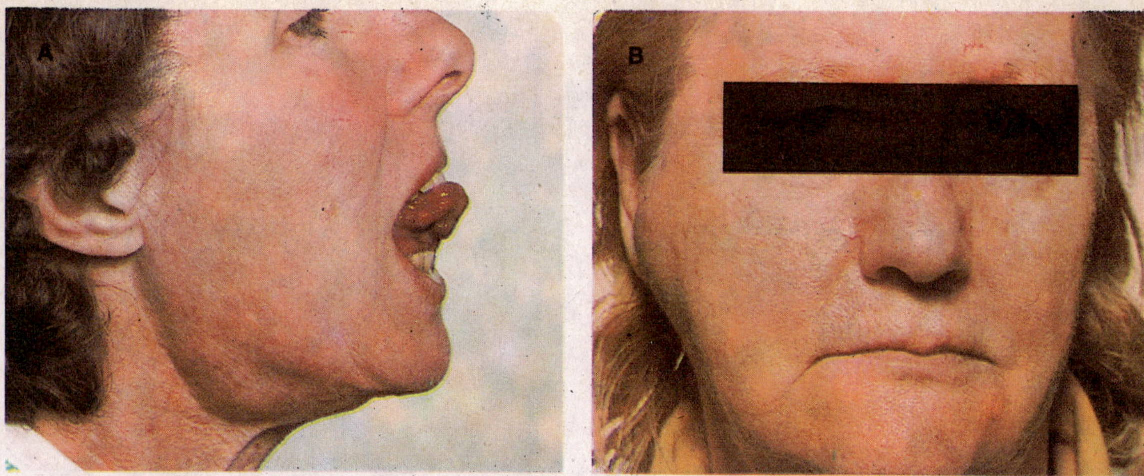

FIG. 9.10 Not all swellings in the parotid and submandibular regions are caused by salivary gland enlargement. **A**: The submandibular swelling in this woman was a lymph gland enlarged by secondary deposits from a carcinoma of the tongue. **B**: Preauricular lymphadenopathy is a condition which is commonly mistaken for parotid gland enlargement. However, this woman's preauricular swelling was caused by a secondary deposit of carcinoma in the ascending ramus of the mandible

10 The mouth

(lips, teeth, tongue, tonsils, palate and jaw)

Always inspect the mouth with a good light and use a spatula:

- **Retract the lips to see the buccal mucosa.**
- **Push the cheek outwards to see the buccal side of the gum.**
- **Push the tongue away from the inside of the gum and the floor of the mouth.**
- **Push the tongue to one side to see the lateral aspect of its posterior third.**
- **Depress the tongue to look at the fauces, tonsils and pharynx.**

Always remember to **palpate the structures in the mouth bimanually**; one finger inside and one outside.

Always wear a finger cot, or, if there is any possibility that the lesion is contagious, a glove.

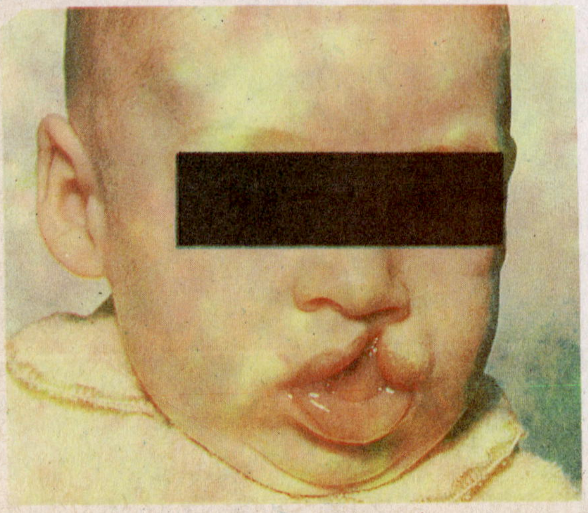

FIG. 10.1 A child with a simple cleft lip

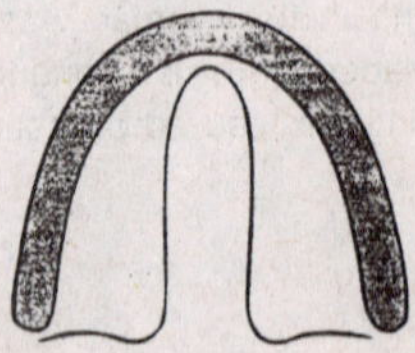

A partial cleft of the hard and soft palate

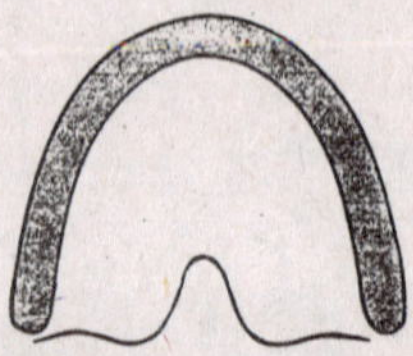

A partial cleft of the soft palate

FIG. 10.2 THE VARIETIES OF A SIMPLE CLEFT PALATE

CONGENITAL ABNORMALITIES OF THE LIPS AND PALATE

The face, jaw and palate are formed by the fusion of the frontonasal, maxillary and mandibular processes:

- The *frontonasal process* forms the nose, the nasal septum, the nostrils, the philtrum of the upper lip and the premaxilla.
- The *maxillary processes* form the cheek, the upper lip (except the philtrum), the upper jaw and palate.

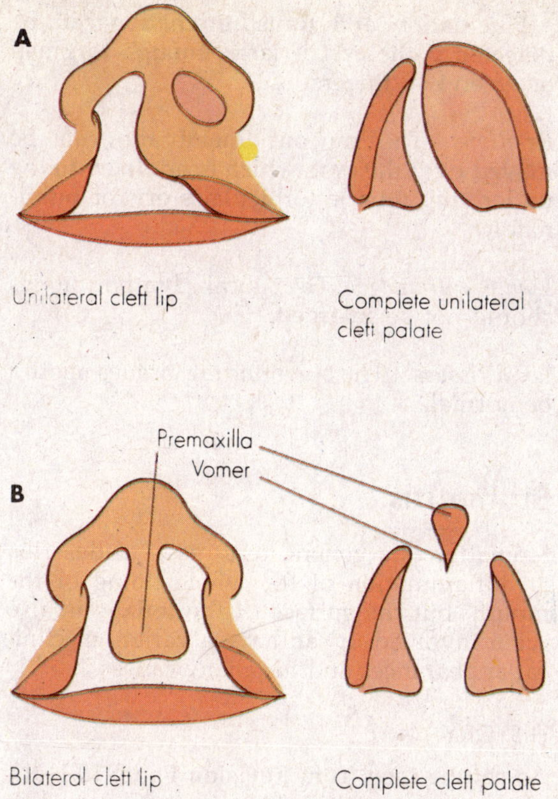

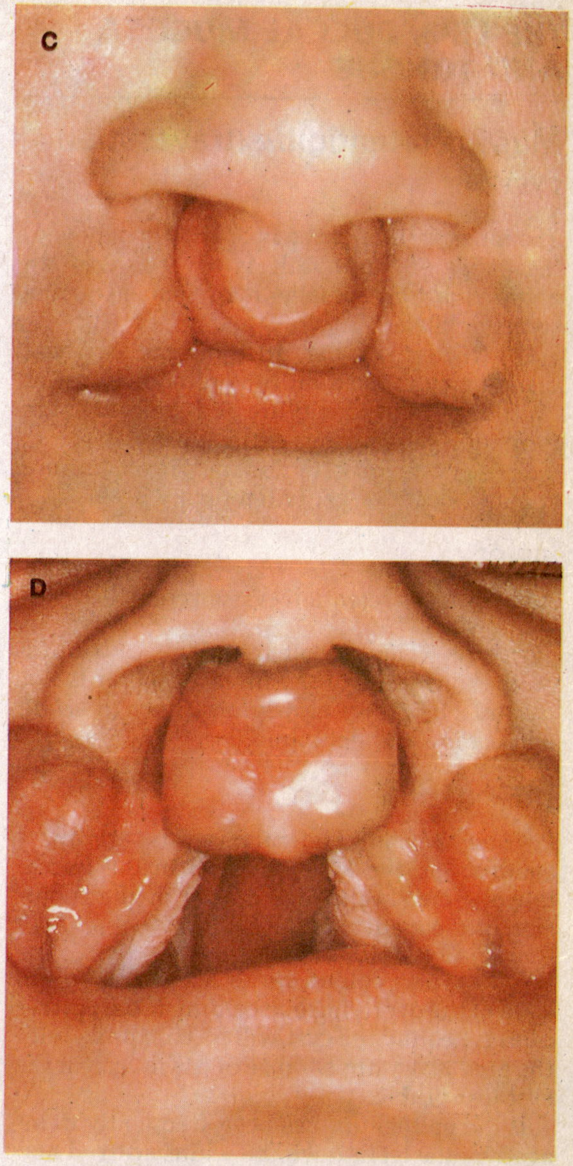

FIG. 10.3 Cleft lip and cleft palate combined. **A**: Complete unilateral cleft lip and palate. **B**: Complete bilateral cleft lip and palate. **C & D**: A baby with a bilateral cleft lip and cleft palate. Note the way in which the premaxilla protrudes

The *mandibular processes* form the lower jaw and lip.

Failure of these processes to meet and fuse produces a group of congenital abnormalities: cleft lips, cleft palates and facial clefts.

Half of the infants with a cleft lip also have a cleft palate.

Complete failure of fusion causes a bilateral cleft lip, a cleft palate and a protuberant premaxilla. The diagnosis is apparent from inspection of the lip and palate.

Partial failure of fusion causes unilateral cleft lip and a unilateral cleft of the palate which may be complete or partial.

Rare varieties of failure of fusion may cause a central **cleft of the lower lip** and jaw, and a **facial cleft** between the maxilla and the side of the nose.

The symptoms of cleft lip and palate, apart from the **disfigurement**, are an **inability to suckle, interference with speech** (particularly the formation of consonants such as D, T and G) and **distortion of the dental arch**.

THE LIPS, BUCCAL MUCOSA AND TONGUE

Mucous retention/extravasation cysts

The inner surface of the lips, and the whole of the inside of the mouth, is covered with an epithelium that contains many small mucus-secreting glands.

Obstruction of the duct of one of these glands may cause a mucous retention cyst or cause the gland to rupture and so initiate the formation of a mucous extravasation cyst.

These cysts are common and often rupture spontaneously or get bitten through.

HISTORY

Age Mucous retention cysts occur at all ages.

Symptoms The patient complains of a lump on the inner side of the lip or cheek. It is **not** painful but grows slowly and may interfere with eating and get bitten.

EXAMINATION

Position Mucous retention cysts are most common on the lower lip and in the buccal mucous membrane at the level of the occlusion of the teeth.

Colour Their colour varies according to the state of the overlying epithelium. If the epithelium is healthy the cyst will be pale pink, with the grey glairy appearance of the mucus in the cyst just visible.

If the epithelium has been frequently damaged by the teeth it will be white, scarred and slightly boggy, and will obscure the colour of the underlying cyst.

Shape These cysts are spherical.

Size They vary in size from 0.5 to 2 cm in diameter.

Surface Their surface is smooth.

Composition Their consistence varies from soft to hard, depending upon the tension of the fluid within them.

Fluctuation and transillumination can be detected if the cyst is large enough to grasp between two fingers.

Relations The mucous membrane can be moved over the cyst, which is not fixed to the underlying muscle (orbicularis oris or buccinator).

Lymph drainage The local lymph nodes should not be enlarged.

Local tissues The surrounding tissues should be normal.

Stomatitis

Stomatitis is a general term used to describe an inflammation of the whole lining of the mouth, but the surface of the tongue is also often involved. It can have a variety of clinical appearances and has many causes.

HISTORY

As can be seen from Revision Panel 10.1, the causes of stomatitis are many and varied. It occurs in all age groups and equally in both sexes.

Symptoms The patient complains of **soreness** in the mouth. The mouth may feel **dry**. Movements of the tongue and cheeks are painful and individual ulcers are very painful. Mastication is difficult.

The patient may also have the symptoms of a generalized condition that is causing the stomatitis.

EXAMINATION

The physical appearances vary according to the cause.

Catarrhal stomatitis

This is often associated with an acute upper respiratory tract infection and acute specific fever. The whole of the mucous membrane of the mouth is oedematous and red. Small ulcers may appear and coalesce to become an ulcerative stomatitis.

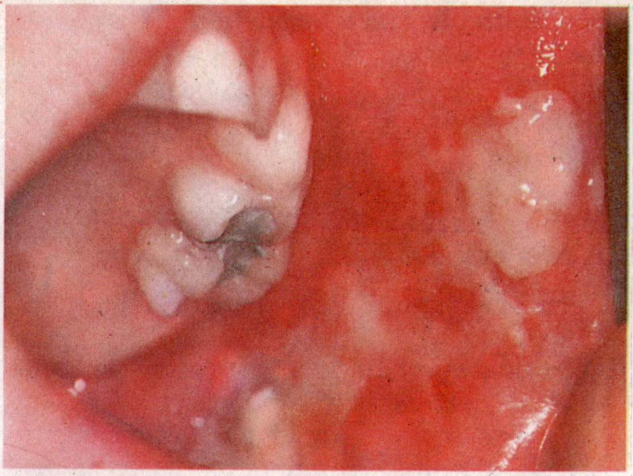

Multiple aphthous ulcers of the buccal mucosa

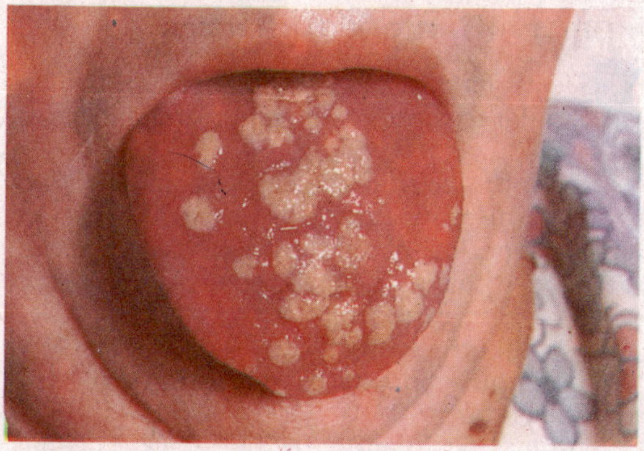

Monilial stomatitis. The colonies of monilia on the tongue and mucous membranes look like patches of cream-coloured paint

FIG. 10.4 STOMATITIS

Aphthous stomatitis

The inside of the mouth becomes covered with small, tender vesicles which have a thickened hyperaemic base. When a vesicle breaks it leaves a small, white, circular, deep, very painful ulcer. The cause of these ulcers is not known.

Recurrent solitary aphthous ulcers are commonplace in normal people. Multiple ulcers are very painful and often associated with a generalized debilitating disease.

Acute monilial stomatitis (Thrush)

Infection of the alimentary tract by the fungus *Candida albicans* is common in children and in people with debilitating disease, and as a complication of any antibiotic therapy which changes the balance of the bacteria in the alimentary canal.

Small red patches appear on the buccal mucosa and tongue which then turn **white**. The white appearance is caused by a layer of oedematous desquamating epithelium, heavily contaminated with the fungus.

The mouth is **painful**, and **salivation is excessive**. This induces frequent swallowing, which is also painful if the infection has spread into the pharynx.

Revision Panel 10.1

The causes of stomatitis

Local trauma
- Poorly fitting dentures
- Sharp teeth
- Excessive smoking
- Radiotherapy

Local infection
- Herpes
- Monilia
- Vincent's angina
- Glandular fever
- Foot and mouth disease

General conditions
- Stevens–Johnson syndrome
- Behçet's syndrome
- Aphthous ulceration

Vitamin deficiencies
- Vitamin C (scurvy)
- Vitamin B and C (coeliac disease, pellagra, pernicious anaemia, kwashiorkor)

Blood diseases
- Acute leukaemia
- Agranulocytosis
- Aplastic anaemia
- Purpura

Immunosuppression
- AIDS
- Chemotherapy

Drugs
- Phenytoin
- Lead, mercury and bismuth poisoning

Debility
- Tuberculosis
- Carcinomatosis

Acute ulcerative stomatitis
(Vincent's angina)

This usually follows a severe gingivitis, but may complicate catarrhal stomatitis. It is caused by an infection (*Borrelia vincenti*) and is often known as **Vincent's angina**.

The **gums are swollen**, inflamed, painful and peppered with small ulcers that are covered by a **yellow slough**. These changes may spread to the tonsils, the fauces and the buccal mucosa.

The gums bleed, there is excessive salivation and a marked foetor oris.

The cervical lymph nodes are enlarged and tender.

The patient feels ill, has a fever and loss of appetite.

Gangrenous stomatitis (Cancrum oris)

Gangrenous stomatitis is now a rare condition except in countries with a high incidence of starvation. It is an uncommon but not rare complication of measles and other specific fevers in malnourished children, and it is occasionally seen in a child with leukaemia.

It begins as an area of oedema and induration on the lip, which becomes ischaemic and necrotic. The area of necrosis spreads steadily, and as the dead tissue separates so the contours of the mouth and face are destroyed.

The process is extremely painful, and the patient is very ill with anorexia, prostration and a pyrexia.

Anguiar stomatitis (Perlèche)

This term describes inflamed red–brown fissures at the corners of the mouth. Its common cause is the dribbling of saliva through the corners of the mouth which follows overclosure of the bite caused by loss of the teeth. Most elderly edentulous patients have some degree of angular stomatitis.

A similar condition occurs in children who rub and lick the corners of their mouth.

The cracks may become infected by *Candida albicans*.

Rhagades is the name given to the small radiating cracks in the corners of the mouth that develop in patients in the **secondary stage of syphilis** (see below). They are sore and uncomfortable, and when they heal they leave fine linear scars.

Syphilis

All three stages of syphilis can cause abnormalities in the mouth.

1 Primary syphilis: chancre on the lip or tongue.
2 Secondary syphilis: 'snail track' ulcers, 'mucous patches', Hutchinson's wart.
3 Tertiary syphilis: gummata, chronic superficial glossitis, gummatous parenchymal infiltration.

Primary (Hunterian) chancre

The features of a primary chancre on the lip are similar to those of one on the genitalia (see page 347).

The initial lesion is an elevated but flat, pink, painless macule. This grows slowly into a hemispherical papule, the mucosal covering of which breaks down to leave a superficial, slightly painful ulcer. The ulcer may be covered with a thick crust.

The papule and its base are rubbery hard and discrete.

The lymph glands in the neck become enlarged and tender, 1–2 weeks after the appearance of the lump.

Ultimately, the ulcer heals, the lump dissolves and the only permanent remnant is a fine superficial scar.

Chancres are **highly contagious**.

The mucous patch

Mucous patches are grey–white or pearl-coloured raised patches which appear on the inside of the lips and cheeks and on the pillars of the fauces. They vary in size, from 3 to 20 mm in diameter. The whiteness is caused by oedema and desquamation of the epithelium. When the grey patch of dead epithelium separates, the underlying mucosa is left raw and bleeding.

Mucous patches are highly contagious.

The patient's main complaint is of a **sore throat**.

'Snail track' ulcers

'Snail track' ulcers are long, narrow ulcers which are covered with transparent glistening mucus or a white boggy epithelium which makes them look like snail tracks. They are commonly seen on the pillars of the fauces.

They form from the coalescence of a number of small mucous patches.

Gummata

Gummatous degeneration may be nodular or infiltrating. Both varieties affect the tongue. Gummata of the lips and cheeks are uncommon.

Gummata also develop in the hard palate and nasal septum, causing perforation of the palate and nasal septum, and collapse of the bridge of the nose.

A gumma in the tongue presents as a painless, hard, discrete mass. It usually develops in the anterior two-thirds of the tongue and, unless there is a history of syphilis or other physical signs of the disease, is indistinguishable from an interstitial carcinoma or a secondary deposit.

Gummatous parenchymal infiltration makes the tongue big, stiff, thick and irregular.

Hutchinson's wart

This is a mid-line condyloma of the tongue. A condyloma is an area of hypertrophic epithelium, broad based and flat topped. It is highly contagious.

Chronic superficial glossitis

This condition is commonly caused by syphilis. Its final stage is leukoplakia, which is a precancerous condition. As it is also caused by other conditions, it is described fully below.

Chronic superficial glossitis

This is a condition in which a sequence of chronic inflammatory, degenerative and hypertrophic changes occur in the tongue, which terminate in the development of a carcinoma.

The causes of chronic superficial glossitis are usually remembered as six Ss:

- Syphilis
- Smoking
- Sharp tooth
- Spirits
- Spices
- Sepsis

The only conditions which can be definitely incriminated are syphilis and recurrent trauma from a tooth or pipe. The role of the other factors is open to doubt.

HISTORY

Age The conditions which predispose to the development of glossitis need to be present for many years before they have any effect. Thus most patients with this disease are over the age of 50 years.

Sex More men are affected than women.

Symptoms The patient has remarkably few symptoms. The condition is not painful and does not interfere with eating. The common complaint is that the tongue has become shiny or white, or developed a lump.

Revision Panel 10.2

Chronic superficial glossitis

Causes

Syphilis
Recurrent trauma:
  Pipe smoking
  Sharp tooth
Spices
Spirits
Sepsis

Clinical features

Thin milky film
↓
Thick white paint (leukoplakia)
← →
Nodules ↓ Cancer
Red, shiny atrophic patches

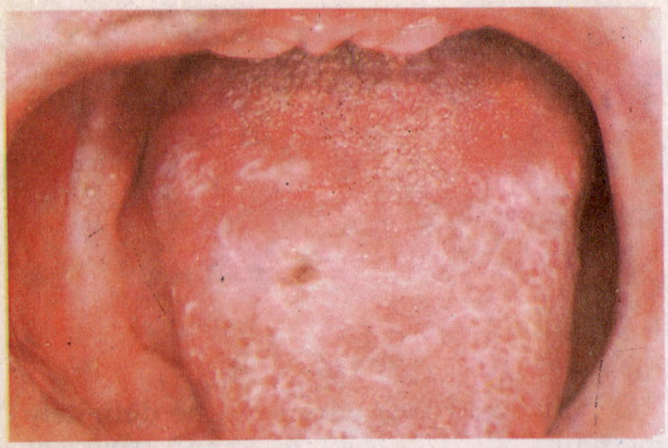

The early stage when the tongue is covered with a transparent grey film and loses its papillae

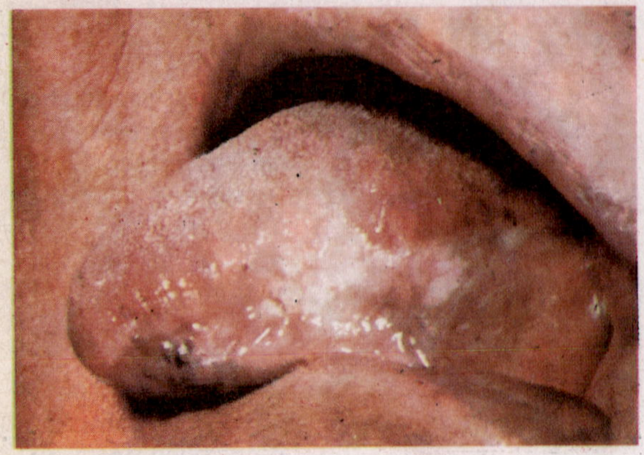

The advanced stage with hard white plaques, nodules and fissures

FIG. 10.5 CHRONIC SUPERFICIAL GLOSSITIS

EXAMINATION

The surface of the tongue passes through a series of changes as the epithelium thickens. The prickle cell layer hypertrophies (acanthosis) and swollen cells with nuclei reach the surface (spongiosis and parakeratosis). These changes are patchy, and all clinical stages may coexist on different parts of the tongue.

First stage The first abnormality is the appearance of a thin, grey, transparent film on a part of the tongue.

Second stage This thin film turns opaque and white. This is **leukoplakia.** Young leukoplakia looks like fresh, soft, semi-matt paint. Old leukoplakia cracks and gets slightly yellow so that it looks like old, cracking, wrinkled, white gloss paint.

Third stage Beneath the white patches the epithelium becomes hyperplastic. Small nodules and warty outgrowths appear which may eventually become overt carcinomata.

The areas of very active cellular division are visible as smooth, red, shiny patches.

Fourth stage The fourth stage is the appearance of clinically detectable carcinomata. The lesions have all the features of a primary carcinoma of the tongue.

Many small cancers may appear together and the cervical lymph nodes may be enlarged. Change identical to chronic superficial glossitis can occur on the lips and any part of the buccal mucosa – cheek, gums and palate. Leukoplakia of the lips and cheeks is now more common than leukoplakia of the tongue.

Carcinoma of the lip

Carcinoma of the lip is no longer common in Great Britain since the reduction of the incidence of syphilis and leukoplakia of the lip. The factors which produce premalignant changes in the epithelium of the lip are leukoplakia and its causes, and recurrent trauma from pipes and prolonged exposure to sunlight.

Since the reduction in the incidence of syphilis, exposure to sunlight, especially the ultraviolet part of sunlight, is the commonest cause of carcinoma of the lip.

HISTORY

Age Most of the patients with carcinoma of the lip are over the age of 60 years.

Sex Men are affected more than women.

Occupation It is particularly common in men with outdoor occupations and is sometimes called 'countryman's lip'; but remember that there are many men with outdoor occupations living in towns.

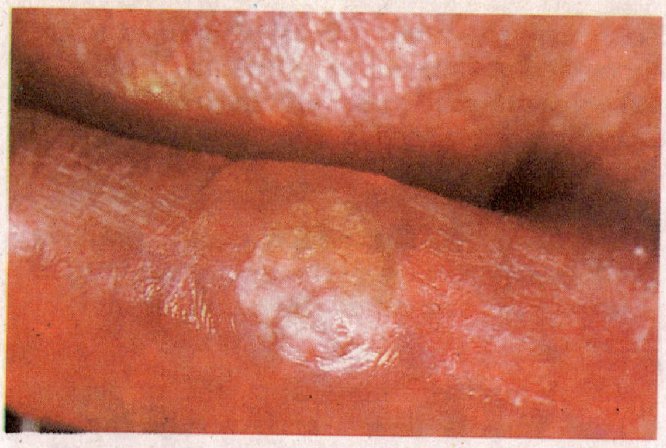

A small, early lesion that has just ulcerated

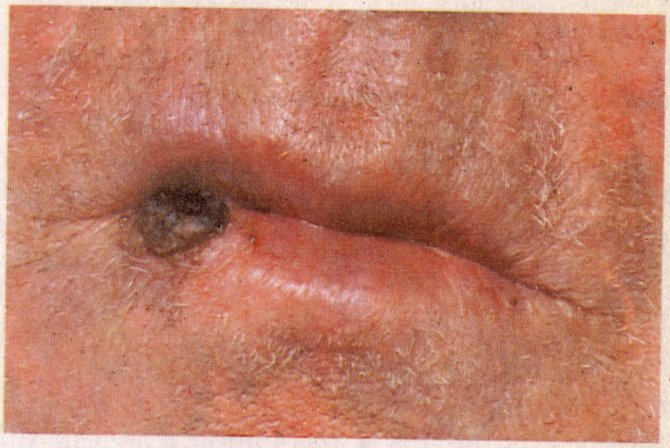

An ulcerating lesion covered with a black slough

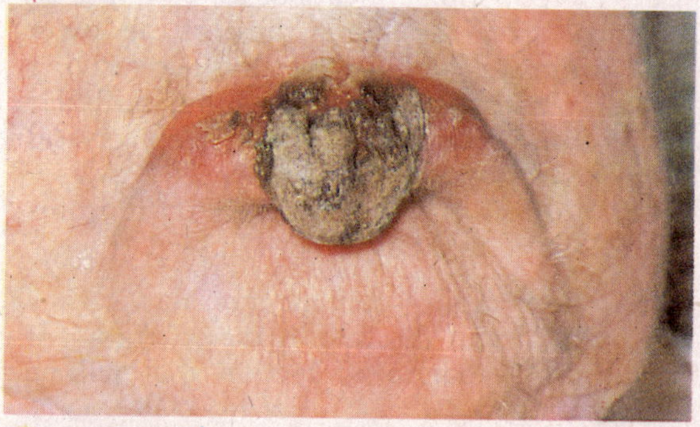

A large proliferating and infiltrating carcinoma distorting the whole lower lip

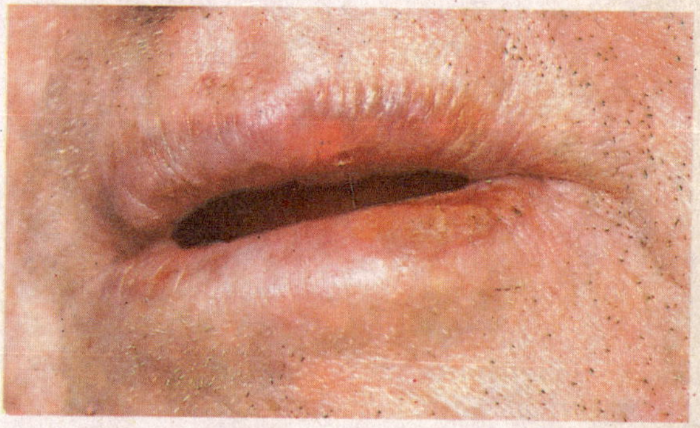

Solar keratoses on the lower lip – a premalignant change

FIG. 10.6 CARCINOMA OF THE LIP

Ethnic group Negroes are less susceptible but not immune to diseases induced by sunlight.

Geography All sunlight exposure conditions are more frequent in countries with a tropical or semi-tropical climate, and populated by white Caucasians, such as Australia.

Symptoms When the premalignant changes are developing in the lip the patient complains of blistering, thickening (keratosis), and white patches (leukoplakia).

A carcinoma causes a **lump**, or **an ulcer which fails to heal.**

As the ulcer grows it interferes with speech and eating, **bleeds** and produces an **offensive discharge**, but is not always painful.

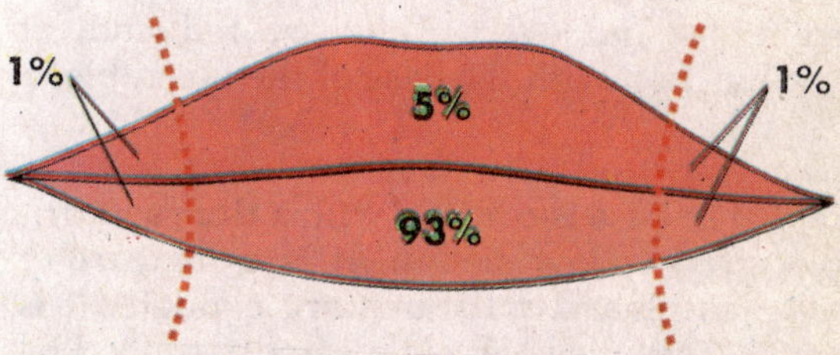

FIG. 10.7 The distribution of carcinoma of the lips

The patient may notice **lumps under his chin.** Although small lumps and sore spots on the lips are common, be suspicious of any lump that does not heal quickly.

Previous history It is important to ask about previous diseases, especially syphilis and conditions caused by exposure to sunlight.

Habits Ask if the patient smokes a pipe. Carcinoma of the lip was common when clay pipes were in common use.

EXAMINATION

Position The lower lip is affected over ten times more than the upper lip. Carcinoma in the angle of the lips is uncommon. The lesion is usually to one side of the mid-line.

Colour The skin over the lump or round the ulcer may show evidence of a premalignant condition: blistering, thickening and pigmentation, or white boggy patches.

Tenderness A cancer of the lip, nodular or ulcerative, is **not always tender**. The absence of tenderness should alert your suspicions because most ulcers in the mouth are very painful and tender.

Shape The cancer starts as a small lump or nodule which ultimately ulcerates in its centre and develops the typical everted edge of a carcinoma.

The initial lesion is small, just a few millimetres across, but can become large if not treated.

Edge Once the lump has ulcerated, the edges proliferate and evert. They are red and, at their junction with the base of the ulcer, bleed easily.

Base The base is covered with a thin, soft, friable, grey–yellow slough. It is a mixture of dying tissue and inflammatory exudate. It is thin because the ulcer is repeatedly rubbed by the tongue.

Depth The ulcer is initially shallow, but can erode deep into the lip, destroying the epithelium and the underlying muscle.

Discharge The discharge is thin, watery and slightly blood-stained. It is usually infected but rarely purulent.

Relations The lump is invariably fixed to the subcutaneous structures of the lip but can be moved, with the lip, separately from the jaw. Only very advanced lesions are fixed to the gum and jaw.

Lymph drainage The lymph glands draining the diseased portion of the lip are likely to be enlarged by secondary infection, if not by tumour.

1. The lymph draining from the upper lip passes across the face and over the angle of the jaw to the upper deep cervical glands.
2. Lymph from the centre of the lower lip drains to the submental glands and then to the lower deep cervical nodes.
3. Lymph from the lateral third of the lower lip drains to the lymphoid tissue overlying and sometimes within the submandibular gland and then to the middle deep cervical lymph nodes.
4. Lymph from the angle of the mouth drains into the lymphatics of both lips.

If the lymph nodes contain metastases, they will be hard and discrete. If the enlargement is caused by secondary infection, they will be slightly tender.

Surrounding tissues Away from the ulcer the rest of the lip is usually normal or mildly affected by the predisposing causes of cancer already mentioned.

GENERAL EXAMINATION

Disseminated distant metastases are rare.

Carcinoma of the tongue

Like carcinoma of the lip, the prevalence of carcinoma of the tongue has fallen in parallel with the reduction in the prevalence of syphilis, and there is no longer a high incidence of the disease in males.

The important premalignant disease of the tongue is chronic superficial glossitis, especially when it has reached the leukoplakia stage. Thus the causes of chronic superficial glossitis, already described, are the causes of carcinoma of the tongue.

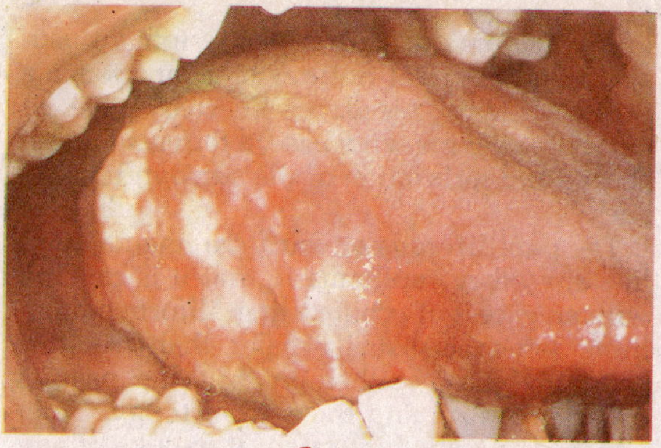

A large ulcer with an everted edge on the side of the tongue

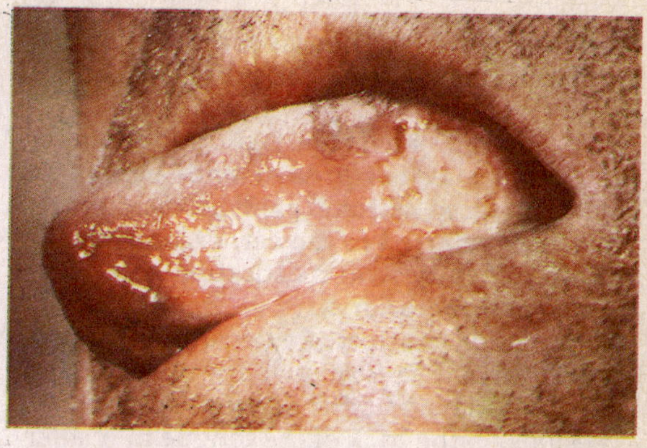

An ulcerated nodule on the side of the tongue

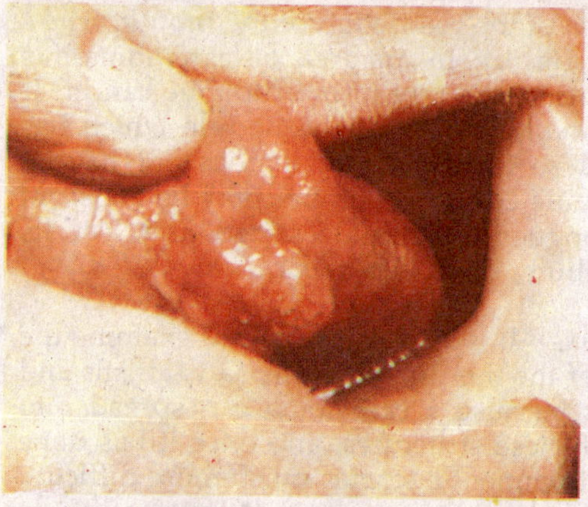

A nodular carcinoma of the tongue

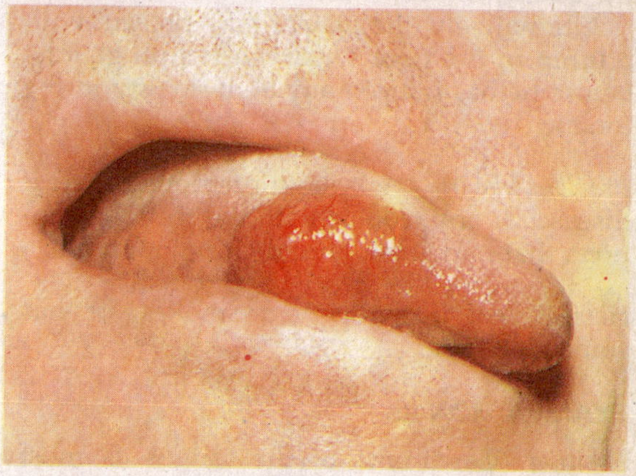

Not all nodules are primary lesions. This one was a metastasis from a carcinoma of the bronchus

FIG. 10.8 CARCINOMA OF THE TONGUE

Carcinoma of the tongue spreads locally and causes death through local complications, and aspiration or obstructive pneumonia. Distant blood-borne metastases are a late and uncommon event.

HISTORY

Age The patients are usually over the age of 50 years. The peak incidence is between 60 and 70 years.

Sex Males were affected far more than females when syphilis and pipe smoking were common. Now there are almost as many women affected as men.

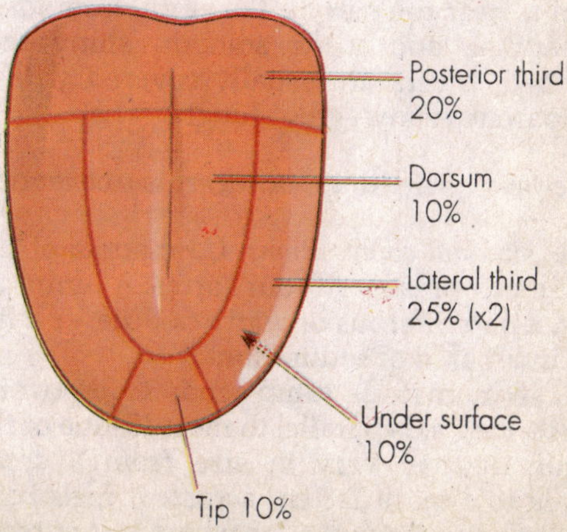

FIG. 10.9 The distribution of carcinoma of the tongue

Symptoms The commonest complaint is of a **painless lump or irregularity** on the surface of the tongue.

If the early lesion is ignored or not noticed, the patient may not present until he has an enlarging ulcer causing pain in the tongue, sometimes **referred to the ear; excessive salivation**; difficulty with mastication and swallowing; and **foetor oris**.

If the lesion has spread extensively before it is noticed it may cause immobility of the tongue (ankyloglossia) and difficulty with speech.

Lesions on the back of the tongue may alter the quality of the voice.

Alternatively, the patient may present with a **lump in the neck** (enlarged lymph glands) before he has noticed any abnormality in the tongue.

Previous history Ask about previous venereal disease, or any trouble with the teeth or dentures that may have caused chronic trauma.

Habits Ask if the patient smokes, or has smoked, a pipe.

EXAMINATION

Position Carcinoma of the tongue is most common on the edge and the lateral surface of the tongue, 20 per cent occur in the posterior third, 20 per cent occur on the dorsum and tip, and 10 per cent occur on the under surface.

Colour The epithelium and papillae over a deep-seated lump look normal, but if the lesion is near the surface the epithelium loses its papillae and looks smooth, shiny and stretched. Ulcers are usually covered with a transparent yellow–grey slough.

Tenderness The lump, or ulcer, is not tender.

Shape, size and composition Carcinoma of the tongue can present in four forms: a lump, an ulcer, a papilliferous or warty nodule, or a fissure in an area of induration.

A **carcinomatous lump** tends to be ovoid, with its long axis parallel to the mid-line of the tongue. It may vary in size from a small nodule to a mass 2–5 cm across. It feels hard and has an **indistinct** edge where it is spreading into the rest of the tongue.

A **carcinomatous ulcer** of the tongue usually has the typical features of a carcinoma: a florid, friable, bleeding, everted edge, a sloughing yellow–grey base, a thin serous discharge and induration of the surrounding tissues.

The **papilliferous or warty** carcinoma looks like any other papilloma in that it is covered with an excess of proliferating filiform epithelium, which is usually paler than the surrounding pink epithelium, but the base is **broad** and **firm** and the area of tongue from which it arises is **indurated**. It may be of any size but rarely juts out far from the tongue because of the restriction of the mouth.

The **fissure in an area of carcinomatous induration** is a rare form of tongue cancer. It is a modified form of the nodule which has spread so diffusely that it does not have a detectable edge. The fissure may be a cleft in the tongue that has deepened and lost its epithelium, or a deep linear ulcer.

Relations It is very important to examine the floor of the mouth, the gums, jaw, tonsils and fauces because a carcinoma can spread into any of these structures, and once it has done so its treatment becomes much more difficult.

Lesions on the side or under surface of the tongue are more likely to spread into the floor of the mouth than lesions on the dorsum.

Spread to the floor of the mouth causes thickening of the tissues and reduces the mobility of the tongue. Infiltration of the gum and jaw fixes the tumour to the bone, and the jaw itself may be swollen. Tumours of the posterior third of the tongue spread into the tonsil and the pillars of the fauces.

Lymph drainage

1 The lymph from the tip of the tongue drains to the submental glands and then to either or both jugular lymph chains.
2 The lymph from the rest of the anterior two-thirds drains to the glands on the same side of the neck, usually the middle and upper deep cervical nodes.
3 Lymph from the posterior third drains into the ring of lymph tissues around the oropharynx and into the upper deep cervical lymph nodes.

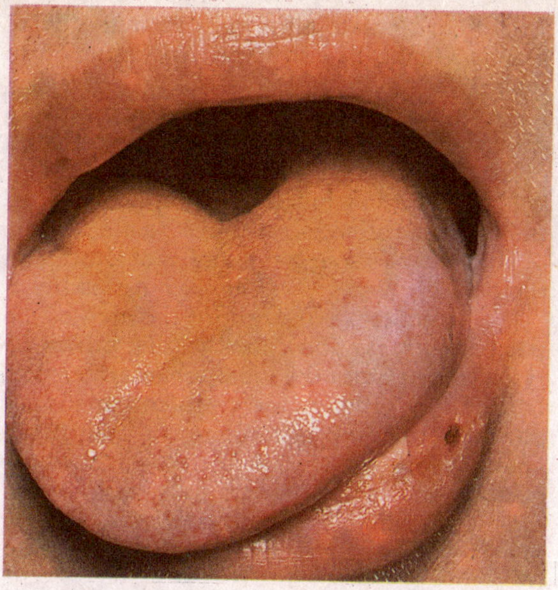

FIG. 10.10 A right hypoglossal nerve palsy. When this patient was asked to protrude his tongue it was wasted on the right and deviated to the right

More than half of the patients who present with a cancer of the tongue have palpable cervical lymph glands, but in some cases the enlargement is caused by secondary infection, not tumour.

State of local tissues Involvement of the lingual nerve causes a pain which is referred to the **ear**, probably through its connections with the auriculotemporal nerve.

Infiltration of the mandible causes pain and swelling of the jaw.

The surface of the tongue around the cancer may be affected by leukoplakia, and there may be other primary tumours.

Differential diagnosis The causes of ulcers on the tongue are given in Revision Panel 10.3.

Macroglossia

Macroglossia is a large tongue. The causes of macroglossia are:

Multiple haemangiomata.
Multiple lymphangiomata.
Plexiform neurofibromatosis.
Amyloid infiltration.
Infiltrating carcinoma.
Muscle hypertrophy (cretins).

Wasting of the tongue

Paralysis of the 12th cranial nerve (the hypoglossal nerve) causes disuse atrophy of one side of the tongue. When the patient is asked to 'put out his tongue' it deviates towards the paralysed side.

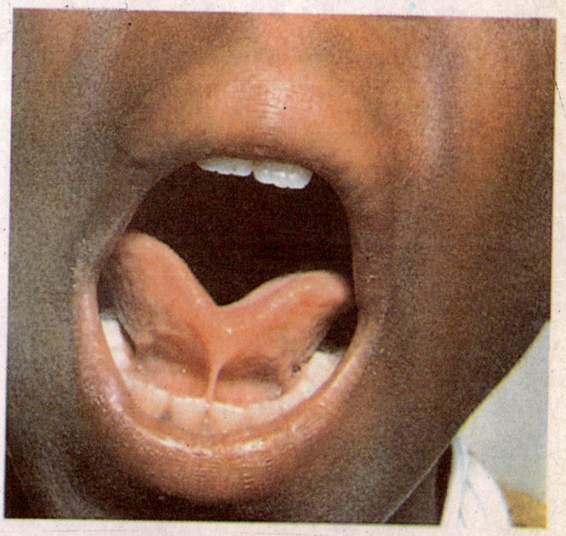

FIG. 10.11 Tongue-tie. A congenitally short frenulum. This rarely causes any significant impairment of speech

Revision Panel 10.3

The causes of ulceration of the tongue

- Aphthous ulcer
- Trauma (dental)
- Non-specific glossitis
- Chancre
- Gumma
- Tuberculosis
- Carcinoma

THE PALATE

The varieties of congenital cleft palate are described on page 234 and 235.

Perforation of the palate

A perforation in the palate can be acquired if disease or trauma destroys the bones of the palate.

When syphilis was common, perforation of the hard palate following **gummatous** destruction of the bone and mucosa was quite common. Nowadays acquired perforation of the palate is rare. It can be caused by:

1. An empyema or tumour of the maxillary antrum bursting through the palate into the mouth.
2. Repeated trauma from poorly fitting dentures.
3. Surgical excision of the palate to approach the maxillary antrum.

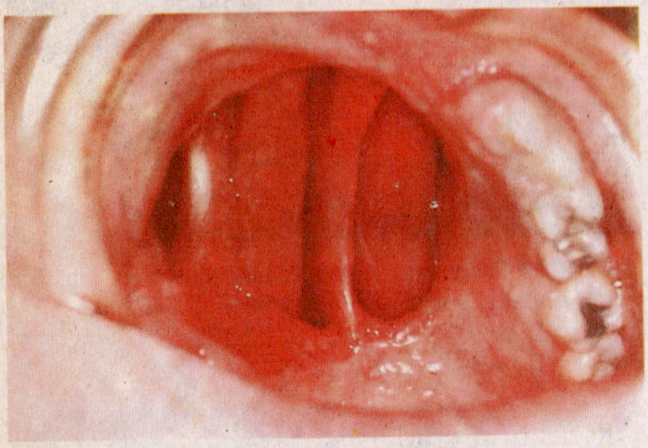

FIG. 10.12 Large perforation of the palate. The nasal septum and turbinate bones are clearly visible

Tumours on the palate

The mucous membrane covering the hard palate is identical to that of the rest of the buccal mucosa. Retention cysts and carcinoma, similar to those of the lips and buccal mucosa, are not uncommon.

The hard palate also contains many small glands identical in structure and function to the salivary glands.

A pleomorphic salivary adenoma (mixed salivary tumour – see Chapter 9) is a common cause of a lump on the palate.

Figure 10.13 includes an example of a small pleomorphic adenomata of the palate.

The patient's sole complaint is of a lump on the palate which grows slowly but steadily.

If it is not treated it can fill the arch of the palate and make speech and eating difficult.

On examination the lump feels smooth and hard. The overlying mucous membrane is not attached to it, and if the lump is small it can be moved over the underlying palate. As the tumour grows it becomes less mobile and more difficult to distinguish from a tumour growing in or above the palate.

THE TONSILS

Tonsillitis is a condition familiar to all because almost everyone has suffered it. It causes a sore throat and pain during swallowing. On examination the tonsils are seen to be enlarged and red, with pus exuding from their crypts. The surrounding pillars of the fauces, soft palate and oropharynx are also red and tender, and may be covered with small yellow-based ulcers.

Bilateral enlargement of the tonsils, together with the above signs, is diagnostic of tonsillitis.

Unilateral enlargement of a tonsil, even if it is red and tender, is not always caused by acute tonsillitis. Remember the other causes of enlargement of the tonsil, described below.

Carcinoma of the tonsil

Carcinoma of the tonsil occurs in the elderly. The enlarging tonsil and deep infiltration by the tumour cells may cause **severe pain** in the throat, which is **referred to the ear**.

The surface of the growth eventually ulcerates to form a deep indolent ulcer, rarely with everted edges, which **bleeds**, causes severe **dysphagia** and a pungent **foetor oris**. The

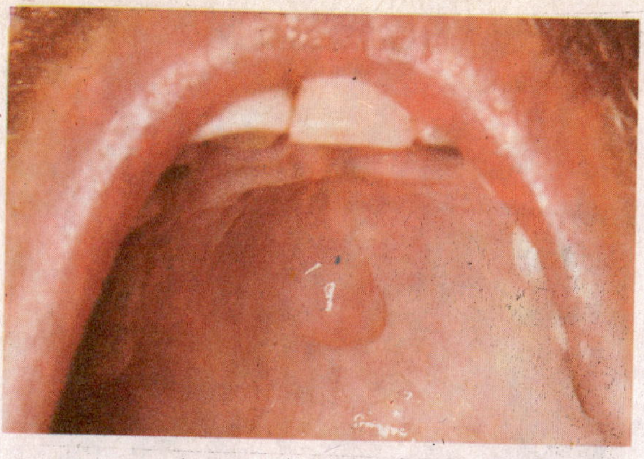

A small pleomorphic adenoma of a salivary gland on the hard palate

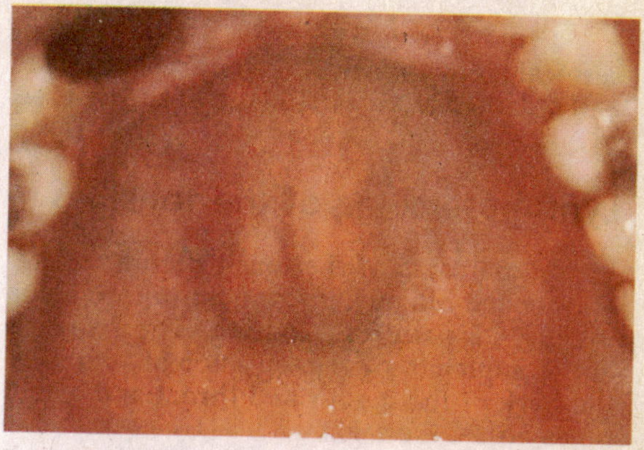

A mid-line bony spur of the hard palate, recognizible by its mid-line cleft, known as a torus palatinus

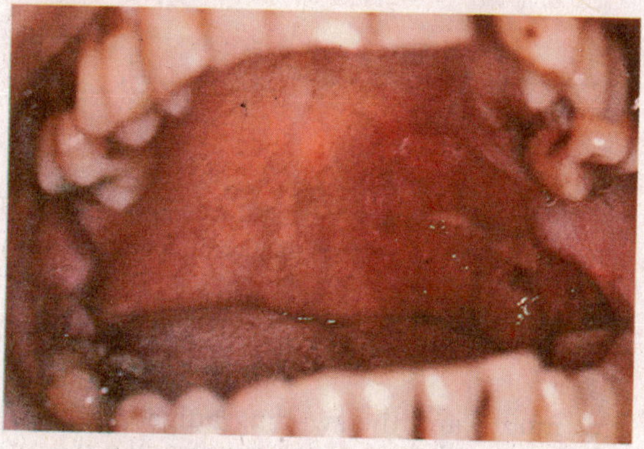

A carcinoma on the side of the hard palate

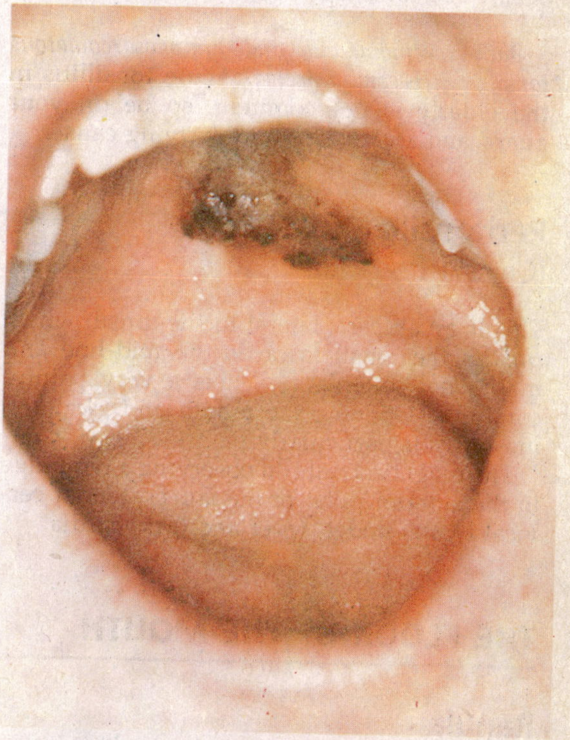

A malignant melanoma of the hard palate. This is a rare condition but included as a reminder that malignant melanoma can arise at the muco-cutaneous junctions, i.e. around the mouth and anus

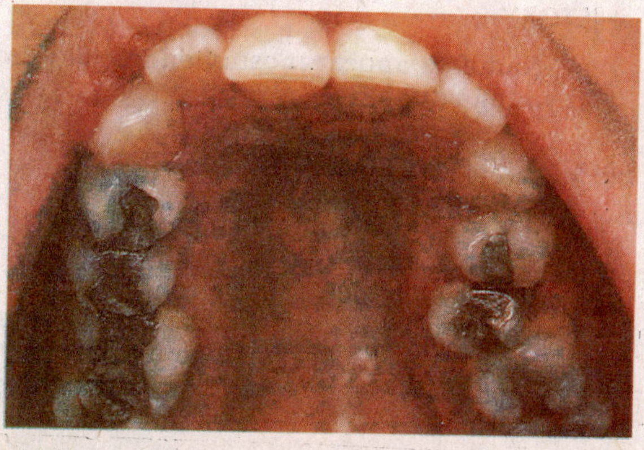

The high-arched palate of Marfan's syndrome

FIG. 10.13 THE HARD PALATE

cervical lymph glands often become involved and enlarged at an early stage of the disease.

Lymphosarcoma of the tonsil

Lymphosarcoma of the tonsil occurs in late-middle and old age. In contrast to carcinoma it causes a **painless swelling**. The patient's only complaints are the sensation of a **lump in the back of the mouth and throat** and sometimes **mild dysphagia**.

Gross swelling may interfere with speech and make the words indistinct.

Enlargement of the cervical lymph nodes occurs at a late stage of the disease.

Both carcinomatous and lymphosarcomatous tonsils can become infected. Acute tonsillitis in the elderly is not common, so be on your guard and search for an underlying cause.

Peritonsillar abscess

(Quinsy)

This is an abscess, lateral to the tonsil, which pushes the tonsil towards the mid-line and makes it look enlarged. It is a very painful condition. Opening the mouth and swallowing saliva is particularly painful.

The diagnosis rests on observing a red bulge in the anterior pillar of the fauces, tender cervical lymph nodes, fever and tachycardia.

THE FLOOR OF THE MOUTH

Ranula

A ranula is a large mucus-containing cyst in the floor of the mouth. The mucus probably comes from acini of the sublingual gland which have ruptured in response to secretory back-pressure secondary to an obstruction of the sublingual duct, or direct injury.

Ranula is the Latin for a small frog. It is said that the swelling was given this name by Hippocrates because he thought it looked like the belly of a frog; but when the patient opens his mouth and the swelling bulges up under the tongue, I think it looks more like the air-filled swelling under the jaw of a frog when it croaks.

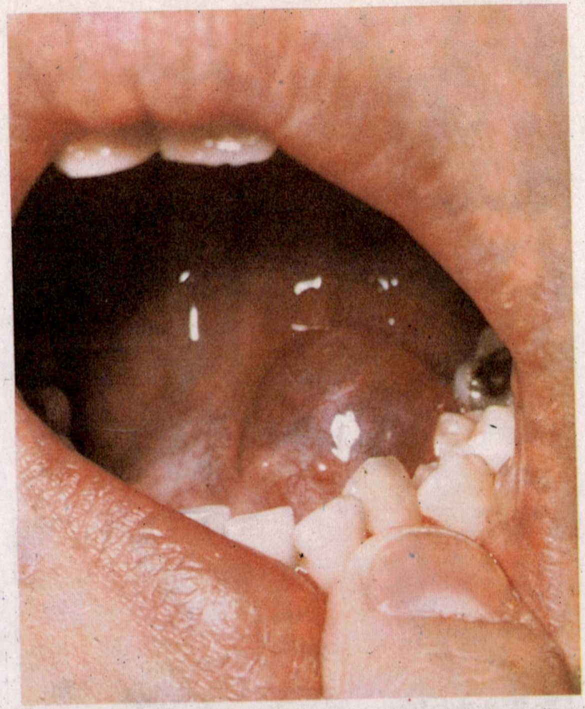

FIG. 10.14 A ranula. A tense, translucent, spherical swelling just below the mucosa of the floor of the mouth

HISTORY

Age Ranulata appear most often in children and young adults.

Sex Both sexes are equally affected.

Symptoms The patient complains of a **swelling in the floor of the mouth**, which has grown gradually over a few weeks.

Some ranulata fluctuate in size, and some swell suddenly and become painful, but they rarely get big enough to interfere with eating or speech.

EXAMINATION

Position The swelling lies in the floor of the mouth, between the symphysis menti and the tongue, just to one side of the mid-line.

Colour The lump has a characteristic semi-transparent grey appearance. The colour and the site are the diagnostic features.

Tenderness The swelling is **not** tender.

Shape Ranulata form spherical cysts but only the top half is visible.

Size They vary from 1 to 5 cm in diameter.

Surface Their surface is smooth but the edge is difficult to feel because it is deep between the arch of the mandible.

Composition The swelling is **soft**, usually **fluctuant** and **transilluminates**, but it cannot be compressed or reduced.

Relations The overlying mucosa is not fixed to the wall of the cyst and the cyst is not fixed to the tongue or the jaw.

The swelling is usually closely related to the duct of the submandibular salivary gland (Wharton's duct), which may be seen running over its surface or alongside it.

Ranulata occasionally extend through the mylohyoid muscle into the neck. This variety is called a 'plunging' ranula.

Lymph drainage The cervical lymph glands should not be enlarged.

The local tissues These should all be normal.

Sublingual dermoid cyst

When the face and neck are formed by the fusion of the facial processes, a piece of epidermis may get trapped deep in the mid-line just behind the jaw, and later form a sublingual dermoid cyst.

Such cysts are in the mid-line, but may be above or below the mylohyoid muscle.

HISTORY

Age The swelling is usually noticed when the patient is between the ages of 10 and 25 years.

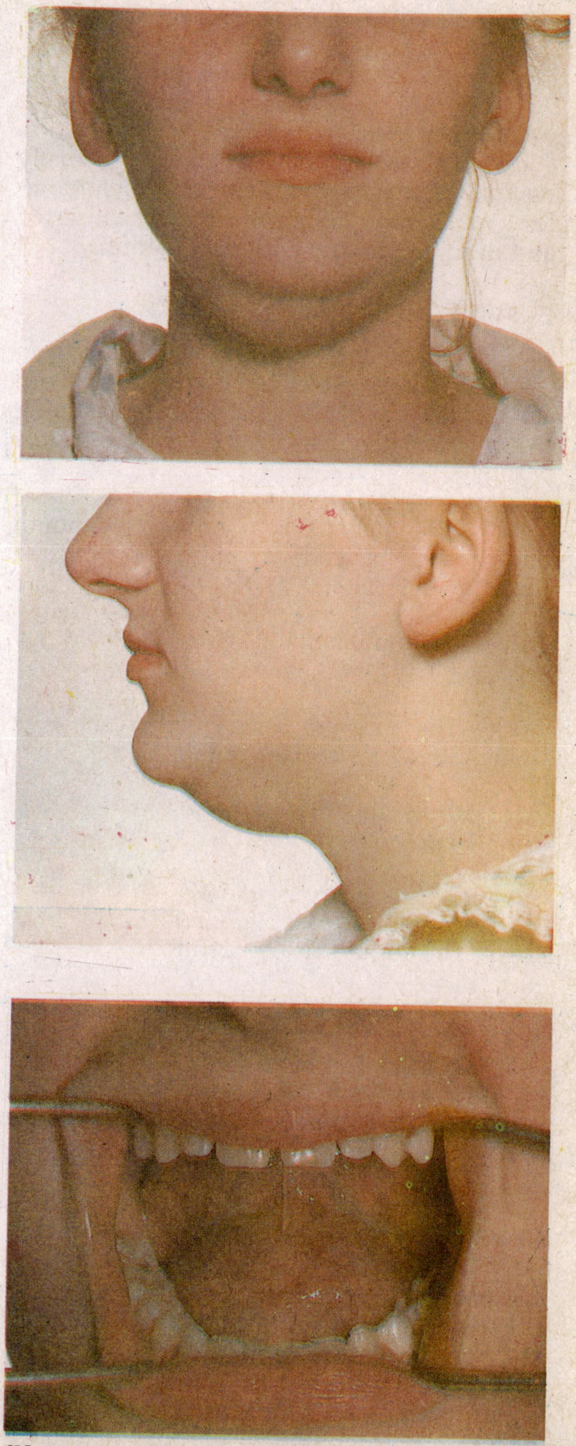

FIG. 10.15 A sublingual dermoid cyst. This cyst was above the mylohyoid muscle but large enough to cause a visible swelling below the chin

Sex Both sexes are equally affected.

Symptoms The patient complains of a **swelling** under the tongue or just below the point of the chin.

It may appear suddenly, when it is usually painful, or gradually. It is otherwise symptomless. Very rarely, the contents become infected and the cyst becomes tense and painful.

EXAMINATION

Position The lump is easily visible, either in the centre of the floor of the mouth between the tongue and the point of the jaw, or bulging down below the chin, looking like a double chin.

Colour The mucous membrane of the mouth and the skin beneath the chin overlying the lump are normal.

Tenderness Sublingual dermoid cysts are not tender.

Shape The cyst is clearly spherical even though its whole surface cannot be felt.

Size By the time these cysts are noticed they are 2–5 cm across.

Surface The surface is smooth.

Edge The edge is clearly defined.

Composition The lump feels **firm**, but bimanual palpation reveals that it **fluctuates**.

These cysts do not usually transilluminate as their contents are often opaque. They cannot be compressed or reduced.

Relations Sublingual dermoid cysts can be felt **bimanually**, with a finger in the mouth and one beneath the chin.

When the tongue is lifted up, the supramylohyoid variety bulges into the mouth.

If the tongue is pushed against the roof of the mouth with the teeth clenched, the submylohyoid variety bulges out below the chin.

Neither variety is attached to the covering buccal mucosa or skin, or the tongue, but the proximity of the tongue muscles and jaw limits their mobility.

Local tissues The nearby tissues should all be normal.

Lymph drainage The local lymph nodes should not be enlarged.

Stone in Wharton's duct

Stones and infection in the submandibular gland and duct are common (see page 222). When such a stone migrates forwards to the mouth of the submandibular duct (Wharton's duct), it forms a lump in the floor of the mouth (see Fig. 9.3, page 225). The lump bulges slightly into the mouth, is tender and, through the surrounding oedema, the centre may feel hard.

Sometimes the surface of the stone can be seen through the open end of the duct.

The submandibular gland is usually swollen and tender.

THE JAW

Retention cysts, carcinoma and salivary tumours can arise from the mucous membrane that covers the jaw, but there are some swellings which are peculiar to the gum. They are called *epulitides*, but this is just a special name to indicate the site of the lump, not its pathology.

An epulis is a swelling that arises from the alveolar margin of the jaw. It can originate from the bone, the periosteum or the mucous membrane.

Fibroma

The commonest variety of epulis is the **fibrous epulis**. This is a fibroma which arises from the gingival tissues, so forming a firm nodule at the junction of gum and tooth. It may bulge out and become polypoid in shape.

Fibrosarcoma

A **fibrosarcomatous epulis** is the malignant variety of the fibrous epulis. It grows rapidly, is soft and friable, and very rare.

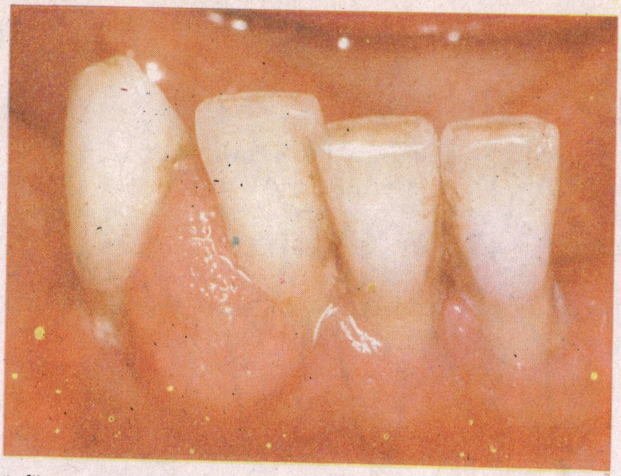

A fibrous epulis

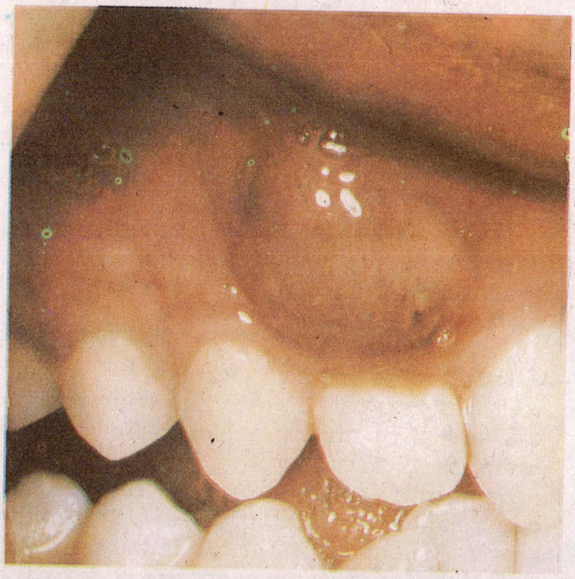

A giant-celled epulis

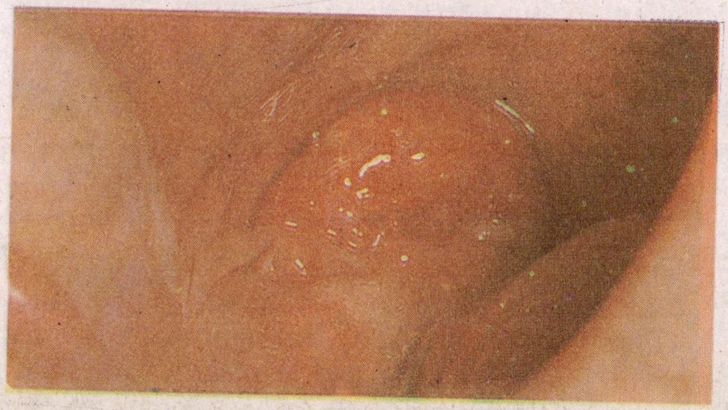

A pyogenic granuloma

FIG. 10.16 SWELLINGS OF THE GUM

Granuloma

A **granulomatous epulis** is a pyogenic granuloma of the mucosa of the gum. It is usually associated with gingivitis or dental caries.

Bone tumour

A **bony epulis** is usually caused by an osteoclastoma (giant cell tumour). Although the underlying mass is hard, the gum covering the mass becomes hyperaemic and oedematous, and may bleed and ulcerate.

Carcinoma

Carcinoma of the gum presents as a lump or an ulcer. It is usually recognizable as a carcinoma, so the description used in some books – carcinomatous epulis – is confusing and unnecessary.

Revision Panel 10.4

The causes of swelling of the jaw

Infections
- Alveolar (dental) abscess
- Acute osteomyelitis
- Actinomycosis

Cysts
- Dental cysts
- Dentigerous cysts
- Other odontogenic cysts and cystic tumours

Neoplasms

Benign
- Fibrous dysplasia
- Giant cell granuloma
- Odontogenic tumours

Locally invasive
- Adamantinoma

Malignant
- Osteogenic sarcoma
- Malignant lymphoma (Burkitt's tumour)
- Secondary tumours (by direct invasion or blood stream spread)

Alveolar (dental) abscess

The commonest cause of swelling of the jaw is a dental or alveolar abscess. This is an abscess which forms at the base of the root of a decaying tooth and tracks outwards, through the external surface of the mandible or maxilla, to form an abscess beneath the cheek or jaw.

HISTORY

Age An alveolar abscess can develop at any age, with the first or the second dentition.

Symptoms The patient complains of a constant **dull ache** in the jaw, which gets gradually worse and becomes **throbbing** in nature.

Soon after the onset of the pain, a **swelling** appears which is very tender.

There is often sweating, general malaise and loss of appetite.

Previous history The patient may know that he has bad teeth, having had toothache and avoided dental care.

EXAMINATION

Position Most alveolar abscesses point to the labial (outer) side of the jaw. Those in the lower jaw also point downwards to the inferior margin of the mandible.

An abscess which points to the lingual (inner) surface causes a swelling on the palate or between the mandible and the tongue.

Colour The overlying skin or mucosa is reddened by the inflammatory hyperaemia.

Temperature and tenderness The swelling is hot and acutely tender.

Shape The abscess takes the form of a flattened hemisphere, but its edges merge into the surrounding tissues, so it does not have a clear-cut shape or edge.

Surface The surface is indistinct.

Composition It is difficult to assess the composition of the swelling because it is so tender.

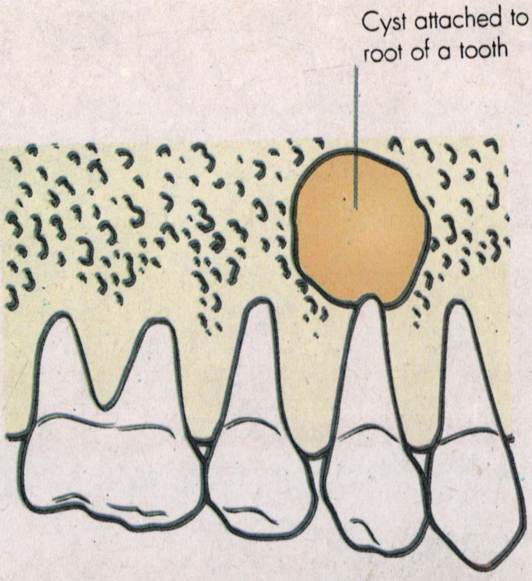

FIG. 10.17 The site of origin of a dental cyst

The deep part of the mass feels firm, but the overlying tissues may be soft and boggy with oedematous fluid. Large abscesses may fluctuate.

Relations The mass is clearly fixed to, and feels as if it is part of, the underlying bone.

The skin or mucosa move freely over the lump until they become involved in the oedema or the inflammatory process. The precise relations depend upon the site of the abscess. The commonest site is the posterior part of the lower jaw in relation to caries in the molar teeth or failure of their eruption.

An alveolar abscess in the upper jaw, pointing medially, causes swelling of the palate and fauces.

Lymph drainage The upper cervical lymph glands are usually enlarged and tender.

State of local tissue The arteries and nerves of the face, jaw and tongue should be normal. There may be visible evidence of neglect of the teeth, such as caries and gingivitis, and there may be unerupted teeth. If an alveolar abscess points and discharges it may become a chronic discharging sinus.

Cysts of the jaw

A swelling of the whole jaw may be caused by infection, a cyst, or a tumour. These are classified in Revision Panel 10.4.

There are two common benign cysts of the jaw.

Dental cyst

This is a cyst attached to the root of a normally erupted but usually decayed and infected tooth.

The epithelial cells that form the cyst are thought to be derived from the enamel organ.

They are more common in the upper jaw. They grow steadily, expanding the jaw and filling the maxillary antrum.

Clinical examination can get no further than detecting that the swelling is in the bone. Sometimes the bone is so thin that it 'crackles' when touched, like a broken eggshell.

Dentigerous cyst

A dentigerous cyst is a cyst containing an unerupted tooth.

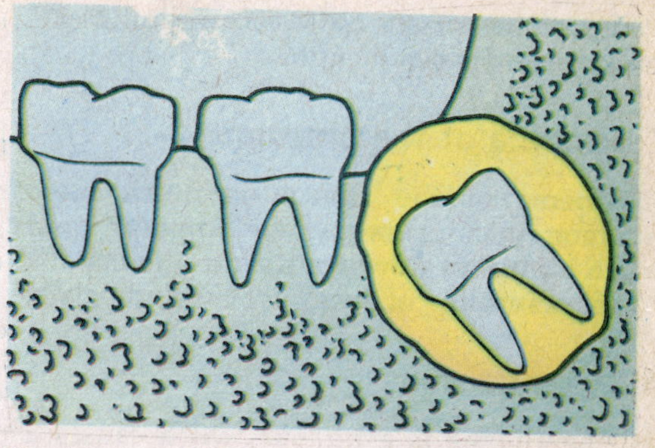

FIG. 10.18 A dentigerous cyst

The cyst can enlarge and cause swelling of the jaw.

Tumours of the jaw

Many types of benign and malignant tumours of the jaw are listed in Revision Panel 10.4. They all present as a bony swelling which grows steadily, and usually painlessly.

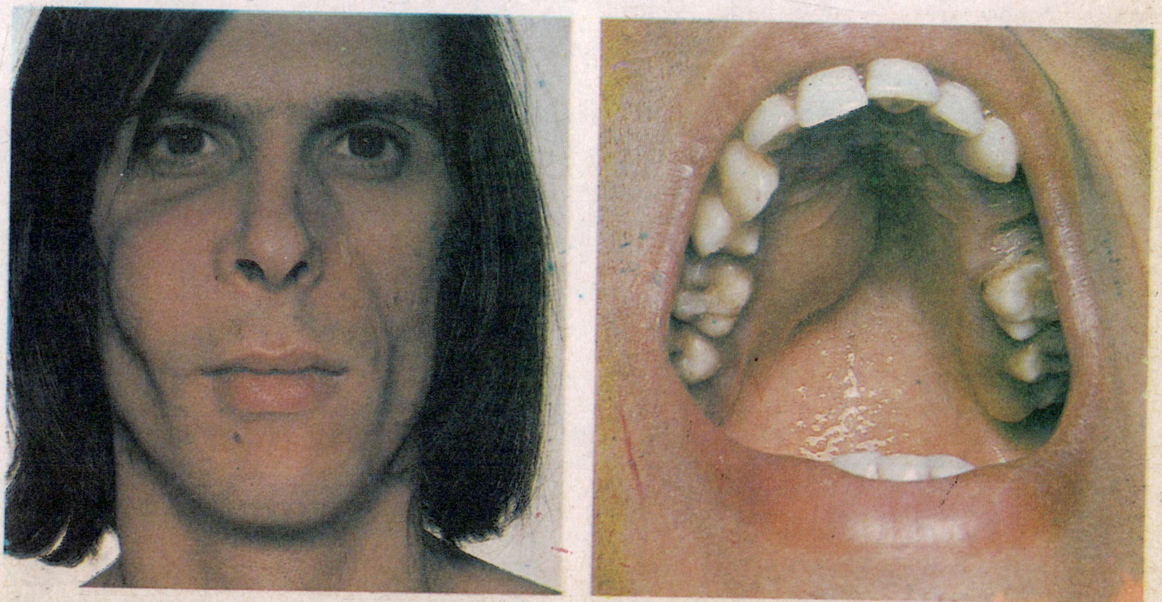

FIG. 10.19 A large dental cyst expanding the maxilla and bulging into the roof of the mouth. The palate crackled when it was palpated because the bone was so thin

The four neoplastic causes of swelling of the jaw deserve special mention.

Carcinoma of the antrum

Carcinoma of the antrum is much more common than primary bone tumours, and when it invades downwards into the maxilla it causes swelling of the upper jaw and palate.

Adamantinoma

Adamantinoma is a tumour which causes a painless, progressive swelling of the jaw, but it is *locally invasive* and tends to recur.

Osteosarcoma

Osteosarcoma can occur in both the upper and the lower jaw.

Malignant lymphoma

(Burkitt's lymphoma)

Burkitt's lymphoma is a malignant tumour of B lymphocytes associated with EB virus infection. In 80 per cent of patients it presents as a tumour in the jaw. In its endemic form it affects children below the age of 12 years and occurs in those areas of sub-Saharan Africa and the coastal regions of New Guinea that have a warm, wet climate and endemic malaria. It is believed that the latter causes immune depression of T suppressor cells which permits the uncontrolled proliferation of EB-virus-infected B cells to form the tumour. Sporadic cases of Burkitt's lymphomata also occur throughout the world.

The child presents with a progressive, painless swelling of the jaw which distorts the face, may displace the eye and partially occludes the mouth.

Other lymphomatous tissue may be present in the retroperitoneal tissues, kidneys, ovaries and spine, and cause abdominal and skeletal symptoms.

Revision Panel 10.5

Remember when the teeth erupt

Primary dentition (months)

7	9	18	22	24
6	9	18	22	24

Incisors Canine Milk molars

Permanent dentition (years)

7	8	11	11	11	6	12	18
7	8	11	11	11	6	12	18

Incisors Canine Premolars Molars

The neck

11

THE HISTORY AND EXAMINATION OF SWELLINGS IN THE NECK

The majority of surgical conditions which arise in the neck present as a swelling. The history and physical examination follow the standard pattern, but there are some important features that deserve special attention.

The history of swellings in the neck

Because the commonest cause of a swelling in the neck is an enlarged lymph gland, and because the commonest causes of enlarged lymph glands are infection and secondary tumour deposits, you must remember to ask about symptoms which might help you decide the cause of the swelling.

Systemic illness

Symptoms such as general malaise, fever, rigors, and contact with persons with infectious diseases, may indicate an infective cause of the swelling.

Loss of appetite, loss of weight, pulmonary, alimentary or skeletal symptoms may suggest the site of a neoplasm.

Irritation of the skin associated with enlarged cervical lymph glands is often seen with lymphoma.

Head and neck symptoms

Ask about: pain in the mouth, sore throats or ulceration; nasal discharge, pain or blockage of the airway; pain in the throat, dysphagia, changes in the voice and difficulty with breathing; and lumps or ulcers on the skin of the head and face that have changed size or begun to bleed.

The skin, mouth, nose, larynx and pharynx are common sites for neoplasms, and whereas head and neck cancer commonly presents with metastases in lymph glands it is not usually associated with general malaise and loss of weight.

Examination of swellings in the neck

Site

It is essential to define the site of a lump in the neck.

The neck is divided into two triangles. The **anterior triangle** is bounded by the anterior

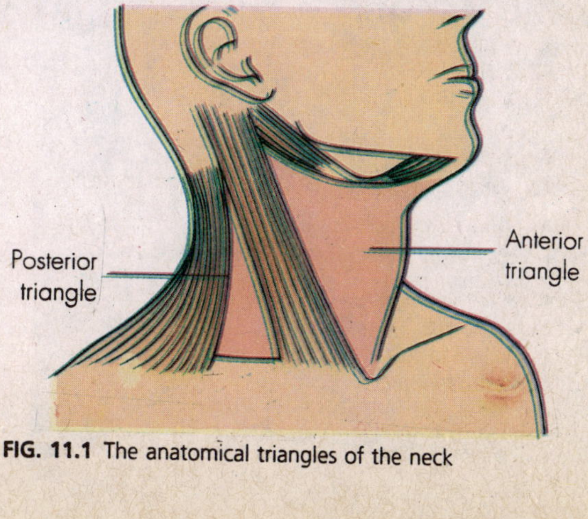

FIG. 11.1 The anatomical triangles of the neck

border of the sternomastoid muscle, the lower edge of the jaw and the mid-line. In clinical practice the structures deep to the sternomastoid muscle are considered to be inside the anterior triangle.

The upper part of the anterior triangle, below the jaw but above the digastric muscle, is sometimes called the digastric or submandibular triangle.

The **posterior triangle** is bounded by the posterior border of the sternomastoid muscle, the anterior edge of the trapezius muscle and the clavicle.

To define the triangles it is necessary to get the patient to tense the neck muscles:

The **sternomastoid** is made to contract by putting your hand under the patient's chin and asking him to nod his head against the resistance of your hand. This tightens both sternomastoids.

The **trapezius** is made to contract by asking the patient to shrug (elevate) his shoulders against resistance.

Relation to muscles

Always feel lumps in the neck with the muscles relaxed and then with them contracted. If the lump is deep to a muscle it will become impalpable when the muscle contracts.

> **Revision Panel 11.1**
> **Causes of cervical lymphadenopathy**
>
> *Infection*
> Non-specific
> Glandular fever
> Tuberculosis
> Syphilis
> Toxoplasmosis
> Cat-scratch fever (*Rochalimaea henselae*)
>
> *Metastatic tumour*
> From head, neck, chest and abdomen
>
> *Primary reticuloses*
> Lymphoma
> Lymphosarcoma
> Reticulosarcoma
>
> *Sarcoidosis*

Relation to trachea

Swellings that are fixed to the trachea will move when the trachea moves. The trachea is elevated during swallowing. Assess the relationship to the trachea of every lump in the neck by watching to see if it moves with the trachea during swallowing.

Relation to the hyoid cartilage

The hyoid cartilage moves only slightly during swallowing but ascends when the tongue is protruded. Ask the patient to open his mouth. When the jaw is still, ask him to protrude his tongue. If the swelling in the neck moves as the tongue protrudes it must be fixed to the hyoid cartilage.

CERVICAL LYMPHADENOPATHY AND OTHER NECK SWELLINGS

Causes of cervical lymph node enlargement

Enlargement of the cervical lymph nodes is the most common cause of a swelling in the neck. Even when only one node is palpable, the adjacent nodes are invariably diseased.

The four main causes of cervical lymph node enlargement are as follows:

Infection: non-specific tonsillitis, glandular fever, toxoplasmosis, tuberculosis, cat scratch fever.

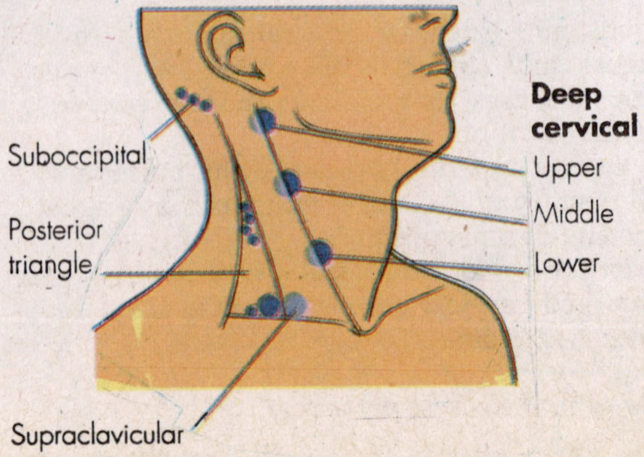

FIG. 11.2 The anatomy of the cervical lymph nodes

Metastatic tumour from the head, neck, chest and abdomen.
Primary reticuloses: lymphoma, lymphosarcoma, reticulosarcoma.
Sarcoidosis.

The diagnosis of lymphadenopathy caused by systemic illnesses such as glandular fever, toxoplasmosis and sarcoidosis depends upon finding lymphadenopathy elsewhere, other evidence of the underlying disease, and special blood tests.

Non-specific inflammatory lymphadenopathy

This commonly follows recurrent bouts of tonsillitis, especially if the attacks have been treated inadequately. The upper deep cervical nodes are most often affected.

In a healthy child, small normal lymph glands are often palpable, especially in the posterior triangle.

HISTORY

Age The majority of patients are below the age of 10 years.

Symptoms The common presenting symptom is a **painful lump** just below the angle of the jaw.

The severity of the pain varies. It is usually a discomfort which becomes acute when the patient has a **sore throat**.

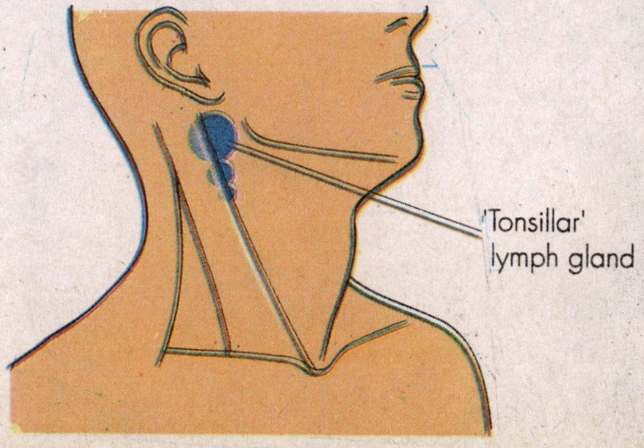

FIG. 11.3 The site of the 'tonsillar' lymph gland

The lump may be large enough to be **visible** or **felt** by the child's mother when she is washing the neck.

The child may **snore** at night, have **difficulty in breathing**, have a **nasal speech** because of tonsillar and adenoid hyperplasia, and suffer from recurrent chest infections.

Cause The child and the parents frequently appreciate the relationship between the appearance of the lump and an episode of tonsillitis.

Systemic effects When the lump is tender the patient often feels ill, has a sore throat and a pyrexia and does not want to eat.

Recurrent episodes can cause loss of weight and slow down the rate of growth and body maturation.

Social history Recurrent sore throats and upper respiratory tract infections are more common in malnurtured children living in substandard, cold, damp houses.

EXAMINATION

Position The tonsils drain to the upper deep cervical lymph nodes. The node just below and deep to the angle of the mandible is often called the tonsillar node. This node and those just below it are likely to be enlarged.

Tenderness If the infection is active the enlarged nodes will be tender.

Shape and size The tonsillar node is usually spherical and approximately 1–2 cm in diameter. It is rarely bigger than this. The nodes below it are usually smaller.

Composition and relations Each node is firm in consistence, solid and discrete, not fixed but not very mobile.

Local tissues The tonsils are likely to be enlarged and hyperaemic. Pus may be seen exuding from the surface crypts.

The nodes on the other side of the neck are often just as large but may not have been noticed by the parents.

GENERAL EXAMINATION

Look for the presence of enlarged lymph nodes elsewhere. They should not be enlarged.

Recurrent chest infections may have damaged the lungs – look for collapsed lobes, bronchiectasis and lung abscess. These are rare complications nowadays.

Tuberculous cervical lymphadenitis and abscess

The **human** tubercle bacillus can enter the body via the tonsils, and from there move to the cervical lymph nodes. The upper deep cervical nodes are most often affected. There is no generalized infection, so there is little systemic disturbance of health. Infection with bovine tuberculosis ceased in the United Kingdom when the control and testing of dairy cattle was introduced.

HISTORY

Age and ethnic groups Tuberculous lymphadenitis is common in children and young adults, and in the elderly. The incidence in the young has diminished since the introduction of BCG vaccination, mass radiography screening and the discovery of effective antituberculosis antibiotics; but the prevalence of cervical lymph node enlargement caused by anonymous mycobacteria is increasing. In Great Britain tuberculous lymphadenitis is found most often in young immigrant adults.

Symptoms The patient complains of **a lump in the neck** (see Fig. 11.4). This appears gradually, sometimes with, sometimes without, pain.

The pain can be intense if the nodes grow rapidly and necrose.

Systemic symptoms are unusual in the young but the elderly sometimes have anorexia and slight weight loss.

If the nodes turn into an abscess the swelling **increases in size**, becomes more **painful** and the patient notices **discolouration of the overlying skin.**

When the glands are very painful, neck movements and swallowing may be painful.

Previous history The elderly patient often has a history of swollen neck glands when young

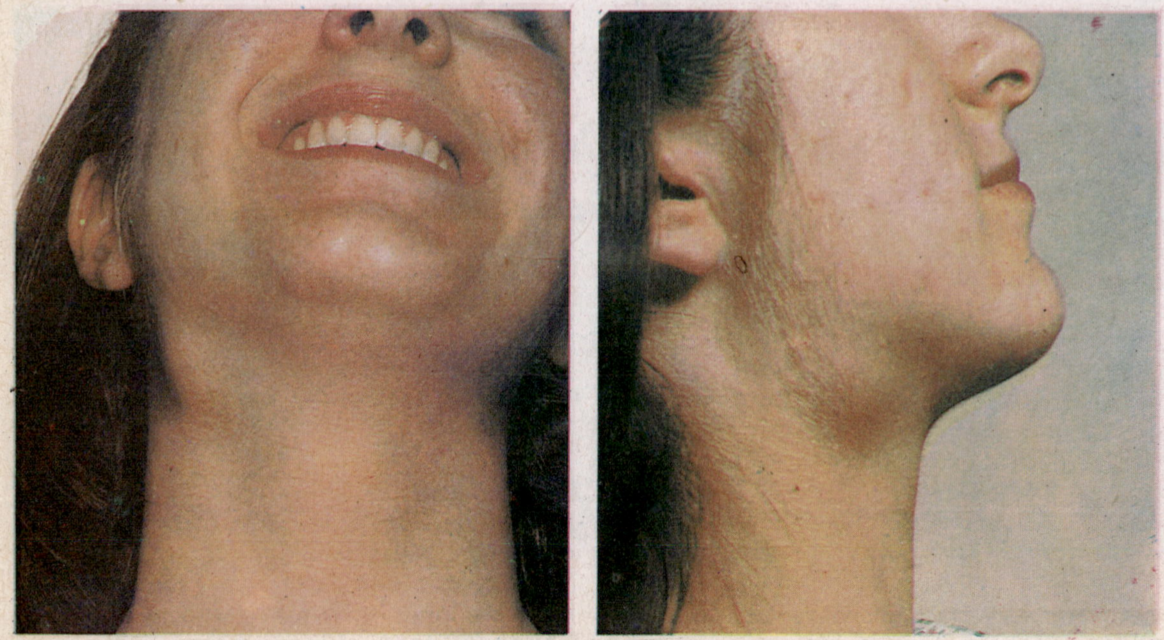

FIG. 11.4 Enlargement of the upper deep cervical lymph glands caused by tuberculosis

– sometimes treated at that time by surgical excision.

Immunization Ask whether the patient has been vaccinated with BCG.

Family history Check that none of the family has had tuberculosis.

Social history Tuberculosis is more common in the underprivileged.

EXAMINATION

The signs of tuberculous lymphadenitis

Position The upper and middle deep cervical nodes are the nodes most often involved.

Temperature The mass of nodes does **not** feel hot.

Tenderness Although the temperature of the skin is normal and the nodes are often slightly tender, pain and tenderness are not prominent features of tuberculous lymphadenitis.

Colour If there is no abscess present the overlying skin should look normal.

Shape, size and consistence In the early stages the nodes are firm, discrete and between 1 and 2 cm in diameter.

As caseation increases and the nodes necrose, the infection spreads beyond the capsule of the nodes. This makes the lumps get bigger and coalesce.

A typical patch of tuberculous lymphadenitis is an **indistinct, firm mass** of nodes which occupies the upper half of the deep cervical lymph chain, partly beneath and partly in front of the sternomastoid.

The nodes are commonly described as **matted together**, but there may be some discrete nodes above or below the matted mass.

Local tissues Other cervical lymph nodes may be palpable. The tonsils and the other tissues in the neck should be normal.

The signs of a tuberculous abscess

When an infected lymph node caseates and turns into pus it becomes, by definition, an abscess. The natural tendency of an abscess is to weaken the overlying tissues until it bursts through them, ultimately to reach and burst through the skin. This is known as **pointing**. At the stage when a tuberculous abscess has burst through the deep cervical fascia into the subcutaneous tissues, it has two compartments, one on either side of the deep fascia, connected by a small central track. This is called a **collar-stud** abscess.

Position Because a tuberculous abscess forms in tuberculous lymph glands, it is most often found in the upper half of the neck.

Colour When the pus reaches the subcutaneous tissues the overlying skin turns reddish-purple.

Temperature The skin temperature is normal because the process of caseation and pus formation is slow and does not stimulate excessive hyperaemia. Hence the name **cold abscess**.

Tenderness The mass is tender, sometimes exquisitely so if the abscess is tense.

Shape The deep part of the abscess tends to be sausage shaped, with its long axis parallel to the front edge of the sternomastoid muscle. The superficial pocket of the abscess is usually lower than the deep part.

Size Most tuberculous abscesses are 3–5 cm across but they can be much larger.

Surface The surface is irregular and indistinct.

Edge The edges are moderately well defined if the abscess is tense, but you will not be able to feel a definite surface or edge if the pocket of pus is lax.

Composition The abscess feels firm and rubbery, and if there is sufficient pus present it will **fluctuate**. This latter sign cannot be elicited if the abscess is small and deep to the sternomastoid muscle.

The subcutaneous part of a collar-stud abscess should be clearly fluctuant, but it is not usually possible to reduce the superficial pocket of pus into the deep pocket.

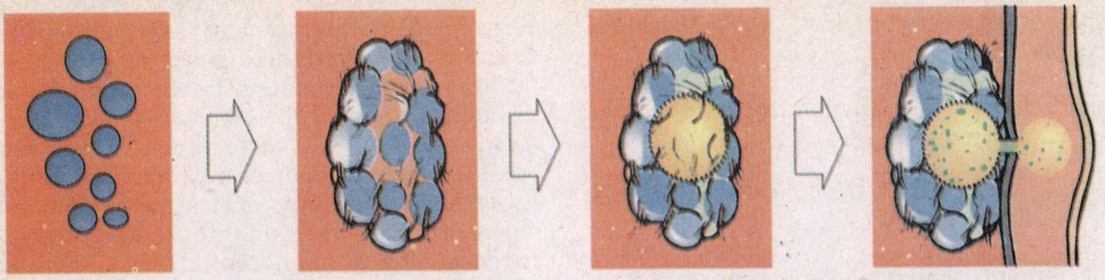

Enlarged discrete glands

'Matted' glands

Abscess forms in the centre of the glands

Abscess bursts through the deep fascia and becomes 'collar stud' in shape

The development of a 'collar-stud' abscess

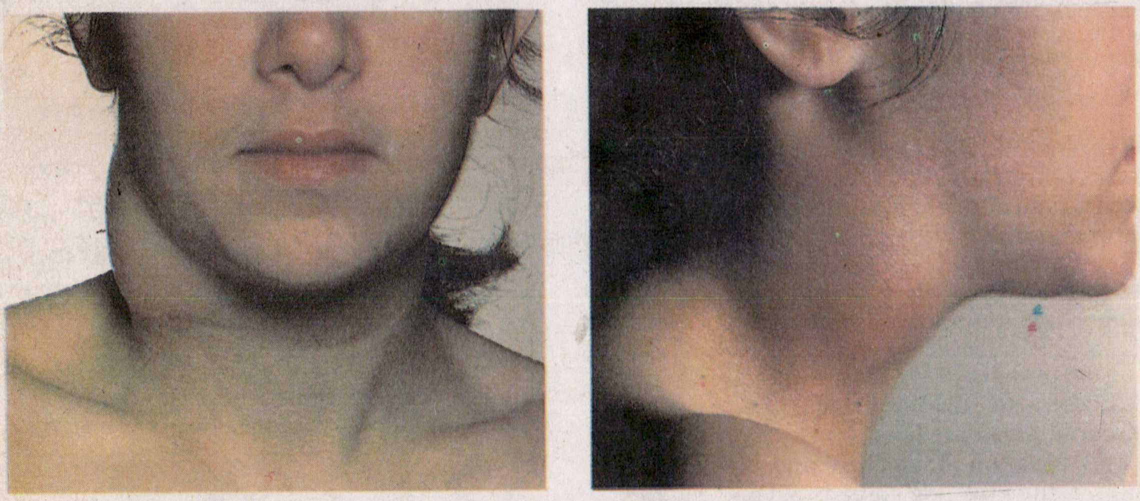

A large tuberculous 'collar-stud' abscess

FIG. 11.5 THE TUBERCULOUS ABCESS

Relations The original abscess is deep to the deep fascia, partly under the sternomastoid muscle, and fixed to surrounding structures. The superficial part of a collar-stud abscess is immediately below the skin and becomes more prominent when the sternomastoid muscle is contracted.

The other lymph nodes in the neck near the abscess may be enlarged.

GENERAL EXAMINATION

When the patient has tuberculous lymphadenitis there are often no systemic abnormalities; but when a tuberculous abscess develops there may be tachycardia, pyrexia, anorexia and general malaise.

There may be signs of tuberculosis in the lungs, in other lymph nodes and in the urinary tract.

Carcinomatous lymph nodes

Metastatic deposits of cancer cells in the cervical lymph nodes are the commonest cause of cervical lymphadenopathy in adults.

The primary cancer is most often in the buccal cavity (tongue, lips and mucous membrane) and larynx, but every possible primary site must be examined when cervical nodes are thought to be enlarged by secondary deposits.

HISTORY

Age Most head and neck cancers occur in patients over the age of 50. The commonest age of patients presenting with metastatic deposits in their cervical lymph nodes is between 55 and 65 years.

The exception is papillary carcinoma of the thyroid, which occurs **in children and young adults**.

Sex Most of the head and neck cancers are more common in men than women.

Local symptoms The patient complains of a **painless lump** in the neck, which he has seen or felt by chance.

It is uncommon for carcinomatous nodes to be tender or to become so large that they interfere with neck movements before being noticed.

The lump **grows slowly**, and **new lumps may appear**.

General symptoms The patient may have symptoms from a primary lesion in the head or neck, such as a sore tongue or a hoarse voice. If the primary is in the chest he may have a cough, or haemoptysis; if it is in the abdomen he may have dyspepsia or abdominal pain.

Generally speaking, head and neck cancers do not cause anorexia and weight loss, whereas cancers in the lungs and abdomen do.

LOCAL EXAMINATION

Site The site of the affected nodes gives a crude indication of the site of the primary. Lesions above the hyoid bone drain to the upper deep cervical nodes. The larynx and thyroid drain to the middle and lower deep cervical nodes. An enlarged supraclavicular lymph node commonly indicates intra-abdominal or thoracic disease. When enlarged by metastases this node is called **Virchow's node**; its presence is **Troisier's sign**.

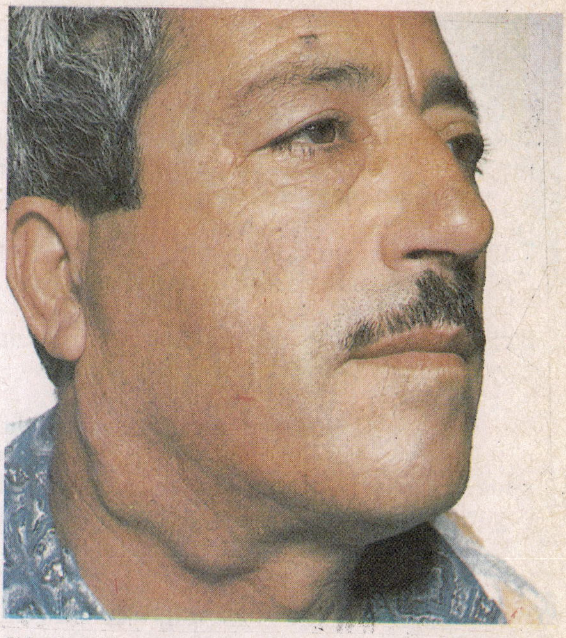

FIG. 11.6 This patient presented with hard, enlarged lymph glands in the neck. The primary lesion was the insignificant mole above his right eyebrow

Colour The overlying skin is a normal colour unless the mass is so large that it stretches or infiltrates the skin. This makes the skin pale or a blotchy red.

Temperature The skin temperature will be normal unless the tumour is very vascular.

Tenderness Nodes containing secondary deposits are **not tender**.

Shape and size Nodes containing metastases vary in size and shape. Both features depend upon the amount of tumour within them and the rate of its growth. At first the nodes are **smooth, discrete** and a **variety of sizes**. As they grow they may coalesce into one large mass.

Composition Nodes containing tumour are **hard**, often stony hard. Rarely, a very vascular tumour deposit will be soft, pulsatile and compressible.

Relations The nodes are tethered to the surrounding structures, so they can usually be moved in a transverse direction, but not vertically.

Their relation to the sternomastoid muscle varies according to the group to which they belong. Secondary cancer is more common in the nodes of the anterior than the posterior triangle. These nodes are deep to the anterior edge of the sternomastoid.

If the tumour spreads beyond the capsules of the glands the mass becomes completely fixed.

Local tissues The overlying skin and muscle may be infiltrated with tumour.

Lymph drainage Other lymph nodes on the pathway between the primary lesion and the node complained of by the patient, and beyond it, may be enlarged.

GENERAL EXAMINATION

Examine all the sites which might contain the primary lesion, in particular:

- The skin of the scalp, the ear and the external auditory meatus.
- The lips, tongue, buccal mucous membrane and tonsils.
- The nose, maxillary antra and nasopharynx.
- The thyroid gland.
- The skin of the upper limb.
- The breasts.
- The lungs.
- The stomach, pancreas, ovaries and testes.

Revision Panel 11.2

Plan of examination for source of secondary cervical lymphadenopathy

(Start at the top and work downwards.)

Examine the *skin* of the scalp, face, ears and neck.

Look in the *nose*.

Look in the *mouth* at the tongue, gums, mucosa and tonsils.

Palpate the parotid, submandibular and thyroid glands.

Examine the arms and the chest wall – including the breast.

Examine the abdomen and genitalia.

Transilluminate the air sinsuses.

Examine the nasopharynx and larynx with mirrors.

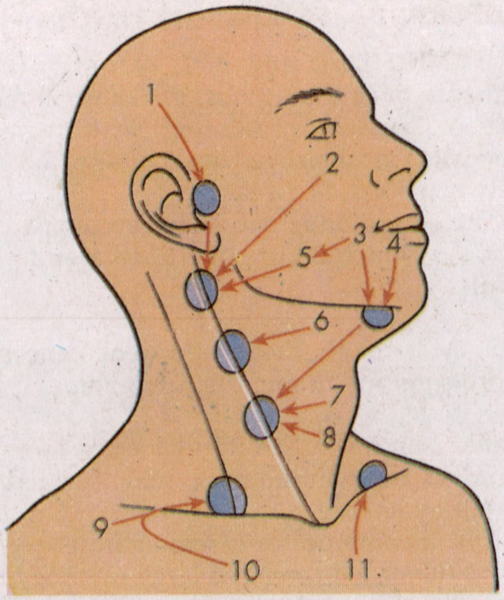

1 Scalp (sometimes via the preauricular node)
Parotid gland
Upper face
Ear
2 Maxillary antrum and other air sinuses
Nasal cavity and nasopharynx
3 Tongue
Buccal mucosa
Floor of mouth
Mandible
4 Lips
5 Tonsil
Base of tongue
Oropharynx
6 Submandibular gland
Skin of neck
7 Larynx and laryngopharynx
8 Thyroid
Upper oesophagus
9 Upper limb and both sides of the chest wall
10 Breast
11 Lungs, stomach and all the viscera

FIG. 11.7 Sites of primary neoplasms that metastasize to the cervical lymph nodes

The symptoms and signs of these organs are discussed in the appropriate chapters.

Some of this examination requires special instruments; for example, a head mirror and light and a laryngeal mirror.

Primary neoplasms of the lymph nodes

(Reticuloses, lymphoma)

The most common primary tumour of lymphoid tissue is the malignant lymphoma. There are many histological varieties of lymphoma, but they are often collectively and loosely divided into **Hodgkin's** and **non-Hodgkin's lymphoma**.

HISTORY

Age The reticuloses are common in children and young adults.

Sex Males are affected more than females.

Symptoms The most common presenting symptom is a **painless lump** in the neck, which is noticed by chance and grows slowly.

Malaise, weight loss and **pallor** are common symptoms.

Itching of the skin (pruritus) is an unexplained but distinctive complaint.

There may be **fever with rigors**, occurring in a periodic fashion (Pel–Ebstein fever).

Lymphomatous infiltration of the skeleton may cause **pains in the bones**, and there may be **abdominal pain after drinking alcohol**.

If there are large masses of lymph nodes in the mediastinum they may occlude the superior vena cava, causing **venous congestion in the neck** and the development of collateral veins across the chest wall.

Large masses in the abdomen can obstruct the inferior vena cava and cause oedema of both legs.

LOCAL EXAMINATION

Site Any of the cervical lymph nodes can be affected. Lymphoma is one of the few conditions, apart from infection, that often causes lymphadenopathy in the **posterior triangle**.

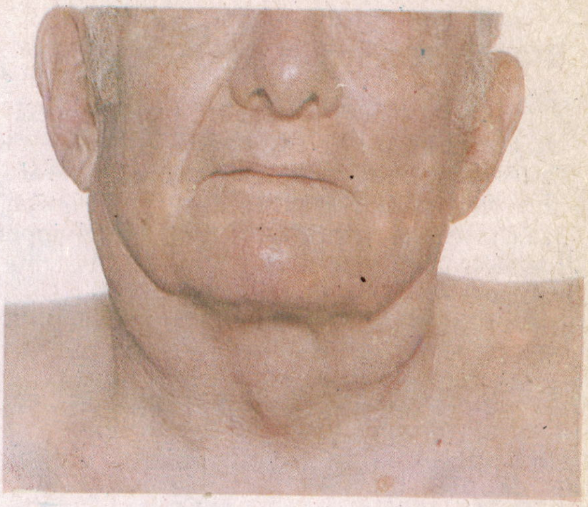

FIG. 11.8 Bilateral cervical lymphadenopathy caused by Hodgkin's lymphoma

Tenderness The nodes are **not tender**.

Shape, size and surface Hodgkin's lymph nodes are ovoid, **smooth** and **discrete**.

It is possible to define individual nodes even when they become large. This is the opposite to tuberculosis, in which the lymph nodes become matted and indistinct.

Consistence Nodes infiltrated by lymphoma are solid and **rubbery** in consistence.

Relations Although tethered to nearby structures, these nodes can usually be moved from side to side and rarely become completely fixed.

Local tissues The surrounding tissues should be normal.

GENERAL EXAMINATION

Other groups of lymph nodes may be enlarged. **The liver and spleen** may be palpable. The patient is often **anaemic** and may be **jaundiced**.

Spread to the skin produces elevated, reddened, scaly patches of skin known as **mycosis fungoides**.

Branchial cyst

A branchial cyst is a remnant of a branchial cleft, usually the second cleft. It is therefore lined with squamous epithelium, but there are also patches of lymphoid tissue in the wall which are connected with the other lymph tissue in the neck and which can become infected.

HISTORY

Age Although these cysts are present at birth they may not distend and cause symptoms until adult life. The majority present between the ages of 15 and 25 years, but a number appear in the 40s and 50s.

Sex Males and females are equally affected.

Symptoms The common presenting complaint is a **painless swelling** in the upper lateral part of the neck.

The lump may be painful when it first appears and later cause attacks of pain associated with an increase in the size of the swelling. The pain is usually caused by infection in the lymphoid tissue in the cyst wall.

A severe throbbing pain, exacerbated by moving the neck and opening the mouth, develops if the contents of the cyst become infected and purulent.

General effects These cysts have no systemic effects and are not associated with any other congenital abnormality.

EXAMINATION

Position A branchial cyst lies behind the anterior edge of the upper third of the sternomastoid muscle, and bulges forwards. Very rarely the cyst can bulge backwards behind the muscle.

Colour and tenderness The overlying skin may be reddened and the lump may be tender if the cyst is inflamed.

Shape The cyst is usually ovoid, with its long axis running forwards and downwards.

Size Most branchial cysts are between 5 and 10 cm long.

Surface Their surface is smooth and the edge distinct.

Composition The consistence varies with the tension of the cyst. Most cysts are hard, but a lax cyst feels soft. They are dull to percussion.

The lump **fluctuates**. This sign is not always easy to elicit, especially if the cyst is small and the sternomastoid muscle thick.

The lump is usually **opaque** because it contains desquamated epithelial cells that make its contents thick and white. Sometimes the fluid is golden yellow and shimmers with fat

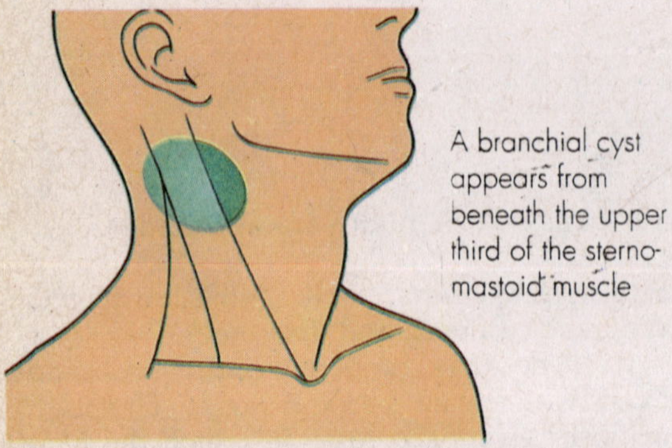

FIG. 11.9 The site of a branchial cyst

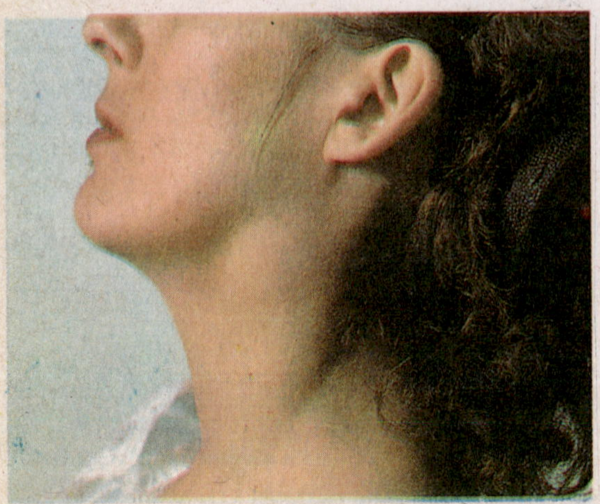

FIG. 11.10 A branchial cyst which presented in adult life. The back of the swelling is clearly deep to the sternomastoid muscle

globules and cholesterol crystals secreted by the sebaceous glands in the epithelial lining. Such cysts may transilluminate.

The cyst cannot be reduced or compressed.

Relations It is important to ascertain that the bulk of the mass is deep to the upper part of the sternomastoid muscle. It is not very mobile because it is closely tethered to the surrounding structures.

Lymph drainage The local deep cervical lymph nodes should not be enlarged. If they are palpable you should reconsider your diagnosis in favour of a tuberculous abscess rather than a branchial cyst.

Local tissues The local tissues should be normal.

If the cyst has turned into an abscess the surrounding tissues will be oedematous and the skin hot and red.

Branchial fistula (or sinus)

This is a rare congenital abnormality. It is the remnant of a branchial cleft, usually the second cleft, which has not closed off.

The patient complains of a small dimple, in the skin at the junction of the middle and lower third of the anterior edge of the sternomastoid muscle, that discharges clear mucus, and sometimes becomes swollen and painful and discharges pus.

When the whole branchial cleft stays patent, the fistula connects the skin with the oropharynx, just behind the tonsil. In most cases the upper end is obliterated and the track should really be called a **branchial sinus**.

Swallowing accentuates the openings on the skin.

Carotid body tumour

This is a rare tumour of the chemoreceptor tissue in the carotid body. It is therefore a chemodectoma. It is usually benign but can become quite large and occasionally becomes malignant.

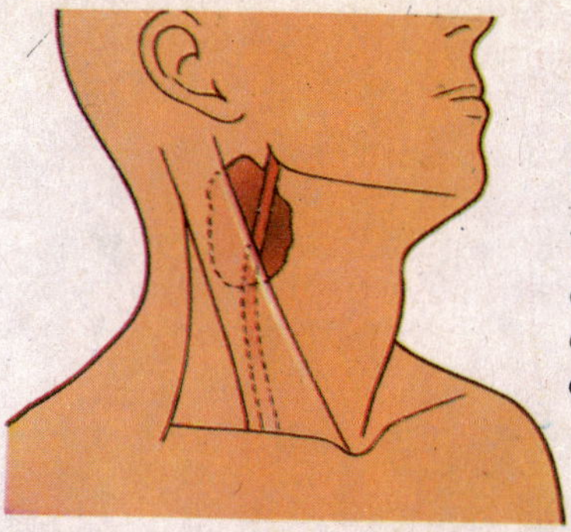

FIG. 11.11 The site of a carotid body tumour

HISTORY

Age Chemodectomas commonly appear in patients between the ages of 40 and 60 years.

Symptoms The common presentation is **a painless, slowly growing lump**. The patient may notice that the lump pulsates, and he may also suffer from symptoms of **transient cerebral ischaemia** (blackouts, transient paralysis or paraesthesia). These symptoms are unusual because the increasing compression of the carotid artery by the tumour is a very slow process.

Development The lump grows so slowly that many patients ignore it for many years.

Multiplicity Carotid body tumours may be bilateral.

EXAMINATION

Always be especially gentle when palpating a lump close to the bifurcation of the carotid artery. Pressure in this area can induce a vasovagal attack.

Position The carotid bifurcation is at, or just below, the level of the hyoid bone. Carotid body tumours are therefore found in the upper part of the anterior triangle of the neck, level with the hyoid bone and beneath the anterior edge of the sternomastoid muscle.

Tenderness, colour and temperature These tumours are not tender or hot, and the overlying skin should be normal.

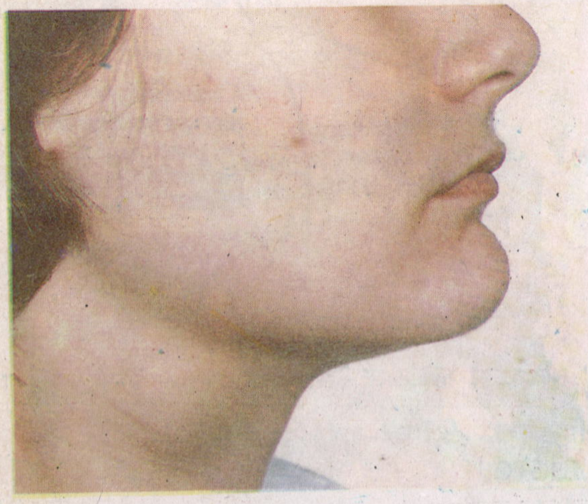

Note that the visible mass is lower than that of a branchial cyst (Fig. 11.10) but indistinguishable on inspection from an enlarged cervical lymph gland. Most carotid body tumours are initially mistaken for enlarged lymph nodes

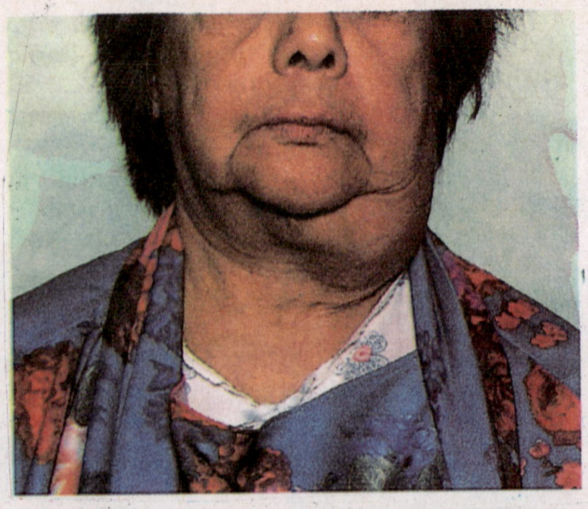

A very large, firm, bosselated carotid body tumour – hence the term 'potato tumour'

FIG. 11.12 TWO CAROTID BODY TUMOURS

Shape The lump is initially spherical but as it grows it becomes irregular in shape, often narrower at its lower end, where it is caught between the bifurcation of the common carotid artery.

Size Carotid body tumours may vary from 2–3 cm to 10 cm in diameter.

Composition The majority of these tumours are solid and hard. They are dull to percussion and do not fluctuate. They are often called **potato tumours** because of their consistence and shape.

Sometimes these tumours **pulsate**. This is either a transmitted pulsation from the adjacent carotid arteries, or a palpable external carotid artery running over the superficial aspect of the lump, or a true expansile pulsation from a soft, or very vascular tumour.

It is surprising that in spite of their vascularity most of these tumours are hard. Those which are soft and very vascular not only have an expansile pulsation, but can also be **compressed**.

Relations The lump is deep to the cervical fascia and beneath the anterior edge of the sternomastoid muscle.

The common carotid artery can be felt below the mass, and the external carotid artery may pass over its superficial surface. Without this close relationship to the arteries this tumour is indistinguishable from an enlarged lymph node.

Because of their intimate relationship with the carotid arteries these tumours can be moved from side to side but not up and down.

Cystic hygromata

(Lymph cysts, lymphangiomata)

A cystic hygroma is a collection of lymphatic sacs which contain clear colourless lymph. They are congenital and are probably a cluster of lymph channels that failed to connect into the normal lymphatic pathways. Lymph cysts commonly occur near the root of the arm and the leg (i.e. in the anatomical junction between the limbs and head and the trunk).

HISTORY

Age The majority of cystic hygromata present at birth or within the first few years of life, but they occasionally stay empty until

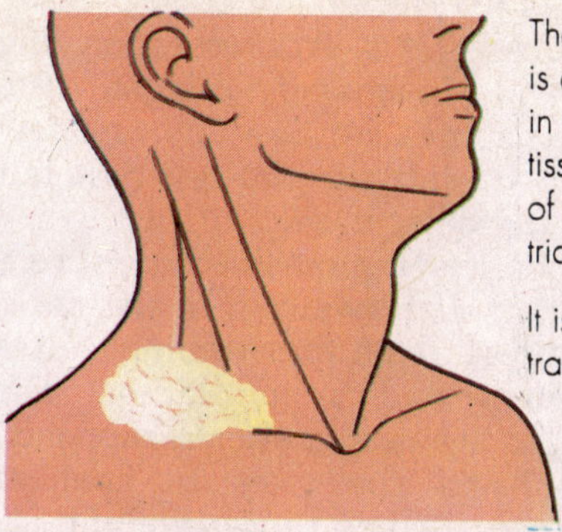

FIG. 11.13 The site of a cystic hygroma

infection or trauma in adult life causes them to fill up and become visible.

Symptoms The only symptom is the complaint about the **lump**, but the child's parents are usually more concerned about the **disfigurement** caused by the cyst.

Family history This condition is not familial.

EXAMINATION

Position Cystic hygromata are commonly found at the base of the neck, in the posterior triangle, but they can be very big and occupy the whole of the subcutaneous tissue of one side of the neck.

Temperature and tenderness They are not hot or tender, and the overlying skin is normal.

Shape A cystic hygroma is a mixture of soft uni- and multilocular cysts, so the whole mass looks **lobulated and flattened.**

Size The small cysts are a few centimetres across. Large cysts can extend over the whole of one side of the neck.

Surface If the cysts are close to the skin it may not be possible to feel a distinct surface. Deep cysts feel smooth, but because they are lax their edges are often indistinct.

Composition Cystic hygromata are soft and dull to percussion. They **fluctuate** easily but, because they are close to the skin and contain clear fluid, their distinctive physical sign is a **brilliant translucence.**

Large cysts will conduct a **fluid thrill**, and in some multilocular swellings the fluid in one loculus can be **compressed** into another.

They cannot be reduced.

Relations Cystic hygromata develop in the **subcutaneous tissues**. Thus they are superficial to the neck muscles and close to the skin but are rarely fixed to the skin. However, it is essential to perform a thorough examination of the oropharynx as a cyst in the posterior triangle may extend deeply beneath the sternomastoid muscle into the retropharyngeal space.

Lymph nodes The local lymph nodes should not be enlarged and, as the lymph drainage of

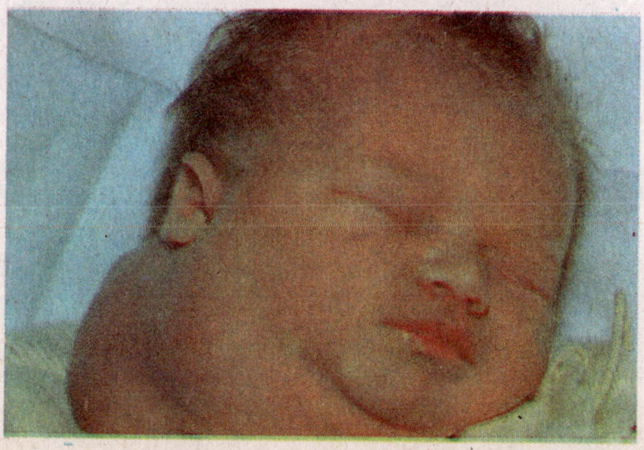

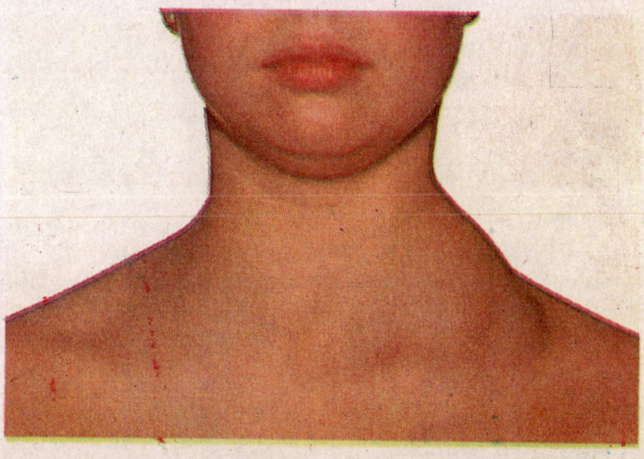

FIG. 11.14 Two examples of cystic hygroma: one in a very young child – the common age of presentation – and the other which presented in adult life

the tissues around the cyst is normal, there is no lymphoedema.

Local tissues The local tissues are normal.

Pharyngeal pouch

A pharyngeal pouch is a pulsion diverticulum of the pharynx through the gap between the lowermost horizontal fibres and the higher oblique fibres of the inferior constrictor muscle. If swallowing is uncoordinated so that the lower sphincter-like fibres of the inferior constrictor do not relax, the weak unsupported area just above these fibres (known as Killian's dehiscence) bulges out. Eventually the bulge grows into a sac which hangs down and presses against the side of the oesophagus.

HISTORY

Age Pharyngeal pouches appear in middle and old age.

Sex They are more common in men.

Symptoms The patient often has a long history of halitosis and recurrent sore throats before noticing the common presenting symptom of **regurgitation of food**. The regurgitated food is undigested and comes up into the mouth at any time. There is no bile or acid taste to it.

Regurgitation at night causes **bouts of coughing and choking,** and if pieces of food are inhaled a **lung abscess** may develop.

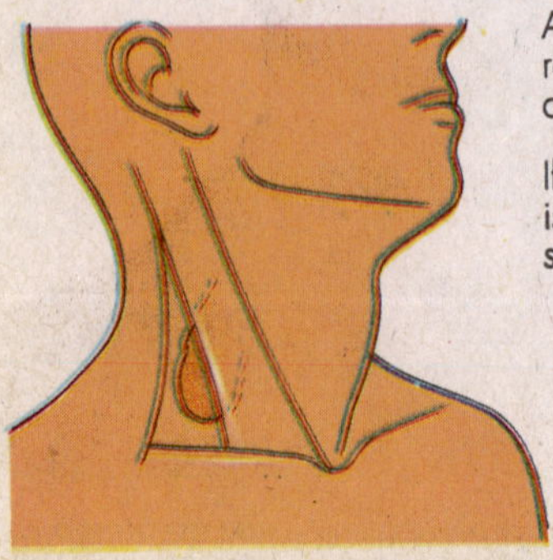

FIG. 11.15 The site of a pharyngeal pouch

As the pouch grows it presses on the oesophagus and causes **dysphagia.** The patient can sometimes swallow his first few mouthfuls of food (until the pouch is full), but thereafter has difficulty in swallowing.

By the time these symptoms become severe he may have noticed a **swelling in the neck,** and find that pressure on the swelling causes **gurgling sounds** and regurgitation. The swelling changes in size and often disappears.

If the dysphagia continues the patient becomes **malnourished** and **loses weight.**

EXAMINATION

Position The swelling caused by a pharyngeal pouch appears **behind the sternomastoid muscle**, below the level of the thyroid cartilage.

Shape Its shape is indistinct because only part of its surface is palpable. It feels like a bulging deep structure.

Size Most pouches only cause a swelling of 5–10 cm diameter. The pouch is not palpable when it is smaller, so **many patients have symptoms but no abnormal physical signs.**

Surface and edge The surface is smooth, but the edge is not palpable.

Composition The lump is **soft** and sometimes **indentable.** It is dull to percussion and does not fluctuate or transilluminate.

It can be **compressed** and sometimes **emptied.** Compression may cause regurgitation. Although the mass may disappear with compression, not to return until the patient eats again, it cannot be said to have been reduced in the usual meaning of the word.

Relations A pharyngeal pouch lies deep to the deep fascia, behind the sternomastoid muscle, and is fixed deeply. Its origin from a structure behind the trachea can be appreciated during palpation but the neck of the pouch and its attachment to the oesophagus cannot be felt.

It cannot be moved about in the neck.

Lymph nodes The cervical lymph nodes should not be enlarged.

Local tissues The surrounding tissues feel normal. Indeed, when the pouch is empty the whole neck feels normal.

GENERAL EXAMINATION

Pay special attention to the chest as there may be an aspiration pneumonia, collapse of a lobe or a lung abscess.

Sternomastoid 'tumour'

(Ischaemic contracture of a segment of the sternomastoid muscle)

This is a swelling of the middle third of the sternomastoid muscle. In neonates it consists of oedema around an infarcted segment of the muscle, caused by the trauma of birth. As the patient grows, the lump disappears and the abnormal segment of muscle becomes fibrotic and contracted.

HISTORY

Age The lump is noticed at birth or in the first few weeks of life.

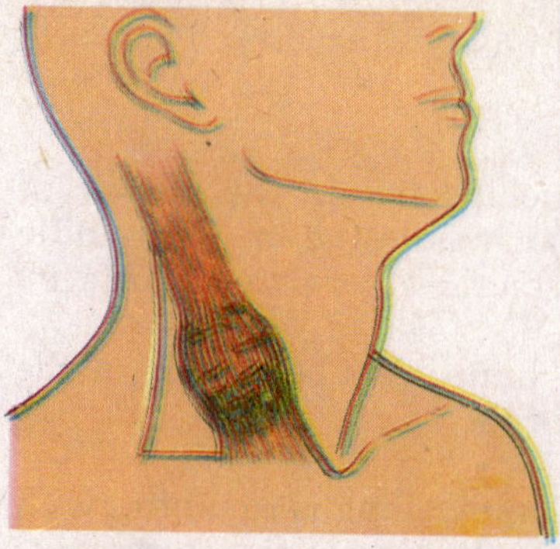

A 'sternomastoid tumour' is an area of oedema and necrosis in the lower third of the sternomastoid muscle

FIG. 11.16 The site of a sternomastoid tumour

Symptoms The mother may notice **the lump** or that the child keeps his head turned to one side – **torticollis**. Attempts to turn the head straight may cause **pain or distress**.

If the muscle is not extensively damaged the swelling slowly subsides, the muscle spasm relaxes and the torticollis disappears. If the muscle damage becomes an area of permanent fibrosis the twist and tilt of the head to one side becomes more noticeable as the child grows.

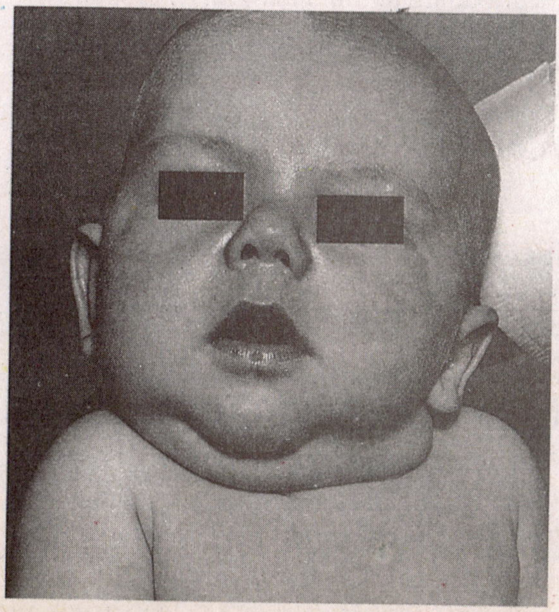

This baby's torticollis is caused by ischaemia of the sternomastoid muscle

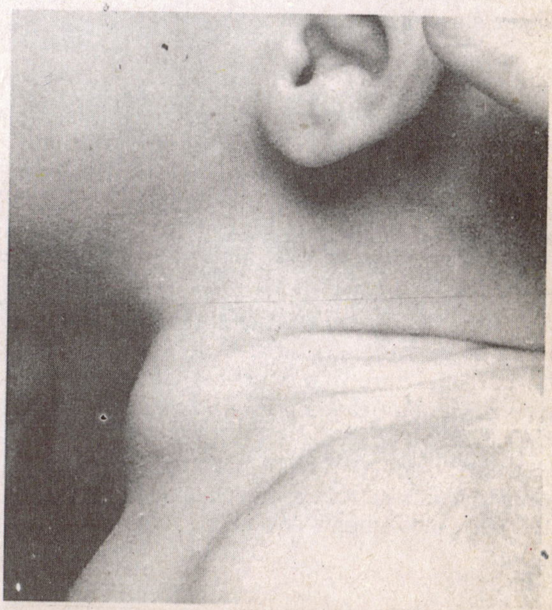

A localized, swollen, segment of sternomastoid muscle with a slight torticollis, in an older child, caused by ischaemia and fibrosis of the muscle after birth. A typical sternomastoid 'tumour'

FIG. 11.17 TORTICOLLIS

EXAMINATION

The lump

Position The swelling lies in the middle of the sternomastoid muscle (i.e. in the middle third of the neck on the anterolateral surface).

Tenderness The lump may be tender in the first few weeks of life.

Shape and size The swelling is fusiform, with its long axis along the line of the sternomastoid muscle. It is usually 1–2 cm across.

Surface The surface is smooth.

Edge The anterior and posterior edges of the lump are distinct but the superior and inferior edges, where the lump becomes continuous with normal muscle, are indistinct.

Composition At first the lump is firm and solid and easy to feel, but as it gradually becomes harder it begins to shrink and may become impalpable.

Surrounding structures and local lymph nodes These should be normal.

The neck

Examine the movements of the neck. As the child is too young to obey commands, you must watch how he moves his head when lying in his cot, and then manipulate the head and neck very gently.

The sternomastoid muscles rotate and tilt the head. Contraction of the left sternomastoid **turns the head towards the right,** but **tilts the head to the left.** Both these deformities may be present. Forced movement to correct the deformity may cause pain and be resisted by the child.

Apart from the restriction of movement caused by spasm of the sternomastoid muscle, the neck movements should be normal.

The eyes

Look at the eyes and watch their movements to detect any **squint**. Torticollis can be a means of correcting a squint. Move the head into a vertical and central position and watch the eyes. If the torticollis is secondary to a squint and not a sternomastoid tumour, the squint will appear as the head is straightened.

The head

An uncorrected torticollis may affect the growth of the facial bones and cause facial asymmetry.

Cervical rib

Although the cervical rib can cause serious neurological and vascular symptoms in the upper arm, clinical examination of the neck usually reveals no abnormalities. The abnormal rib is usually detected with an x-ray. Sometimes there is a fullness at the root of the neck but it is rarely distinct enough to justify a firm clinical diagnosis of cervical rib.

The common neurological symptoms caused by a cervical rib are pain in the C8 and T1 dermatomes, and wasting and weakness of the small muscles in the hand. Vascular symptoms such as Raynaud's phenomenon, trophic changes, even rest pain and gangrene, may occur but are uncommon.

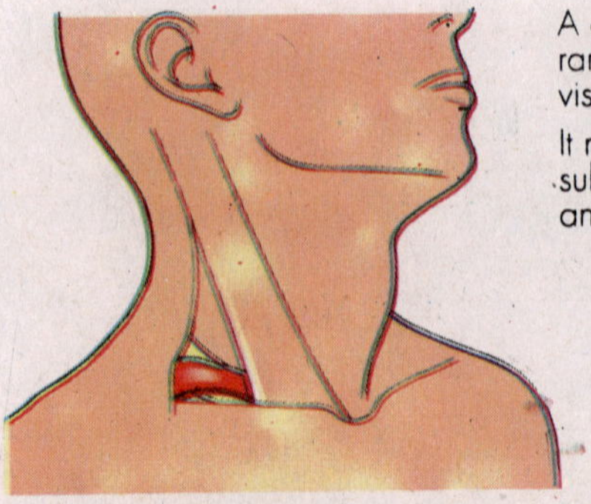

FIG. 11.18 The site of a cervical rib

Thyroglossal cyst

The thyroid gland develops from the lower portion of the thyroglossal duct, which begins at the foramen caecum at the base of the tongue. If a portion of this duct remains patent it can form a thyroglossal cyst.

Theoretically, thyroglossal cysts can occur anywhere between the base of the tongue and the isthmus of the thyroid gland, but they are commonly found in two sites: between the isthmus of the thyroid gland and the hyoid bone, and just above the hyoid bone. Thyroglossal cysts within the tongue and in the floor of the mouth are rare.

HISTORY

Age Thyroglossal cysts appear at any age, but the majority are seen in patients between 15 and 30 years old.

Sex They are more common in women than men.

Symptoms The commonest symptom is **a painless lump** in a prominent and noticeable part of the neck. **Pain, tenderness** and **an increase in size** occur only if the cyst becomes infected.

Duration of symptoms The lump may have been present for many years before the patient complains. In these circumstances it is usually an increase in size that changes the patient's attitude to her lump.

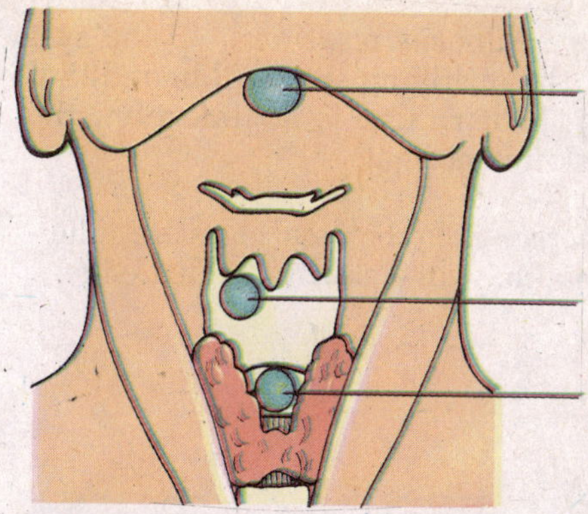

FIG. 11.19 The sites of a thyroglossal cyst

Systemic symptoms There are no systemic symptoms associated with this condition.

EXAMINATION

Position Thyroglossal cysts lie close to the mid-line, somewhere between the chin and second tracheal ring. In the fetus the thyroglossal duct is in the mid-line, but when a cyst forms in adult life it often slips to one side of the mid-line, especially if it develops in front of the thyroid cartilage.

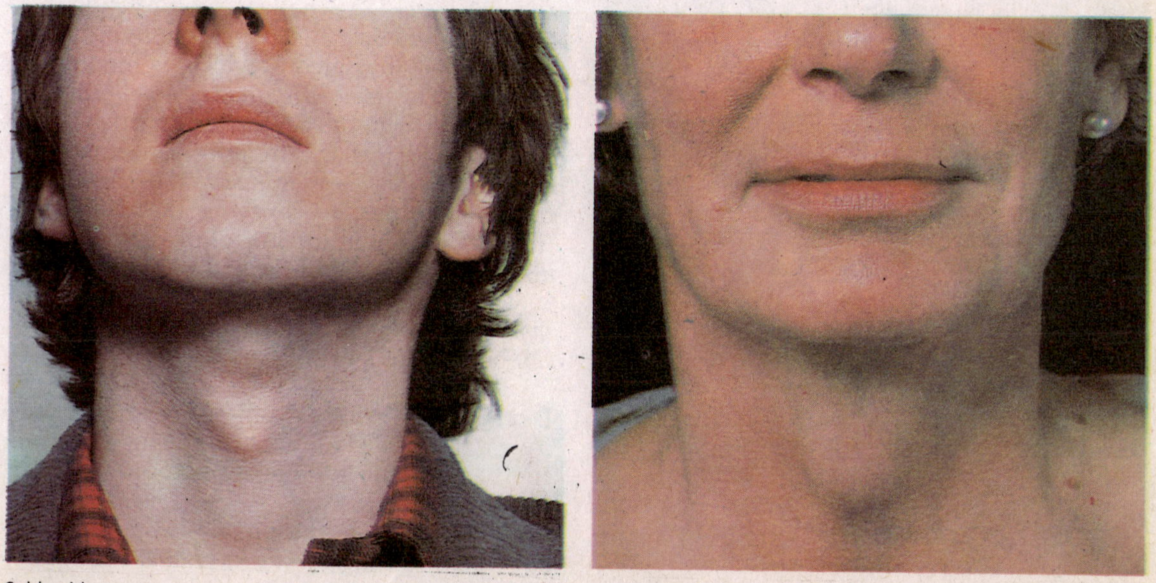

Subhyoid

Pretracheal

FIG. 11.20 TWO THYROGLOSSAL CYSTS

Colour, temperature and tenderness If the cyst is infected, the overlying skin will be red, hot and tender. When there is no infection, the overlying skin is normal.

Shape and surface Thyroglossal cysts are spherical and smooth, with a clearly defined edge.

Revision Panel 11.3

A scheme for the diagnosis of swellings in the neck

(Deep to the deep fascia)

After your examination you should be able to answer four critical questions: Is there one or more than one lump? Site? Solid or cystic? Does it move with swallowing?

Multiple lumps are invariably *lymph nodes*

A single lump:

In the anterior triangle that does not move with swallowing
- Solid:
  - A lymph node
  - Carotid body tumour
- Cystic:
  - Cold abscess
  - Branchial cyst

In the posterior triangle that does not move with swallowing
- Solid:
  - A lymph node
- Cystic:
  - Cystic hygroma
  - Pharyngeal pouch
- Pulsatile:
  - Subclavian aneurysm

In the anterior triangle that moves with swallowing
- Solid:
  - Thyroid gland
  - Thyroid isthmus lymph node
- Cystic:
  - Thyroglossal cyst

Size They vary from 0.5 to 5 cm in diameter. Because of the prominence of a lump in the front of the neck, patients often complain of these cysts when they are very small.

Composition Thyroglossal cysts have a firm or hard consistence, depending upon the tension within the cyst. Some cysts are too tense and others too small to fluctuate, but the majority of thyroglossal cysts are between these extremes and **fluctuate** with ease. Some cysts transilluminate but many do not, because the contents have become thickened by desquamated epithelial cells or the debris of past infection. Many cysts are too small to transilluminate.

Relations to nearby structures Thyroglossal cysts are tethered by the remnant of the thyroglossal duct. This means that they can be moved sideways, but not up and down.

The thyroglossal duct is always closely related, usually fixed, to the hyoid bone. When the hyoid bone moves the cyst also moves.

The hyoid bone moves upwards when the tongue is protruded. First, ask the patient to open her mouth and keep the lower jaw still, hold the cyst with your thumb and forefinger, and then ask the patient to protrude her tongue. If the cyst is fixed to the hyoid bone you will feel it **tugged** upwards as the tongue goes out. This is a difficult sign to elicit.

Do not expect to see much movement. It is far easier to feel the tugging sensation. Although this test is diagnostic, the absence of movement does not exclude the diagnosis. Indeed this sign is absent from most cysts that are below the level of the thyroid cartilage.

Lymph nodes The local lymph nodes should not be enlarged.

Local tissues Whenever there is an abnormality of thyroid gland development, **examine the base of the tongue** for ectopic (lingual) thyroid tissue.

A lingual thyroid looks like a flattened strawberry sitting on the base of the tongue.

Revision Panel 11.4

Physiology of the thyroid gland

Changes in hormone activity can be assessed by:

- Clinical examination
- Measuring circulating T3 and T4
- Measuring the rate and quantity of radioactive iodine taken up by the gland

Hormone secretion can be suppressed by:

- Iodine, which inhibits hormone release
- Potassium perchlorate, which interferes with iodine trapping
- Carbimazole and thiouracil, which inhibit the iodination of tyrosine and the coupling of tyrosines to make thyronines
- Destroying the gland surgically or with radiotherapy
- Giving thyroid hormones

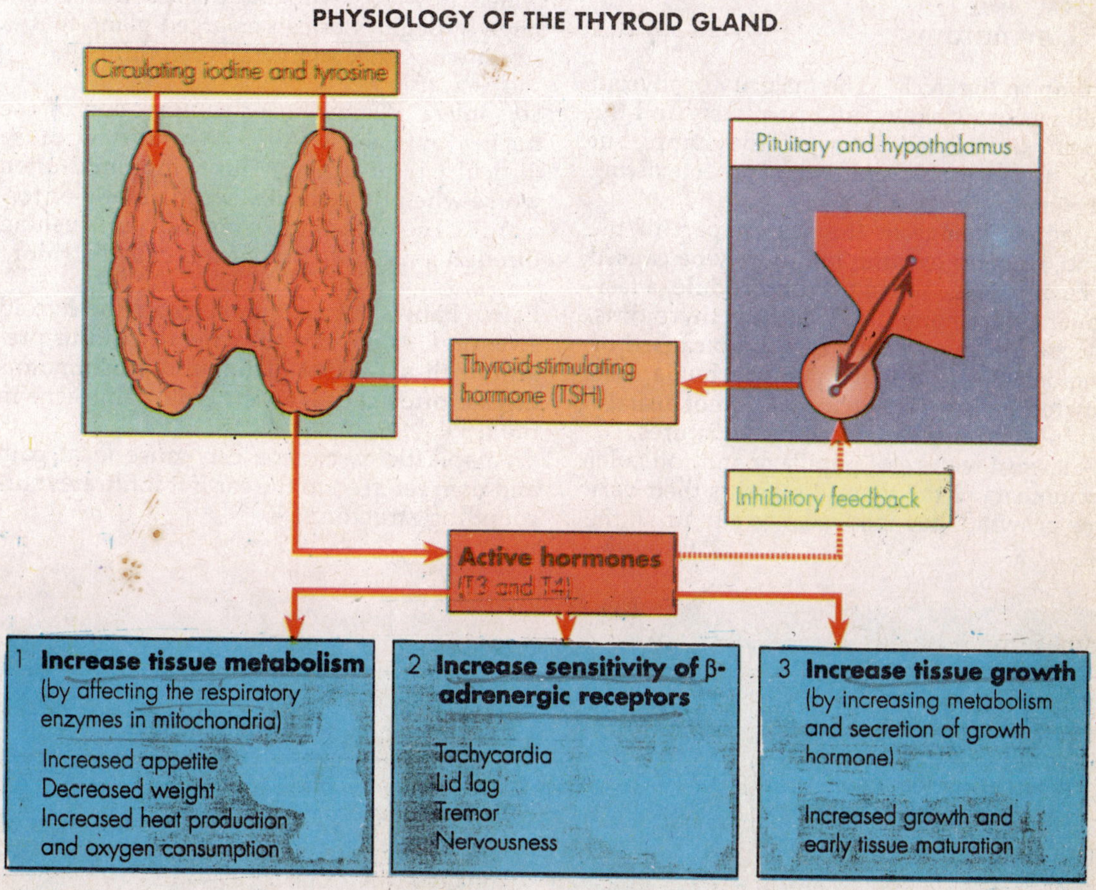

FIG. 11.21

The thyroid gland

SYMPTOMS OF THYROID DISEASE

The thyroid gland can cause two groups of symptoms: those connected with the swelling in the neck, and those related to the endocrine activity of the gland. The history and examination must detect local and general symptoms and signs.

Neck symptoms

A lump in the neck The majority of thyroid swellings grow slowly and painlessly and the patient simply complains of the lump; but some lumps appear suddenly, and an existing lump may enlarge quickly.

A rapid change in the size of part of the gland, or of an existing lump, may be caused by haemorrhage into a necrotic nodule, a fast-growing carcinoma, or subacute thyroiditis. The sudden enlargement of a lump caused by haemorrhage is usually painful, but a fast-growing anaplastic carcinoma is not usually painful until it invades nearby structures.

A special feature of papillary and follicular carcinomata of the thyroid gland is their very slow growth. They may exist as a lump in the neck for many years before metastasizing. Thus the age of a lump is no indication of its nature.

Discomfort during swallowing Large swellings give the patient a tugging sensation in the neck when she swallows. This is not true dysphagia. Thyroid swellings rarely obstruct the oesophagus because the oesophagus is a muscular tube which is easily stretched and pushed aside. However, because the thyroid has to be pulled upwards with the trachea in the first stage of deglutition, an enlarged gland makes swallowing uncomfortable, even difficult.

Dyspnoea Deviation or compression of the trachea by a mass in the thyroid may cause difficulty in breathing. This symptom is often worse when the neck is flexed laterally or forwards. The whistling sound of air rushing through a narrowed trachea is called **stridor**.

Pain Pain is not a common feature of thyroid swellings. Acute and subacute thyroiditis present with a painful gland, and Hashimoto's disease often causes an uncomfortable ache in the neck.

Anaplastic carcinoma can cause local pain and pain referred to the ear if it infiltrates surrounding structures.

Revision Panel 11.5

Plan for the examination of a patient with a goitre

Look at the whole patient for agitation, nervousness or lethargy.

Examine the hands for sweating, tremor, tachycardia.

Examine the eyes for exophthalmos, lid lag, ophthalmoplegia, chemosis.

Examine the neck. Always check that the lump moves with swallowing.

Palpate the cervical lymph nodes.

Revision Panel 11.6

The eye signs of thyrotoxicosis

Lid retraction and lid lag

Exophthalmos, which also causes difficulty with convergence and absent forehead wrinkling when looking upwards

Ophthalmoplegia, particularly of the superior rectus and inferior oblique muscles (cannot look 'up and out')

Chemosis

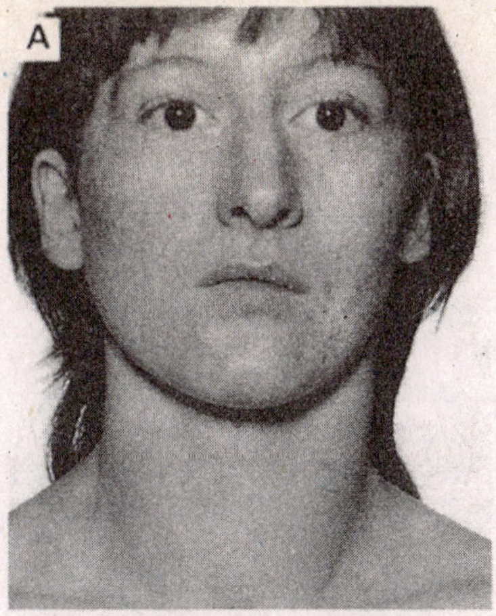

Look at the eyes and the neck

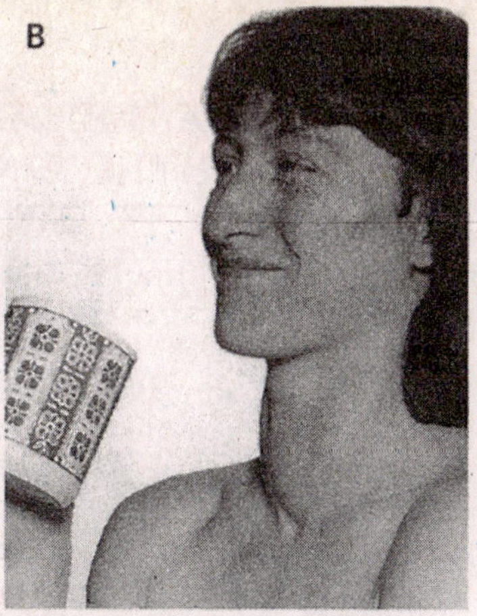

Ask the patient to swallow

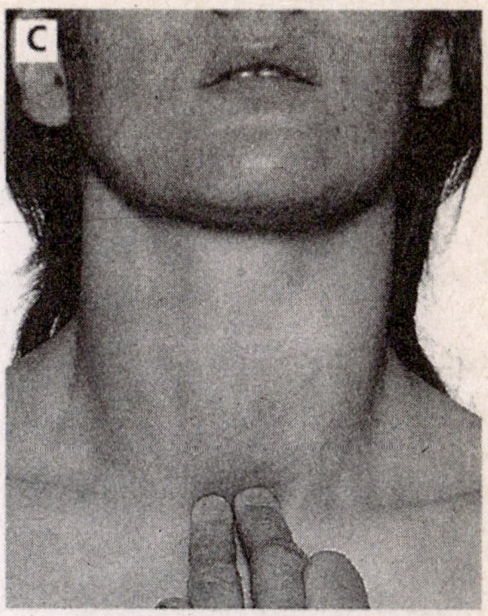

Feel the trachea

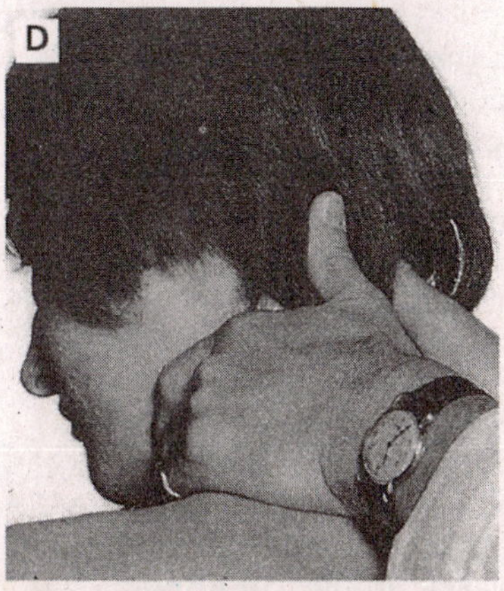

Palpate the neck from behind, with the thumbs pushing the head forwards to flex the neck slightly

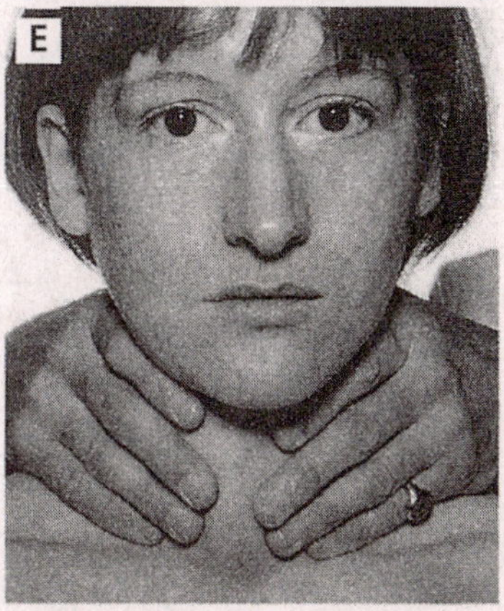

Palpate both lobes and the isthmus with the fingers straight and flat

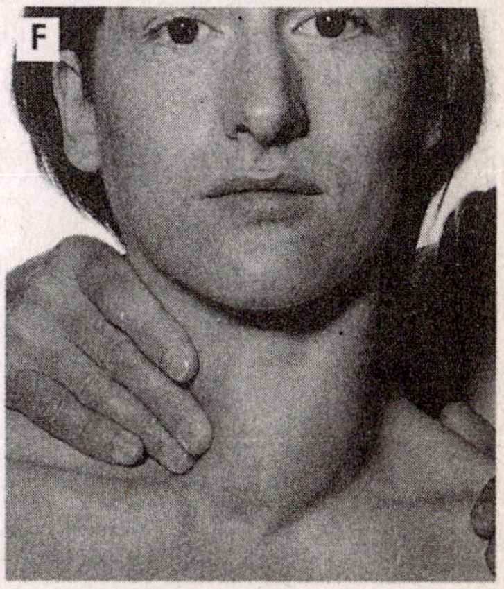

If one lobe is difficult to feel, make it more prominent by pressing firmly on the opposite side

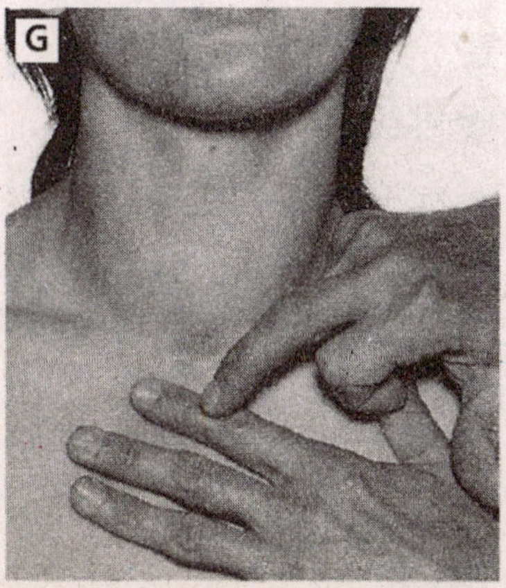

Percuss the lower limit of the gland

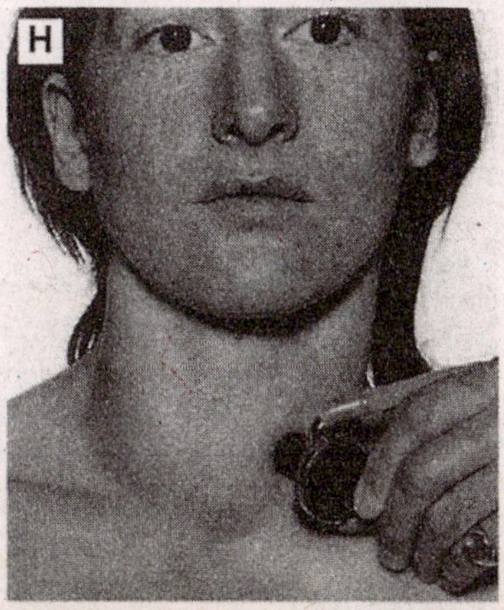

Listen over the lateral lobes for a systolic bruit

Try to decide if there is:

- one lump
- two lumps
- diffuse enlargement

FIG. 11.22 THE EXAMINATION OF THE THYROID GLAND

Hoarseness A change in the quality of the voice of a patient with a lump in the neck is a very significant symptom because it is probably caused by a paralysis of one recurrent laryngeal nerve, which means that the lump is likely to be an anaplastic carcinoma infiltrating the nerve.

Eye symptoms

The patient may complain of **staring or protruding eyes and difficulty in closing her eyelids** (exophthalmos), **double vision** caused by muscle weakness (ophthalmoplegia), and swelling of the conjunctiva (chemosis). She may get **pain** in the eye if the cornea ulcerates.

Symptoms of thyrotoxicosis

Nervous system Symptoms are **nervousness**, irritability, insomnia, nervous instability and **tremor** of the hands; occasionally a thyrotoxic psychosis.

Cardiovascular system Symptoms are **palpitations**, dyspnoea on exertion, swelling of the ankles and chest pain.

Metabolic and alimentary systems There is **an increase in appetite but loss of weight**, and sometimes a change of bowel habit, usually diarrhoea. Proximal muscle myopathies occur with **wasting** and **weakness**. The patient has **a preference for cold weather**, with excessive **sweating** and an intolerance of hot weather. Some women have a change of menstruation, usually **amenorrhoea**.

Symptoms of myxoedema

There is **an increase of weight**, with deposition of fat across the back of the neck and shoulders. Symptoms also include: **slow thought, speech and action; intolerance of cold weather; loss of hair**, especially the outer third of the eyebrows; **muscle fatigue**; a dry skin and 'peaches and cream' complexion; and constipation.

EXAMINATION OF THE THYROID GLAND

Although this should be part of the general examination, the method of examining the neck is described in detail because it is so important. The important features of the general and eye examination are also reiterated.

Concentrate upon the state of the gland and its endocrine activity. It is easiest to assess both aspects in a combined approach, rather than try to assess each separately.

Inspection

First confirm that the swelling in the neck is in the thyroid gland by watching to see **if it moves when the patient swallows**. Then **look at the whole patient**.

Is she sitting still and composed, or fidgeting about, constantly moving her fingers and looking nervous and agitated?

Is she thin or fat? Where is the wasting or the fattening? Patients with thyrotoxicosis have a generalized loss of weight, especially about the face, but may also get wasting of their hand, face and shoulder muscles.

Is she under-clothed and sweaty, or wrapped up in a large number of jumpers but still cold?

LOOK AT THE HANDS

Feel the pulse Tachycardia suggests thyrotoxicosis; bradycardia suggests myxoedema. In middle-aged and elderly patients thyrotoxicosis may cause atrial fibrillation.

Are the palms moist and sweaty?

Is there a tremor? Test for a tremor by asking the patient to hold her arms out in front of her, elbows and wrists straight, fingers straight and separated. Thyrotoxicosis causes a fine, fast tremor. If in doubt, hold out your own hand beside the patient's for comparison.

EXAMINE THE EYES

There are four important changes that can occur in the eyes in thyrotoxicosis. Each one may be unilateral or bilateral.

Lid retraction and lid lag This sign is caused by over-activity of the involuntary (smooth muscle) part of the levator palpebrae superioris muscle. If the upper eyelid is higher than normal and the lower lid is in its correct position, the patient has **lid retraction**. Do not be deceived into thinking this abnormality is due to exophthalmos.

When the upper lid does not keep pace with the eyeball as it follows a finger moving from above downwards, the patient has **lid lag**.

Exophthalmos If the eyeball is pushed forwards by an increase in retro-orbital fat, oedema and a cellular infiltration, the normal relationship of the eyelids to the iris is changed. Sclera becomes visible below the lower edge of the iris (the inferior limbus).

Because the eyes are pushed forwards the patient can **look up without wrinkling her forehead**, but will have **difficulty in converging**. In severe exophthalmos the patient cannot close her eyelids and may have a corneal ulcer.

Ophthalmoplegia Although exophthalmos stretches the eye muscles, it does not usually affect their function. The cause of the weakness of the ocular muscles associated with severe exophthalmos is oedema and cellular infiltration of the muscles themselves and the oculomotor nerves. The muscles most often affected are the superior and lateral rectus and inferior oblique muscles. Paralysis of these muscles prevents the patient looking upwards and outwards.

Chemosis Chemosis is oedema of the conjunctiva. The normal conjunctiva is smooth and invisible. A thickened, crinkled, oedematous and slightly opaque conjunctiva is easy to recognize.

Chemosis is caused by the obstruction of the normal venous and lymphatic drainage of the conjunctiva by the increased retro-orbital pressure.

INSPECT THE NECK

After checking that the lump is in the anatomical site of the thyroid gland, **ask the patient to swallow**. The patient may need a sip of water to help deglutition. **All thyroid swellings ascend during swallowing.**

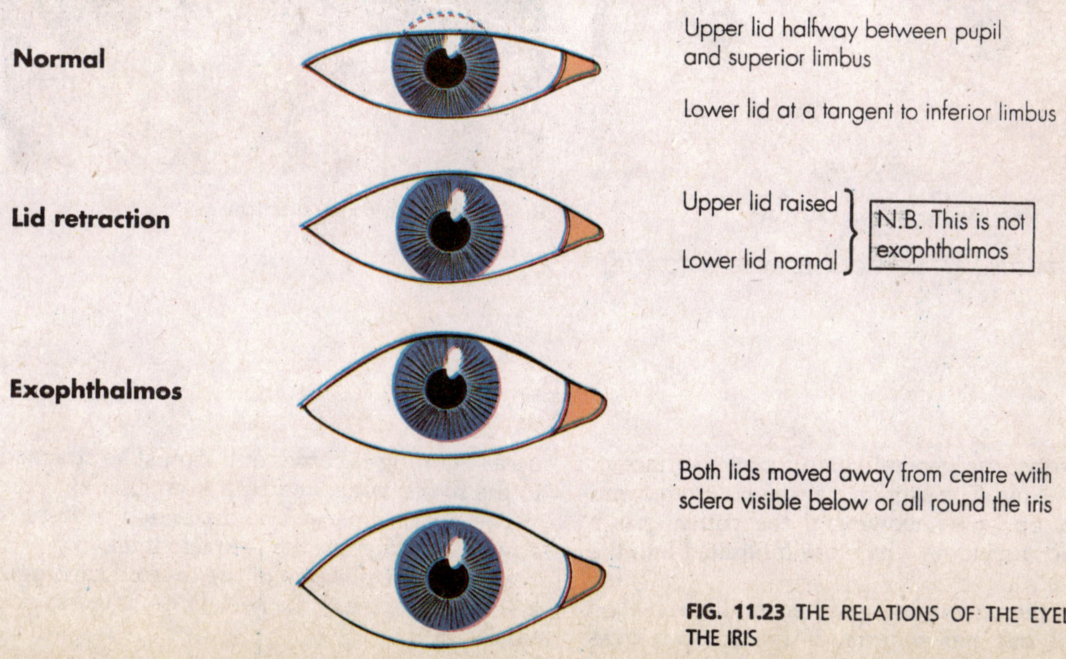

FIG. 11.23 THE RELATIONS OF THE EYELIDS TO THE IRIS

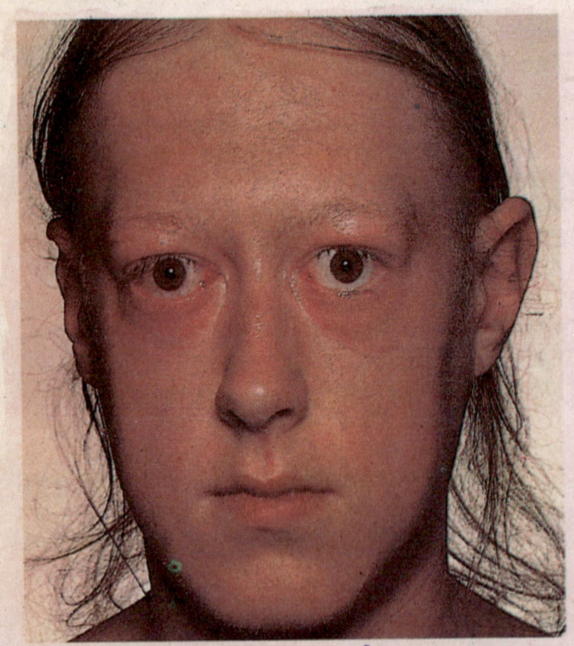

Exophthalmos ē lid retraction

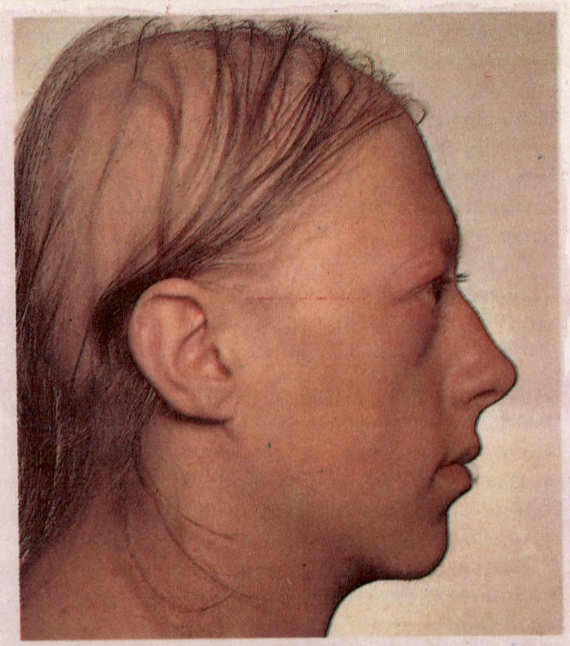

Note also the wasting and loss of hair

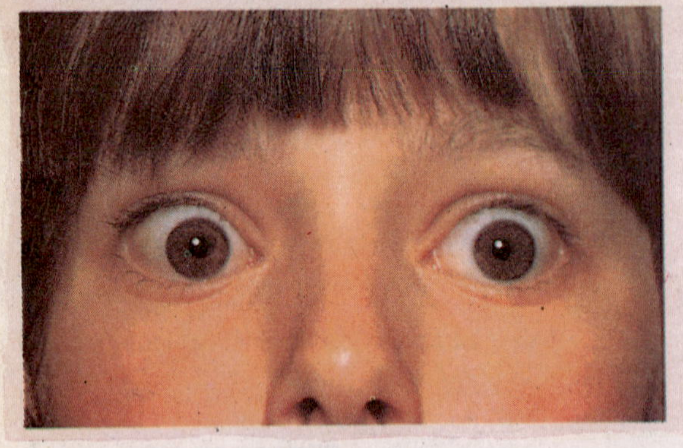

Severe lid retraction but no exophthalmos

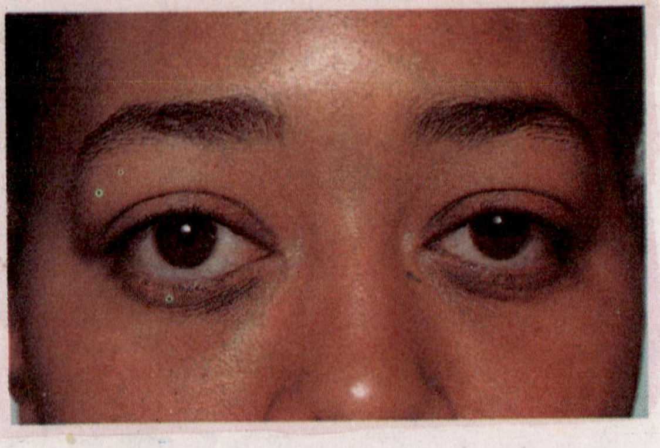

Exophthalmos but no lid retraction

FIG. 11.24 SOME EYE SIGNS CAUSED BY THYROTOXICOSIS

Observe the general contours and surface of the swelling. The skin may also be puckered and pulled up by swallowing if the patient has a thyroid carcinoma which has infiltrated into the skin.

Ask the patient to open her mouth and then to **put out her tongue**. If the lump moves up as her tongue comes out, it must be attached to the hyoid bone, and be a thyroglossal cyst.

The neck veins will be distended if there is a mass obstructing the thoracic inlet.

Look at the position of the thyroid cartilage. Is it in the centre of the neck or deviated to one side?

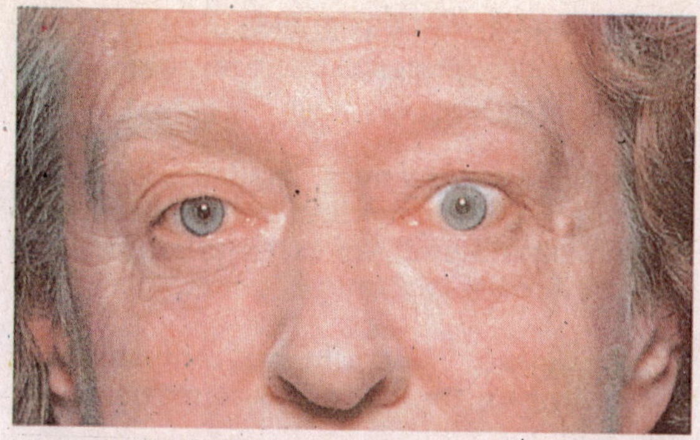

Unilateral lid retraction. Unilateral eye signs are usually due to generalized disease, i.e. thyrotoxicosis

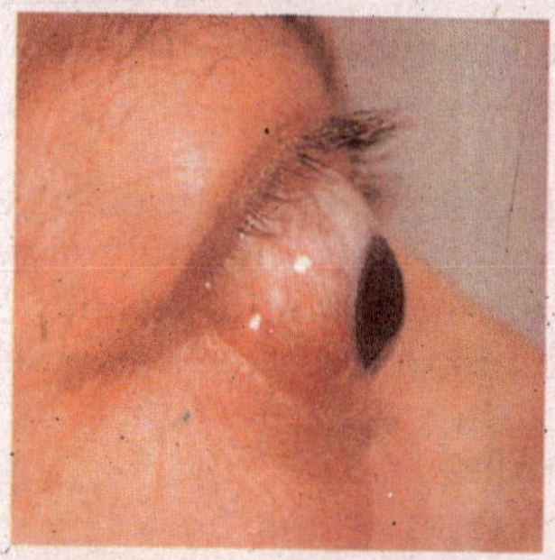

Chemosis. The conjunctiva is hyperaemic and bulging over the eyelids. There is exophthalmos, lid retraction, and periorbital oedema

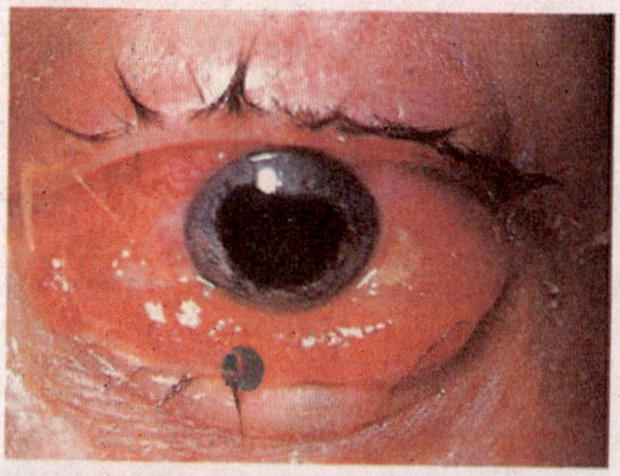

This patient had gross chemosis and exophthalmos but the eye was pulsating and the cause of these abnormalities was a carotid artery–cavernous sinus fistula

Palpation

PALPATE THE NECK FROM THE FRONT

The most important part of palpation is done from behind, but it is worthwhile placing your hand on any visible swelling while standing in front of the patient, to confirm your visual impression of its size, shape and surface, and to find out if it is tender. It is sometimes helpful to measure and record the circumference of the neck with a tape measure.

Check the **position of the trachea**. This is best done by feeling with the tip of two fingers in the suprasternal notch. The trachea should be exactly central at this point. When a thyroid mass extends below the suprasternal notch and obscures the trachea you must examine the thyroid cartilage. A mass which is displacing the trachea will tilt the thyroid cartilage laterally.

PALPATE THE NECK FROM BEHIND THE PATIENT

Stand behind the patient. Place your thumbs on the ligamentum nuchae and tilt the head slightly forwards to relax the anterior neck muscles. Let the palmar surface of your fingers rest on each side of the neck. They will be resting on the lateral lobes of the thyroid gland. A small lobe can be made prominent and easier to feel by pressing firmly on the opposite side of the neck.

If you are still doubtful about the origin of the lump, ask the patient to swallow while you are palpating the gland to confirm that it moves with swallowing. This manoeuvre also lifts up lumps that are lying behind the sternum, into the reach of your fingers.

At the end of palpation you should know the following facts about the gland and/or the lump: tenderness, shape, size, surface and consistence.

A normal thyroid gland is not palpable.

Palpate the whole of the cervical and supraclavicular lymph chains.

Percussion

Percussion is used to define the lower extent of a swelling that extends below the suprasternal notch by percussing along the clavicles and over the sternum and upper chest wall. This can be done when standing in front of or behind the patient. Percussion of the lump in the neck itself is rarely helpful.

Auscultation

Listen over the swelling. Vascular glands and lumps may have a systolic bruit.

General examination

Pay particular attention to the cardiovascular and nervous systems for any evidence of hyper- or hypothyroidism, the signs and symptoms of which are described on pages 283–287.

GOITRES

Simple hyperplastic goitre

Simple enlargement of the thyroid gland is invariably caused by excess stimulation by thyroid-stimulating hormone (TSH), the production of which is stimulated by low levels of circulating thyroid hormone. Iodine deficiency is the commonest pathological cause for a low level of thyroid hormone production. Physiological states, such as puberty and pregnancy, which require an increased activity of the thyroid gland, are also associated with enlargement of the gland.

The term **colloid goitre** is used to describe the late stage of diffuse hyperplasia, when all the acini are distended with colloid which has not been released because the stimulation by TSH has dropped off.

HISTORY

Age In areas where goitre is endemic (prevalent in the local population), hyperplastic goitres appear in **childhood**.

Sporadic physiological hyperplastic goitres appear at puberty, during pregnancy, and during severe illnesses and emotional disturbances, so they commonly occur at **puberty** and in **young adult life**.

Sex Hyperplastic goitres are five times more common in women than men.

Geography Endemic goitre is common in places where the drinking water has a low iodine content, such as the habitable valleys of the Alps, Andes, Himalayas and Rocky Mountains, and the lowland areas that depend upon water from mountain ranges, such as the Nile Valley, Congo Delta and Great Lakes of the USA. The rain that falls on the mountains has a normal iodine content, but it is filtered out by the time it reaches the springs and streams of the highland valleys.

Diet Some vegetables contain chemicals which are **goitrogens** (i.e. they interfere with hormone synthesis). An excess of cabbage and kale in the diet can cause a goitre.

Local symptoms The principal complaint is of **a swelling in the neck**. This appears slowly and without pain.

If it becomes large – especially if it remains as a colloid goitre after the initial stimulus has gone – it can cause pressure symptoms such as **dyspnoea, venous engorgement** and mild **discomfort during swallowing**.

General symptoms Diffuse hyperplastic goitres are not usually associated with clinically significant hyper- or hypofunction of the gland.

Long-standing colloid goitres often become nodular goitres and then thyrotoxicosis or myxoedema may develop.

LOCAL EXAMINATION

Position The swelling occupies the anatomical site of the thyroid gland.

Tenderness It is not tender.

Shape The swelling can usually be seen to have two lobes and an isthmus.

Size Physiological goitres are only two or three times larger than a normal gland, but iodine-deficiency goitres can become very large.

Surface The surface of a hyperplastic goitre is **smooth**. If it turns into a colloid goitre its surface becomes bosselated and, as the years pass by, nodular.

Composition The gland feels **firm and is dull** to percussion. Hyperaemic physiological goitres may have a very soft systolic bruit.

Relations The gland **moves upon swallowing**. The other tissues in the neck should be normal.

Lymph nodes The deep cervical lymph nodes should not be palpable.

The eyes The eyes should be normal.

GENERAL EXAMINATION

The patient is usually euthyroid.

Multinodular goitre

Multinodular goitres develop spontaneously, and in glands subjected to prolonged stimulation (i.e. hyperplastic glands). They are therefore **endemic** (in iodine-deficient areas) and **sporadic** (occurring haphazardly).

A nodular goitre results from a disorganized response of the gland to stimulation, and contains areas of **hyperplasia** and **hypoplasia**, side by side.

The cut surface of a nodular goitre reveals nodules with haemorrhagic, necrotic centres, separated by normal tissue. The normal tissue contains normally active follicles; the nodules contain both hyperactive and necrotic, involuting follicles.

When the nodules are hyperplastic the patient may become thyrotoxic.

In long-standing nodular goitres, most of the nodules are inactive and the quantity of normally active follicles so reduced that thyroid hormone production is inadequate and myxoedema develops.

HISTORY

Age In **endemic** areas, nodular goitres appear in **early adult life** (15–30 years). **Sporadic** nodular goitres appear later, between the ages of 25 and 40 years.

Sex Nodular goitres are six times more common in women than men.

Geography These goitres are common in the areas where the drinking water is deficient in iodine (see hyperplastic goitre).

Symptoms The commonest presenting symptom is an **enlarging painless lump in the neck.**

The lump may cause **dyspnoea, discomfort when swallowing, stridor,** and **engorged** neck veins.

Sudden enlargement and pain can occur if there is haemorrhage into a necrotic nodule. Necrotic nodules are not cysts, and it is wrong to call this event a haemorrhage into a cyst.

Thyrotoxicosis occurs in a considerable proportion (approximately 25 per cent) of patients with nodular goitres. The symptoms of thyrotoxicosis are listed on page 283.

Myxoedema As the follicular hyperplasia and its stimulation subside, the patient is left with a devastated gland that has little normal tissue. Ultimately, its endocrine secretions are inadequate and the patient has a considerable chance of becoming myxoedematous by the time she reaches 60 or 70 years of age. The symptoms of myxoedema are described on page 286.

LOCAL EXAMINATION

Position The swelling is in the lower third of the neck in the anatomical site of the thyroid gland and is usually asymmetrical.

Tenderness A nodular goitre is only tender when there has been a recent haemorrhage into a nodule.

Shape and size The nodules are asymmetrical and the gland can become any shape. Nodules in the isthmus are prominent. The nodules may extend below the clavicles and the sternal notch, into the superior mediastinum.

Surface The surface of a nodular goitre is **smooth** but **nodular**. Frequently, **only one nodule may be palpable**, even though the rest of the gland is grossly diseased.

Composition The consistence of the nodules varies. Some feel hard, others feel soft. There is an old saying 'Solid lumps in the thyroid feel cystic, whereas cystic lumps feel solid'. The explanation is that a nodule composed of thyroid tissue is soft, whereas a nodule full of blood and liquefied necrotic tissue becomes tense and feels hard.

The nodules of a nodular goitre do not fluctuate, or transilluminate, and are dull to percussion.

There should be **no bruit** over the gland.

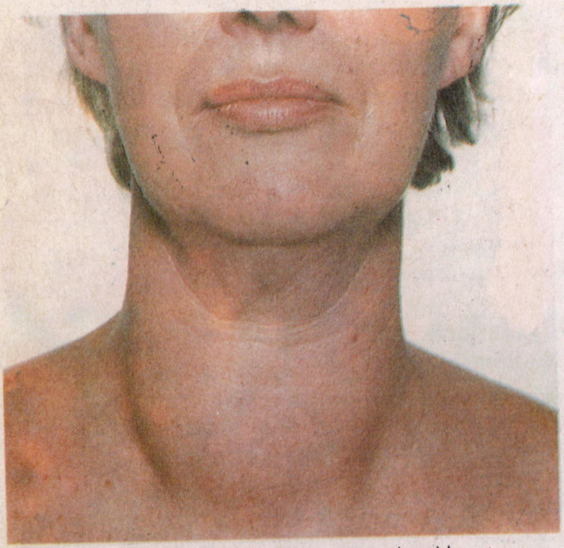

A large colloid goitre. The patient was euthyroid

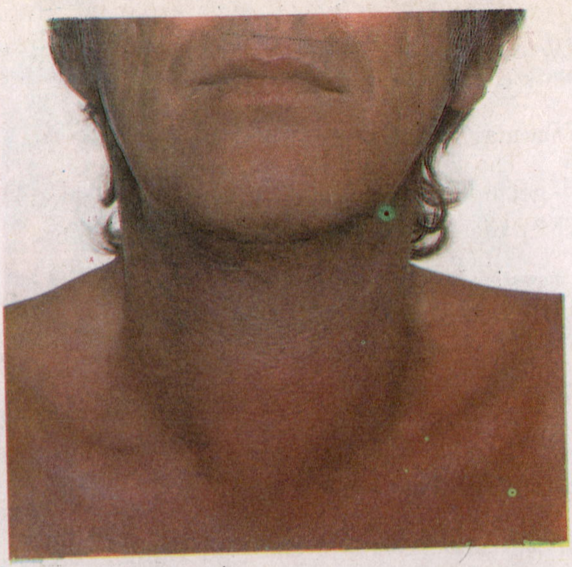

A large solitary nodule

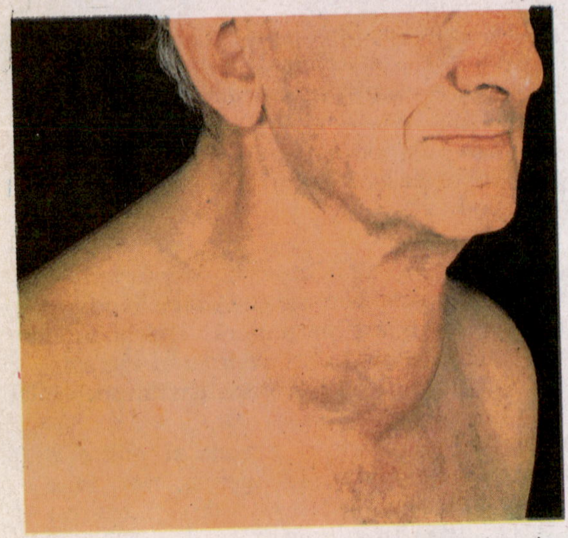

A nodular goitre extending below the sternum and causing venous obstruction. Distended veins are visible above the right clavicle. The patient was euthyroid

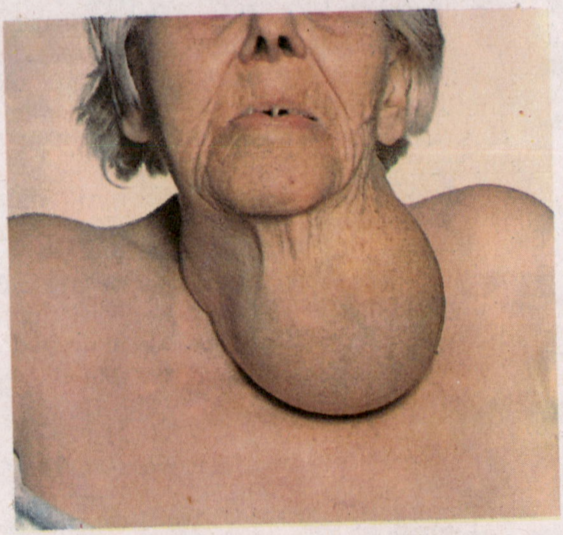

Beware! Not all lumps in the neck are goitres. This mass was soft and did not move with swallowing. It was a lipoma. Never make a spot diagnosis. Examine every lump carefully and completely

FIG. 11.25 GOITRES

Relations The lump will **move upon swallowing,** indicating that it is fixed to the trachea. It should not be fixed to any other nearby structures.

Lymph drainage The cervical lymph nodes should not be palpable.

State of local tissues The trachea may be **compressed** and/or **deviated**, depending on the site of the nodules. Bilateral nodules will compress the trachea into a narrow slit, causing dyspnoea and stridor – especially during lateral flexion of the neck. Large unilateral nodules will push the trachea laterally.

When the trachea is pushed to one side the *larynx* is tilted away from the mid-line.

If the gland is jammed in the thoracic inlet it may obstruct and distend the jugular veins.

The *eyes* should be normal. It is unusual to get neurological or eye changes with thyrotoxicosis associated with a nodular goitre – often called secondary thyrotoxicosis. These systems are affected more often in primary thyrotoxicosis.

GENERAL EXAMINATION

There may be the general signs of thyrotoxicosis – especially the **cardiovascular** signs, or in elderly patients with very long-standing nodular goitres, the signs of myxoedema.

The solitary nodule

Although only one nodule may be palpable, **approximately one-half of the patients who present with a solitary nodule actually have a multinodular goitre**.

It is unusual to be able to determine the pathology of a solitary nodule by clinical examination. Thus, although the majority of solitary nodules are benign, they must all be investigated.

Thyrotoxicosis caused by a solitary adenoma is rare and never (well, hardly ever) caused by a solitary malignant nodule.

The causes of a solitary nodule in the thyroid gland are:

- Multinodular goitre.
- Haemorrhage into, or necrosis of, a hyperplastic nodule.
- Adenoma.
- Carcinoma (papillary or follicular).
- Enlargement of the whole of one lobe by a thyroiditis.

THYROTOXICOSIS AND MYXOEDEMA

Thyrotoxicosis is caused by an excess of circulating thyroid hormone. The gland may be hyperplastic, nodular, or the site of disease such as thyroiditis, adenoma or carcinoma.

The terms 'primary' and 'secondary' thyrotoxicosis are used to describe thyrotoxicosis arising in a previously normal or previously abnormal gland, respectively. They are confusing terms.

The thyroid hormones tri-iodothyronine (T3) and thyroxine (T4) have three effects:

1. They increase the metabolic rate of all cells.
2. They increase the sensitivity of beta-adrenergic receptors.
3. They stimulate all cells to grow, but the effect on growth is only significant before natural growth has finished.

The increased tissue metabolism causes an increased appetite, a decrease in weight and an increased heat production.

The increased adrenergic receptor sensitivity causes tachycardia, extrasystoles, atrial fibrillation, tremor and nervousness, and lid retraction and lid lag.

Stimulation of growth, during childhood, produces early maturation and a slight increase in the rate of growth.

In myxoedema all of these symptoms are reversed. The lack of growth stimulation in a child causes dwarfism.

The history of thyrotoxicosis

Age Primary thyrotoxicosis occurs most often in young women, between 15 and 45 years of age. Toxic nodules can occur at any age.

Secondary thyrotoxicosis (from a nodular goitre) occurs in middle age – between 45 and 65 years.

Revision Panel 11.7

Causes of a 'solitary' nodule in the thyroid gland

- Multinodular goitre
- Haemorrhage into a nodule
- Adenoma
- Carcinoma (papillary or follicular)
- Enlargement of the whole of one lobe (usually Hashimoto's disease)

Sex Primary thyrotoxicosis is ten times more common in women than men.

Geography Secondary thyrotoxicosis is more common in those areas where simple hyperplastic goitre, and nodular goitre, is endemic.

Metabolic symptoms The patient complains of a **ravenous appetite**, but in spite of eating excessively she **loses weight**. She also finds that she is always warm, so that she **likes cold weather and dislikes hot weather**. There may be **excessive sweating**.

Cardiovascular symptoms The patient complains of **palpitations, shortness of breath** during exertion, missed and irregular heartbeats (extrasystoles and atrial fibrillation) and **tiredness**. Cardiovascular symptoms are often the presenting symptoms of secondary thyrotoxicosis.

Neurological symptoms Symptoms such as **nervousness, irritability, insomnia**, depression and excitement, even mania and melancholia, may be noticed by close relatives long before the patient appreciates them.

There may be hyperaesthesia, headaches, vertigo and tremors of the hands and tongue.

The patient may complain that her eyes have become more protuberant and that some eye movements are difficult.

Alimentary symptoms The changes in appetite and weight have been mentioned under metabolic symptoms. There is often a slight change in bowel habit – usually mild diarrhoea.

Genital tract symptoms Most women have a reduction in the quantity of their menses; some have amenorrhoea.

Musculoskeletal symptoms In addition to generalized weight loss, there may be specific wasting and weakness of the small muscles of the hand, shoulder and face. These muscles rarely become completely paralysed.

Cause The patient with primary thyrotoxicosis may relate the onset of her symptoms to puberty, pregnancy, an illness or a sudden emotional upset. Although it is difficult to be certain that events of this sort are the prime cause of hypersecretion of the thyroid gland, they undoubtedly exacerbate any hidden or developing abnormality. They are sometimes remembered as the three Ss – **sex** (puberty and pregnancy), **sepsis** and **psyche**!

The signs of thyrotoxicosis

SIGNS IN THE NECK

The thyroid gland is usually enlarged, but thyrotoxicosis can be present without any enlargement of the gland.

The enlargement may be diffuse, nodular, or tender, depending upon the local pathology.

A diffusely enlarged hyperaemic gland usually has a **systolic bruit** audible over its lateral lobes.

SIGNS IN THE EYE

Thyrotoxicosis is associated with four groups of physical signs in the eyes.

1 *Lid retraction and lid lag* These are common signs. In lid retraction the upper eyelid crosses the eye above its usual level (mid-way between the pupil and the superior limbus of the iris) because the autonomic part of the levator palpebrae superioris muscle is hypertonic.

Ask the patient to follow your finger as you move it slowly from above downwards. If the upper eyelid does not keep pace with the eye, the patient has **lid lag**. This is also caused by the increased tone of the levator palpebrae superioris muscle.

The patient may blink less frequently than normal.

2 *Exophthalmos* Oedema of the retro-orbital tissues pushes the eye forwards. The first abnormality is the appearance of sclera **below the inferior limbus**, but when the condition is extreme the eye appears to be popping out and the eyelids cannot be completely closed.

Exophthalmos **makes convergence difficult** and allows the patient to look up without raising her eyebrows or wrinkling her forehead. **Corneal ulceration** may complicate severe exophthalmos.

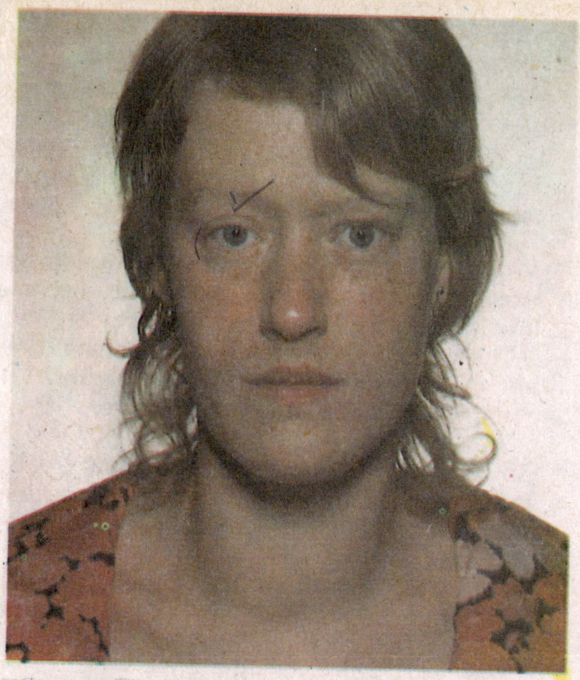

A small goitre, nervousness and agitation, beginning to lose weight, left lid retraction and very early exophthalmos (sclera visible below right inferior limbus)

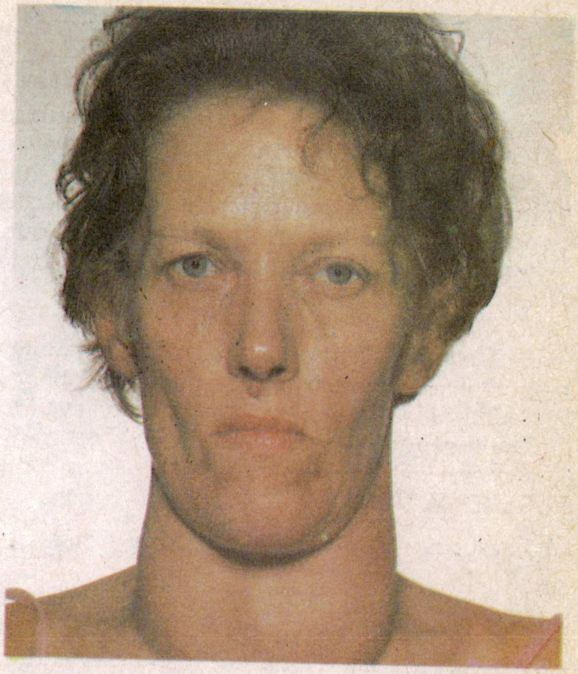

A large goitre, increasing appetite, but loss of weight – particularly of face and shoulder girdle – no eye signs

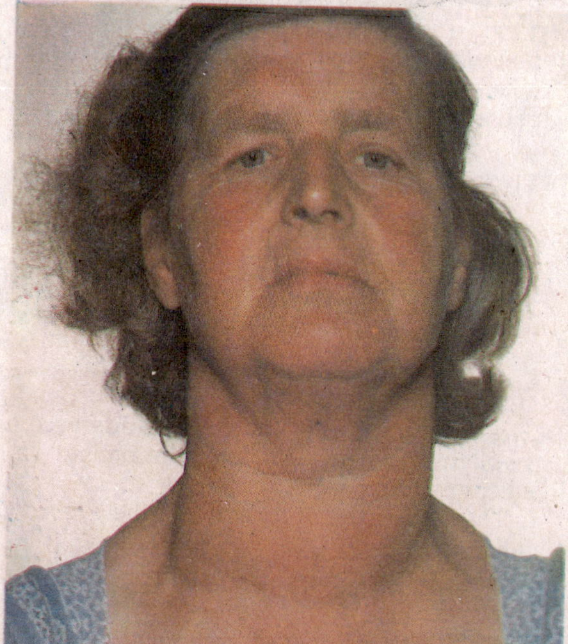

A nodular goitre. No eye or nervous system signs. Palpitations, breathlessness and atrial fibrillation

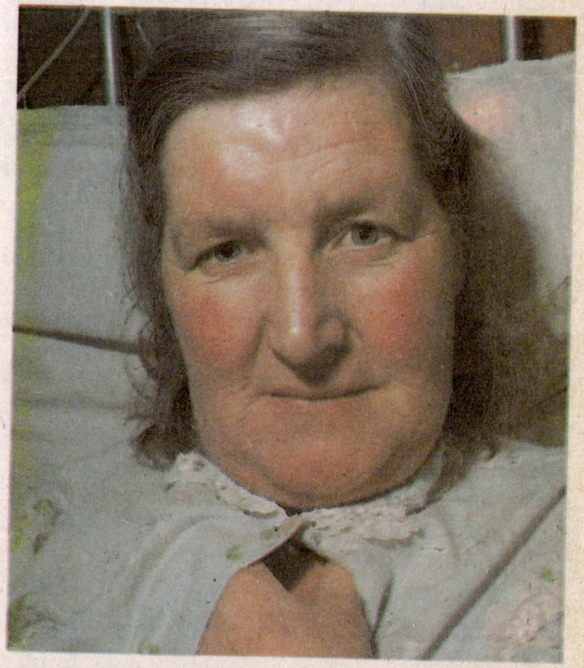

Myxoedema. Thinning of the hair, loss of outer third of the eyebrows, 'peaches and cream' complexion, thickening and heaviness of the eyelids

FIG. 11.26 THE FACIES OF THYROTOXICOSIS AND MYXOEDEMA

3 *Ophthalmoplegia* Infiltration of the ocular muscles weakens the eye muscles and diminishes the eye movements. The muscles most often affected are the superior rectus and inferior oblique muscles. As these muscles normally turn the eye upwards and outwards, this is the first movement to become weak.

4 *Chemosis* This is oedema of the conjunctiva. The conjunctiva becomes thick, boggy and crinkled and may bulge over the eyelids. The eyes water excessively.

GENERAL SIGNS

These are best described in bodily systems.

Metabolic signs The patient looks thin and her face and hands may be particularly wasted. She may look hot and be sweating, even in a cold room.

Cardiovascular signs There is a **tachycardia**, of 90 beats/minute or more, **at rest**, which **persists during sleep**.

If there are **extrasystoles** or **atrial fibrillation** the pulse will be irregular.

If there is mild heart failure there may be râles at the bases of the lungs and oedema of the ankles.

Neurological signs The patient looks worried and nervous and moves about in an agitated, jerky way. She often twists and twines her handkerchief between her fingers.

When she holds her hands outstretched there is a **fine tremor**. A similar tremor may be present in the protruded tongue.

Musculoskeletal signs The muscles of the hands, shoulders and face may be wasted and weak and the finger tips enlarged.

The history of myxoedema

Myxoedema is the clinical state which follows a severe lack of thyroid hormone. The term means 'mucous swelling' because when it was first described it was believed that the increase in weight and body swelling was caused by a new form of oedema.

Age Myxoedema appears in middle and old age.

Sex It is more common in women than in men.

Metabolic symptoms The patient complains of **tiredness** and **weakness** which become intense physical and mental **lethargy**.

The patient always **feels cold**, so she **likes hot weather and dislikes cold weather**. She gains weight but has a poor appetite.

Cardiovascular symptoms **Dyspnoea** and ankle **oedema** indicate the onset of cardiac failure.

Neurological symptoms The patient finds it difficult to think and to speak quickly and clearly. Hallucinations and dementia can occur ('myxoedema madness').

Alimentary symptoms Progressive and obdurate **constipation** is common.

Genital tract symptoms Menorrhagia is common when myxoedema occurs before the menopause.

The signs of myxoedema

SIGNS IN THE NECK

The thyroid gland may be enlarged by long-standing disease such as a nodular goitre, but in many cases the neck is normal.

SIGNS IN THE EYES

The eyes are normal but the eyelids become swollen and heavy, making the patient look sleepy and lethargic.

The hair of the outer third of the eyebrows falls out.

GENERAL SIGNS

General appearance and metabolic signs The complexion of a white-skinned patient with myxoedema is said to resemble **peaches and cream**. The skin is **smooth** and has a **pale yellow** (the cream) **colour**. The cheeks are often slightly flushed and have a pink–orange tinge (the peaches).

The patient is overweight, with excess connective tissue and fat in the supraclavicular fossae, across the back of the neck and over the shoulders.

The hair looks thin and ragged and falls out.

The skin is **dry and inelastic** and does not sweat. Although it may look oedematous it does not pit after prolonged pressure.

The hands are **puffy and spade-like.**

The tongue **enlarges** and seems to fill the mouth during speech and interfere with the articulation of words. The voice becomes **deep and hoarse.**

Cardiovascular signs The pulse rate is slow (40–60 beats/minute) and the blood pressure is low. Both these changes may be reversed if heart failure develops.

The **hands are cold** and the finger tips blue.

Neurological signs Mental alertness and the ability to respond to questions and solve problems are noticeably retarded. Conversation is also hampered by the difficulty in articulation caused by the enlargement of the tongue.

All movements are slow and deliberate.

The reflexes are sluggish and their relaxation period prolonged.

Cretinism

A cretin is a child whose mental and physical development has been retarded by a lack of thyroid hormone. Nowadays cretins are rare because the hormone deficiency can be replaced.

Cretinism is likely to occur in those places where goitre is endemic. The child may have a goitre.

The cretin has an underdeveloped skeleton (a dwarf), a large protruding tongue, the eyes are wide apart, and the skull is also wide. The limbs and neck are short and the hands spade-like.

The skin is dry and there are supraclavicular pads of fat.

The abdomen is distended and protuberant and there is often an umbilical hernia.

There is mental retardation, even imbecility.

When hypothyroidism occurs in older children they develop a mixture of the symptoms of cretinism and myxoedema.

CARCINOMA OF THE THYROID GLAND

The thyroid gland is a very vascular organ, and secondary tumour deposits from primary lesions in the breast, stomach, colon and lung are often found at autopsy. However, these secondary deposits rarely become large and noticeable. The majority of the neoplasms in the thyroid gland that present as a lump in the neck are primary thyroid tumours.

There are three varieties of carcinoma of the thyroid follicles:

- Papillary carcinoma.
- Follicular carcinoma.
- Anaplastic carcinoma.

The parafollicular (C) cells can also undergo malignant change, and this cancer is called:

- Medullary carcinoma.

The lymphoid tissue in the gland can also undergo malignant change to become a lymphosarcoma, but this is not a true thyroid tissue neoplasm. Lymphosarcoma is more common in patients with Hashimoto's disease.

Papillary carcinoma

This tumour contains a few formed follicles, but its bulk consists of hyperplastic follicular epithelium with a papilliferous configuration which sometimes produces a small quantity of colloid. This tumour spreads in the lymphatics. The lymph nodes may be palpable long before the primary lesion in the thyroid gland becomes palpable.

HISTORY

Age Papillary carcinoma is a tumour of **children and young adults**. Because it occurs in young children, the metastases in the lymph nodes were once thought to be clusters of aberrant normal thyroid tissue. They are not. They are true metastases.

Sex Females are affected three to four times more than males.

Symptoms The common presenting symptom is a **lump in the neck**. The lump may be in the region of the thyroid gland, or, if it is caused by secondary deposits in the lymph glands, in the anterolateral part of the neck.

Distant secondary deposits or a change in thyroid function are very uncommon with papillary carcinomata.

Duration of symptoms The lump may have been present for many years before the patient seeks advice, because these tumours are slow growing, and slow to spread beyond the thyroid gland and its draining lymph nodes.

Cause The patient will have no idea of the cause of the lump, but it is important to ask her if she has had any **radiation** to the neck or mediastinum. There is a greater incidence of papillary carcinoma in children who have had their neck or chest irradiated for conditions such as asthma, tuberculosis, enlargement of the thymus, tonsillitis and acne – a form of treatment no longer practised.

LOCAL EXAMINATION

The principal, and usually the only, abnormality is the lump or lumps in the neck.

Position The lump may be in the region of the thyroid gland or deep to the sternomastoid.

Temperature and tenderness The skin of the neck should be normal, provided the tumour has not infiltrated into it. The lumps are usually **not tender**.

Shape and size The primary nodule in the thyroid gland may vary in size from a minute, impalpable nodule to a nodule 3–5 cm in diameter. It is usually spherical, smooth and clearly defined, but its surface may be bosselated.

Lymph nodes containing thyroid carcinoma metastases are ovoid or nodular, and usually smooth and clearly defined. The thyroid gland lymph first drains to the pre- and paratracheal lymph glands and then to the lower deep cervical lymph nodes which lie beneath the anterior edge of the lower third of the sternomastoid muscle.

Composition The consistence of both the primary nodule and the secondary lymph nodes is hard or firm. Both are dull to percussion, do not fluctuate and do not cause a bruit.

Relations The primary nodule in the thyroid gland will move upon swallowing and is not usually fixed to superficial structures.

Enlarged lymph nodes move more easily in a transverse than a vertical plane and do *not* move with swallowing. They are not usually attached to the skin.

Lymph drainage If you feel a nodule in the thyroid gland, examine all the lymph nodes in the neck with care.

GENERAL EXAMINATION

The patient usually appears fit and well, without any of the systemic signs which suggest a disseminated neoplasm or thyroid dysfunction.

Follicular carcinoma

The cells in this well-differentiated thyroid cancer retain their normal follicular configuration. Most of the follicles contain a small amount of colloid, which implies that the cells are synthesizing hormone. This has an important bearing on treatment, because the tumour cells will take up radioactive iodine. This tumour spreads by the blood stream.

HISTORY

Age Follicular carcinomata occur in adults between the ages of 20 and 50 years.

Sex Women are affected more than men.

Symptoms The common presenting symptom is a **lump in the neck**, which may have been present for many years.

If the tumour has spread beyond the thyroid, the patient may complain of breathlessness, chest pain or **pain or swelling in a bone**, caused by lung and bone metastases, respectively. In these circumstances the pathologist usually finds that the tumour has a thin capsule and has spread into the substance of the gland – the 'invasive' variety of follicular carcinoma.

Multiple lumps in the neck caused by metastases in lymph nodes do occur, but not as frequently as with papillary carcinoma.

Systemic effects These patients are euthyroid.

LOCAL EXAMINATION

The principal, and often the only, abnormality is the lump in the neck.

Position Follicular carcinoma usually arises in one of the lateral lobes of the thyroid gland.

Temperature and tenderness The overlying skin is not hot and the lump is not tender.

Shape and size The lump is usually spherical and smooth with distinct edges. Even the invasive variety feels as if it has a distinct surface.

Composition The lump is hard, does not fluctuate, is dull to percussion and has no bruit.

Relations The lump moves with swallowing, but is not attached to overlying structures.

Lymph nodes The deep cervical lymph nodes may be enlarged and hard.

Local tissues The local tissues are usually normal.

GENERAL EXAMINATION

Examine **the chest** carefully for any evidence of consolidation or collapse. Pulmonary secondary deposits are quite common but may not cause any abnormal physical signs.

Metastases in the **skeleton** are often painful and tender. If a bone near to the skin contains a metastasis it may be visibly deformed, swollen and hot. Some thyroid cancer metastases are so vascular that they are **soft** and **pulsatile** and have an audible **bruit**.

Anaplastic carcinoma

This is the worst variety of thyroid cancer because it spreads rapidly. Most patients with this disease are dead within 1 year of diagnosis. Its cells do not synthesize thyroid hormone.

HISTORY

Age Anaplastic carcinoma of the thyroid gland appears between the ages of 60 and 80 years.

Sex Females are affected more often than males.

Symptoms The common complaint is a **swelling of the neck** rather than 'a lump'. The patient complains of swelling because the tumour is diffuse and infiltrating, not localized.

A dull **aching pain** in the neck is quite common.

Dyspnoea occurs when the tumour begins to compress the trachea, especially when the neck is flexed.

Dyspnoea may also occur if there are multiple pulmonary metastases.

Hoarseness or a **change in the quality of the voice** is a diagnostic symptom because it implies infiltration of the recurrent laryngeal nerve.

Pain in the ear, caused by infiltration of the vagus nerve, is not uncommon.

There may be **bone pain**. Any bone can be the site of a secondary deposit and **pathological fractures** can occur.

General malaise and weight loss appear when there is disseminated disease.

Duration of symptoms The symptoms of an anaplastic carcinoma often develop rapidly as this carcinoma grows quickly and is highly invasive. Local invasion and compression of the trachea can lead to death from asphyxia or precipitate a fatal pneumonia.

EXAMINATION

The swelling in the neck

Position The swelling is in the region of the thyroid gland. At first this is in one lobe but in advanced cases the whole gland may be enlarged.

Colour The overlying skin often has a red–blue tinge because the underlying infiltration interferes with its venous drainage.

Temperature The skin temperature is normal, or slightly raised.

Tenderness The mass often becomes tender as the tumour infiltrates beyond the thyroid gland.

Shape The mass in the neck has no definable shape once it has spread beyond the thyroid gland, and before this stage it is not easy to define because the surface is so indistinct.

Size The mass may become so big that it interferes with neck movements.

Surface and edge The surface is irregular and indistinct and the lump often has no palpable edge.

Composition The mass is hard and solid. It does not fluctuate, is dull to percussion and has no bruit.

Relations Provided the mass is not infiltrating the whole neck, it will move during swallowing.

It may be fixed to the sternomastoid muscles and the overlying skin as well as to the trachea. When the sternomastoid muscle is contracted, the movement of the lump during swallowing is limited and the skin becomes puckered.

The skin may be infiltrated with tumour, making it thick, nodular and a reddish-brown colour.

Lymph nodes Although the deep cervical lymph nodes are invariably involved in the disease, their enlargement may be obscured by the primary mass in the gland.

If the local lymph nodes are palpable they feel hard and fixed. At first they are smooth and discrete, but they become irregular and indistinct when the tumour begins to spread through their capsules.

State of local tissues The skin of the neck may be tethered or fixed to the lump or even infiltrated with tumour.

The *trachea* is often compressed and deviated, causing stridor.

One vocal cord may be paralysed by infiltration of the recurrent laryngeal nerve. This may be suspected if the patient has a hoarse voice, but must be confirmed by indirect laryngoscopy.

All the soft tissues of the neck may be fixed and hardened by infiltrating tumour.

GENERAL EXAMINATION

The patient is often breathing with difficulty, and has stridor. There may be basal pneumonia or collapse caused by pulmonary secondary deposits or the restriction of lung expansion by the narrowed trachea.

There is often wasting and anaemia.

There may be evidence of skeletal metastases – even pathological fractures.

In advanced cases the liver may be enlarged, and secondary deposits occasionally appear in the skin.

Medullary carcinoma

This is a rare condition but is mentioned briefly because it can sometimes be diagnosed before operation. It is a neoplasm of the parafollicular (C) cells.

The common presentation is a firm, smooth and distinct lump in the neck, indistinguishable from any other form of thyroid solitary nodule.

The majority of patients are between the ages of 50 and 70 years, but the condition can occur in young adults (20–30 years) and these sometimes have a family history of the same condition or associated conditions such as:

- Neuromas of the tongue, lips and conjuctiva.
- Pale brown birthmarks.
- Phaeochromocytoma.
- Parathyroid tumours.

The symptoms which should make you think of medullary tumour, apart from a lump in the neck and the presence of the above lesions in the patient or her family, are **diarrhoea** and flushing. Diarrhoea occurs in one-third of the patients. The fluidity of the stool and the frequency of defaecation are both increased.

If this tumour is suspected it is worthwhile measuring the serum calcitonin level.

THYROIDITIS

There are three varieties of thyroiditis which can be diagnosed clinically: Hashimoto's disease, de Quervain's thyroiditis and Riedel's thyroiditis.

The term 'thyroiditis' is a non-specific description of the histological changes occurring in the gland. Although the aetiology of these conditions is partly understood, the eponyms are useful because they do not imply an aetiology but a clinical description (provided you ignore the aetiologies proposed by the three gentlemen who made the original descriptions!).

Hashimoto's disease

This is an autoimmune thyroiditis. The body fails to recognize part of itself – in this case both the mitochondria of the thyroid cells and the thyroglobulin they produce – and sets up an immune response against its own tissues. The result is a lymphocyte and plasma cell infiltration of the gland which ultimately destroys the thyroid cells. In the first instance the thyroid cells respond by becoming hyperplasic, causing thyrotoxicosis, but eventually and inevitably the gradual destruction of the thyroid cells causes myxoedema.

HISTORY

Age and sex Hashimoto's disease is most common in middle-aged women, especially those near the menopause; but it can occur in men, and at any age.

Symptoms in the neck The patient usually complains of a **swelling** or **lump in the neck**. This lump may appear gradually or rapidly, and is often **painful**, particularly when it appears rapidly.

The swelling, or lump, fluctuates in size, and the pain is often intermittent. The symptoms are worse when the patient is tired, or run down, or has an intercurrent illness.

The voice should not alter.

Systemic effects The symptoms of mild **thyrotoxicosis** or **myxoedema** may be present.

The common course of events is for the mild symptoms of thyrotoxicosis, which appear at the onset of the disease, to gradually die out and become replaced by the opposite symptoms of myxoedema.

The majority of patients are euthyroid when they complain of the lump, having ignored or not had any symptoms of thyrotoxicosis, and not reached the myxoedematous phase.

This variability of the local and systemic effects of the disease makes the diagnosis difficult.

Family history Other members of the family may have suffered from the same or other forms of autoimmune disease, such as pernicious anaemia and autoimmune gastritis.

EXAMINATION

The main complaint is usually the lump in the neck.

Position The swelling is in the region of the thyroid gland and may be uni- or bilateral.

Temperature In the initial acute phase – if it occurs – the overlying skin may feel warm.

Tenderness The swelling is often slightly tender.

Shape The swelling may be any shape – a solitary nodule, the whole of one lobe, or the whole gland. When one lobe or more is involved the swelling is usually lobulated.

Size Hashimoto's disease usually causes a moderate swelling of the gland, easily visible but rarely gross.

Surface The swelling has a smooth surface and the edge is distinct.

A SCHEME FOR THE DIAGNOSIS OF THYROID SWELLINGS

Once you have examined the patient you should be able to draw one of the following conclusions about the gland and one about its activity

The gland
1 Contains one palpable nodule
2 Contains more than one palpable nodule
3 Is diffusely (evenly) enlarged

Activity of the gland
1 Normal
2 Hypersecretion
3 Hyposecretion

It is simpler to classify swellings according to their pathology. If you try to classify according to the activity of the gland you will get hopelessly confused with needless repetition.

First try to decide the pathology and then remember that any thyroid abnormality can be associated with hyper-, normal, or hypofunction, even though some abnormalities are more likely to be associated with one type of malfunction than others.

⊕ = may be associated with thyrotoxicosis
⊖ = may be associated with myxoedema

If only one lump is palpable it may be:

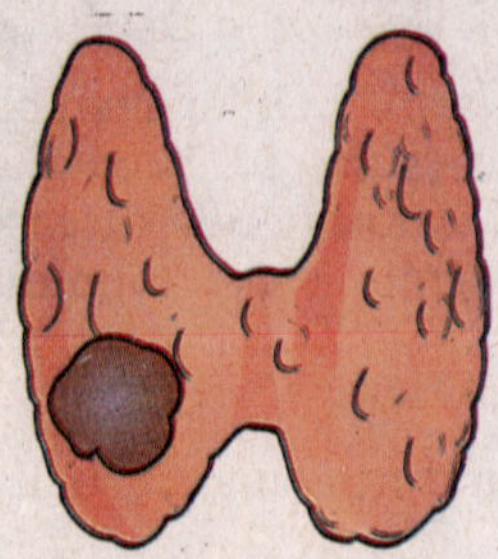

The only palpable nodule of a **multinodular goitre**

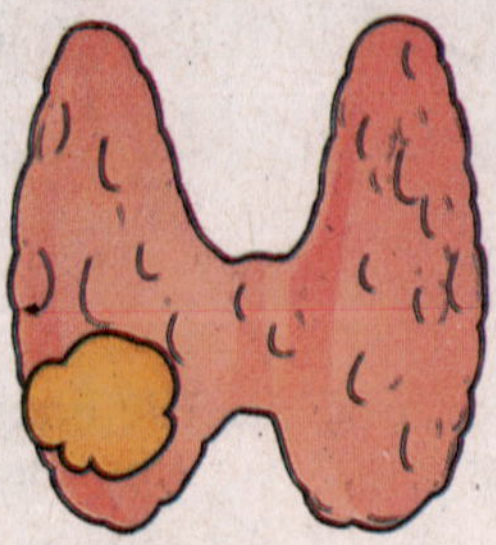

A **'cyst'** caused by haemorrhage into a necrotic nodule

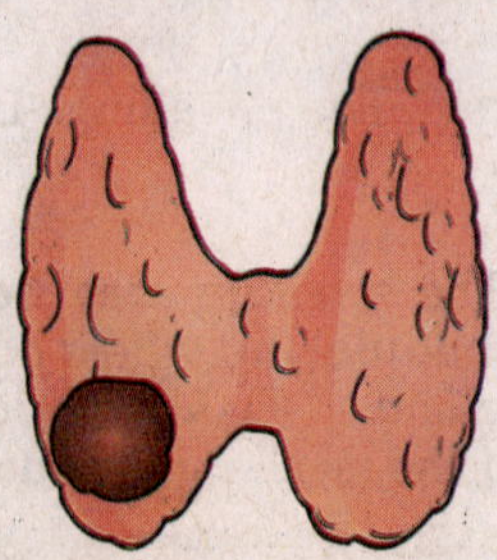

● A benign **adenoma**

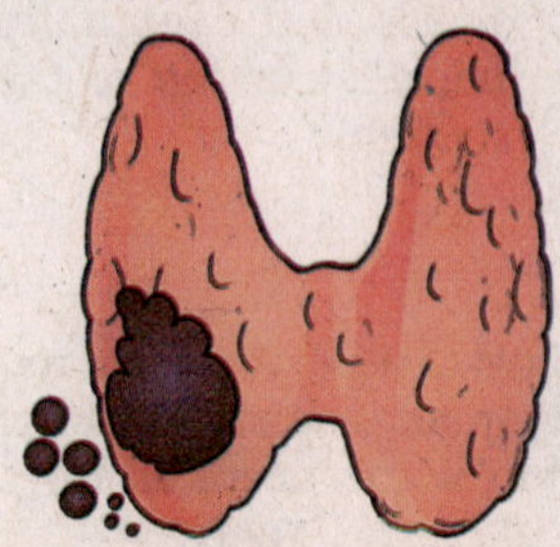

Carcinoma (papillary, follicular or medullary). The lymph nodes may be palpable, especially with the papillary type

FIG. 11.27

If more than one lump is palpable the swelling may be:

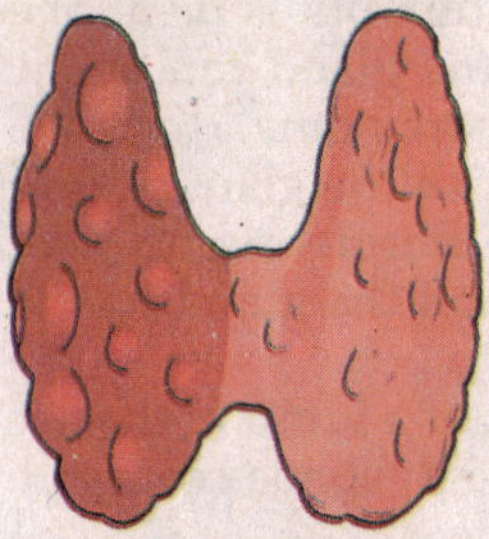

⊕ ↓ ⊖ The **whole of one lobe**, usually involved by Hashimoto's thyroiditis

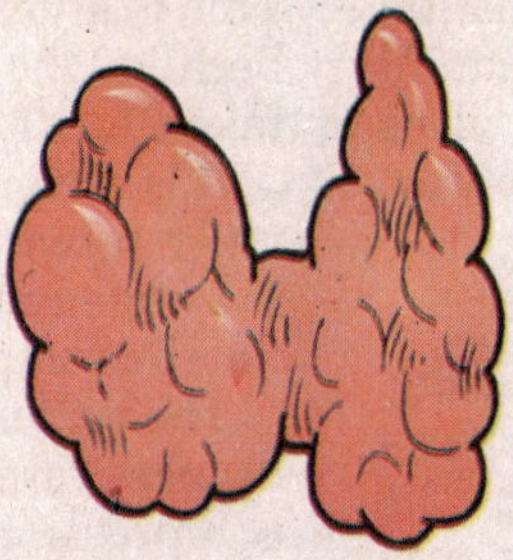

⊕ or ⊖ **A multinodular goitre**

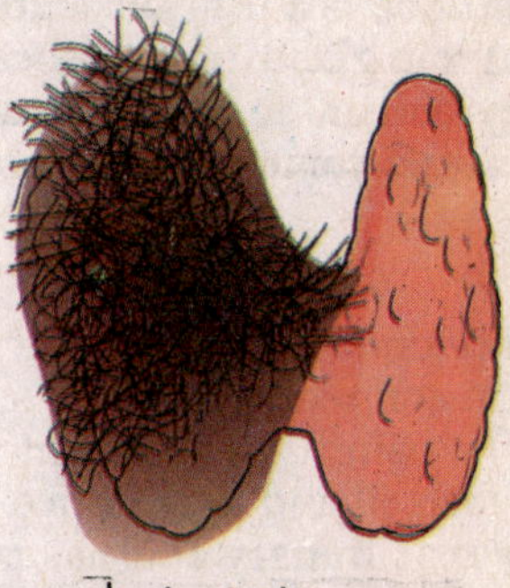

An **anaplastic carcinoma**, especially if the voice is hoarse and the mass fixed to the surrounding tissues

If there is diffuse, homogeneous enlargement of the whole gland the swelling may be:

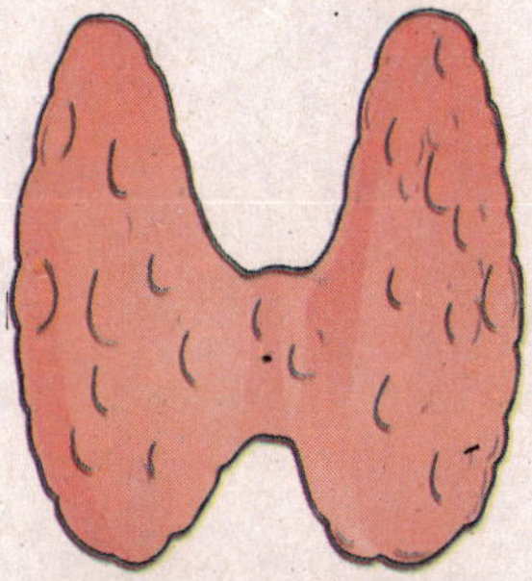

⊕ Graves' disease.
Primary thyrotoxicosis
Slight to moderate enlargement.
Soft, smooth with a bruit

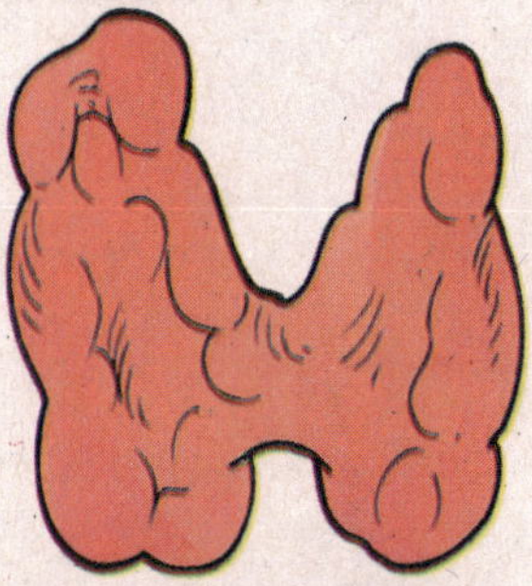

Hyperplastic (colloid) goitre.
Moderate to gross enlargement.
Bosselated. No bruit

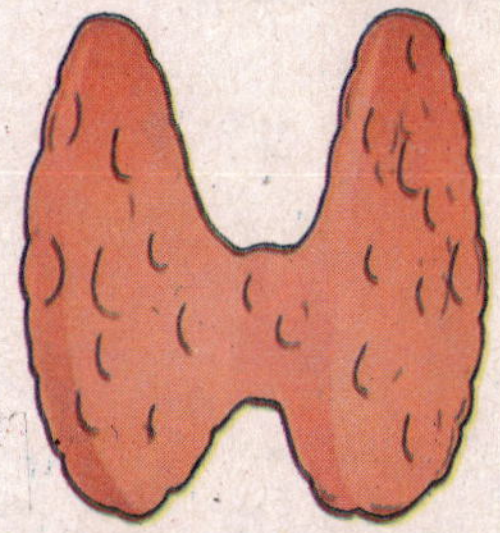

⊕ ↓ ⊖ **Thyroiditis.** Hashimoto's, de Quervain's or Riedel's
Moderate or small.
Hard, tender

FIG. 11.27 *Continued*

Composition The swelling has the texture of firm rubber. This texture is homogeneous, in spite of the lobulated shape, which helps distinguish the swelling from a nodular or colloid goitre.

There is no bruit.

The composition and mild tenderness are the features most likely to alert you to the possibility of the diagnosis.

Relations The swelling moves with swallowing but is not fixed to any other structures.

Local tissues All the local tissues should be normal.

Lymph glands The nearby lymph nodes should not be enlarged.

GENERAL EXAMINATION

The majority of patients are euthyroid, but some will have the signs of mild thyrotoxicosis and others early myxoedema.

De Quervain's thyroiditis

This condition is a true subacute inflammation of the thyroid gland, often associated with mild hyperthyroidism. It may be caused by a virus infection, and sometimes occurs in epidemics.

HISTORY

De Quervain's thyroiditis occurs in adults. The main complaint is of the sudden appearance of a painful swelling in the neck. The patient feels ill and may notice that he is anxious, sweaty, hungry and has palpitations.

EXAMINATION

Examination reveals a diffuse, firm, **tender** swelling of the whole of the thyroid gland.

There may be signs of mild thyrotoxicosis – nervousness and agitation, lid lag and tachycardia.

De Quervain's thyroiditis is self-limiting. It disappears in 1–3 months.

Riedel's thyroiditis

This is a very rare condition but is mentioned because the changes in the gland can be mistaken for the signs of a carcinoma.

It is a condition in which the gland is gradually replaced by dense fibrous tissue which may even infiltrate beyond the gland into the nearby strap muscles.

The patient complains of a lump in the neck or, very rarely, increasing dyspnoea caused by compression of the trachea.

Examination reveals a stony hard swelling of the thyroid gland, at first of one lobe, but eventually both lobes and the isthmus.

The lump moves with swallowing but may be fixed to the surrounding tissues, which are otherwise normal.

When both lobes are involved, the smooth discrete surface usually excludes the diagnosis of carcinoma, but when one lobe is involved it is impossible to make a firm diagnosis.

The breast

12

Many women come to the surgical outpatient department complaining of pain or a lump in the breast, so you must be able to examine the breast thoroughly and be able to make a reasonably accurate clinical diagnosis of any abnormality that you find.

When I ask a student the question 'What is that lump in the breast?' I am usually answered with the phrase 'A carcinoma until proved otherwise'. That is the **wrong answer** but the **correct management**. A correct management decision does not release you from the obligation of making a clinical diagnosis on the basis of the history and physical signs. It is bad practice to avoid making a clinical diagnosis by assuming that every lump in the breast is a carcinoma until proved otherwise. Examine each lump carefully and make a reasoned guess as to its nature. You will find that you will be right on three out of four occasions.

THE HISTORY AND EXAMINATION OF BREAST DISEASE

The history of breast disease

The majority of patients with breast disease complain of either a lump, pain and tenderness, a change in breast size, or a discharge from the nipple. The history that you must obtain about these complaints is no different from that of any other lump or pain (see Chapter 1); but it is also important to record the history of the development of the breasts, the endocrine state of the patient, and the relationship of the patient's symptoms to the normal physiological variations of ovarian activity that accompany menstruation and pregnancy, drug ingestion (particularly the contraceptive pill) and any family history of breast carcinoma.

Breast development

The breast usually begins to develop a few months or years before the menarche. Lack of breast development associated with other female endocrine deficiencies is significant; but if menstruation and hair distribution is normal then lack of breast development, which may be fortunate or unfortunate depending upon the current fashion, has no clinical significance.

Normal changes in the breast during the menstrual cycle

The breasts increase in size in the second half of the menstrual cycle, after ovulation, and often become tender and slightly painful. Pain or tenderness caused by pre-existing disease in the breast is likely to get worse in this period, and lumps often get bigger or become palpable.

To ascertain the relationship of any symptoms to the menstrual cycle it is obviously necessary to take a careful history of the onset, development, frequency, duration and quantity of menstruation.

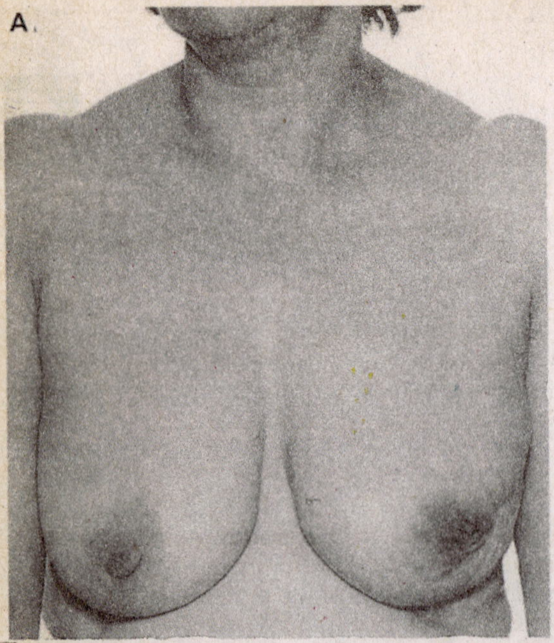

Look at the breast for asymmetry, changes in the skin and the nipple

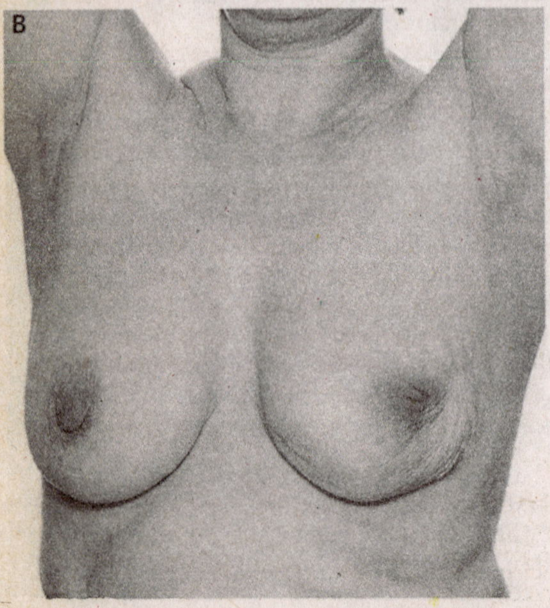

Ask the patient to raise her hands above her head. This exaggerates asymmetry and skin tethering

FIG. 12.1 THE EXAMINATION OF THE BREAST

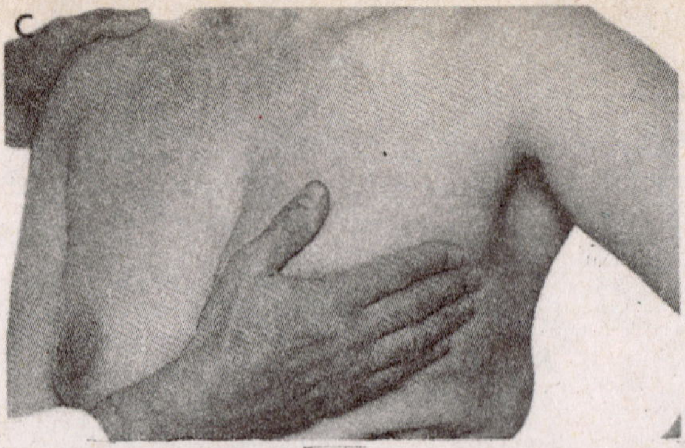

Feel the breast with your fingers flat

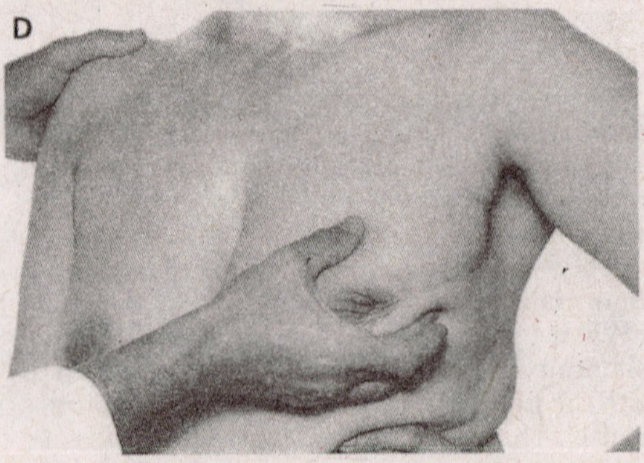

Test the mobility of every lump in two directions, with the pectoralis muscle relaxed and tense

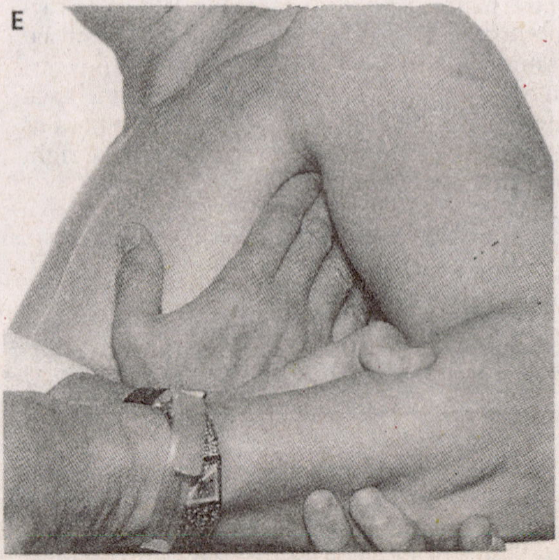

When you palpate the axilla hold the patient's arm to relax the muscles that form the axillary folds

Pregnancy

Profound changes occur in the breast during pregnancy in preparation for lactation, which may affect the incidence of breast disease. Record the number and dates of the patient's pregnancies and the occurrence of any complications during pregnancy, such as nipple soreness, cracks, retraction or breast abscess.

Lactation

Lactation is a hazardous period for the breasts. Cracks in the nipple, milk retention and breast abscesses are common and may be the cause of abnormalities which can present months or years later. Since breast-feeding may affect the infant as well as the mother, the infant's records in the mother's notes may provide helpful information many years later. If lactation was suppressed, record the indications and complications.

Examination of the breast

POSITION

Expose the whole of the upper half of the patient. You must be able to see both breasts, the neck, all of the chest wall and the arms. You cannot examine a breast if it is still half covered or partly trapped and distorted in an incompletely removed brassière.

Relax the patient in a semi-recumbent (45°) position. This position is the best compromise between lying flat, which makes the breasts flatten out and fall sideways, and sitting upright, which makes the breasts pendulous and bulky. Sometimes it is necessary to feel the breasts in all three positions, but for the majority of patients the 45° position is best for the examiner and the most comfortable for the patient.

It is the natural response of a modest woman to fold her arms across her chest; persuade her to let them rest comfortably at her sides.

INSPECTION

Look at both breasts

Stand squarely in front of the patient and observe the following features.

Size The breast may be under- or overdeveloped. The extremes of this very broad range are usually obvious. Complaints about small variations from the norm may reflect the patient's psyche and fashion consciousness more than pathology.

Symmetry and contour Any change in one breast is likely to make the breasts asymmetrical. Pathological changes, especially those which involve the skin, are the commonest

> **Revision Panel 12.1**
>
> **Points to remember when examining the breast**
>
> *History*
> Menarche, Development, Menopause, Changes during menstrual cycle, Pregnancies, Lactation, Family and drug history.
>
> *Examination*
> *Expose* all of the top half of the trunk.
>
> *Inspect* the breasts at rest and ask the patient to raise her arms above her head.
>
> *Look at*:
> - size
> - symmetry
> - skin:
>   - puckering
>   - peau d'orange
>   - nodules
>   - discolouration
>   - ulceration
> - nipples and areolae
> - axillae, arms and neck.
>
> *Feel the normal side first.*
>
> *Examine the axillae and arms.*
>
> *Examine the supraclavicular fossae.*
>
> *Palpate the abdomen for*:
> - hepatomegaly
> - ascites
> - nodules in the pouch of Douglas.
>
> *Examine the lumbar spine*:
> - percussion
> - movements
> - straight-leg raising
> - ankle jerks.

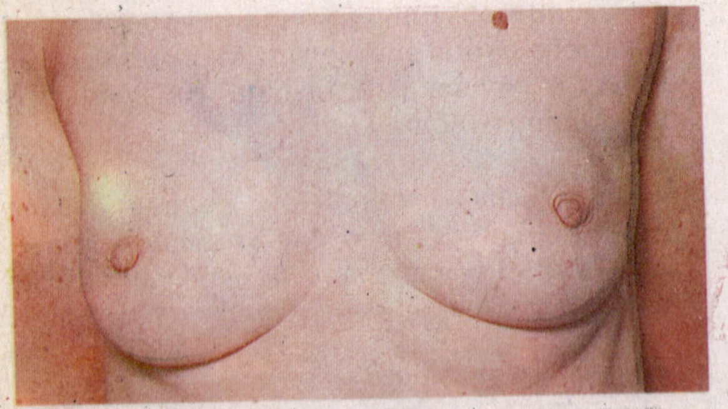

Displacement and deviation. The left nipple is elevated (displaced) and pointing downwards and inwards, not downwards and outwards (deviation). The tumour can be seen just above the areola

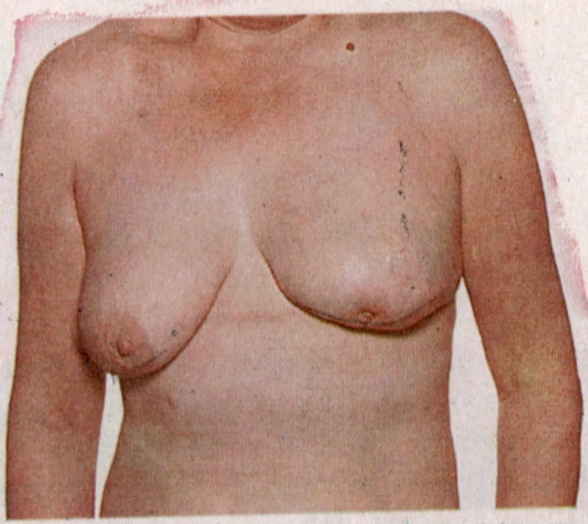

Retraction and displacement. The left nipple has been pulled into the breast (retraction) and pulled upwards (displacement) by the underlying carcinoma

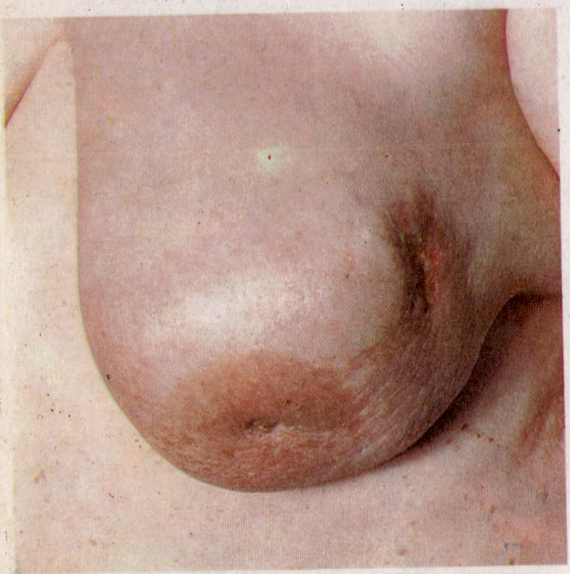

Retraction and peau d'orange. This carcinoma has invaded the skin and ulcerated. The skin of the lower part of the breast is oedematous and looks like the skin of an orange

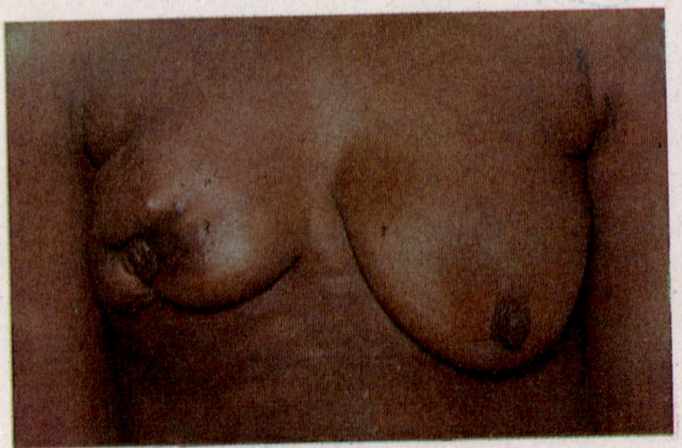

Destruction. The right nipple and areola have been invaded and destroyed by the underlying carcinoma

FIG. 12.2 CHANGES IN THE NIPPLE THAT MAY BE CAUSED BY AN UNDERLYING CARCINOMA

causes of a change in shape, but asymmetry can also be caused by simple unilateral under- or overdevelopment.

Skin The skin may be pulled in and **puckered** by an underlying neoplasm.

Oedema of the skin gives it an 'orange peel' appearance (**peau d'orange**) because the oedema deepens the mouths of the sweat glands and hair follicles.

There may be **nodules** visible in the skin or loss of the normal skin **texture** if it is diffusely infiltrated with tumour.

Areas of skin may be made red by eczema or infection, or **discoloured** by infiltration with underlying malignant disease.

There may be an **ulcer**. All its features – position, colour, shape, size, edge and base – must be noted.

Look at the nipples and areolae

Presence Are both nipples present? If one (or both) is absent it might be inverted (**retracted**) or **destroyed**.

Colour The skin of the areola of young white girls is pale pink, but it becomes slightly darker in adult life and much browner during and after pregnancy.

Areola The normal areola is slightly corrugated and contains a few small nodules – Montgomery's glands. These glands become much larger during pregnancy when they are known as Montgomery's tubercles.

Asymmetry Changes deep in the breast may displace the nipple long before the patient notices any changes in the substance of the breast.

The nipples are usually at the same horizontal level and point downwards and outwards. If the deep attachments of the nipple are altered by disease, it may be deviated so that it points upwards or inwards. This change often precedes **retraction**, which is the commonest cause of asymmetry.

Discharge Look for any discharge on the surface of the nipple and look at the patient's underclothes. The colour of the stain may indicate the nature of the discharge.

Duplication Supernumerary nipples are quite common. They can occur anywhere along the mammary line, which runs from the axilla to the groin.

Look at the axillae, arms and supraclavicular fossae

There may be swelling of the arm, localized swellings caused by enlarged axillary or supraclavicular lymph nodes, distended veins and wasted muscles.

Ask the patient to slowly raise her arms above her head

The change in the shape of the breasts caused by abducting the arms often reveals lumps, puckering and distortion not visible when the arms are by the sides.

This action also usually reveals the lower surface of the breasts. If the skin in the submammary fold is still not visible, lift up the breast and inspect it.

When the arms are above the head inspect the axillae for swelling, skin puckering and ulceration.

The shoulder movements may be affected by disease in the axilla.

Ask the patient to press her hands against her hips

This changes the shape of the breasts and may reveal lumps that were not visible when the pectoral muscles were relaxed. It will also accentuate any depressions in the skin caused by tethering or fixity to underlying lumps.

PALPATION

Keep the patient in the semi-recumbent, 45° position, and ask her to point to the site of the pain or the lump.

Feel the normal side first. The texture of the breast varies from woman to woman. In some it is so soft and smooth that it is not possible to distinguish the glandular tissue from the subcutaneous tissue; in others it is firm, fibrous and granular. Unless the patient is complaining of trouble in both breasts it is very important to determine the texture of the normal breast before feeling the breast that is abnormal.

Feel the breast with the palmar surface of the fingers (i.e. with the **hand flat**). The expression found in many textbooks, 'The breast should be palpated with the flat of the hand', is *wrong*. The flat of the hand is the palm of the hand and quite unsuitable for feeling lumps.

Feel the **whole** of the breast. Do not forget the axillary tail which runs upwards and laterally over the edge of the pectoralis major muscle towards the axilla.

If you find a lump, ascertain its **Position, Tenderness, Temperature, Shape, Size** (measure it), **Surface, Edge** and **Composition**.

To do this you will also need to feel the lump with the pulps of your fingers, which may mean that you have to hold the lump steady with your other hand.

Remember that a very large lump can fill the whole breast and can easily be missed if it is not causing generalized enlargement of the breast.

Once you have elicited the physical characteristics of the lump you must ascertain its relations to the overlying skin and the underlying muscles.

If a woman of cancer age says she can feel a lump and you cannot, remember *she is probably right* and you wrong. The older she is, the more likely she is to be right, especially if she has large breasts.

Relations to the skin

Lumps are often described as being attached to the skin. I would advise you not to use this expression because it gives no idea about the degree or extent of the attachment. Lumps in the breast can be related to the skin in two ways: they may be **tethered** to it, or **fixed** to it. The clinical significance of these two varieties of attachment is different.

Tethering When malignant disease in the breast begins to spread, it grows along the fine fibrous septae that pass from the skin through the subcutaneous fat and the lobules of the breast. These are called (Astley) Cooper's ligaments. Infiltration of these strands by tumour makes them shorter and inelastic. This pulls the skin inwards, puckering the skin surface. The underlying lump can still be moved independently of the skin for a limited distance, so it is described as **tethered** to the skin.

Thus, tethering of a lump to the skin can be demonstrated by moving the lump from side to side and watching to see if the skin dimples at the extremes of movement. Raising the arms above the head can have a similar effect (see Fig. 12.1B).

Fixation When a lump is fixed to the skin the two structures (lump and skin) cannot be moved separately. Whenever one is moved the other goes with it.

Fixity means that there is direct, continuous and widespread infiltration of the skin by the underlying disease, with the implication that the disease has actually spread far beyond the visible area of fixation. Tethering does not have this implication. Tethering implies that the disease is on its way to the skin but has not necessarily reached and spread into it.

Relations to the muscle

The same definitions apply to the deep attachments of a lump in the breast, but it is more difficult to distinguish between tethering and fixation because you cannot see puckering or movement of the muscle.

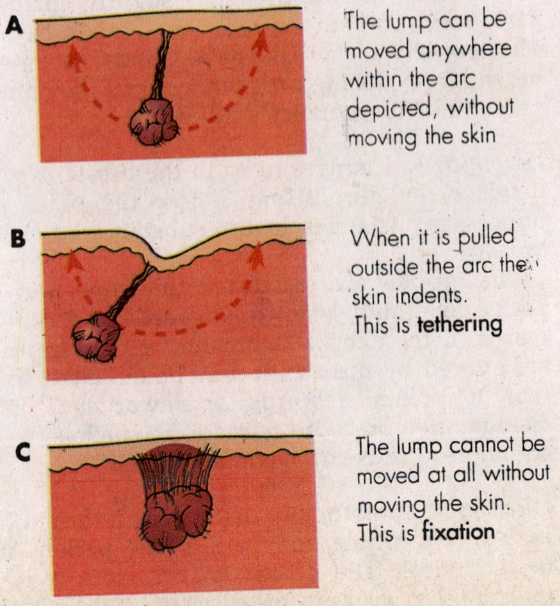

FIG. 12.3 Tethering and fixation

Ask the patient to rest her hand on her hip with the arm relaxed. Hold the lump between your thumb and fingers and estimate its mobility in two directions at right-angles to each other. Lumps that are attached to the underlying muscle can be moved quite a long way when the muscle is relaxed but are immobile if the disease has spread through the muscle to the bony chest wall.

Now ask the patient to press her hand against her hip to contract the pectoralis major muscle and re-estimate the mobility of the lump. If the lump is less mobile it must be tethered or fixed to the muscle. The less the movement, the more likely the lump is fixed rather than tethered.

Palpate the nipple

If the nipple is retracted, press gently on each side of it to see if it will evert. If the nipple has retracted spontaneously it can be everted by gentle pressure. If it has been pulled in by underlying disease it cannot be everted. Feel the breast deep to the nipple. If there is a palpable lump, see if moving it increases or causes nipple retraction.

If there is a discharge from the nipple, find its source by gently pressing on each segment of the breast and areola. Note whether it appears from one or many ducts. If the discharge is visible, try to decide if it is blood, serum, pus or milk. Test it for blood and take a bacteriological swab for culture.

Palpate the axilla and supraclavicular fossa

The axillary lymph nodes form a three-sided pyramid whose apex is in the narrow gap between the first rib and the axillary vessels.

Stand on the patient's right side. Take hold of her right elbow with your right hand and let her forearm rest on your right forearm. Persuade her to allow you to hold the weight of her arm. (Patients always want to help by holding their arm away from their side, but this tenses the muscles in the anterior and posterior axillary folds and makes palpation of the lymph nodes impossible.) Place your left hand flat against the chest wall and feel for any nodes that may lie in the central or medial aspects of the right axilla by sweeping the tips of your fingers across and from the top to the base of the axilla to catch the nodes against the chest wall.

To reach the apex of the axilla you will have to push the tips of your fingers upwards and inwards and this often causes discomfort. Explain to the patient that you must push firmly to examine thoroughly.

Next move your left hand anteriorly over the edge of the pectoralis minor muscle and downwards into the axillary tail and behind the edge of the pectoralis major. Turn your hand (or change hands) to feel the subscapular nodes on the posterior wall of the axilla, and finally feel the lateral aspect of the axilla, in case there are any brachial nodes level with the neck of the humerus.

Revision Panel 12.2

The changes which can occur in the nipple

- Destruction
- Depression (retraction or inversion)
- Discolouration
- Displacement
- Deviation
- Discharge
- Duplication

Revision Panel 12.3

The types of discharge from the nipple

Colour	*Cause*
Red (blood) Pink (serum + blood) Clear pale yellow (serum)	Duct papilloma Duct carcinoma Duct ectasia
Brown Green Black (breast secretions and debris)	Duct ectasia Cysts
Creamy white or yellow (pus)	Duct ectasia
Thin white (milk)	Lactation

To palpate the left axilla lean across the patient, hold her left elbow with your left hand and use your right hand to feel the axilla. If it is difficult to feel the axilla in this way move round to her left side.

In a fat patient it is sometimes easier to feel the posterior and apical nodes when standing behind the patient.

Remember that it is often possible to feel small, soft normal nodes in thin young women.

Palpate for glands in the **supraclavicular fossae** and in the lower deep cervical lymph chain.

Record the number, size, consistence and fixity of any glands that you can feel.

Examine the arms

Check that there is no swelling of the arms and that there are no venous, arterial or neurological abnormalities.

General examination

A full general examination is essential, but in a busy outpatient clinic concentrate on the abdomen for hepatomegaly and ascites, and the lumbar spine for pain and limitation of movement.

PRESENTATION OF BREAST DISEASE

Breast disease presents in six common ways:

1 A painless lump.
2 A painful lump.
3 Pain and tenderness but no lump.
4 Nipple discharge.
5 Changes in the nipple and areolar.
6 Changes in breast size.

The common conditions which cause these symptoms will be described individually, but the likely diagnoses when the patient presents with one of the above symptoms are:

A painless lump

Carcinoma.
Cyst.
Fibroadenoma.
Nodularity (fibroadenosis).

A painful lump

Cyclical nodularity (fibroadenosis).
Cyst.
Abscess (usually lactational).
Periductal (plasma-celled) mastitis.
Carcinoma (rare).

Pain and tenderness but no lump

Cyclical mastalgia
(including premenstrual tension).
Non-cyclical mastalgia.
Pregnancy mastitis.

Nipple discharge

Duct ectasia.
Duct papilloma.
Duct carcinoma.
Cysts.

Changes in the nipple and/or areola

Nipple retraction.
Congenital inversion.
Duct ectasia with periductal fibrosis.
Carcinoma.
Paget's disease.
Eczema.
Mammary duct fistula.

Changes in breast size

Pregnancy.
Carcinoma.
Benign hypertrophy.
Giant fibroadenoma.
Phylloides tumour.
Sarcoma.

The fact that many diagnoses are repeated in different sections explains why it is often difficult to make a definite clinical diagnosis.

Carcinoma of the female breast

Cancer of the breast is an adenocarcinoma, but one of its interesting histological features is the variable quantity of fibrous tissue that surrounds the cancer cells. Sometimes 90 per cent of the mass is fibrous stroma with just a few cancer cells scattered through it. This is the atrophic scirrhous' variety of cancer which is very slow growing and occurs in elderly women. At the other end of the spectrum there is the cancer with no fibrous reaction which may be so cellular, vascular and fast growing that it is clinically indistinguishable from acute inflammation.

The cut surface of a carcinoma is concave, rough, gritty and pale grey with prominent yellow and white flecks. The cut surface of benign lesions bulges out to become convex, is white rather than grey, and feels smooth and rubbery, not gritty.

HISTORY

Age Carcinoma of the breast can occur at any age after the menarche but is not very common in women under 30 years of age. Thereafter the incidence steadily increases to reach a peak in the mid-fifties.

Ethnic group There are unexplained geographical variations in the incidence of the disease. It is much less common in Japan.

Symptoms The presenting symptoms may be related to the primary lesion or rarely to the effects of secondary deposits.

The patient often notices **a painless lump** when washing or looking into a mirror. The size of the lump when first noticed does not give an accurate indication of its age.

Occasionally the patient notices **mild aches and pricking sensations** in the breast and finds a lump when feeling the painful area. This is an uncommon presentation for a carcinoma.

The shape and size of the breast may be distorted by an enlarging lump. Skin tethering and fixation can also distort the shape of the breast.

The nipple may be deviated, displaced, retracted, or destroyed.

The patient may notice a mass underneath the arm, caused by enlarged axillary lymph nodes.

Swelling of the arm, caused by lymphatic or venous obstruction in the axilla, is an uncommon presentation.

Backache, caused by infiltration and collapse of lumbar vertebrae, with nerve root pains radiating down the back of the legs, is a common symptom of advanced disseminated disease, but an uncommon mode of presentation.

There may be **general malaise and loss of weight; dyspnoea or pleuritic pain**, from extensive lung or pleural secondary deposits, and pleural effusions; **nodules in the skin; jaundice** from secondary infiltration of the liver; **mental changes and fits** from cerebral secondaries; and **pain from pathological fractures**.

Family history It is not uncommon to find that other female members of the family have suffered from the same disease. Rarely, all the female members of a family are afflicted.

Parity Carcinoma of the breast is more common in nulliparous women, and less common in women who have had many children and breast-fed them.

LOCAL EXAMINATION

A technique for examining the breast is described at the beginning of this chapter.

Site Approximately one-half of carcinomata of the breast occur in the upper outer quadrant. This quadrant includes the axillary tail, so do not forget to feel the axillary tail when palpating the breast. The axillary tail often extends a long way over the lateral edge of the pectoralis major muscle, up into the axilla.

Colour If the tumour is close to the surface the overlying skin may be discoloured. At first the hyperaemia around the tumour cells gives

Revision Panel 12.4

The cardinal signs of a late cancer of the breast

- Hard, non-tender, irregular lump
- Tethering or fixation of the lump
- Palpable axillary lymph nodes

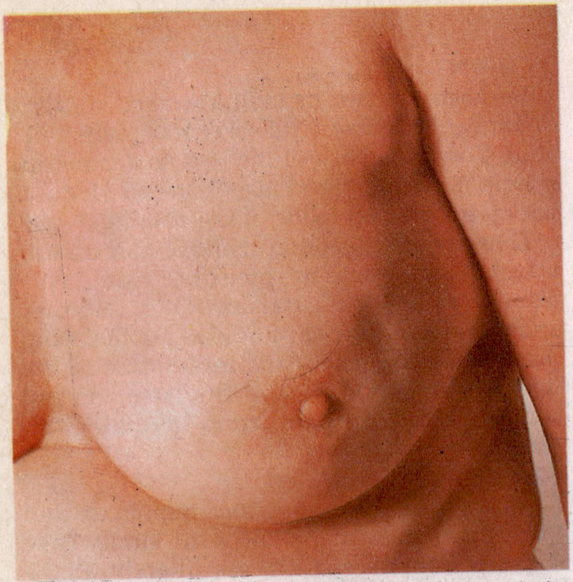

Retraction, deviation and displacement of the nipple. Puckering and tethering of the skin

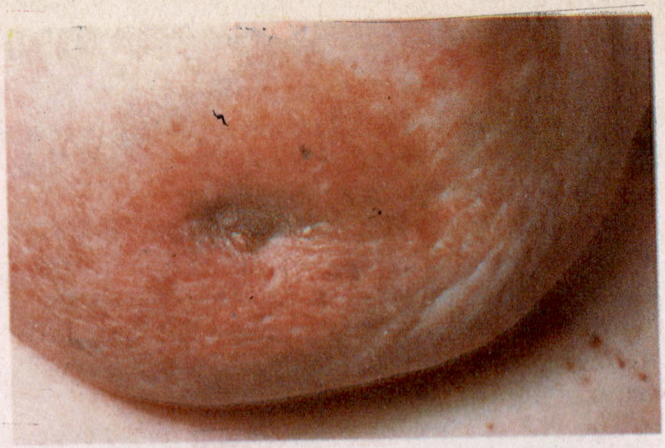

Peau d'orange

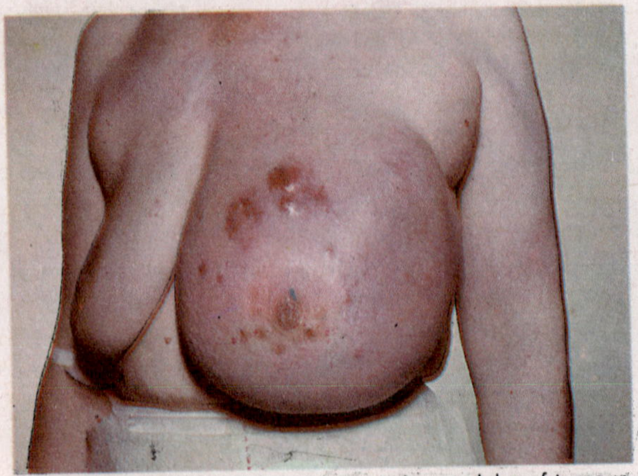

Enlargement of the breast with secondary nodules of tumour in the skin

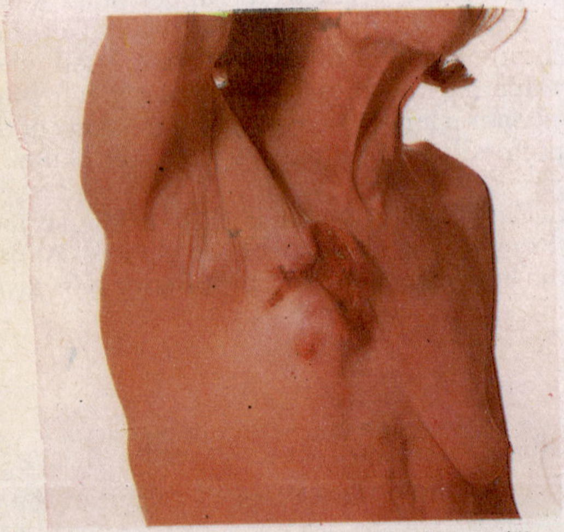

A fungating, foul-smelling ulcer with an everted edge, and enlarged, fixed axillary lymph glands

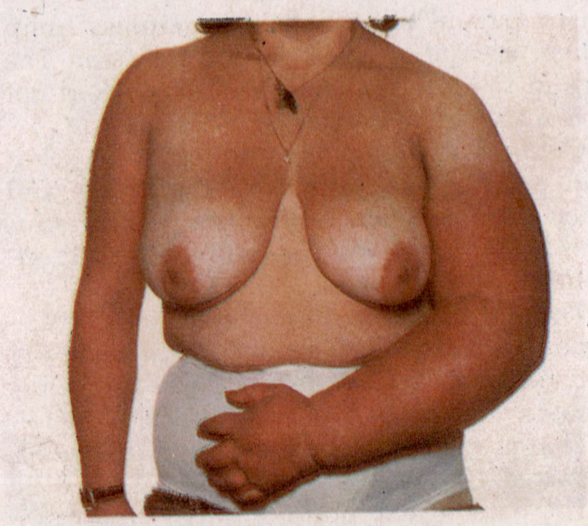

Secondary lymphoedema of the left arm caused by metastases in the lymph glands

FIG. 12.4 SOME DIAGNOSTIC FEATURES OF ADVANCED CARCINOMA OF THE BREAST

The Manchester classification

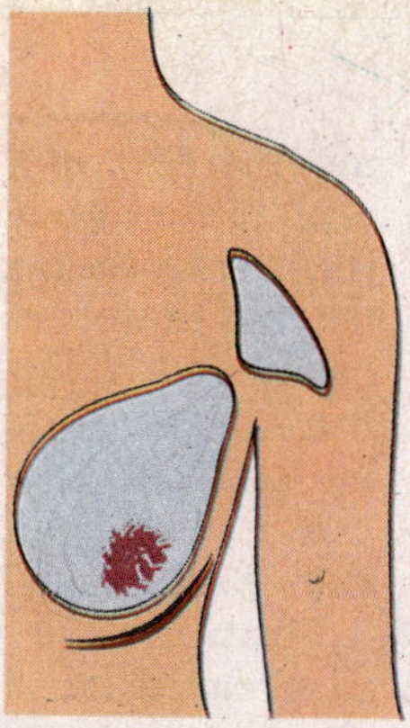

Stage I
A mobile lump in the breast.
No palpable axillary lymph glands

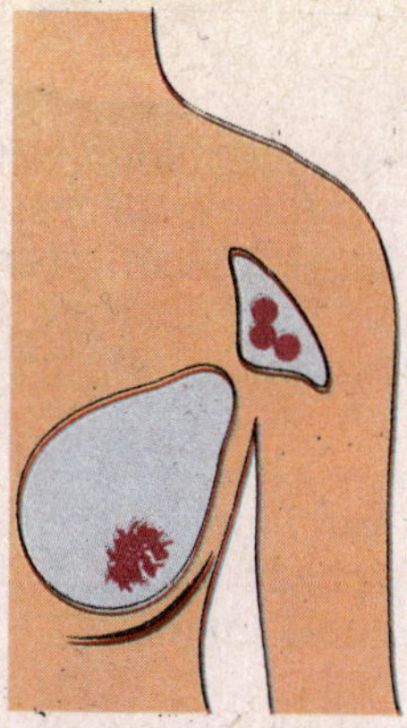

Stage II
A mobile lump in the breast ± some tethering.
Palpable mobile axillary lymph glands

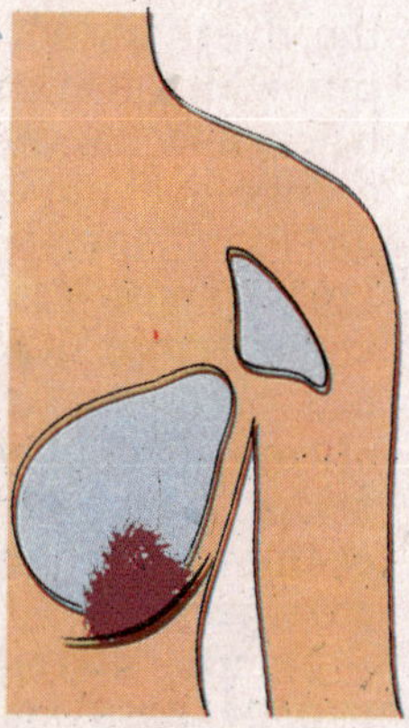

Stage III
A fixed lump in the breast with or without palpable mobile axillary glands

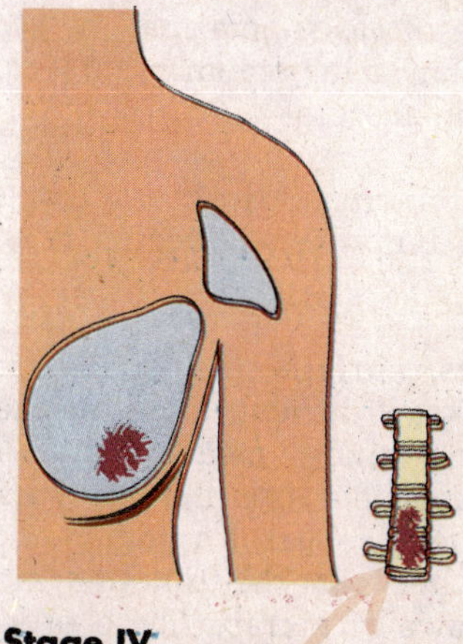

Stage IV
Distant metastases.
State of lump in breast irrelevant

The International TNM classification

T = Tumour

- T_1 2cm diameter or less. No fixation or tethering
- T_2 2–5cm diameter (or less than 2cm) with tethering or nipple retraction
- T_3 5–10cm diameter (or less than 5cm) with infiltration, ulceration or peau d'orange over the tumour, or deep fixation
- T_4 Any tumour with infiltration or ulceration wider than its diameter. Tumours larger than 10cm

N = Nodes

- N_0 No palpable axillary nodes
- N_1 Mobile palpable axillary nodes
- N_2 Fixed axillary nodes
- N_3 Palpable supraclavicular nodes. Oedema of the arm

M = Metastases

- M_0 No evidence of distant metastases
- M_1 Distant metastases

FIG. 12.5 The basic features of the two common classifications of carcinoma of the breast

the skin a reddish-purple colour, but once the skin is completely infiltrated it becomes less vascular and looks yellow or pearly white. The degree to which these changes are visible also depends upon the amount of skin oedema.

Tenderness Most carcinomata are not tender, but palpation may produce a mild discomfort, not bad enough to call a pain.

Temperature The temperature of the lump and the overlying skin depends upon the rate of growth of the tumour and its vascularity. The common scirrhous carcinoma is not vascular and has the same temperature as the surrounding tissue, but the anaplastic 'encephaloid' type of carcinoma may be so hot and make the skin so hyperaemic that it can be mistaken for an abscess.

Shape Carcinoma of the breast can grow into any shape but when it begins it is roughly spherical.

Surface Its surface is usually indistinct, which makes it difficult to define the shape.

The word 'cancer' means a crab. The comparison arose because the cut surface of a cancer usually reveals a number of processes extending out from the tumour which resemble the claws of a crab. These processes are masses of invading tumour cells and it is their presence which makes the surface indistinct.

A few carcinomata are encapsulated and have a smooth surface.

Composition Carcinomata are solid so they do not fluctuate, transilluminate or have a fluid thrill. Their consistence is normally **very hard**. The term **stony hard** gives a good impression of the typical texture of a carcinoma. However, the cellular, vascular tumours are soft, so do not attribute too much significance to the absence of a stony hard consistence.

Relations to surrounding structures The terms 'tethering' and 'fixation' have already been defined.

If a lump is tethered to the skin it behaves as if it is tied to it by a piece of string. It can move freely and independently of the skin within the limits determined by the length of the string, but pulls the skin when moved beyond these limits. If a lump is fixed it cannot be moved independently. Carcinoma of the breast can be tethered or fixed to the overlying skin or to deep structures.

It may infiltrate through the muscle into the chest wall. Such a cancer will be fixed.

Fixation of a lump to the skin **is almost diagnostic** of a carcinoma. Only chronic abscesses and fat necrosis can have the same sign. Nowadays both these conditions are relatively uncommon.

When a tumour spreads along the fibrous septa of the breast it blocks the lymphatics which run with them. This causes oedema of the overlying skin between the many small pits which mark the openings of the hair follicles and sweat glands. The result is an orange-peel appearance – **peau d'orange**.

Lymph drainage The axillary and supraclavicular lymph nodes are often enlarged (but not necessary involved with tumour). But always remember that the internal mammary nodes, which are beyond the reach of your examining fingers, are also likely to be enlarged.

Lymph nodes containing metastases are usually hard and discrete. As they enlarge they may mat together and become adherent to nearby structures such as the skin, axillary vessels and nerves.

Nearby tissues Extensive involvement of the axillary nodes may cause **lymphoedema of the arm** or venous thrombosis and **venous oedema**.

The other breast may contain a lump which the patient has not noticed. Such a lump may be a secondary deposit or another primary lesion. The lymph nodes in the **opposite axilla and supraclavicular fossa** may also be enlarged.

General examination

A full general examination is essential to detect the presence of metastases. The common sites for metastases from the breast are:

- *The skeleton* – especially the lumbar spine, causing backache, reduced spine and hip movements, lumbago and sciatica, and pathological fractures.
- *The lungs* – causing pulmonary consolidation and collapse, and pleural effusions.
- *The liver* – making it palpable and nodular, and causing jaundice and ascites.
- *The skin* – causing multiple hard nodules.
- *The brain* – causing motor, sensory and psychological defects.

Painful nodularity

For many years this condition was called 'chronic mastitis'. It is now generally accepted that that was a bad name because there is no clinical or microscopical evidence of an inflammatory process; but the name is still sometimes used.

The same is true for many other names used for the same condition, such as fibroadenosis, fibrocystic disease and cystic hyperplasia. These names are derived from the histological features of breast biopsies, such as fibrosis, adenosis, microcyst formation, epithelial hyperplasia and lymphocytic infiltration. However, studies of normal breasts have shown that all these changes are non-specific and often present in women without breast complaints. They simply represent the histological appearances of the dynamic changes that occur throughout normal reproductive life – during breast development, cyclical menstrual change and pregnancy, and menopausal involution.

In fact most of the conditions which lead a woman of reproductive age to seek medical advice in relation to her breasts are merely minor variations (or, in severe cases, aberrations) of normal processes. These aberrations are believed to be caused by very minor hormonal imbalances during the multiple menstrual cycles of the reproductive period of her life.

The terminology now used is one which describes the clinical presentation – **mastalgia** (if it is pain), **nodularity** and **macrocysts**. Histological descriptions are used only when the changes are outside the range of normality (e.g. epithelial hyperplasia with atypical cells) and when they describe a particular appearance, such as sclerosing adenosis.

A generic term which recognizes the pathogenesis of these conditions but introduces no inaccurate terminology, and is currently gaining acceptance, is Aberrations of Normal Development and Involution (ANDI), used in conjunction with the simple descriptive terms, mastalgia and nodularity.

The commonest manifestation of ANDI is cyclical pain and nodularity seen in the premenstrual period. Although pain (mastalgia) and nodularity frequently coexist, they are best considered and assessed separately when one or other dominates. Cysts are the third important element. **Microcysts** are an extremely common variant of normal involution and are clinically unimportant, but a macrocyst is the commonest cause of a discrete lump in the 35–55 age group.

Nodularity (diffuse or local) and macrocysts

HISTORY

Age The symptoms of nodularity and macrocysts occur during the years of ovarian activity, from menarche to menopause. They commonly begin in the early twenties and reach a peak between the ages of 35 and 55 years. A few symptoms may persist for a short time after the menopause.

Symptoms Most patients present complaining of one or more **lumps in the breasts**. The majority also complain of **mild tenderness**, which may be periodic, becoming worse just before menstruation (*premenstrual tension*), and there may be other signs of premenstrual water retention, such as oedema of the ankles, thirst and irritability. It is often the tenderness which draws the patient's attention to the lump because these nodules are often in the upper outer quadrant of the breast where, because they are rubbed by clothing or arm movements, they are noticed earlier than lumps in the centre or inner half of the breast.

Sometimes nodularity causes **enlargement of the breast** without pain. This change is also often periodic and maximal just before menstruation, but it can be unrelated to menstruation and slowly progressive for weeks or months.

Many patients have had their symptoms for months or years before they see a doctor because they ignore minor symptoms in the breast associated with the menstrual cycle. Some patients may even have had a lump for a long time but ignored it because it only appears for a few days before each menstruation and then disappears.

A history which suggests that the lump **fluctuates in size** is typical of cyclical nodularity and almost excludes the diagnosis of carcinoma.

LOCAL EXAMINATION

The most important decision to be made on examination is whether the nodularity is focal (when it must always be taken seriously) or diffuse. The latter is very common since most women experience some degree of tenderness and nodularity in the upper outer quadrant of the breast in the premenstrual week.

Diffuse cyclical nodularity can occur anywhere in the breast, but is most commonly bilateral and found mainly in the upper outer quadrant and axillary tail. If the patient is first seen in the premenstrual period, it is useful to examine her again in the first half of the cycle, when the changes may be much less obvious.

Focal nodularity is an area of nodularity which is different from the rest of the breast (a 'dominant' nodule) and is always significant, no matter how diffusely nodular the rest of the breast may be.

Position Nodularity and macrocysts may occur in any part of the breast, but the **upper outer quadrant and axillary tail** are the areas most often affected.

Colour The colour of the skin over the lump is normal. The subcutaneous veins may be engorged in breasts which have an exaggerated premenstrual change.

Large cysts, close to the skin, have a bluish-green tinge – the blue-domed cyst of Bloodgood.

Tenderness The tenderness of a patch of nodularity is very variable. It is usually possible to palpate the breast firmly without causing much discomfort.

Shape, surface and composition The contour and surface of simple nodularity differs from those of a cyst.

Focal (solid) nodularity has no characteristic size, shape or surface. It is of moderate (rubbery) hardness, moderately mobile within the breast and lacks skin or deep attachment and significant lymphadenopathy.

A solitary cyst is smooth, spherical and of variable consistence – varying from soft and cystic to a hardness equal to cancer. It is rarely possible to elicit fluctuation, a fluid thrill or transillumination. The clinical diagnosis of a cyst usually rests upon its smooth spherical shape.

Multiple macrocysts may be sufficiently discrete to feel like a bunch of grapes, but more often form an irregular mass with a distinct surface and outline in some parts, and an indistinct outline in others.

Relations to surrounding structures Macrocysts and patches of focal nodularity are not fixed or tethered to the skin or the underlying muscle and are usually moderately mobile within the breast.

Local lymph nodes The axillary nodes should not be enlarged.

Local tissues The tissues of the chest wall, arm and neck should be normal. The other

Revision Panel 12.5

The causes of cystic swellings in the breast

- Simple macrocyst
- Galactocele
- Chronic abscess
- Haematoma
- Cystic degeneration of a colloid carcinoma
- Hydatid cyst
- Lymph cyst

breast may be affected by diffuse subclinical disease, giving it a granular, 'shotty' texture.

GENERAL EXAMINATION

Although the changes in the breast may be caused by minor variations in hormone balance, these variations affect only the breast and there are never any systemic signs of abnormal hormone secretion.

Mastalgia

Where pain is a dominant symptom it needs to be assessed apart from nodularity. The history is explored to divide it into cyclical (premenstrual) and non-cyclical (irregular or continuous) mastalgia.

Cyclical mastalgia is one facet of the cyclical pain and nodularity complex described above and rarely, if ever, reflects any serious underlying condition. If it extends beyond the common 10 days premenstrually, its severity should be assessed in relation to the interference it causes in quality of life related to work and family, since severe cases may warrant treatment.

Non-cyclical mastalgia is a poorly defined condition. Some cases have a musculoskeletal origin from the chest wall; other cases seem to be associated with inflammatory episodes caused by duct ectasia or periductal mastitis. But remember, a persistent, localized pain or discomfort can be a symptom of cancer.

Fibroadenoma

A fibroadenoma is a benign neoplasm of the breast in which the fibromatous element is the dominant feature. The cut surface of a fibroadenoma reveals lobules of whorled, white fibrous tissue which bulge out of their capsules.

There are two histological varieties of fibroadenomata. **Pericanalicular** fibroadenomata mainly consist of fibrous tissue surrounding a few small tubular glands. They tend to be small and hard. **Intracanalicular** fibroadenomata contain more glands which are indented by the fibrous tissue and stretched into elongated, spidery shapes. They are usually larger and softer than the pericanalicular type.

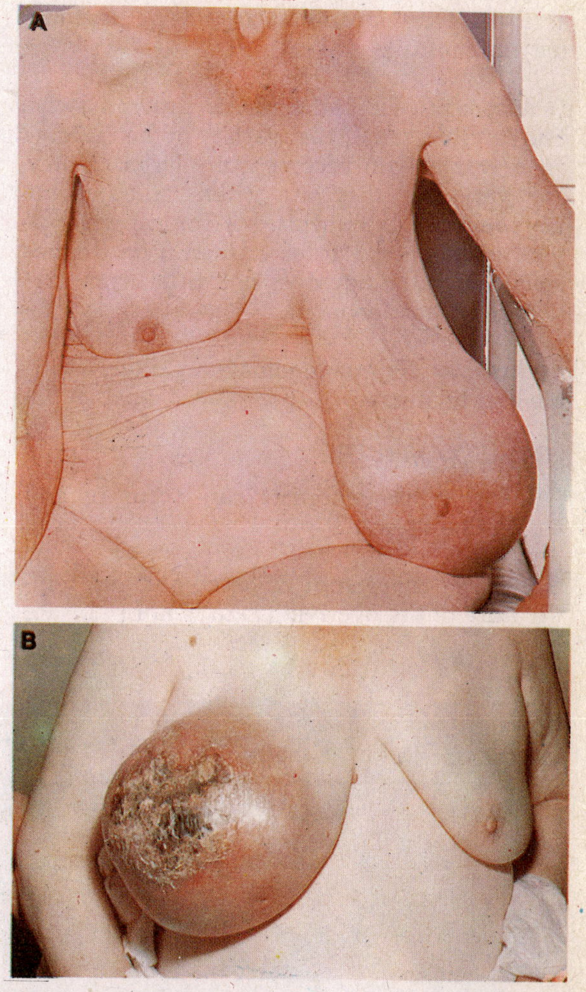

FIG. 12.6 **A**: A giant fibroadenoma of the left breast. **B**: A large phylloides tumour (Brodie's tumour) causing necrosis of the overlying skin (see page 313)

HISTORY

Age The small, hard fibroadenoma is found in young women between the ages of 15 and 30 years. The larger softer fibroadenoma is found in women at the extremes of reproductive life, just after the menarche or in the perimenopausal period.

Symptoms The patient presents with a lump in the breast which she has usually noticed by accident. Fibroadenomata are **not painful** but may be multiple.

Development Fibroadenomata grow slowly. The soft intracanalicular variety in the middle-aged woman can become quite large. If they are very big they are often called **giant fibroadenomata** but this is a clinical description based on size (greater than 5 cm diameter); their pathology does not differ from that of other fibroadenomata.

Multiplicity Fibroadenomata are often multiple and bilateral.

LOCAL EXAMINATION

Position Fibroadenomata can occur in any part of the breast.

Colour and temperature The colour and temperature of the overlying skin is normal.

Tenderness Fibroadenomata are not tender.

Shape These tumours consist of whorls of fibrous tissue which form separate lobules, making them spherical, ovoid or knobbly. They are usually 1–3 cm in diameter.

Surface The surface is **smooth and bosselated.** Only the smallest tumours consist of one lobule and are spherical. The edge of the lump is quite distinct.

Composition Fibroadenomata are **solid** tumours with the consistence of **firm rubber**. They are dull to percussion and do not fluctuate.

Relations to surrounding tissues These tumours are not fixed to the skin or the deep structures. Although they lie within the breast and are derived from breast tissue they are **highly mobile**. It is often necessary to get the patient to find and fix the lump for you, before you can examine it. Such mobility, without tethering,

Revision Panel 12.6

A comparison of the clinical features of four common breast lumps

Type of lump	*Age (years)*	*Pain*	*Surface*	*Consistence*	*Axilla*
Solitary cyst	35–55	Occasionally	Smooth	Soft to hard	Normal
Nodularity	20–55	Occasionally	Indistinct	Mixed	Normal
Fibroadenoma	15–55	No	Smooth and bosselated	Rubbery	Normal
Carcinoma	35+	No	Irregular	Stony hard	Nodes may be palpable

Revision Panel 12.7

A simplified plan for the diagnosis of the common breast lumps

Define the surface and shape and then define the consistence.

- Irregular and indistinct
  - Hard → Carcinoma
  - Rubbery → Nodularity
- Smooth and well defined
  - Hard → Cyst
  - Rubbery → Fibroadenoma

excludes carcinoma from the differential diagnosis and has given rise to the colloquialism *breast mouse.*

Lymph nodes The axillary lymph nodes should not be enlarged.

Local tissues Apart from the possibility of finding a similar lump in the other breast, all the adjacent tissues should be normal.

GENERAL EXAMINATION

Fibroadenomata are not associated with any other abnormalities.

Acute breast abscess

Bacteria can enter and infect the breast through the lactiferous ducts that open on the nipple, or through the blood stream. The former is the common route, especially during pregnancy and lactation when the breasts are engorged and hyperaemic, and the nipples are subjected to the trauma of suckling.

HISTORY

Age Breast abscess is uncommon outside the childbearing age.

Symptoms The commonest presenting symptom is **pain**. At first it is a dull ache, but as the pus forms it becomes a **severe, continuous throbbing** pain and the painful area becomes very tender.

The patient may feel **a lump** or notice a diffuse swelling in the breast and redness of the overlying skin. She may also complain that the breast feels **hot**, internally and externally, when she palpates it.

The general symptoms of infection, **malaise, night sweats, flushes and rigors**, may be present.

Development If untreated, the symptoms get progressively worse until the pus bursts through the skin.

Social history Cracks in the skin of the nipple, which are a common cause of breast abscesses, are more common in women who do not keep the skin of their breasts and nipples spotlessly clean during breast-feeding.

LOCAL EXAMINATION

Position Abscesses can occur in any part of the breast.

Colour and temperature The overlying skin is red and hot, and it may also be oedematous.

Tenderness The whole of the inflamed area is tender but the most tender spot is over the centre of the abscess where the pus is collecting.

Shape, size and surface Most abscesses are spherical but the surrounding oedema and inflammation makes their shape and surface indefinable. They vary in size. Neglected abscesses can become so big that they fill the whole breast.

Composition The composition of an abscess changes with its development. Before any pus forms, when it is an inflammatory mass, it may be soft/solid, tender and diffuse. As the pus collects in its centre it becomes harder and more tender. Ultimately, the volume of pus may become large enough and sufficiently close to the skin to be fluctuant; but it will not transilluminate, and the outer surface of the mass will still be indistinct.

Relations to surrounding structures As the abscess grows it becomes fixed to the skin, which turns red and shiny, and may also become fixed deeply.

Lymph drainage The axillary lymph nodes will probably be enlarged, firm and tender.

State of local tissues The whole of the breast is likely to be engorged and slightly tender. If the **nipple** was the site of entry of the infection it may still be tender, thickened and cracked.

GENERAL EXAMINATION

There will be a tachycardia and pyrexia.

Recurrent and chronic breast abscess

Most recurrent and chronic breast abscesses occur in association with the duct ectasia or periductal mastitis complex. In this condition stagnant secretions from the dilated ducts (similar to bronchiectasis) leak out and cause a chemical and/or bacterial periductal mastitis. The inflammatory infiltrate often contains a predominance of plasma cells ('plasma cell mastitis') or foreign-body giant cells (often misdiagnosed in the past as fat necrosis). The associated **periductal fibrosis** often leads to **nipple retraction.**

The inflammatory process develops and regresses very rapidly (within a few days) but recurs frequently, each time more severe, eventually to present as an abscess at the edge of the areola. A common subgroup occurs in young women with congenitally inverted nipples.

Simple drainage of the abscess leaves a fistula into the affected duct – a **mammary duct fistula**. This has a very characteristic appearance – an **inverted nipple** with **distortion of the areola** and a **sinus** at its edge. Abscesses will keep recurring until the fistula is excised.

Periductal mastitis will sometimes develop into a chronic abscess (again, usually para-areola) which presents as a tender mass with a thick wall, skin fixity, oedema, nipple retraction and enlarged axillary lymph glands – features which make it indistinguishable, clinically, from cancer.

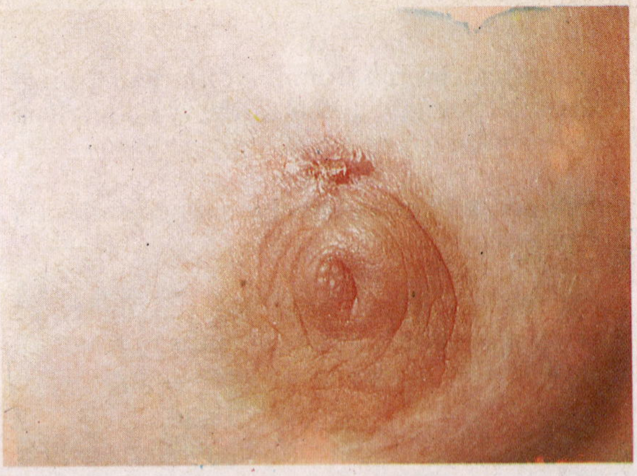

FIG. 12.7 A mammary fistula. This tract connects with a mammary duct. Recurrent infection causes recurrent acute breast abscesses

Fat necrosis

This is a rare condition in which an injury to the breast may cause death of some of the fat cells and saponification of their fat, which turns into a cyst containing thick oily fluid. Rarely the damaged fat turns into a small, hard mass resembling a cancer.

In the past fat necrosis was thought always to form a hard mass fixed to the skin, with nipple inversion (resembling cancer), but most times these were probably cases of misdiagnosed periductal mastitis.

Most cases of 'fat necrosis' first noticed after injury, which the patient thinks has stimulated cancer, prove to have been cancer all the time! The solid form of fat necrosis is very rare and should not be diagnosed except by biopsy.

Revision Panel 12.8

The breast changes of pregnancy

- Fullness and pricking sensations
- Enlargement
- Distended subcutaneous veins
- Increased nipple and areolar pigmentation
- Circumareolar pigmentation
- Hypertrophy of subareolar sebaceous glands (Montgomery's tubercles)
- A clear, expressible secretion (colostrum)

Pregnancy

Pregnancy is the commonest cause of changes in the breast.

Within a few weeks of the ovum being fertilized the breasts become tense, heavy and slightly uncomfortable. Many women notice pricking sensations deep inside the breast.

By 2 months the breasts are enlarged and feel granular – even 'lumpy' in texture. The subcutaneous veins dilate and become prominent, and the skin of the breasts is warm. The nipples enlarge and the areolae become darker. The skin around the areolae may also become slightly pigmented. The sebaceous glands of the areolae become larger and the skin over them appears stretched and pale. The lumps they form are called Montgomery's tubercles.

By the fourth month a thin clear secretion can be expressed from the nipple.

Duct papilloma and carcinoma

A benign or malignant papilliferous tumour may grow in a collecting duct and, long before it becomes big enough to form a palpable lump, may ulcerate, bleed and cause a blood-stained discharge from the nipple. If it blocks the duct it may cause a retention cyst.

HISTORY

Age Duct papillomata are most common in women 30–40 years old. Over the age of 40 years the chance of papilliferous lesions in the lactiferous ducts being malignant increases significantly.

Symptoms The commonest symptom is a **bloody or serous discharge from the nipple**. Although the blood loss is small, often just enough to stain the patient's underclothes, it is usually dark red or pink coloured and coagulates so the patient recognizes it as blood.

The patient may notice a **swelling, deep to, or just lateral to, the areola**. The lump may fluctuate in size and be painful as it enlarges. Pressure on the lump may produce the discharge from the nipple.

Rarely, the primary lesion is symptomless and the patient presents with enlarged axillary nodes or the symptoms of distant metastases.

EXAMINATION

The discharge The discharge may be visible on the patient's clothes or appear when the breast is squeezed. Try to find out which part of the breast is producing the blood by gently compressing each quadrant of the breast, and then small sections of the areola.

Always confirm that the discharge is blood by testing it with one of the commercial tests used for urine analysis or by inspecting a smear of the discharge with a microscope.

The lump If a lump is present it can be solid and have all the features of a carcinoma (already described), or be fusiform, tense and fluctuant, with its long axis lying radially to the nipple – the signs of a retention cyst of a lactiferous duct.

Axilla The axillary lymph nodes may be enlarged if the lesion is a duct carcinoma.

Phylloides tumour (Brodie's disease)

Brodie gave the name cystosarcoma phylloides to a large tumour of the breast which was cystic, had a cut surface resembling a leaf or fern (phylloides) and which he believed to be sarcomatous. This name has been discarded in favour of phylloides tumour (benign or malignant) because most are benign and many are not cystic; nor do they all show the leaf-like appearances.

The clinical features do not differ from those of a giant fibroadenoma – the differentiation from phylloides tumour is made only on histology. Both are tumours showing mixed epithelial and connective tissue elements. The epithelial element is benign in both (if it were malignant it would be a cancer). When the connective tissue (fibrous stroma) element is bland it is called a fibroadenoma (whether it is large or small). When the connective tissue element is abnormal it is called a phylloides tumour (again, whether it is large or small). The degree of histological abnormality of the connective tissue determines whether it is benign or malignant. Even the very large, characteristic tumours described by Brodie are commonly benign. These very large tumours are so characteristic that their clinical features warrant description, but it should be remembered that they represent just one end of a clinical spectrum which covers all sizes of tumours.

HISTORY

Age Brodie's (phylloides) tumour usually presents between the ages of 50 and 70 years.

Symptoms The patient may notice a large **lump in the breast**, but more often complains of **enlargement of the whole breast**. Brodie's disease is one of the causes of massive enlargement of the breast.

The skin is usually white and stretched; rarely it is reddened and contains a **small ulcer** from pressure necrosis of the overlying skin. The ulcer produces a serosanguinous discharge.

Pain is an uncommon symptom.

LOCAL EXAMINATION

(see Fig. 12.6, page 309)

Site The lump may be in any part of the breast.

Colour The overlying skin may be shiny, red or bluish. Necrotic patches will be black.

Temperature The temperature of the skin over the lump is normal.

Tenderness The lump is not tender but the edges of the ulcer, if present, are tender – unlike the edges of a fungating carcinoma.

Shape and size The lump is basically spherical but is often lobulated. These tumours grow slowly to a large size, 20–30 cm in diameter.

Surface Their surface is smooth and distinct.

Composition As the tumour is solid with areas of cystic degeneration it has a variable texture – spongy in places, hard in others. It is dull to percussion and does not fluctuate.

Ulcer If there is an ulcer present it will have a punched-out edge of healthy sensitive skin and a base of grey–white tumour covered with poor-quality granulation tissue.

Because the tumour is encapsulated there is sometimes a plane of cleavage between it and the subcutaneous tissue. A probe can be passed easily under the edge of the ulcer into this gap. This never occurs with a carcinoma.

Relations to surrounding structures While the tumour remains encapsulated it is not fixed to the skin or the underlying muscles, but it may be so big that the absence of fixation may not be demonstrable. If the lesion becomes truly sarcomatous it infiltrates the surrounding tissues.

Lymph nodes The axillary nodes are enlarged only if there is secondary infection in an ulcer.

State of local tissues The surrounding tissues are normal.

GENERAL EXAMINATION

There should be no other abnormalities except on the very rare occasion when the lesion has become truly sarcomatous and has spread via the blood stream to the lungs and the liver.

Revision Panel 12.9

The causes of massive enlargement of the breast

- Benign hypertrophy (usually bilateral)
- Giant fibroadenoma
- Phylloides tumour (Brodie's disease)
- Sarcoma
- Colloid carcinoma
- Filarial elephantiasis

Benign hyperplasia of the breast

Sometimes the breasts enlarge to a degree far beyond that which can be considered normal. This is called idiopathic benign hypertrophy. The cause is not known.

At first the breasts feel normal, but as they become gross they become **nodular** and **tender**. The subcutaneous veins become engorged and there is a characteristic grooving of the shoulders from pressure of the brassière straps.

Benign hyperplasia is **disfiguring** and **embarrassing** to the patient. It can be unilateral.

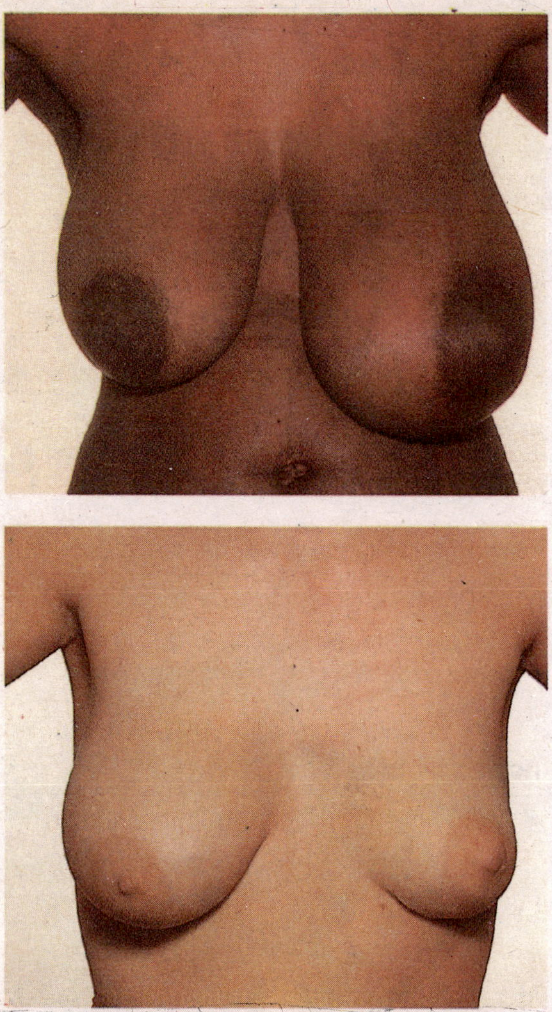

FIG. 12.8 Benign hyperplasia of the breast. This condition is usually bilateral, though often slightly asymmetrical (**A**) but can be unilateral (**B**)

THE NIPPLE

The nipple may undergo a number of changes, many of which have already been described. In many cases the change is diagnostic of the underlying lesion. For example, destruction, retraction, displacement and elevation usually indicate an underlying carcinoma.

Discharge from the nipple is classified in Revision Panel 12.3, page 301.

Paget's disease

Paget's disease of the nipple is caused by an intraduct carcinoma which begins in the epithelium of a main collecting lactiferous duct, and then **spreads within the duct epithelium** up to the skin of the nipple and down into the substance of the breast.

When the intraepithelial carcinoma reaches the skin of the nipple it causes changes similar to an eczema. Patches of skin first become red, and then encrusted and oozy; but the edges of these lesions are distinct, unlike an eczema, and they do not itch (although the patient often complains of abnormal sensations and pricking feelings).

As the months and years pass, the nipple is eventually destroyed, leaving a patch of weeping ulceration.

In the early stages of the disease there may be no other detectable abnormality in the breast, but ultimately a lump develops deep to the nipple. This is the carcinoma spreading into the breast substance.

Revision Panel 12.10

The differences between eczema of the nipple and Paget's disease

Eczema	*Paget's disease*
Bilateral	Unilateral
Commonly occurs at lactation	Occurs at menopause
Itches	Does not itch
Vesicles	No vesicles
Nipple intact	Nipple may be destroyed
No lumps	May be an underlying lump

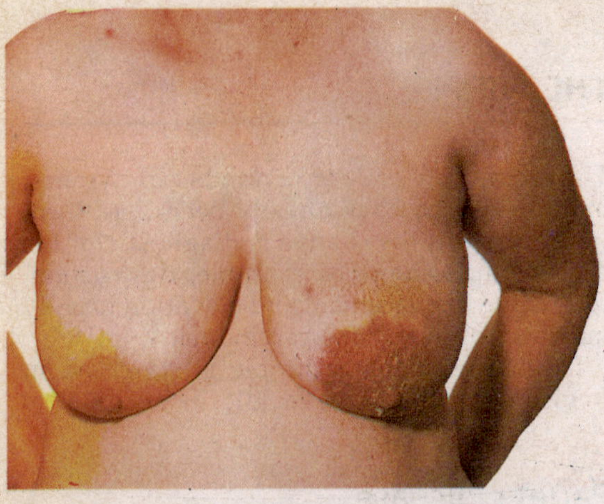

Florid exudative eczema of the left nipple and areola

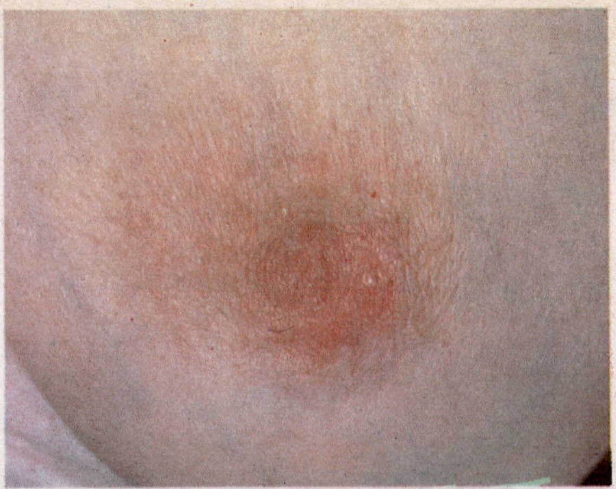

Paget's disease of the left nipple. The skin of the outer lower quadrant of the areola is red and slightly thickened. Careful palpation revealed the mass of a small underlying carcinoma

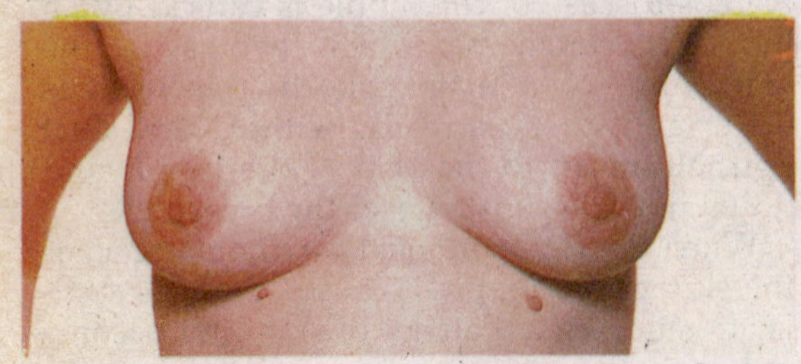

Supernumerary nipples

FIG. 12.9 THE NIPPLE

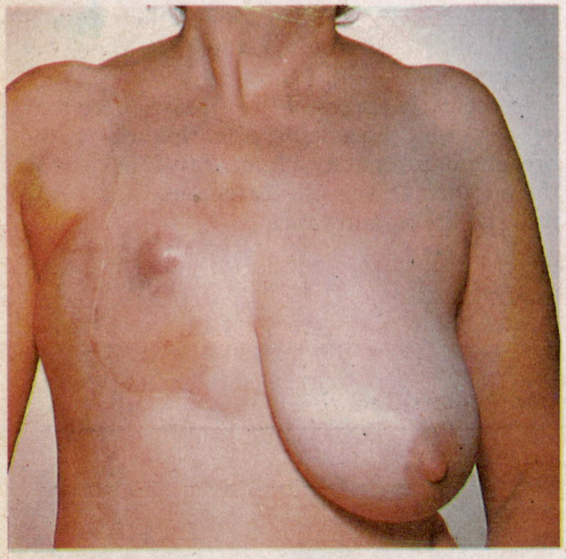

Recurrent nodules in the skin flaps

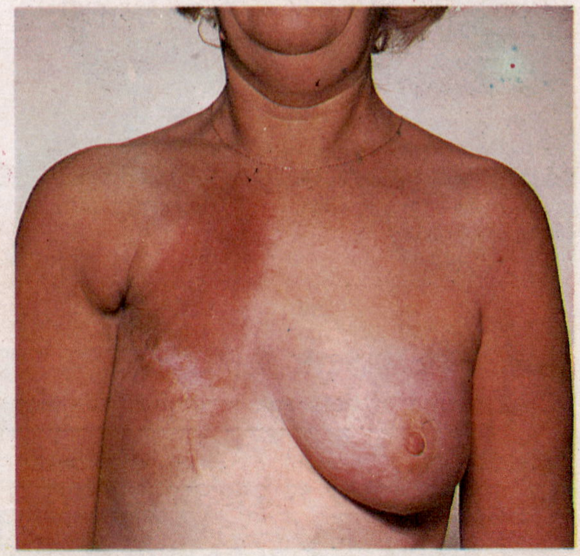

Telangiectases caused by radiotherapy

FIG. 12.10 TWO COMMON APPEARANCES AFTER MASTECTOMY

Many women do not come and complain of the early skin changes because they think they have a mild skin disease. Consequently at least half have a palpable lump in the breast by the time they come to a surgical clinic, and some have palpable axillary lymph nodes.

Apart from its unusual site and presentation, the intraepithelial carcinoma which causes Paget's disease is no different in its general behaviour and prognosis from any other type of cancer of the breast.

THE MALE BREAST

There are two causes of enlargement of the male breast: one is benign and common – gynaecomastia; the other is malignant and rare – carcinoma.

Gynaecomastia

This is a condition in which there is an increase in the ductal and connective tissue elements of the breast. It may be induced by hormones, drugs or general illnesses, but the precise mechanisms by which these stimuli instigate overgrowth of the breast is not known. The majority of cases are idiopathic.

HISTORY

Age The patient may be of any age. The peak incidence of the hard variety is between the ages of 10 and 30 years. The peak incidence of the soft variety is between 60 and 80 years, in men being treated for carcinoma of the prostate gland with oestrogens.

Symptoms The patient complains of painless, or slightly tender, **enlargement of one or both breasts**. Schoolboys with gynaecomastia are often teased by their classmates.

Previous history There may be a history of a recent illness, such as hepatitis, malnutrition or renal failure.

Drug history Ask the patient if he has been taking oestrogens, tranquillizers, diuretics, digitalis, cimetidine or steroids, because all these drugs may induce gynaecomastia.

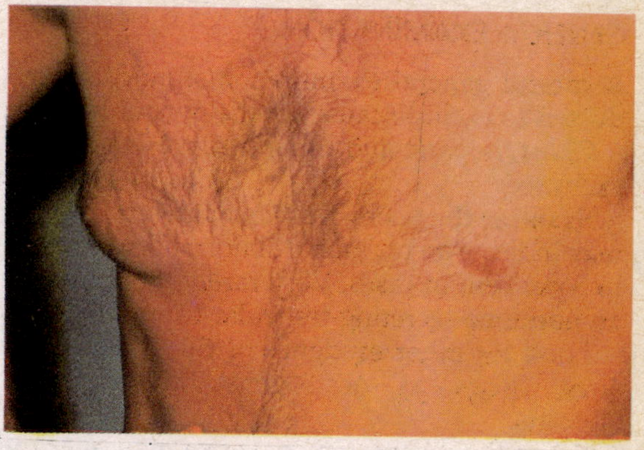

FIG. 12.11 Unilateral 'soft' gynaecomastia in a man taking oestrogens. The bilateral gynaecomastia of adolescents is usually less prominent and 'hard'

LOCAL EXAMINATION

Position One or both breasts may be enlarged.

Tenderness They are not usually tender.

Size The degree of enlargement varies. The breasts may become so large that they look female in character, but more often in the younger age group the enlargement just causes a diffuse fullness deep to the nipple.

Composition The texture of the enlarged breast may be **soft or hard**. These two varieties are sometimes distinguished by calling them 'true gynaecomastia' and 'mammaplasia', respectively. I do not think it worthwhile differentiating them in this way.

Hard enlargement is localized to the subareolar region and causes a firm disc of tissue beneath the areola that may be slightly tender and feels rough and gritty in texture. It is mobile and not attached to the skin or the deep structures. The **hard** enlargement is the variety commonly seen in young pubertal and adolescent boys.

Soft enlargement is most often caused by drug therapy.

Lymph drainage The axillary lymph glands should not be enlarged.

Local tissue All the nearby tissues are normal.

GENERAL EXAMINATION

A careful general examination should be conducted to exclude causes of the gynaecomastia.

Chest, hepatic and renal diseases should be excluded.

Examine the testes. Testicular atrophy, which may indicate an hormonal abnormality, is found in 5 per cent of cases. Very rarely there may be an hormone-secreting testicular tumour.

Look for other evidence of the ingestion of such drugs as oestrogens, digitalis and steroids.

When the disease presents in a man over the age of 30 years it is highly likely that you will find one of the precipitating causes mentioned above. Cases presenting between the ages 12 and 25 years are probably caused by an intrinsic, unimportant change of hormone balance in a completely fit patient.

Revision Panel 12.11

The varieties of true mastitis

- Neonatal (caused by maternal hormones)
- Milk engorgement during lactation
- Diffuse infection during lactation
- Mumps

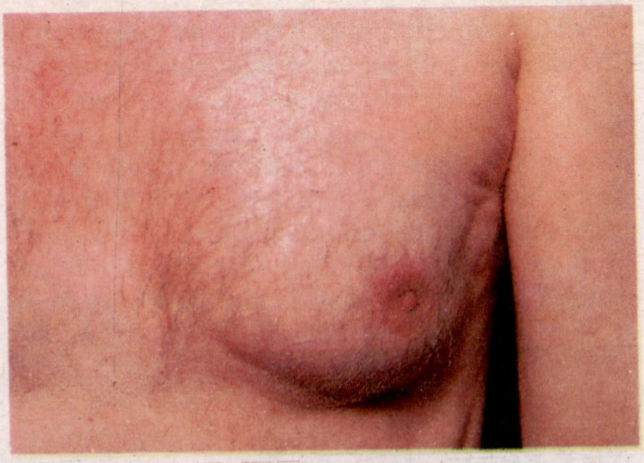

FIG. 12.12 Carcinoma of the male breast. Although the mass of tumour is relatively small it has already caused retraction of the nipple and is fixed to, and dimpling the skin

Carcinoma of the breast

This is an uncommon condition of elderly men. Its symptoms and physical signs are identical to those of carcinoma of the female breast so it does not require a separate description.

Because the male breast is small and not covered by a thick layer of subcutaneous fat the signs of spread of the disease, such as skin fixation, ulceration, peau d'orange and axillary lymphadenopathy, are seen at an early stage.

Abdominal herniae

13

A hernia is the protrusion of an organ through its containing wall. The term can be applied to the herniation of a muscle through its fascial covering, to the herniation of brain through a fracture of the skull or through the foramen magnum into the spinal canal, as well as to the protrusion of an intra-abdominal organ through a defect in the abdominal wall, pelvis or diaphragm.

Before an organ can herniate through its retaining wall there must be a weakness in that wall. This may be a **normal weakness**, found in everyone, and related to the anatomical configuration of the area – for example, a place where a vessel or viscus enters or leaves the abdomen; or an **abnormal weakness**, caused by a **congenital** abnormality or **acquired** as a result of trauma or disease.

This chapter deals with **abdominal herniae**, excluding herniae through and around the oesophageal hiatus. There are a few common varieties and a number of rarities. The common ones are the inguinal, umbilical, femoral and incisional herniae, the order reflecting their frequency in adult life, except in Negroes and in childhood where umbilical hernia is more common than inguinal hernia.

You seldom need to remember rarities, but it is important to know about the rare types of abdominal herniae because failure to diagnose any type of strangulated hernia, common or rare, may lead to the patient's death.

The less common types of herniae are the epigastric, Spigelian, obturator, lumbar and gluteal herniae.

Herniae occur frequently in both sexes. Inguinal hernia is common in men and women. Although femoral hernia is found much more often in women than in men, the commonest hernia in women is still the inguinal hernia.

Certain physical signs are common to all herniae but are not always present:

1 Abdominal herniae occur at congenital or acquired weak spots in the abdominal wall.
2 Most herniae can be **reduced**.
3 Most herniae have an **expansile cough impulse**.

The last two signs may be absent, especially if the hernia is tightly constricted at its neck, so their absence does not exclude the diagnosis of hernia.

The diagnosis of a hernia therefore rests upon the site, the presence of reducibility and an expansile cough impulse, or, when these signs are absent, the exclusion of other causes of a lump.

ANATOMY OF THE INGUINAL REGION

An inguinal hernia is the protrusion of part of the contents of the abdomen through the inguinal region of the abdominal wall. To understand inguinal herniae it is necessary to understand the anatomy of the inguinal canal (outlined in Fig. 13.2).

Surface anatomy

The inguinal ligament stretches between the anterior superior iliac spine and the pubic tubercle. The former is easy to see and feel but most students have difficulty in finding the pubic tubercle. A skin crease runs across the lower abdomen, convex downwards, separating the abdomen from the triangle known as the mons veneris. **The centre of this crease lies over the upper edge of the pubic bones.** The pubic tubercles lie beneath this crease approximately 2–3 cm from the mid-line. To find the pubic tubercle put your finger on the centre of this skin crease, push inwards until you feel the crest of the pubis, and then slide your finger sideways until you reach the tubercle. Confirm this on yourself.

Muscles

Beneath the skin and subcutaneous tissue lies the aponeurosis of the external oblique muscle. The lower edge of this aponeurosis, between the iliac spine and pubic tubercle, forms the inguinal ligament. The fibres of the aponeurosis run parallel to the inguinal ligament but divide above the crest of the pubis to form the external inguinal ring.

Revision Panel 13.1

The basic features of all herniae

They occur at a weak spot.

They reduce on lying down, or with direct pressure.

They have an *expansile* cough impulse.

Revision Panel 13.2

The causes of abdominal herniae

An anatomical weakness where:
- structures pass through the abdominal wall;
- muscles fail to overlap;
- there are no muscles, only scar tissue (e.g. umbilicus).

An acquired weakness following trauma.

High intra-abdominal pressure from:
- coughing;
- straining;
- abdominal distention.

Deep to the external oblique aponeurosis are the lowermost fibres of the internal oblique muscle arising from the lateral third of the inguinal ligament. They run medially in an arch, convex upward, to the edge of the rectus abdominis muscle, where they join the

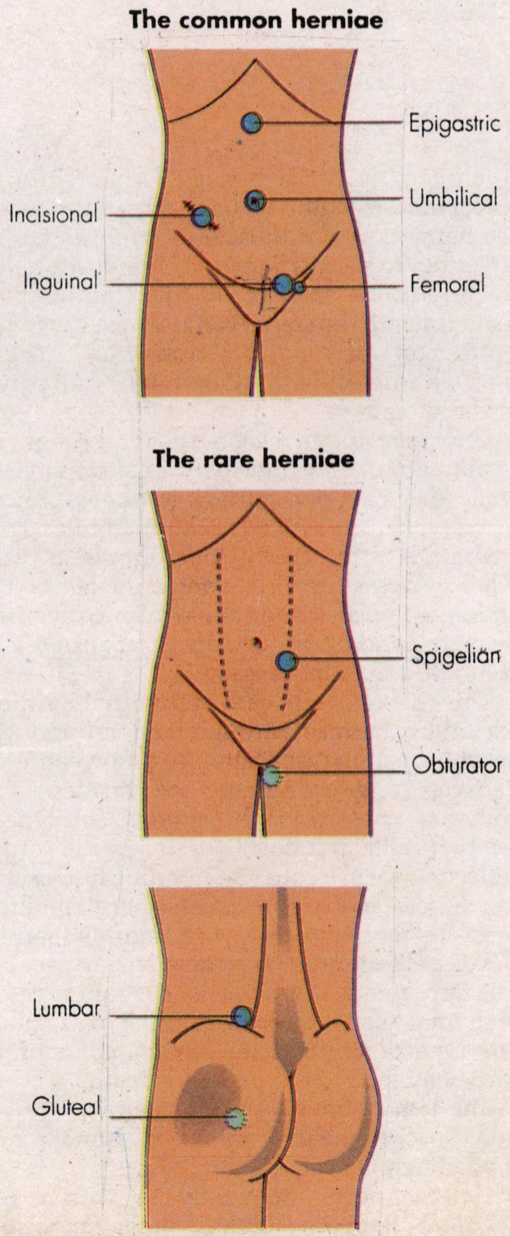

FIG. 13.1 The sites of herniae

THE ANATOMY OF THE INGUINAL REGION

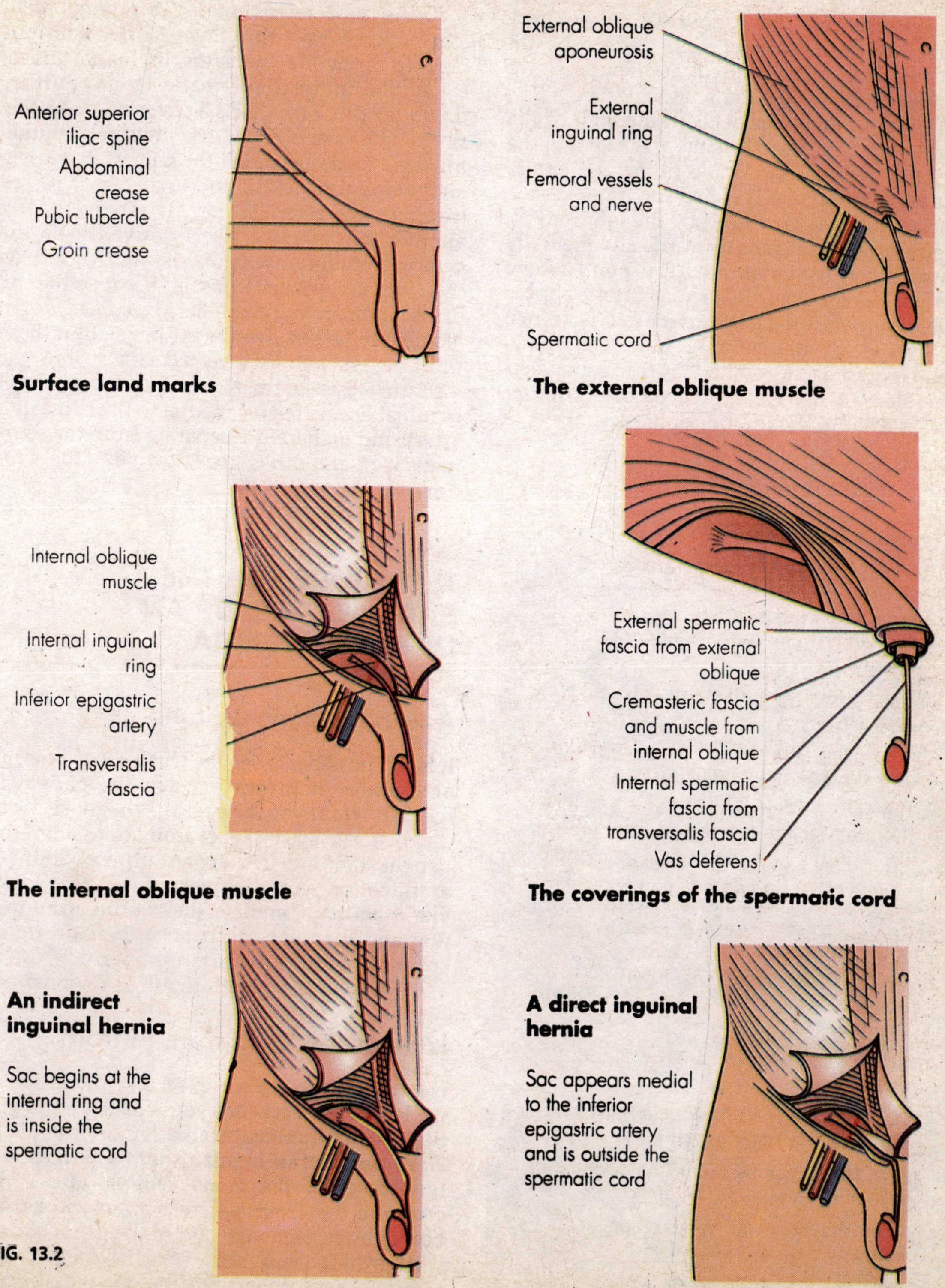

FIG. 13.2

aponeurosis of the transverse abdominal muscle to form the front of the rectus sheath. At this point the united aponeuroses are known as the 'conjoined tendon'.

The half-moon gap beneath the arch of the internal oblique muscle is the weak spot of the inguinal region. The tissue filling the gap is not very strong and is called the transversalis fascia. This area is crossed by the inferior epigastric artery as it runs upwards and medially towards the rectus sheath. The point where the vas deferens and testicular artery appear is lateral to the epigastric artery and is known as the internal inguinal ring. Indirect inguinal herniae start at this point. Direct inguinal herniae start in the weak area of the posterior wall medial to the inferior epigastric artery.

As the vas deferens enters the inguinal canal it is covered by a thin layer of fascia that is derived from the transversalis fascia and is called the internal spermatic fascia. Further down the canal it collects a covering of muscle fibres and fascia from the internal oblique muscle – these are called the cremaster muscle and cremasteric fascia; and finally, as it passes through the external ring, it is covered by another thin layer of fascia derived from the external oblique aponeurosis and known as the external spermatic fascia. Because the sac of an indirect inguinal hernia comes down alongside the vas deferens it lies within these three layers and is directed down into the scrotum. By contrast, the sac of a direct inguinal hernia begins medial to the epigastric artery and is therefore separate from the spermatic cord and rarely goes down into the scrotum.

Revision Panel 13.3

The features of inguinal herniae

Features of an indirect inguinal hernia

Can (and often does) descend into the scrotum.

Reduces upwards, then laterally and backwards.

Controlled, after reduction, by pressure over the internal inguinal ring.

The defect is not palpable as it is behind the fibres of the external oblique muscle.

After reduction the bulge reappears in the middle of the inguinal region and then flows medially before turning down to the neck of the scrotum.

Features of a direct inguinal hernia

Does not (hardly ever) go down into the scrotum.

Reduces upwards and then straight backwards.

Not controlled, after reduction, by pressure over the internal inguinal ring.

The defect may be felt in the abdominal wall above the pubic tubercle.

After reduction the bulge reappears exactly where it was before.

Uncommon in children and young adults.

TECHNIQUE FOR THE EXAMINATION OF AN INGUINAL HERNIA

Ask the patient to stand up

It is not possible to see the true size of a hernia or examine it properly when the patient is lying down. If you suspect the diagnosis from the history, start the examination with the patient standing. If, during routine abdominal examination, you discover a lump that looks like a hernia, complete the routine examination and then ask the patient to stand up in order to examine the lump properly.

Always examine both inguinal regions.

Look at the lump from in front

It is essential to see the exact site and shape of the lump. With practice you will be able to distinguish an inguinal from a femoral hernia at sight because an inguinal hernia bulges into the corner of the mons veneris, **above** the crease of the groin, whereas a femoral hernia bulges into the medial end of the groin crease.

Inspection will also reveal whether the lump extends down into the scrotum, and if

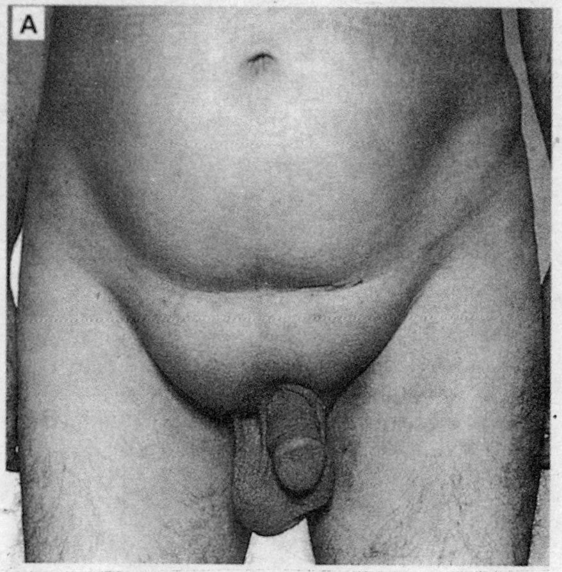

Ask the patient to stand up

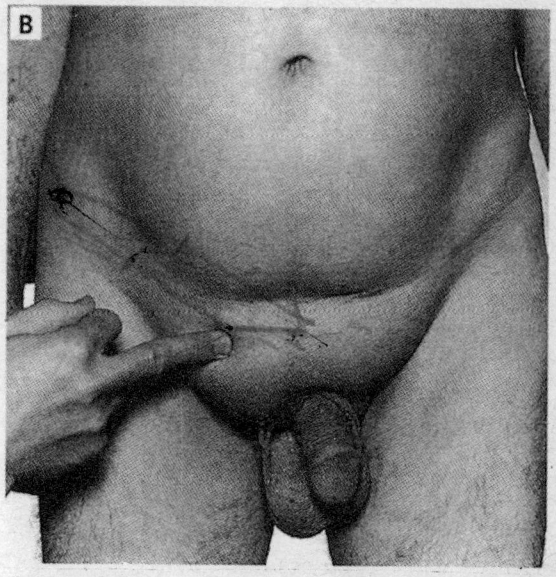

The upper crease of the mons veneris indicates the crest of the pubis and the level of the pubic tubercle. Note that it is not low down in the crease of the groin

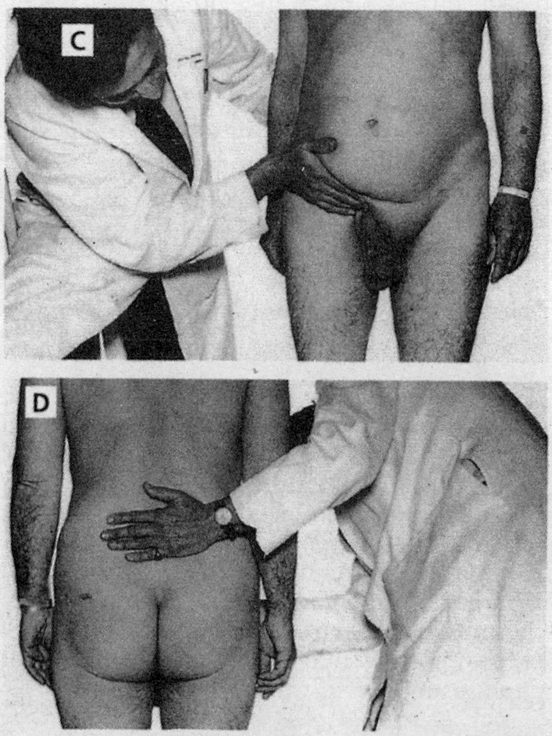

Place your examining hand flat on the groin parallel to the inguinal ligament and your other hand on the patient's back to stop him being pushed over. You will then be able to manipulate and reduce the hernia with ease

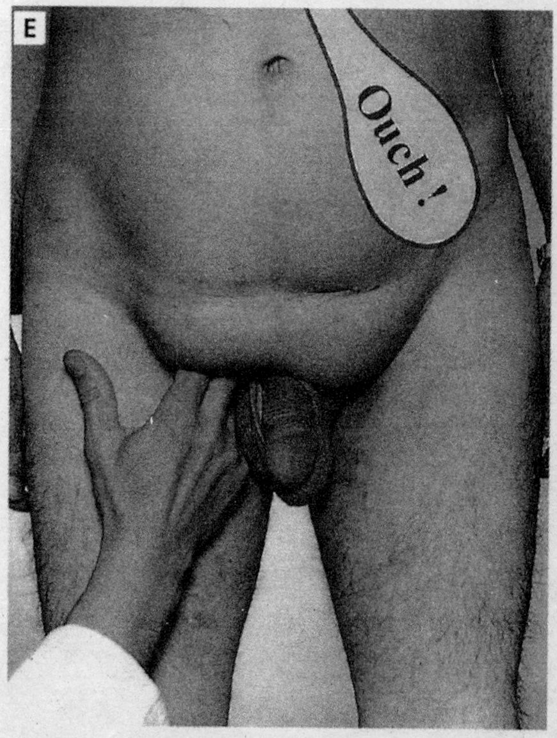

Never feel a hernia this way; it is very painful and uninformative

FIG. 13.3 TECHNIQUES FOR THE EXAMINATION OF AN INGUINAL HERNIA

there are any other scrotal swellings, and any swellings on the 'normal' side.

Feel from the front

1 Examine the scrotum and its contents. It is not unusual to find an epididymal cyst or a hydrocele as well as a hernia because they are all common conditions.

2 In men, first decide if the lump is a hernia or a true scrotal lump by examining its upper edge. If you can 'get above it' (i.e. feel its upper edge between your thumb and index finger and a normal spermatic cord above it) then it must be a scrotal swelling and not a hernia.

If you cannot feel the upper edge of the lump because it passes into the inguinal canal then it is likely to be a hernia, but it might be the rare variety of hydrocele that extends up along the spermatic cord – an infantile hydrocele (see Chapter 14).

3 Do not examine the external ring or palpate the pubic tubercle by pushing a finger up along the spermatic cord into the neck of the scrotum. This is a very painful method of examination and very rarely yields useful information.

Feel from the side

Having examined the scrotal contents and decided that you cannot get above the lump, you can make a provisional diagnosis of inguinal hernia and proceed to examine the lump itself.

Stand at the side of the patient, on the same side as the hernia. Place one hand in the small of the patient's back to support him, and your examining hand on the lump with your fingers and arm roughly parallel to the inguinal ligament.

You must now ascertain the following facts about the lump.

- Position.
- Temperature.
- Tenderness.
- Shape.
- Size.
- Tension.
- Composition (solid, fluid, gaseous).

8 **Expansile cough impulse.** Compress the lump firmly with your fingers; ask the patient to turn his head towards the opposite side, and then to cough. If the swelling **expands** with coughing, it has a 'cough impulse'. Movement of the swelling without expansion or an increase in tension is not a cough impulse. A localized swelling in the spermatic cord or an undescended testis will sometimes move down the inguinal canal and come out through the external ring during coughing, and look exactly like a hernia, but neither will get bigger or more tense during coughing. The presence of an expansile cough impulse is almost diagnostic of a hernia, but the absence of an expansile cough impulse does not exclude a diagnosis of hernia because the neck of the sac may be blocked by adhesions which prevent the movement of additional viscera into the sac during coughing.

9 **Is the swelling reducible?** The main reason for standing at the side of the patient is to be able to place your hand in exactly the same position as the patient places his own hand when he is reducing or supporting the hernia. He puts his hand on the lump and lifts it upwards and backwards. You must do the same. You can only do this if your arm comes from a position above and behind the hernia.

First, press firmly to reduce the tension of the lump. Then gently squeeze the lower part of the swelling. As the lump gets softer, lift it up towards the external ring. Once it has all passed in through this point, slide your fingers upwards and laterally towards the internal ring to see if the hernia can be controlled (kept inside) by pressure at this point. If the lump reduces into or through the abdominal wall at a point **above and medial** to the pubic tubercle it is an **inguinal** hernia. If the point of reduction is below and lateral to the pubic tubercle it is a femoral hernia. Note that this method of differentiation **refers to the point where the lump reduces**, not the position of the unreduced hernia, because once a hernia reaches the subcutaneous tissue it can expand and spread in any direction.

If the hernia can be held reduced only by pressure over the external inguinal ring, it is a direct inguinal hernia. If it can be controlled by pressure over the internal ring it is an indirect inguinal hernia.

10 **Remove your hand and watch the hernia reappear.** The direction of movement of the swelling and the way in which it reappears will help to confirm your deductions about its site of origin.

An indirect hernia will seem to slide obliquely along the line of the canal whereas a direct hernia will project directly forwards. However, particularly in the obese, it may be impossible to differentiate between these two types of hernia with any certainty.

Percuss and auscultate the lump

If there is gut in the sac it may be resonant and there may be audible bowel sounds.

Feel the other side

Move to the other side of the patient and palpate that inguinal region. Bilateral herniae are common. Even when you cannot feel a lump ask the patient to cough whilst feeling the inguinal canal just in case there is an invisible small bulge which is palpable only at the peak of a cough.

Examine the abdomen

Examine the abdomen if this has not already been done. Particularly look for anything that may be raising the intra-abdominal pressure, such as a large bladder, an enlarged prostate, ascites, chronic intestinal obstruction and pregnancy.

Cardiovascular and respiratory assessment

Assess the cardiovascular and respiratory systems with the patient's fitness for operation in mind.

SYMPTOMS AND SIGNS OF AN INGUINAL HERNIA

HISTORY

Age Inguinal herniae occur at *all* ages. They may be present at birth or appear suddenly in an 80-year-old. The peak times of presentation are in the first few months of life, in the late teens and early twenties, and between 40 and 60.

Occupation Heavy work, especially lifting, puts a great strain on the abdominal muscles. If there is an underlying weakness, the appearance of a hernia may coincide with strenuous physical effort. Workmen's compensation laws in most countries accept that herniae can be caused by heavy work.

Local symptoms The commonest symptoms are **discomfort** and **pain**. The patient complains of a dragging, aching sensation in the groin, which gets worse as the day passes.

If the hernia becomes very painful and tender then it is probably strangulated. There may be pain long before the lump is noticed.

On the other hand, many herniae cause no pain and the patient presents because he has noticed a **swelling in the groin** or in the scrotum. He may have noticed that it gets smaller when he lies down and that he can push it away. The patient may complain of lumps on both sides.

Systemic symptoms If the hernia is obstructing the lumen of a loop of bowel the patient may complain of one or more of the four cardinal symptoms of intestinal obstruction: **colicky abdominal pain**, **vomiting**, **abdominal distension** and **absolute constipation**.

It is important to remember that bowel may be obstructed without being strangulated, and that strangulation will only be accompanied by obstruction if the contents of the hernia are bowel.

Cause The patient may relate the onset of the hernia to a particular event, such as lifting a heavy weight. It is usual to ask about other diseases which may have caused him to strain his abdominal muscles, such as chronic bronchitis with persistent coughing, constipation and difficulty with micturition, even though the precise importance of these conditions in the aetiology of inguinal hernia is uncertain.

Social history Find out if the symptoms are affecting the patient's ability to work and whether the possibility of litigation and com-

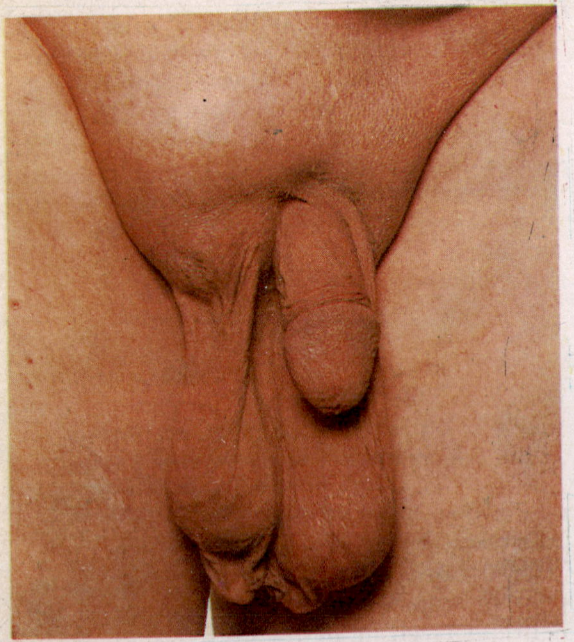

An indirect inguinal hernia. It is obviously coming downwards and medially from the inguinal canal and is just entering the neck of the scrotum

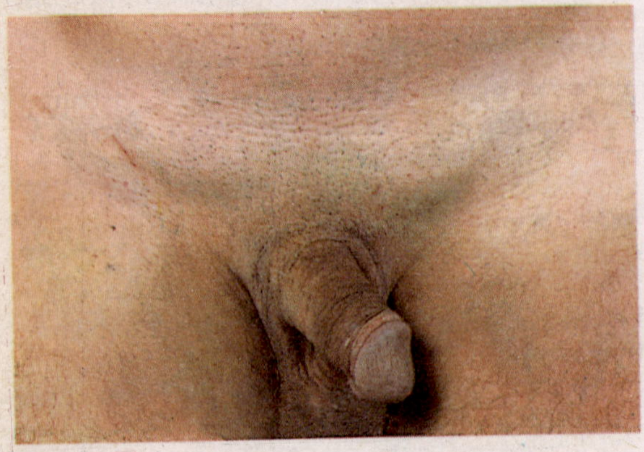

A left direct inguinal hernia. A small bulge coming straight out through the transversalis fascia and external inguinal ring. There is an early bulge on the right

FIG. 13.4 INGUINAL HERNIAE

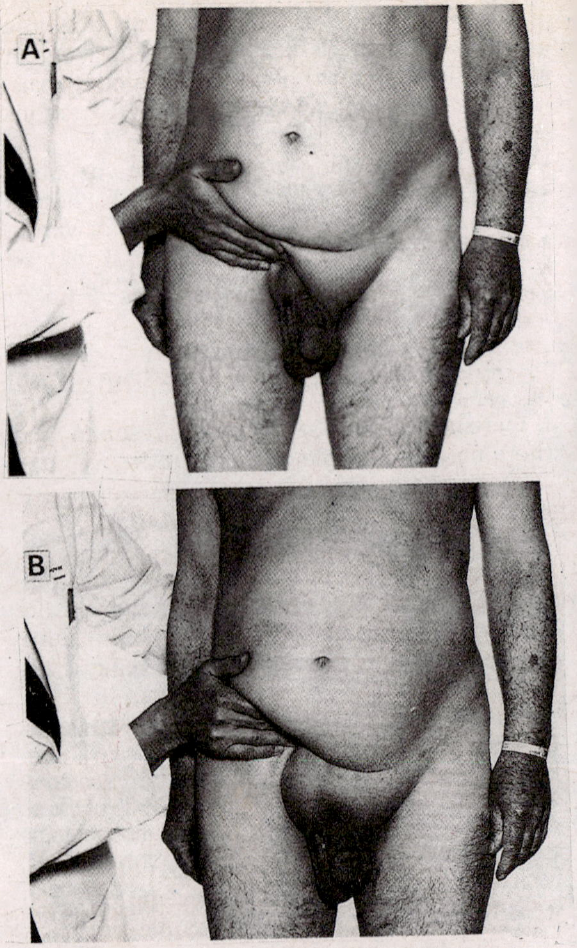

FIG. 13.5 This hernia can be controlled by pressure on the external inguinal ring (**A**) but appears when the fingers are slid laterally so that they cover only the internal ring (**B**). Thus it is a direct inguinal hernia. This is a difficult test to perform and not wholly reliable

pensation are affecting the presentation of the symptoms.

EXAMINATION

The principal features to be determined are the site, size and constituents of the lump together with the two diagnostic signs – reducibility and an expansile cough impulse.

Position All inguinal herniae can be seen as a visible lump when they appear through the superficial inguinal ring. This ring is just above the crest of the pubic bone and the pubic tubercle and is widest medial to the pubic tubercle.

Once the hernia has passed through the ring it spreads out over the whole pubis into the neck of the scrotum, and may descend to fill the scrotum. Thus as it descends into the scrotum it is often not medial to the pubic tubercle. The oft-quoted description 'above and medial to the pubic tubercle' refers to the point at which the hernia reduces into the abdominal wall (i.e. the external inguinal ring), not to the position of the whole hernia.

Colour The skin overlying an inguinal hernia should be normal. If the hernia is strangulated the skin may be a little reddened. If the patient has worn a truss for many years the patch of skin over the external inguinal ring, which has been subjected to years of pressure by the pad of the truss, may be white and scarred and sometimes show streaks of brown pigmentation caused by haemosiderin deposition.

Temperature The temperature of the skin overlying a hernia should be the same as the surrounding skin except when the hernia is strangulated or infected, when it becomes hot.

Tenderness Herniae may contain any viscus and, as all abdominal structures have a visceral sensory innervation, manual pressure is usually uncomfortable but rarely very painful. By contrast a strangulated hernia is very tender. An irreducible, non-strangulated hernia is not tender to light pressure, but any attempt at reduction by excessive pressing and squeezing can cause considerable pain.

Shape Most inguinal herniae resemble a large pear with the 'stalk' at the external inguinal ring. Some also cause a bulge along the line of the inguinal canal, with a narrowing at the external inguinal ring, giving them an hourglass appearance.

Size Inguinal herniae vary from very small bulges, 1–2 cm in diameter, to large masses which extend down to the knee joint.

Surface The surface will vary according to the nature of the contents but is usually smooth and sometimes bosselated.

Composition Herniae that contain gut should be soft, resonant and fluctuant, and may have bowel sounds. If the contents within the sac are tense then the hernia will feel hard, but if it contains bowel it should still be resonant and fluctuant. A large scrotal hernia containing small intestine may show visible peri-stalis.

Many herniae contain omentum; this makes them feel firm (rubbery), non-fluctuant and dull to percussion.

Cough impulse A hernia should become larger and more tense during coughing (i.e. have an **expansile** cough impulse). Most lumps in the groin move with coughing – a transmitted impulse – but only herniae and vascular tumours expand.

Compressibility A hernia can be compressed by steady pressure but, unlike vascular tumours that may have the same physical sign, a hernia will not recur immediately the compression is released unless some force, such as gravity or coughing, forces it out.

Reducibility The diagnostic sign of a hernia is reducibility. This implies that it is possible to return the contents of the hernia to their normal anatomical site – the abdomen. Unlike a compressible lump, a lump which has been reduced does not immediately reappear when the pressure is removed unless forced to do so by gravity or muscle tone. When you reduce a lump you move it to another place; when you compress a lump you just empty its fluid contents to another place.

Relations The relations of the lump will have already been defined when deciding the site and nature of the hernia.

State of local tissues As acquired inguinal herniae are caused by a weakness of the tissues of the inguinal canal, bulging of both inguinal regions with coughing is common. Minor bilateral bulging of the inguinal canal is normal and known as **Malgaigne's bulges**.

Look carefully for any scars near the hernia. It may have been repaired in the distant past.

There is an increased incidence of right inguinal hernia in patients who have had an

SOME DEFINITIONS

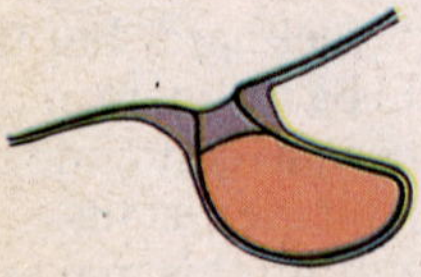

Neck of sac
This tight ring of peritoneum is usually the site of any strangulation

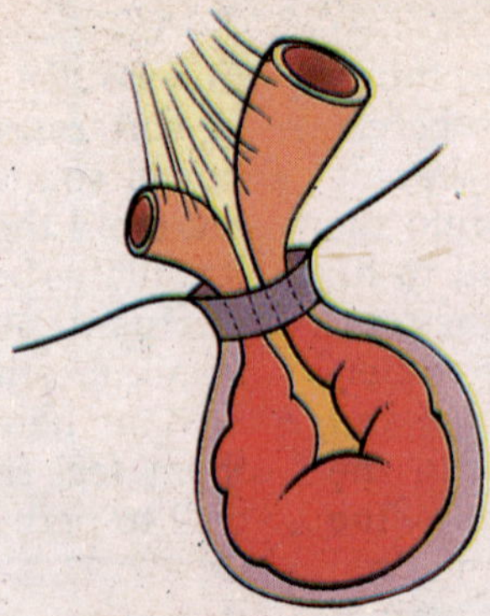

A strangulated hernia
The blood supply of the contents of the hernia is cut off. When a loop of gut is strangulated there will also be intestinal obstruction

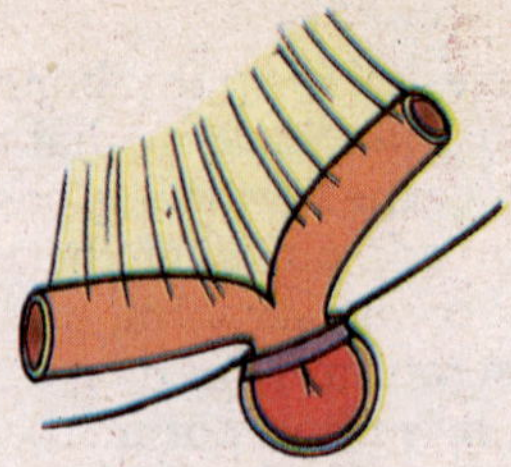

A strangulated hernia
If the sac is small, a knuckle of bowel can be caught in the sac and strangled without causing intestinal obstruction. This is called a *Richter's hernia*

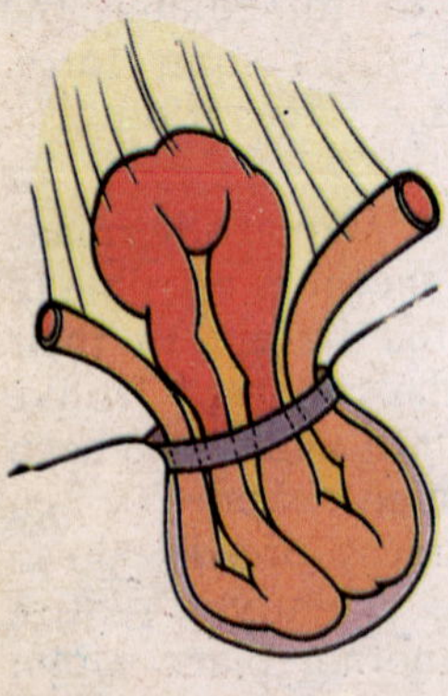

Maydl's hernia
When two adjacent loops of bowel are in the sac, the intervening portion in the abdomen is the first to suffer if the neck of the sac is tight, because it is the centre of the whole loop involved. Thus the strangulated piece is intra-abdominal. This is a rare variety of strangulation

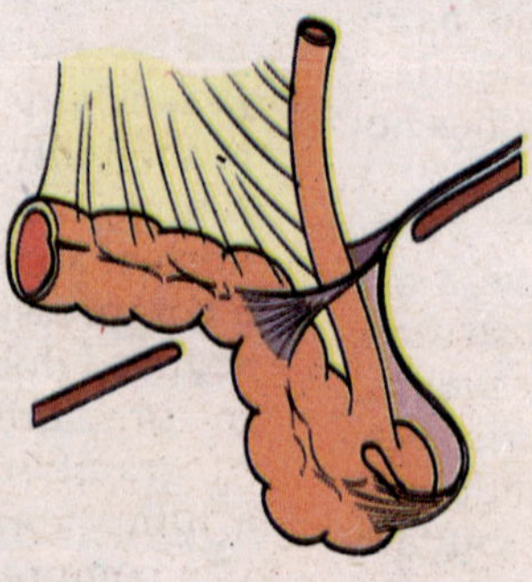

Sliding hernia
If bowel which is normally extraperitoneal forms one side of the sac, it is thought to have slid down the canal pulling peritoneum with it, hence the name *hernia-en-glissade*. The sac can contain other loops of bowel, and the gut forming the wall of the sac can be strangled by the external ring

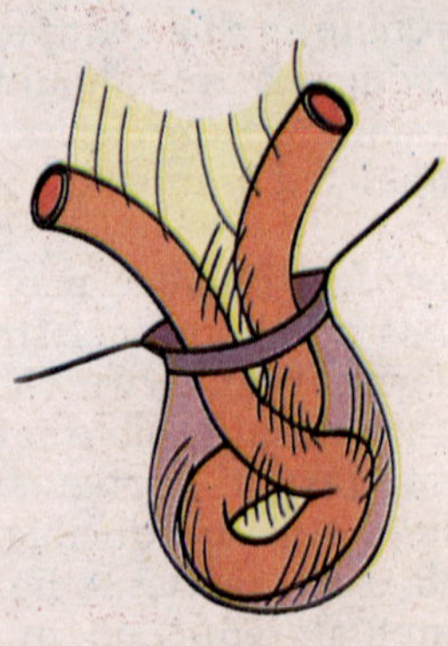

Incarceration
The contents are fixed in the sac because of their size and adhesions. The hernia is irreducible but the bowel is not strangulated or obstructed

FIG. 13.6

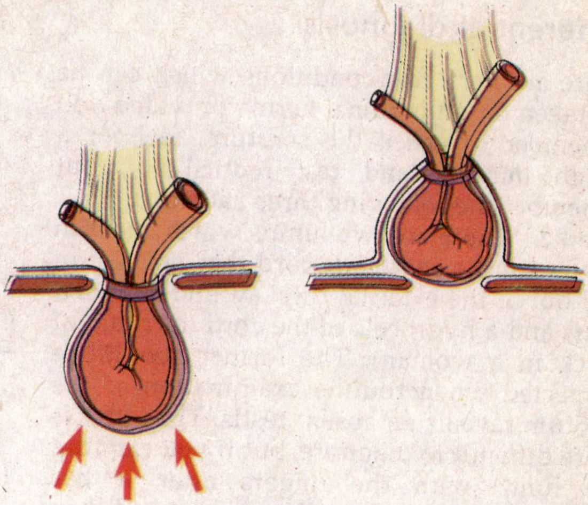

Reduction-en-masse

It is possible to push a hernia back through the abdominal wall, so apparently reducing it, without actually pushing the contents out of the sac. If they were strangulated in the first position they will still be strangulated in the second. Never push hard when trying to reduce a hernia

FIG. 13.6 *Continued*

appendectomy through a right iliac fossa incision because this incision weakens the adjacent muscles and occasionally divides the subcostal or ilioinguinal nerve.

GENERAL EXAMINATION

Look for the common causes of a raised intra-abdominal pressure – chronic bronchitis and coughing, chronic retention of urine, difficulty in micturition, ascites, intra-abdominal masses and chronic constipation. These factors may have caused the hernia.

Look for any signs of intestinal obstruction – distension, increased bowel sounds, visible peristalsis.

Special varieties of inguinal hernia

The differences between a direct and an indirect inguinal hernia are listed in Revision Panel 13.3. From a practical point of view this differentiation is quite irrelevant, but it is important to make yourself decide upon the variety because it makes you examine the hernia more carefully.

The **sliding hernia** is a hernia of a piece of extraperitoneal bowel, usually caecum or sigmoid colon, which slides down into the inguinal canal, pulling a sac of peritoneum on its surface. It is sometimes possible to guess that a hernia is of the sliding variety by the slow way in which it reappears after reduction and the manner in which it slithers down into the scrotum. The clinical differentiation of this variety is purely guesswork and quite unnecessary, although it presents problems to the surgeon who has to repair it.

The other varieties of inguinal hernia shown are defined by their contents and cannot be determined clinically.

Maydl's hernia (hernia-en-W), in which there are two loops of bowel in the sac, can be suspected clinically when it is strangulated because the loop of bowel in the abdomen which connects the two loops in the sac becomes tender before the loops in the hernia. Thus a patient with intestinal obstruction, a tense, slightly tender irreducible hernia and a tender mass **above the inguinal ligament** may well have this variety of hernia.

Revision Panel 13.4

The differential diagnosis of inguinal hernia

- Femoral hernia
- Vaginal hydrocele
- Hydrocele of the cord *or* the canal of Nück
- Undescended testis
- Lipoma of the cord

Differential diagnosis

There are very few conditions which can be mistaken for an inguinal hernia provided you remember to check the scrotum, feel for a cough impulse and test reducibility, but remember the following three catches.

1 and 2 There are two lumps which occur in the line of the spermatic cord that can pop in and out of the external ring: an undescended testis and a hydrocele of the cord (or canal of Nück in a woman). The former should be suspected when routine examination of the scrotum reveals an absent testis. The latter is more difficult to diagnose, but if you can trap the lump with the fingers after it has appeared through the external ring, and then feel its upper edge, it cannot be a hernia. Neither of these lumps has an expansile cough impulse and the latter may fluctuate and transilluminate.

3 An infantile hydrocele (see Chapter 14) looks like a complete scrotal hernia and you cannot feel the spermatic cord above it, but it does not have a true expansile cough impulse, although it will bulge forwards on coughing. It should fluctuate and transilluminate. The testis is not palpable and the mass is irreducible.

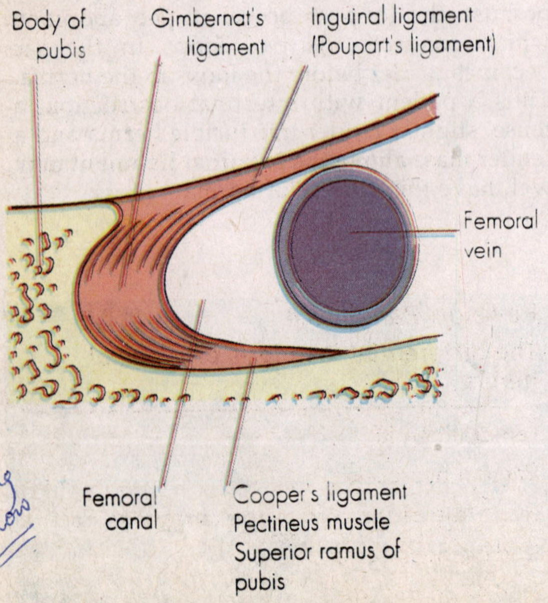

FIG. 13.7 The boundaries of the left femoral canal

FEMORAL HERNIAE

ANATOMY

A femoral hernia is a protrusion of extraperitoneal fat, peritoneum and, sometimes, abdominal contents through the femoral canal. The anatomical margins of this canal are the inguinal ligament superoanteriorly, the pubic ramus and pectineus muscle inferoposteriorly, the pubic part of the inguinal ligament (Gimbernat's ligament) and pubic bone medially, and the femoral vein laterally.

With bone or ligament on three sides, the femoral canal is a rigid opening, so that bowel is more likely to become strangulated if it is pushed through it.

HISTORY

Age Femoral herniae are uncommon in children and do not become common until late middle age, over 50 years. The majority are found in 60–80-year-old women.

Sex Femoral hernia is much more common in women than men. Nevertheless, do not forget that even in women the commonest hernia in the groin region is the inguinal hernia.

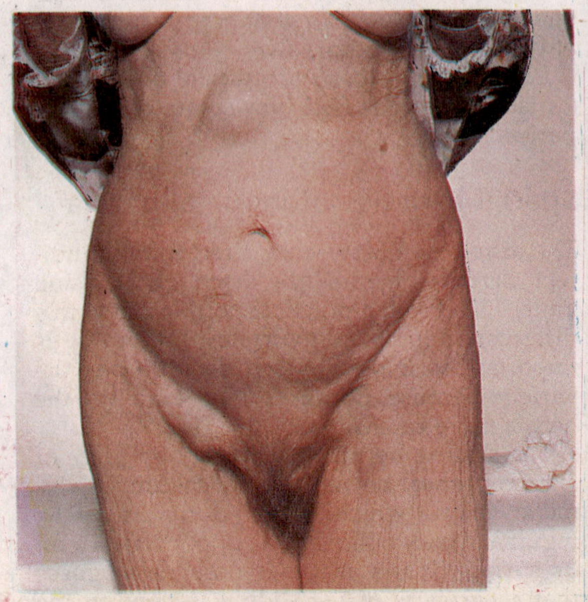

FIG. 13.8 A right femoral hernia. Note that the femoral hernia bulges into the crease of the groin

Symptoms The symptoms of this variety of hernia are similar to those described above for inguinal hernia:

Local – lump in the groin; pain and discomfort.

General – if causing obstruction: colic, distension, vomiting and constipation.

The femoral hernia is renowned for its ability to strangle a part of the wall of the bowel without occluding the lumen and causing intestinal obstruction – Richter's hernia.

Multiplicity Femoral herniae are often bilateral.

EXAMINATION

All the comments made about the examination of inguinal herniae apply to femoral herniae. Ask the patient to stand up, try to determine the exact anatomical relations of the lump to the inguinal ligament and pubic tubercle, and then decide if the lump has a cough impulse and whether it is reducible.

Position The femoral canal is lateral to the body of the pubis and inferior to the tip of the pubic tubercle. Therefore, **the neck** of a femoral hernia, or the point at which it disappears into the abdomen, is **below and lateral** to the pubic tubercle. The main bulk of the hernia may spread in any direction. It usually points downwards and laterally, but it can pass medially and may bulge up and over the inguinal ligament. Normally the bulge appears to be directly behind the skin crease of the groin, whereas the inguinal hernia bulges above the groin crease.

Begin by feeling the lump, and, if it appears to have a neck tethered deeply, feel around the neck very carefully to determine its exact position.

A small hernia in a fat person is very difficult to feel so take great care when palpating this region.

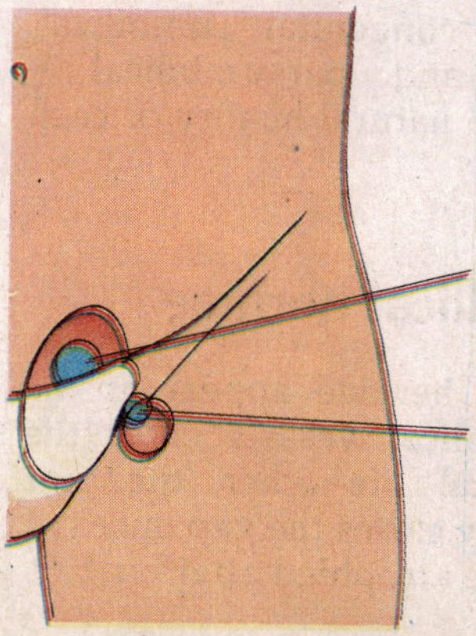

FIG. 13.9 The sites of appearance of inguinal and femoral herniae

Colour The overlying skin should be a normal colour. The skin may become red and oedematous if the hernia is obstructed.

Temperature The skin temperature is normal unless there is hyperaemia caused by underlying inflammation.

Tenderness Femoral herniae are not usually tender unless strangulated, but you may cause pain if your attempts at reduction are too vigorous.

Shape and size The lump is almost spherical with an area above and behind it which is difficult to define, corresponding to the site of the neck at the femoral canal. Most femoral herniae are small. If they do enlarge they tend to flatten and spread in the fold of the groin because downward extension is limited by the attachment of the deep part of the superficial fascia to the deep fascia of the upper thigh.

Surface The surface of the sac is usually smooth.

Composition The majority of femoral herniae feel firm and are dull to percussion because they contain omentum or consist of a very small empty sac surrounded by a lot of extraperitoneal fat. They may contain bladder.

If large enough to contain bowel, they feel soft and may be resonant to percussion.

Reducibility The size of most femoral herniae can be reduced by firm pressure, but often cannot be completely reduced because the contents are often adherent to the peritoneal sac.

Cough impulse For the same reason that they do not reduce easily – adherence of the contents and a narrow neck of sac – many femoral herniae do not have a cough impulse. This makes the differential diagnosis very difficult.

Relations to surrounding structures Because many femoral herniae do not have the two signs diagnostic of hernia – reducibility and a cough impulse – the diagnosis depends upon the **site of the lump**; hence the importance of clearly defining its relations to surrounding structures.

State of local tissues Femoral herniae develop because the femoral canal is a naturally weak spot in the abdominal wall, but the region may have been weakened by injury, the commonest of which is the surgical repair of an adjacent inguinal hernia. Look out for other scars near the hernia and always examine the other groin.

GENERAL EXAMINATION

Look for the causes of a raised intra-abdominal pressure – chronic bronchitis, retention of urine and constipation – and for signs of intestinal obstruction.

Prevascular femoral hernia

This is the only special variety of femoral hernia that you need remember. It is easy to diagnose. Instead of the sac coming through the narrow femoral canal, it bulges down underneath the whole inguinal ligament, in front of the femoral artery and vein. This means that it has a wide neck and a flattened wide sac which bulges downwards and laterally.

Prevascular herniae are usually easy to reduce and have a cough impulse. They rarely get strangulated and, because the femoral vessels lie immediately behind, are difficult to repair.

Revision Panel 13.5

The differential diagnosis of femoral hernia

- Inguinal hernia
- Enlarged lymph gland
- Sapheno-varix
- Ectopic testis
- Psoas abscess
- Psoas bursa
- Lipoma

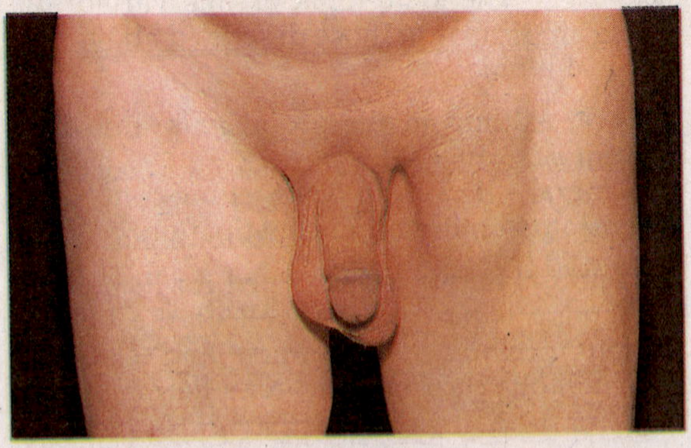

FIG. 13.10 A prevascular femoral hernia

UMBILICAL HERNIAE

All herniae which appear to be closely related to the umbilicus can be called umbilical herniae, but most clinicians subdivide them into three varieties – congenital umbilical, acquired umbilical and paraumbilical – because the cause and natural history of each variety is different.

Congenital umbilical herniae

Congenital umbilical herniae appear at the site where the umbilical vessels enter the abdomen during fetal life when the scar tissue, which normally closes the gap once the umbilical vessels have atrophied after birth, is weak.

A congenital protrusion of bowel through the umbilical defect *without* a covering of skin

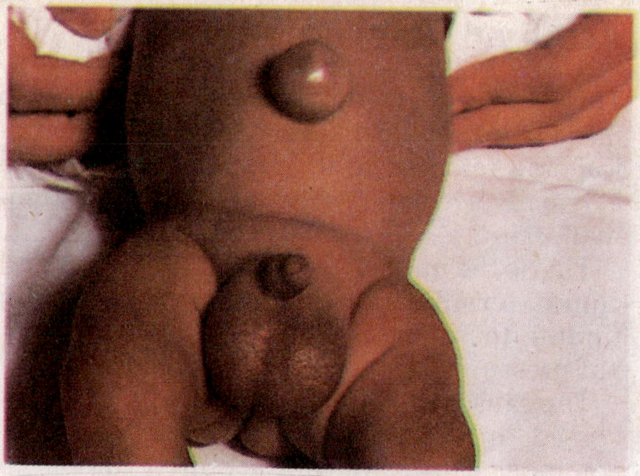

This baby also has a left inguinal hernia and right hydrocele

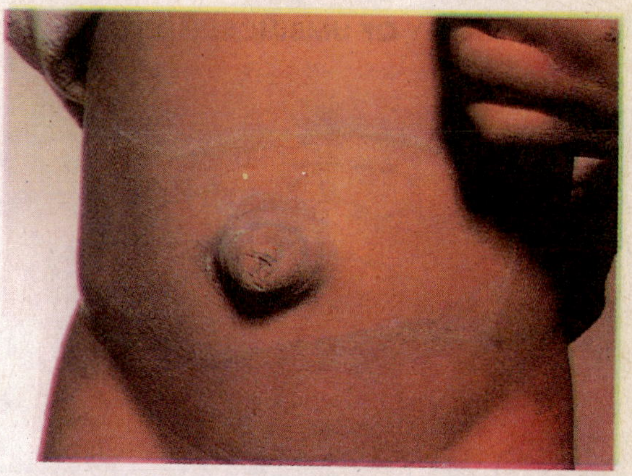

A regressing congenital umbilical hernia. The defect has almost closed and the overlying skin is collapsing inwards to become a normal umbilicus

FIG. 13.11 CONGENITAL UMBILICAL HERNIAE

is called an *exomphalos* and is discussed in Chapter 15.

HISTORY

Age Although the weakness is present at birth, the hernia may not be noticed until the umbilical cord has separated and healed. Even then it may be very small and so not present until it enlarges months later.

Ethnic group Congenital umbilical herniae are more common in Negroes.

Symptoms They rarely cause any symptoms other than parental agitation and distress. They have a wide neck and reduce easily so rarely give rise to intestinal obstruction.

Large herniae are embarrassing to small children when they begin to go to school and occasionally cause aching abdominal pains.

Natural history About 90 per cent of congenital umbilical herniae disappear spontaneously during the first 5 years of life as the umbilical scar thickens and contracts.

EXAMINATION

Position Congenital umbilical herniae appear in the centre of the umbilicus. When they are small they cause only a slight bulge in the centre of the umbilical depression, but when they are large they evert the whole umbilicus.

Shape and size These herniae are usually hemispherical and overlie an easily palpable defect in the abdominal wall. The size of the lump can vary from very small (0.5 cm diameter) to very large (10 cm diameter). Very small herniae can only be diagnosed by carefully exploring the depth of the umbilicus with the tip of your little finger to find the defect in the abdominal wall.

Composition Congenital umbilical herniae are soft, compressible and easy to reduce. They usually contain bowel and so may be resonant to percussion. They reduce spontaneously when the child lies down.

Cough impulse An expansile cough impulse is invariably present.

Relations Once the hernia has reduced it is usually easy to feel the defect in the abdominal wall. The edge of the defect can be made more prominent by asking the patient to cough or tense the abdominal muscles.

The central skin of the umbilicus, which overlies the hernia, is usually attached to the sac.

In neonates the remnants of the umbilical cord, and sometimes a chronic granuloma at the point from which it separated, may be visible.

ANATOMY OF UMBILICAL HERNIAE

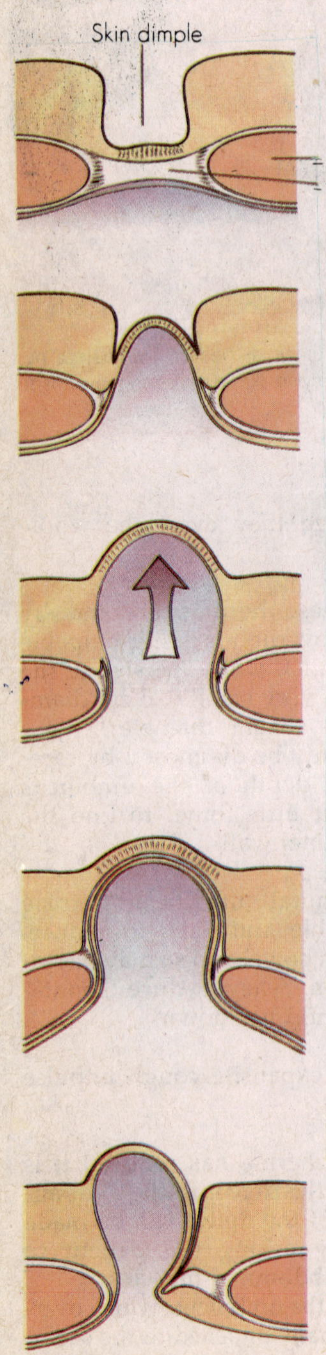

The normal umbilicus

A congenital umbilical hernia

The umbilical scar fails to form or is weak. The abdominal contents bulge through the weak spot and evert the umbilicus

An acquired true umbilical hernia

The umbilical scar is stretched by a raised intra-abdominal pressure and the umbilicus everts

A paraumbilical hernia

The hernial orifice is at the side of the umbilical scar so the sac bulges out beside the umbilicus, turning it into a crescent-shaped slit

FIG. 13.12

Acquired umbilical hernia

This is a hernia through the umbilical scar, so it is a true umbilical hernia and has the umbilical skin tethered to it. It is not common and is usually secondary to a raised intra-abdominal pressure.

This is the important point to remember and clinical examination should concentrate on finding the cause of the raised intra-abdominal pressure.

The causes of abdominal distension are discussed in detail in Chapter 16, but the common causes of an acquired umbilical hernia are pregnancy, ascites, ovarian cysts, fibroids and bowel distension.

The local physical signs of the hernia are identical to those described for the congenital variety.

General examination of the abdomen may reveal one of the causes of distension just mentioned.

Paraumbilical hernia

This is the common acquired umbilical hernia. It appears through a defect which is adjacent to the umbilical scar. That it is truly paraumbilical is clinically apparent because it does not bulge into the centre of the umbilicus and evert it, and the umbilical skin is not attached to the centre of the sac. Why the linea alba should give way so often just adjacent to the umbilical scar is not known.

HISTORY

Age Paraumbilical herniae develop in middle and old age.

Sex They are more common in women than men, especially obese women.

Symptoms The commonest symptoms are **pain** and a **swelling**. Sometimes the swelling is so small that it is not noticed by the patient and she presents complaining of pain or discomfort and tenderness around the umbilicus, made worse by prolonged standing or heavy exercise.

The patient may have the general symptoms of partial or recurrent **intestinal obstruction**.

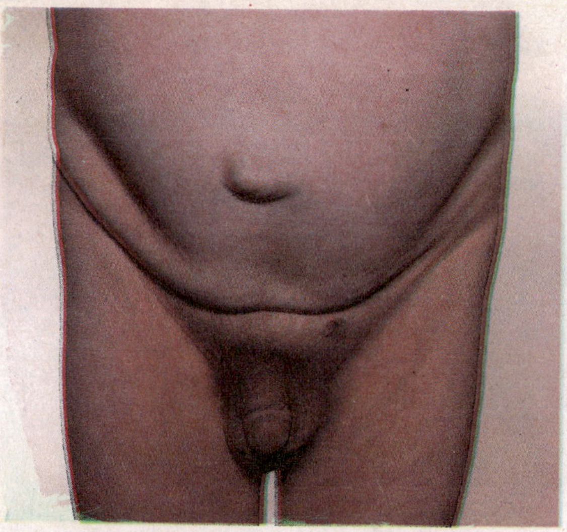

FIG. 13.13 A paraumbilical hernia. Note that the hernia is on one side of the umbilicus, which is stretched into a crescent shape

EXAMINATION

Position The main bulge of the hernia is beside the umbilicus, which is pushed to one side and stretched into a crescent shape.

Surface and edge The surface is smooth and the edge easy to define except when the patient's abdominal wall is very fat.

Composition The lump is firm as it usually contains omentum. If it contains bowel it is soft and resonant to percussion. The majority of paraumbilical herniae are **reducible**, but when the contents are adherent to the sac, or the neck of the sac is very narrow, they are irreducible.

Cough impulse Most of these herniae have an expansile cough impulse.

Relations The skin at the centre of the umbilicus is not attached to the centre of the sac as in the true umbilical hernia, but the umbilical skin is usually firmly applied to the side of the sac and may be fixed to it.

If the hernia can be reduced, the firm fibrous edge of the defect in the linea alba is easy to feel. It may vary in size from a few millimetres in diameter to a defect big enough to admit your fist.

GENERAL EXAMINATION

The patient is quite likely to be obese and may have other herniae and generalized abdominal wall laxity. There may be an apron of pendulous fat across the lower abdomen.

Although abdominal distension usually causes a true umbilical hernia, it can cause a paraumbilical hernia, so examine the contents of the abdomen with care.

Epigastric hernia

An epigastric hernia is a protrusion of extraperitoneal fat, and sometimes a small peritoneal sac, through a defect in the linea alba somewhere between the xiphisternum and umbilicus.

The patient complains of epigastric pain which is localized exactly to the site of the hernia, but often he does not notice the underlying lump.

For some inexplicable reason the pain often begins after eating – possibly because of epigastric distension – and so the patient thinks he has indigestion and makes a self-diagnosis of peptic ulceration. Thus when a patient complains of epigastric discomfort, palpate the abdominal wall in the epigastrium very carefully before concentrating on deep palpation, because all the symptoms may be due to a small, fatty, epigastric hernia.

On examination these herniae feel firm, do not usually have a cough impulse and cannot be reduced. It is sometimes impossible to distinguish them from lipomata, only the typical position suggesting the correct diagnosis.

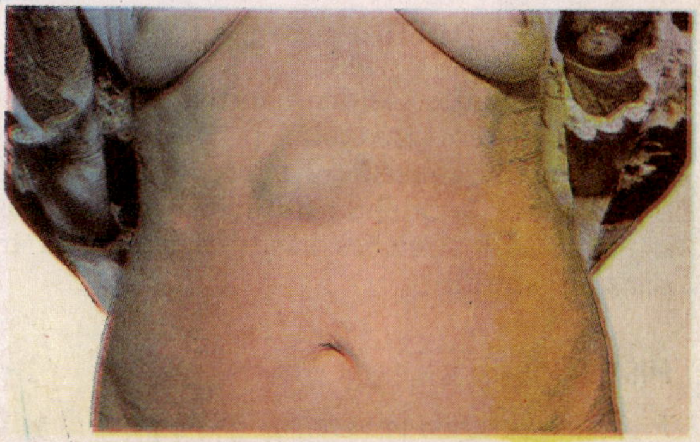

FIG. 13.14 An epigastric hernia in an elderly lady

A

B

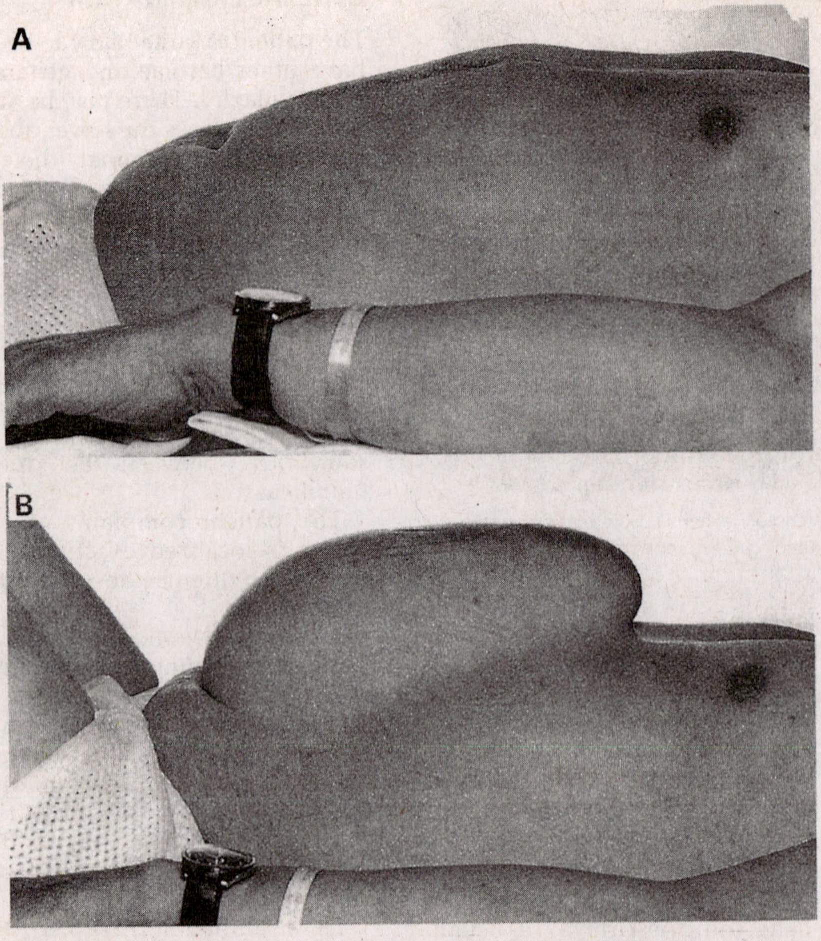

FIG. 13.15 Herniae often reduce and are not visable when a patient lies down (**A**). This patient has a large mid-line incisional hernia which appeared when he tensed his abdominal muscles by lifting his legs up off the couch (**B**)

Incisional hernia

An abdominal incisional hernia is a hernia through an acquired scar in the abdominal wall, usually caused by a previous surgical operation or accidental trauma. Scar tissue is inelastic and stretches easily if subjected to constant strain.

HISTORY

Previous operation or accident The patient will usually remember the trauma that caused the scar, but may not remember any complications in the original wound such as a **haematoma** or **infection**, which weakened it and made it more susceptible to the development of a hernia.

Age Incisional herniae occur at all ages but are more common in the elderly.

Symptoms The commonest symptoms are a **lump** and **pain**. Intestinal obstruction can occur, causing distension, colic, vomiting, constipation and severe pain in the lump.

EXAMINATION

The common findings are a reducible lump, with an expansile cough impulse, underneath an old scar. The defect in the abdominal wall may be palpable.

If the lump does not reduce and does not have a cough impulse, then it may not be a hernia but a deposit of tumour, a chronic abscess or haematoma, or a foreign-body granuloma. All these lesions, except recurrent tumour, occur soon after an incision. Incisional herniae usually appear in the first year after surgery but may develop later than this.

The **local tissues** may be thin and weak because of local damage or general cachexia.

Divarication of the recti

After prolonged abdominal distension, as in multiple pregnancies, and after repeated midline abdominal operations, the linea alba may stretch and allow the two rectus abdominis muscles to separate. These muscles are inserted close together on the pubis but their origins are quite a way apart on the anterolateral aspect of the lower ribs. Thus when both muscles contract there is a tendency for the upper portions to move apart; and when the lateral pull on the rectus sheath from contraction of the oblique and transverse abdominal muscles is added to this, it is not surprising that the recti can separate by several inches if the linea alba is weak.

Revision Panel 13.6

The differential diagnosis of a lump in the groin

- Inguinal hernia
- Femoral hernia
- Enlarged lymph nodes
- Sapheno-varix
- Ectopic testis
- Femoral aneurysm
- Hydrocele of the cord *or* hydrocele of the canal of Nück
- Lipoma of the cord
- Psoas bursa
- Psoas abscess

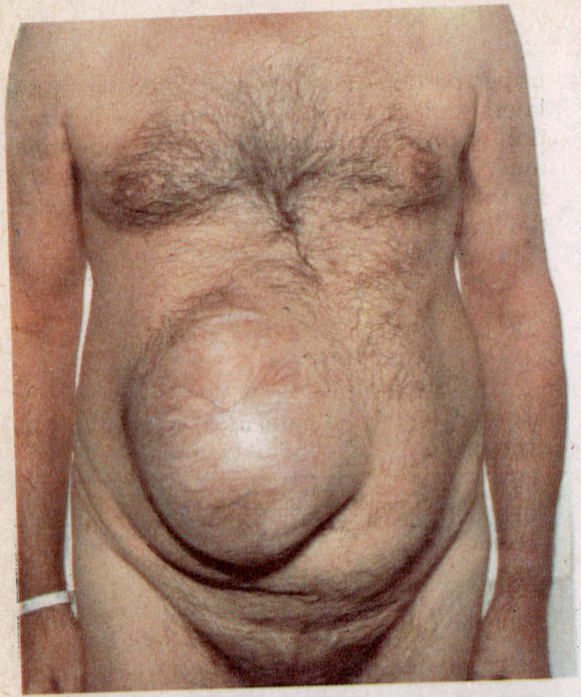

A large incisional hernia

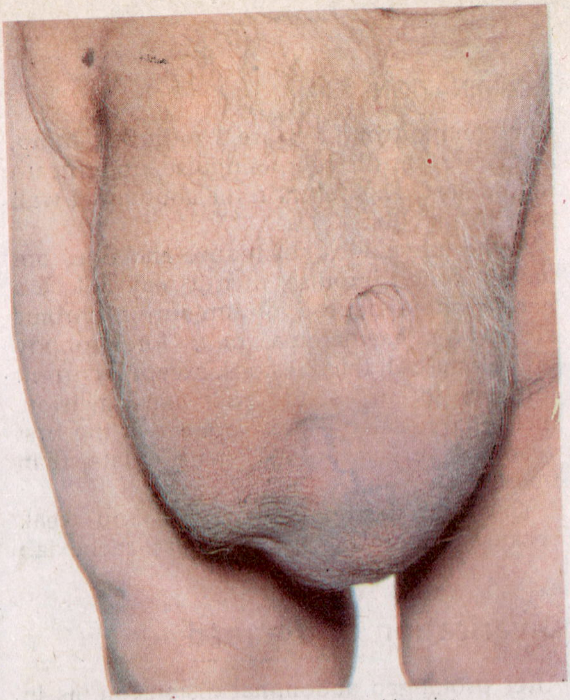

Very large bilateral, irreducible inguinal herniae

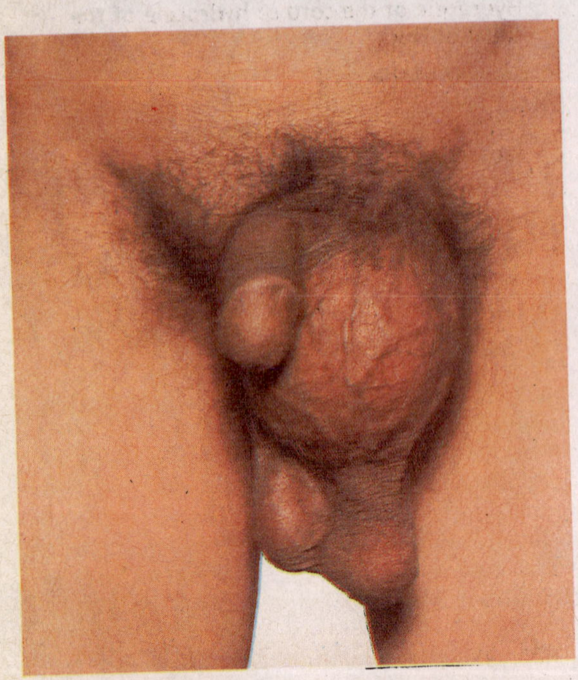

Is this a hernia? No, because it was possible to feel the spermatic cord above the lump and it had no cough impulse. It was a hydrocele of the cord

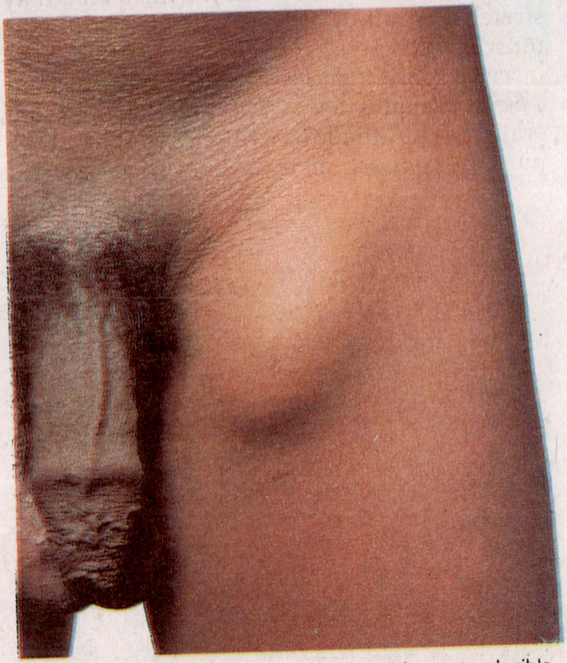

Is this a hernia? No, because it was firm, tender, not reducible and distant from both the inguinal and femoral canals. It was a mass of enlarged inguinal lymph nodes caused by lymphogranuloma

FIG. 13.16 THE OBVIOUS AND THE DECEPTIVE

The external genitalia

The penis and testes are sensitive organs and difficult to examine when they are tender. This is especially true of the testis, and you must be very gentle and careful when examining a tender testis if you wish to gain your patient's confidence and elicit all the abnormal physical signs.

EXAMINATION OF THE MALE GENITALIA

Always put on protective gloves especially if there is any urethral discharge or if you have any suspicion that the patient is suffering from a communicable disease.

The penis (Figs 14.1 and 14.2)

Inspection

Note the size and shape of the penis, the colour of the skin, the presence or absence of the foreskin and any discharge, scaling or scabbing around its distal edge.

Palpation

Assess the texture of the body of the penis and palpate the whole length of the urethra right down to the perineal membrane. Note the state of the dorsal vein and, if indicated, feel the pulses on the dorsal surface.

Always retract the prepuce carefully, to examine the skin on its inner aspect, the glans penis and the external urethral meatus. Look for any secretion or discharge and collect a specimen on a bacteriological swab.

At birth the foreskin is tethered to the glans penis and is slowly separated from it during the first few years of life by the secretion of smegma into the coronal sinus, so do not expect to be able to pull back the prepuce of a tiny baby. Occasionally these adhesions become permanent and prevent retraction of the prepuce in adult life. In these circumstances the glans penis can only be examined fully after surgical division of the adhesions. When there is a tight phimosis, a circumcision or a dorsal slit may be required to permit a proper examination. Although such measures, just to complete an examination, may seem excessive, they are essential to exclude the presence of a hidden condition such as a carcinoma.

The scrotal skin

The skin of the scrotum is usually wrinkled and freely mobile over the testes. If it is reddened, tethered or fixed there is probably a deep abnormality, but do not forget that the conditions which affect hair-bearing skin on any other part of the body – sebaceous cysts, small infected hair follicles, boils and squamous carcinomata – often affect the scrotal skin.

The scrotum is two-thirds of a sphere. Remember it has a back and front. **Always lift up the scrotum and inspect its posterior aspect.**

When you find a lesion in the scrotal skin, elicit all the signs required for a diagnosis of any lump or an ulcer.

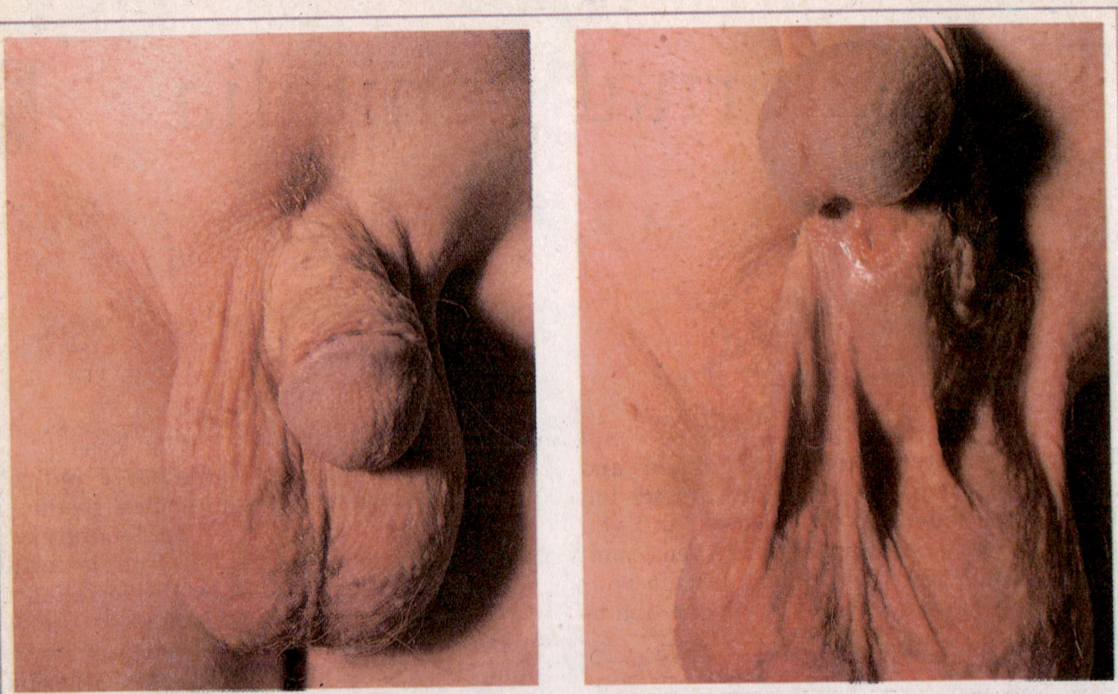

FIG. 14.1 Examination of the penis. **Always look at the ventral surface of the penis**. In this patient it revealed a hypospadias

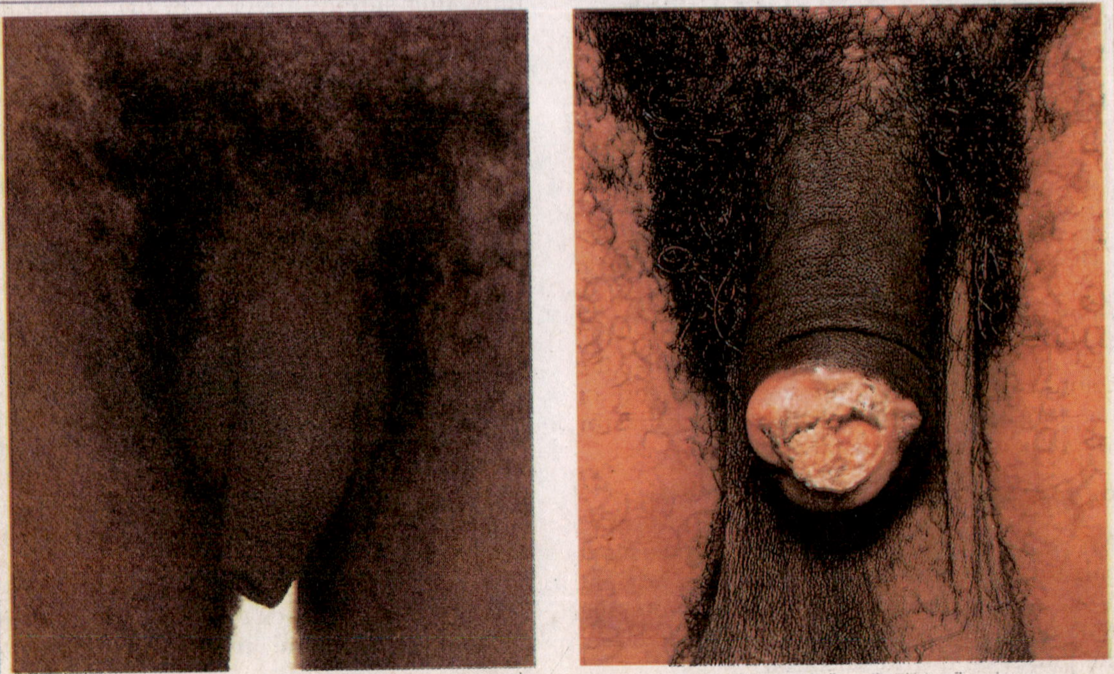

FIG. 14.2 Examination of the penis. **Always retract the prepuce** and inspect its inner surface, and the glans penis. In this patient it revealed a carcinoma

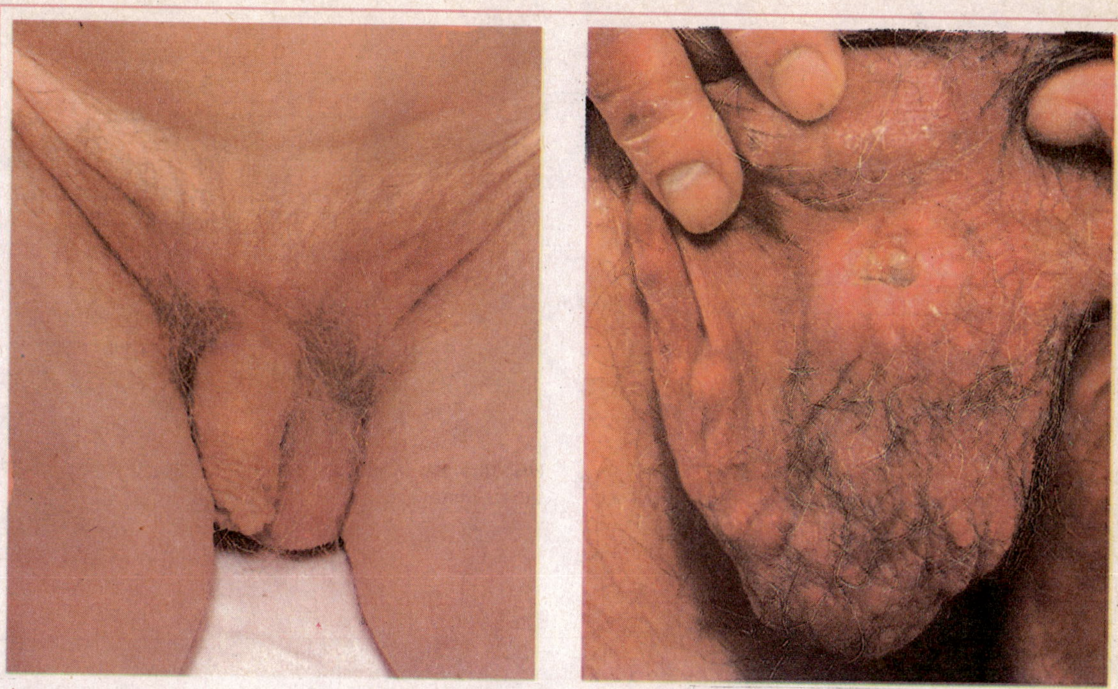

FIG. 14.3 Examination of the scrotum. **Always look at the posterior surface of the scrotum.** In this patient it revealed a carcinoma

The scrotal contents

It is possible to palpate the contents of the scrotum with the patient supine, but the shape of the scrotum and the position of the testes within it can only be observed properly when the patient is standing up.

Some clinicians insist that the scrotum should always be examined with the patient standing, but this overstates the case and it is quite acceptable to perform the major part of the examination with the patient lying supine.

Inspection

Note the size and shape of the scrotum, particularly any asymmetry.

Palpation

The scrotal contents are examined by gently supporting the scrotum on the fingers of one or both hands, while feeling the testis and any other lumps between your index finger, which is behind the scrotum, and the thumb, which is in front. Do not squeeze the testis or a lump between your thumb and index finger – let it slip from side to side so that you can feel its shape and surface.

First, check that the scrotum contains two testes.

Next, decide the position and nature of the body of each testis, the epididymitides and, lastly, the cords; that is, try to define the anatomy of the scrotal contents. As you feel the testes think of the picture that you will draw in your notes, after the examination. If the testis is normal draw it like Fig. 14.4. Unless you continue your examination until you are quite clear about the position of the testes and the epididymis, and their relation to any other masses, you will make many wrong diagnoses.

There are three main characteristics of any scrotal lump which you must determine, and which will be mentioned time and time again in the descriptions of individual diseases:

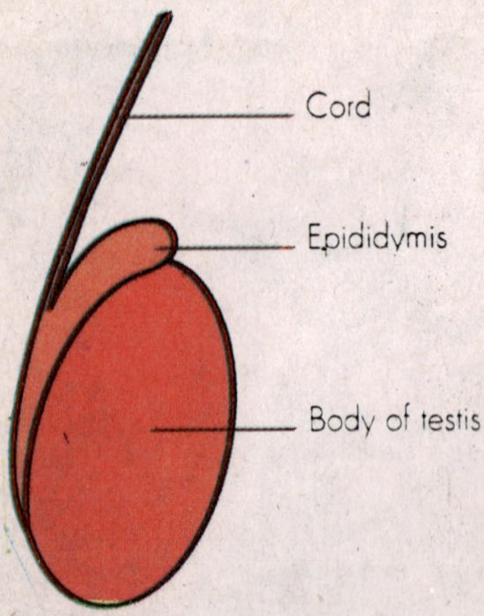

FIG. 14.4 If you think of the way in which you will draw the testes, and any abnormality you find, in your notes, it will help you define the anatomy. Do not stop your examination until you have defined the position and condition of the cord, the epididymis and the body of the testes

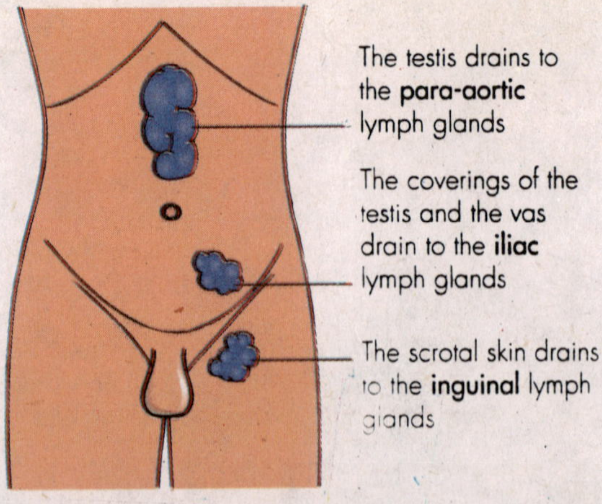

FIG. 14.5 The lymph drainage of the testis, its coverings and the scrotum

1 **Is the lump confined to the scrotum?** (Can you get above it?)
2 **Does the lump transilluminate?**
3 **Does the lump have an expansile cough impulse?**

If you know the answers to these three questions and have defined the physical characteristics of the lump and its relations to each testis and epididymis, you will have no difficulty making the diagnosis.

The perineum and rectum

Examination of the perineum, the anal canal and the rectum, particularly to feel the prostate and seminal vesicles, is an essential part of the examination of the genitalia (and the abdomen).

Lymph drainage (Fig. 14.5)

Remember the general rule that skin lymphatics follow the superficial veins; deep lymphatics accompany the arteries.

Lymph from the skin of the penis and scrotum drains to the **inguinal** glands.

Lymph from the coverings of the testis and spermatic cord (i.e. the tunica vaginalis and the cremasteric and spermatic fasciae) drains to the internal and, then, to the **common iliac** glands.

Lymph from the body of the testis drains to the para-aortic glands.

The aortic bifurcation is at the level of the umbilicus; therefore, the abdominal aorta is above the level of the umbilicus. Thus, enlarged para-aortic nodes are felt in the **upper half** of the abdomen, in the **epigastrium**.

THE PENIS

Phimosis

Phimosis is a narrowing of the end of the prepuce (foreskin), which prevents its retraction over the glans penis. It may be a congenital abnormality or be caused by scarring of the skin following infection or trauma.

HISTORY

Age Congenital phimosis presents in the first few years of life. Acquired phimosis presents in adult life.

Symptoms In the young child there may be **difficulty with micturition**, with **ballooning** of the prepuce as it becomes full of urine.

Recurrent balanitis (see below) causing **pain** and a **purulent discharge** is a common complication, but urinary tract infection is uncommon.

Similar symptoms may occur in the adult, but the commonest complaint is of interference with erection and sexual intercourse. If a tight foreskin does get retracted, it may not be possible to pull it forwards again; the patient then has a **paraphimosis** (see below).

EXAMINATION

A baby may not take kindly to an examination of his penis, so make certain that your hands are warm and that the mother has him as contented and quiet as possible.

It is usually easy to see that the prepuce narrows at its tip, but the only way to prove that the opening is small is to demonstrate that the foreskin cannot be retracted. This is not possible in a baby less than 1 year old because there are still adhesions between the prepuce and glans penis; but it is possible to retract the loose skin until you can see the orifice in the prepuce and assess its size.

If a child will not let you examine him, watch him passing urine. You may see the prepuce balloon out or see a very fine stream of urine. Both signs indicate an orifice narrow enough to justify circumcision.

When an adult has a discharge from the preputial orifice and a phimosis, examine the rest of his genitalia carefully in case the balanitis or its cause is the main problem and the phimosis a coincidental or secondary event.

Paraphimosis

This is common in young men and occurs when the narrowing of the prepuce is insufficient to interfere with micturition but just sufficiently tight to get stuck behind the glans penis after an erection.

In this position it impedes venous blood flow and causes oedema and congestion of the glans, which in turn makes reduction of the prepuce more difficult.

HISTORY

Age Paraphimosis usually occurs in young men between 15 and 30 years old. It is also a common complication of urethral catheterization, at any age, if the foreskin is not pulled forwards over the glans penis after the catheter has been passed.

Duration The condition may pass unnoticed for many hours because it is not painful until the glans begins to swell.

Symptoms If the patient has failed to notice that the foreskin has not returned to its normal position, his first complaint is of **swelling and discomfort** of the glans penis. The skin below the corona becomes red and sore, and the tight constricting band below the corona is painful.

It is uncommon for the urethra to be so compressed that it obstructs micturition.

Past history The patient will not have been circumcised.

EXAMINATION

The diagnosis is usually obvious, especially if you know that the patient has not been circumcised. The glans penis is swollen and oedematous and there is a deep groove just below the corona where the skin looks tight, and may be split and ulcerated.

Long-standing cases can get infection and superficial ulceration of the skin of the glans penis.

Revision Panel 14.1

Age-related incidence of separation/retractability of the foreskin

At birth	4%
At 1 year	50%
At 4 years	90%

Note that the majority of non-retractable foreskins in children do *not* have a phimosis.

FIG. 14.6 HYPOSPADIAS

Note that the external urethral meatus may be on the glans penis, the shaft of the penis or the perineum

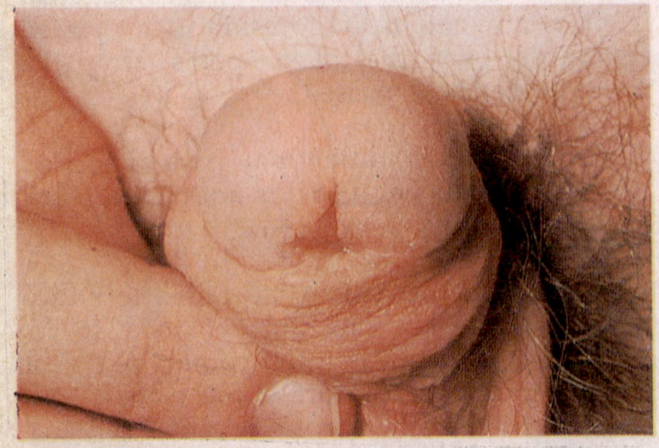

Glandular hypospadias. The urethral opening is on the edge of the glans penis. The pit where the opening should be is also visible

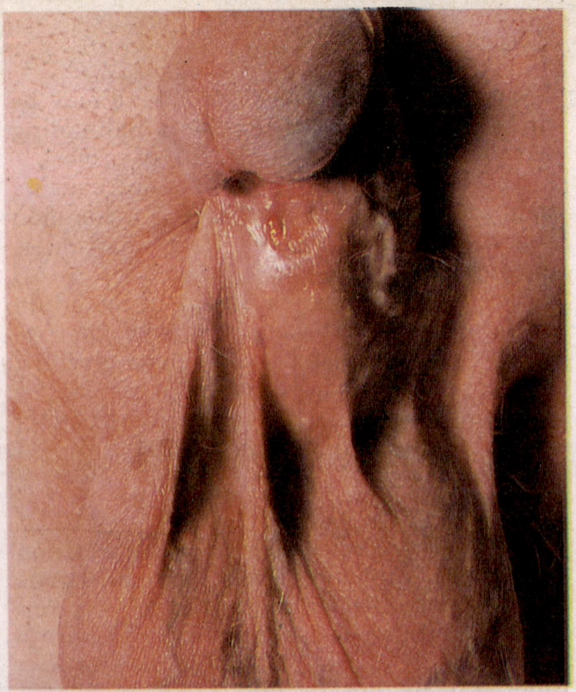

Penile hypospadias. The urethral opening is 1 cm below the edge of the glans

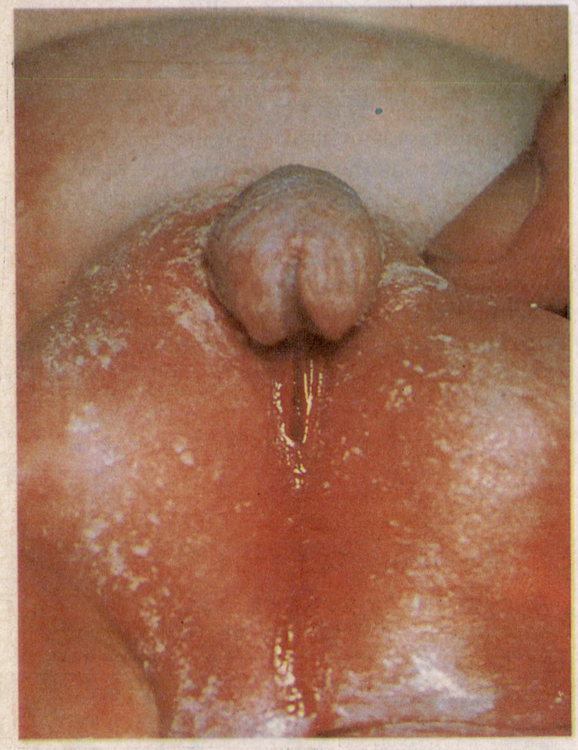

Penoscrotal hypospadias. The urethral opening is at the junction between the shaft of the penis and the scrotum

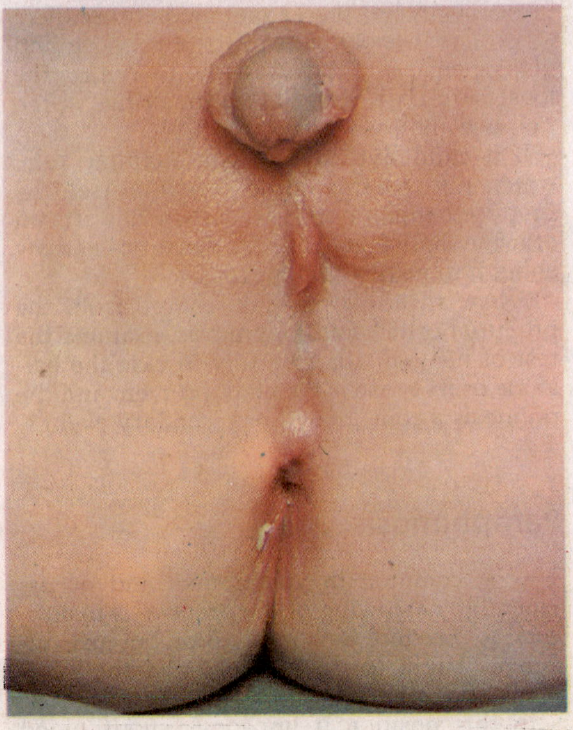

Periheal hypospadias. The urethral opening is in the perineum. The scrotum is bifid

Hypospadias

Hypospadias is a congenital abnormality in which the urethra opens on the ventral surface of the penis (i.e. proximal to its usual position at the tip of the penis).

The opening may be anywhere along the line of the urethra, from a few millimetres from the tip of the penis to the perineum. If the urethral opening is in the perineum the scrotum is bifid. The site of the opening is, therefore, defined as glandular (on the glans), penile (on the shaft) or perineal.

Glandular hypospadias is easy to miss because it causes no symptoms and there is a deceptive small pit at the normal site of the urethral opening, so always inspect the urethral surface of the shaft of the penis.

Chordee is commonly associated with hypospadias. It is a descriptive term for a curved penis. A normal penis, even when flaccid, is usually straight, but if there is a urethral abnormality, or fibrosis of the corpora cavernosa (Peyronie's disease), the penis becomes curved. This curvature is increased during an erection.

Epispadias is the opposite of hypospadias the urethral opening is on the dorsal surface of the glans penis. It is rare.

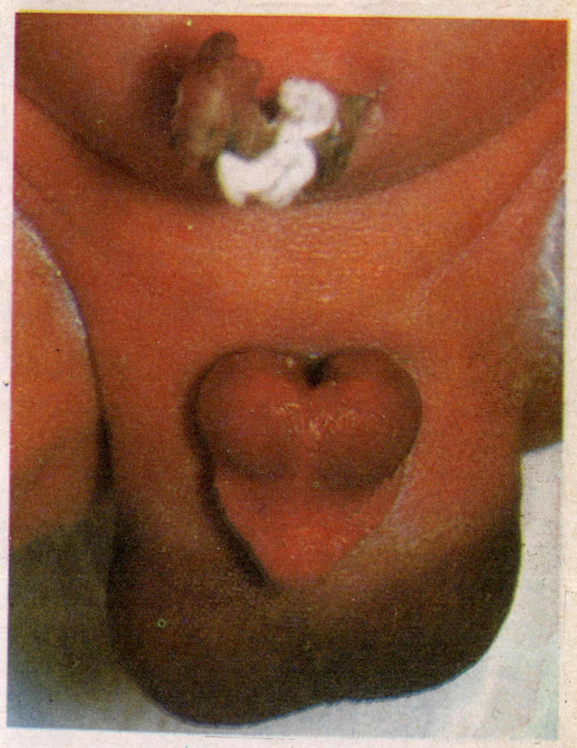

FIG. 14.7 Epispadias. The urethra opens on the dorsum of the glans penis, almost on the dorsal aspect of the shaft of the penis

Balanoposthitis

Strictly speaking, balanitis is an inflammation of the prepuce, but the word is commonly used to describe inflammation involving the glans penis (posthitis). If both prepuce and glans are involved, the correct name is balanoposthitis.

The patient may complain of itching, pain, or discharge from the subpreputial space. There may be difficulty in retracting the foreskin.

The important points in the clinical examination are:

1 First palpate the glans through the foreskin.
2 Next retract the foreskin and examine the inside of the prepuce and glans for discharge, erosion or tumour.
3 If the foreskin cannot be retracted, it may be necessary to arrange for a surgeon to perform a dorsal slit or circumcision.
4 Palpate the inguinal lymph glands.
5 Search for a cause of balanoposthitis (this will vary with the patient's age):
   (a) *Candida albicans* is common in sexually active persons and diabetics;
   (b) herpes genitalis;
   (c) carcinoma of the penis;
   (d) primary chancre (syphilis);
   (e) fixed drug eruption;
   (f) dirt.

Candidal balanoposthitis The glans penis will show red patches which may be itchy. The foreskin has a white appearance with longitudinal fissuring, particularly at the tip.

Herpes genitalis This recurrent infection can involve the shaft, glans or foreskin. The initial itchy vesicles are soon replaced by shallow, painful erosions. Particularly in the primary attack, there may be painful inguinal lymphadenopathy.

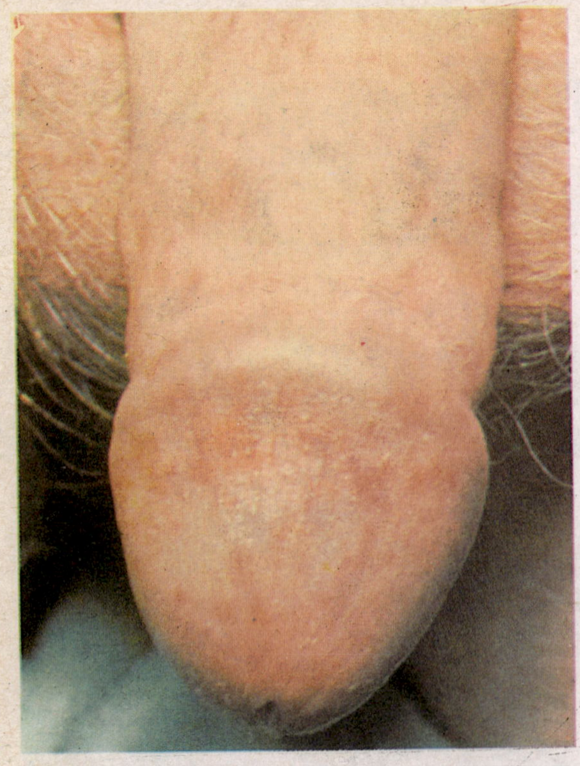

Monilial balanoposthitis

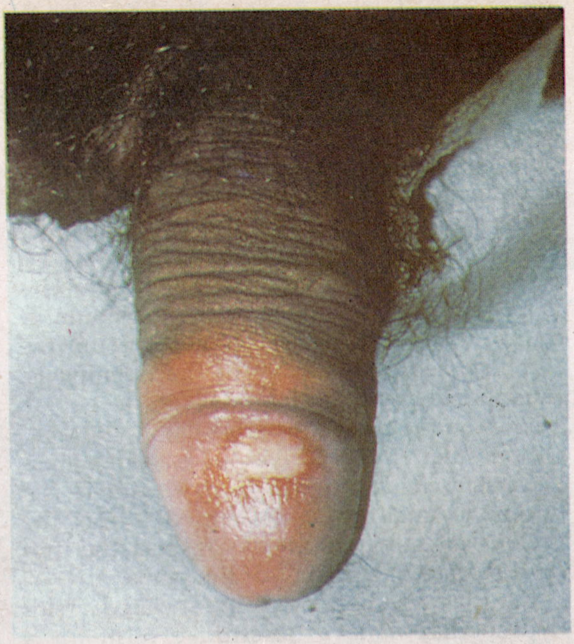

A drug eruption. This ulcer was part of a reaction to Septrin

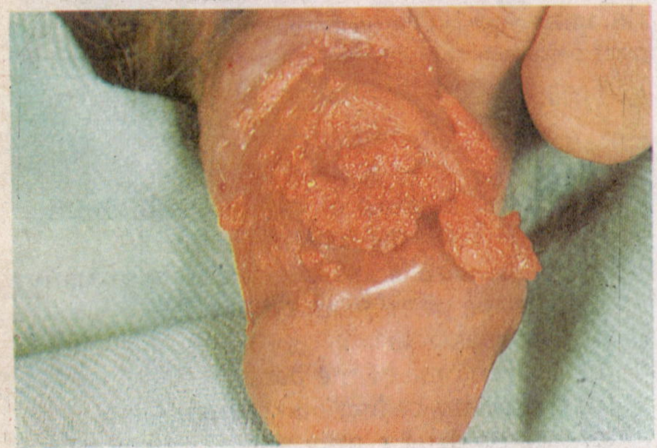

Penile warts

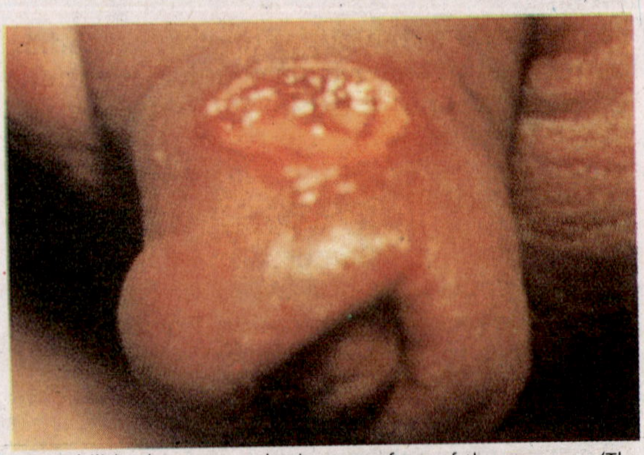

A syphilitic chancre on the inner surface of the prepuce. (The ungloved hand is that of the patient)

FIG. 14.8 FOUR COMMON PENILE CONDITIONS

Fixed drug eruptions These are painless discolourations, most often seen on the glans penis, which are sometimes the only manifestation of drug hypersensitivity.

Dirt Poor personal hygiene, surroundings with a high concentration of dust and dirt, and phimosis can all encourage the accumulation of debris beneath the prepuce. The resulting irritation may cause non-specific inflammation. Coexisting diseases, such as **diabetes**, which render patients more susceptible to infection, increase the risk of secondary infection.

Syphilitic chancre

In many parts of the developed world, syphilis is now rare. The primary sore (chancre) is usually **solitary** and **painless**. It usually occurs in the **coronal sinus**, the prepuce, and fraenum, and produces a serosanguinous discharge.

Beneath an area of **superficial ulceration** is an indistinct, indurated lump, 5–10 mm in diameter. The ulcer is usually covered with a slough and has a sloping, indolent edge. It is not fixed to deeper structures.

The inguinal lymph glands are invariably enlarged, often mainly on one side, rubbery and discrete but **not tender**.

General examination may reveal no other abnormalities, but a primary sore may still be present when the secondary manifestations of the disease appear, 4–6 weeks after the appearance of the chancre.

Carcinoma of the penis

Carcinoma of the penis is a squamous cell carcinoma. It is exceedingly rare in men who are circumcised at birth or in adolescence (e.g. Jews and Muslims).

It may be preceded by a number of premalignant conditions described later. It invades the tissues of the shaft of the penis and spreads beyond the penis via the lymphatics.

HISTORY

Age Carcinoma of the penis commonly presents in middle or old age, but it can occur in young men.

Ethnic group Religious and other practices are closely linked to race. Carcinoma of the penis is more common in cultures that do not practice ritual circumcision, so it is commonly found in India and the Far East; but whether this geographical distribution is related solely to circumcision is not clear.

Symptoms Most patients present with a **lump** or an **ulcer**, representing the papilliferous or ulcerating varieties of skin carcinoma.

The lesion may be **painful**, especially if it is infected.

There is usually a **purulent discharge**, which may be blood-stained.

The patient may also complain of a **phimosis**. In these circumstances the primary lesion can become quite advanced before it is detected.

The **inguinal lymph nodes may be enlarged** by secondary infection or secondary deposits and be the first abnormality noticed by the patient.

Presentation with malaise due to distant metastases is rare.

EXAMINATION

The prepuce

The patient is most unlikely to have been circumcised. There may be a serous, purulent or sanguinous **discharge** coming from beneath the prepuce. If the foreskin cannot be retracted it must be slit surgically, to allow a full examination of its inner surface and the glans penis.

Deformity

The penis may be swollen at its tip owing to the mass beneath the prepuce. In the advanced stages the tumour may appear through the opening in the prepuce or erode through the preputial skin.

The carcinoma

Position The lesion may be anywhere on the skin of the prepuce or the glans penis.

Tenderness The lump or ulcer is not usually tender.

Shape Carcinoma of the penis tends to adopt one of two macroscopic forms: a classic carcinomatous ulcer with a **raised everted edge** and necrotic base, or a **papilliferous tumour** with a wide sessile pedicle and an **indurated base**.

Size Most patients appear early in the course of the disease provided they can retract the prepuce. If they have a phimosis, and have grown accustomed to an occasional discharge, they may not present until the tumour is large and appearing through the preputial opening or eroding through the skin of the prepuce.

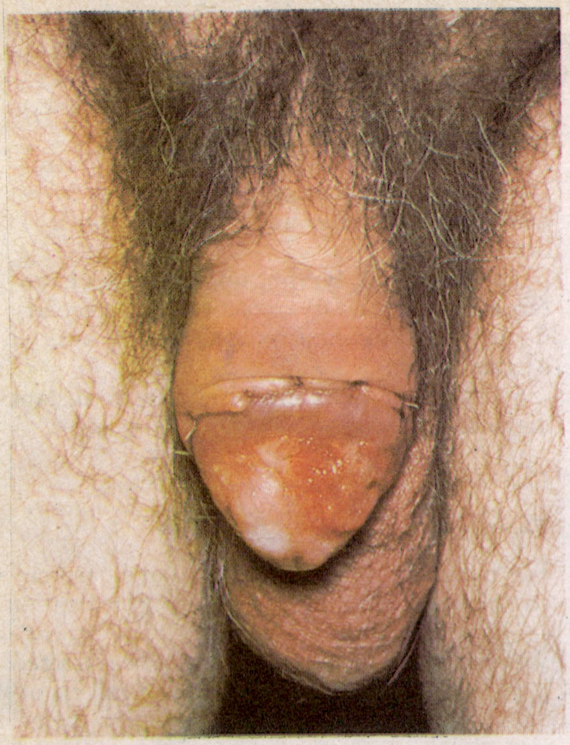

An early carcinomatous ulcer on the glans penis, exposed by a circumcision

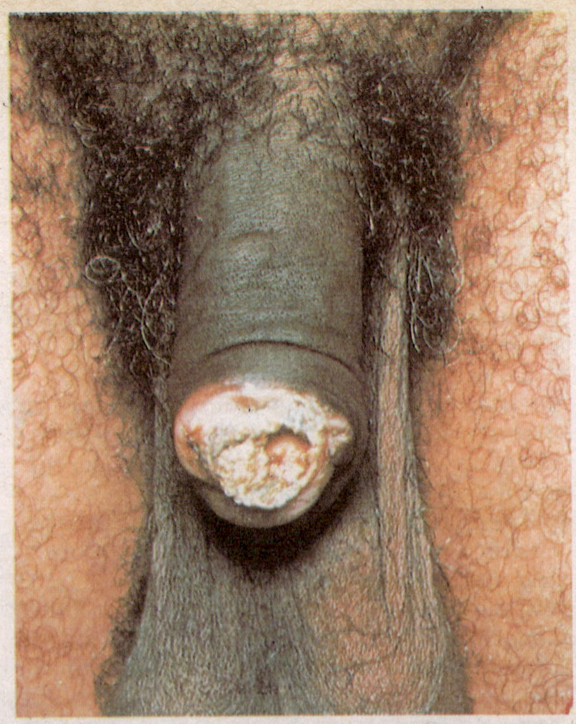

A papilliferous carcinoma arising in the coronal sulcus

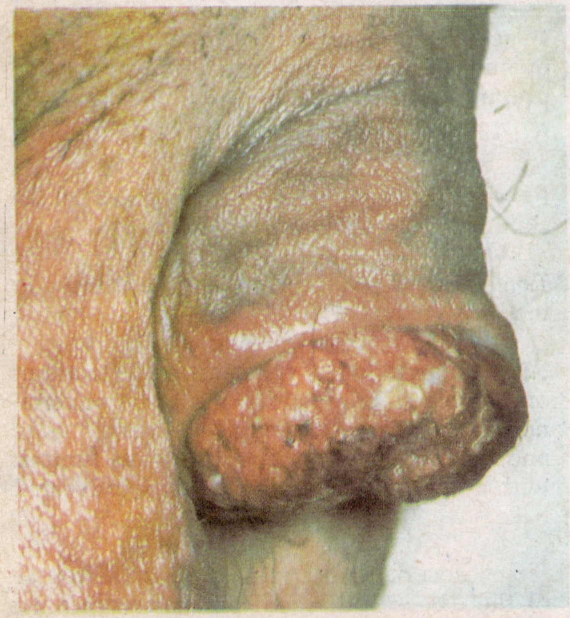

An advanced infiltrating carcinoma which has invaded the whole thickness of the prepuce

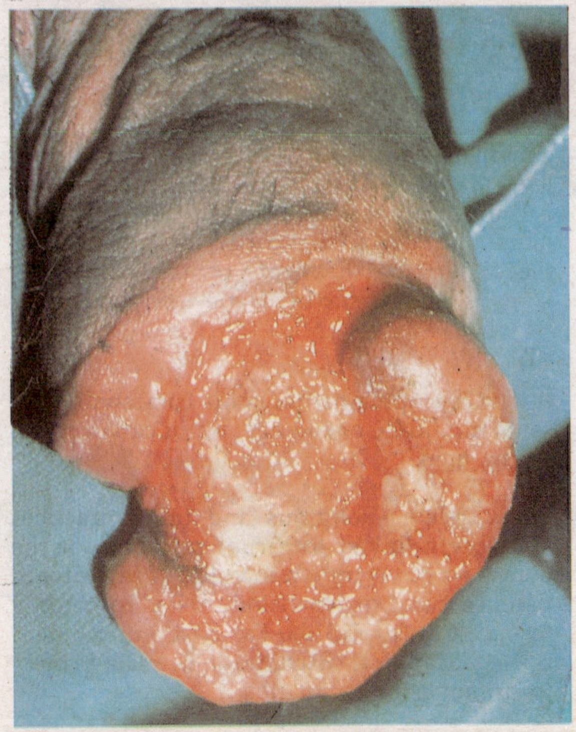

An ulcerating carcinoma that has destroyed half of the glans penis

FIG. 14.9 CARCINOMA OF THE PENIS

Composition The tumour has a **hard consistence**, especially at its base. Any part of the penis which is infiltrated also feels hard. The surface of the papilliferous variety is soft and friable. It often looks like poor-quality granulation tissue, and bleeds easily.

Relations In the early stages the tumour is confined to the skin, but it may invade and spread through the whole corpus cavernosum, making it stiff and hard, and if it begins on the inner side of the prepuce it may spread to and through the outer layer of skin.

Lymph drainage The inguinal lymph nodes of both groins are likely to be enlarged, by infection or secondary deposits. The tumour may have spread from these nodes all the way up the iliac and lumbar lymph chain and reached the supraclavicular nodes.

GENERAL EXAMINATION

It is not uncommon to find that the patient is elderly, dirty and malnourished.

Premalignant conditions of the penis

Three diseases are definitely associated with an increased incidence of carcinoma of the penis.

Leukoplakia

This term describes areas of white, boggy epithelium (identical to the appearances of leukoplakia on the tongue, vulva and vagina), which are definitely premalignant.

It is the visible evidence of hyperkeratosis; the epithelial cells are hypertrophic (acanthosis) and there is infiltration of the dermis with lymphocytes.

Figure 14.10 show very clearly how leukoplakia resembles patches of greyish-white paint. It is **painless**.

Paget's disease

This is an area of chronic, red eczema on the glans penis or inside of the prepuce which alternately oozes and crusts over. If the patient is not circumcised the skin beneath the

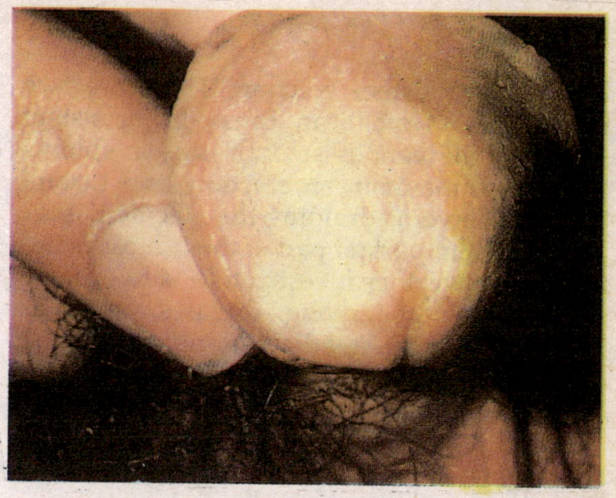

FIG. 14.10 Leukoplakia of the glans penis, showing the typical 'patches of white paint' appearance

prepuce never dries out and the patches of Paget's disease may become 'boggy'.

Paget's disease is the intraepithelial stage of a squamous carcinoma, very similar to the condition with the same eponym that occurs on the nipple of the breast. It is rare.

Erythroplasia of Queyrat

This condition occurs most often on the penis, but it can occur on the vulva and in the mouth. It causes a dark red, flat but slightly indurated patch of skin on the glans penis or inner side of the prepuce. It may occasionally be slightly raised and nodular.

Two other conditions may predispose to cancer of the penis but the association is not so certain – **chronic balanitis** and **chronic papillomata**.

Revision Panel 14.2

Diseases associated with precancerous changes of the penis

- Leukoplakia
- Paget's disease
- Erythroplasia of Queyrat
- [Chronic papilloma]
- [Chronic balanitis]

Priapism

This is a persistent erection. There are two mechanisms which can cause it: persistent spasm of the venous smooth muscle sphincters which maintain an erection, and thrombosis of the veins draining the erectile tissue.

The most important part of the clinical examination and further investigation is to exclude any serious underlying diseases, such as **leukaemia, sickle-cell disease** and other blood diseases associated with a thrombotic tendency, and local prostatic and pelvic disease.

On rare occasions persistent priapism is neurogenic in origin and secondary to disease of the spinal cord.

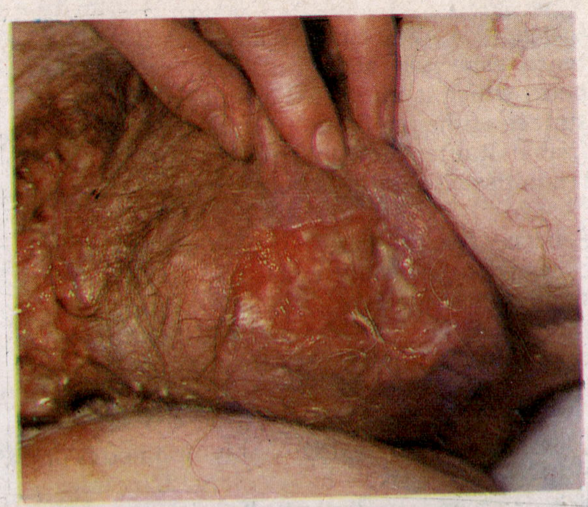

FIG. 14.11 A carcinoma of the scrotal skin. Note that it is on the posteromedial surface of the scrotum

THE SCROTAL SKIN

Sebaceous cysts

Sebaceous cysts are common in the scrotal skin. They have all the features described in Chapter 3 but are mentioned here because it is surprising how often they are misdiagnosed.

Occasionally they can become infected, discharge and produce so much granulation tissue that they look like a carcinoma.

Carcinoma of the scrotal skin

This is a squamous carcinoma. It can be caused by frequent contact with soot (chimney sweep's cancer), tar or oil (mule spinner's cancer). The skin must be exposed to these irritants for many years before a cancer develops.

HISTORY

Age Carcinoma of the skin of the scrotum is uncommon below the age of 50 years.

Occupation The patient's occupation may be responsible for frequent soiling of the scrotal skin with oil and other carcinogenic hydrocarbons. Even today, the clothes of garage mechanics and machine operators become soaked in oil which percolates through to their underclothes.

Symptoms The commonest presenting symptoms are an **ulcer** or a **lump** in the scrotal skin. A **purulent discharge** may appear, and if the ulcer is hidden in the cleft between the scrotum and leg the discharge may be noticed before the ulcer.

The patient may notice **lumps in the groin** if the inguinal lymph nodes are involved.

EXAMINATION

Position A carcinomatous ulcer can occur on any part of the scrotal skin, but industrial cancers are often high up in the cleft between the leg and the scrotum, where there is repeated friction and persistent traces of oil.

Tenderness The ulcer is usually painless and not tender.

Shape In its early stages the ulcer is small and circular, but it usually enlarges in an irregular fashion and develops an irregular outline.

Edge The edge is reddish, friable and typically everted.

Base The base is covered with yellow-grey, infected, necrotic tumour.

Discharge There is often a purulent, bloody, offensive discharge.

Relations In the early stages the skin and ulcer are freely mobile, but if the tumour cells spread deep to the skin the ulcer may become tethered to the underlying testis. At this stage it may be difficult to decide whether the lesion is a primary skin cancer or a testicular tumour ulcerating through the skin.

Lymph drainage The inguinal nodes may be enlarged by secondary deposits or inflammation.

GENERAL EXAMINATION

Distant metastases are a late complication of cancer of the scrotum, but lymph nodes in the iliac, para-aortic and supraclavicular regions may be enlarged by secondary deposits.

Tinea cruris

Common conditions present in diverse clinics. Tinea cruris is a fungus infection (*Epidermophyton*) of the skin of the upper medial aspect of the thigh and the adjacent scrotal skin.

The first symptom is itching, but this is soon followed by the appearance of a dry erythematous rash with a sharply defined edge on the thigh and scrotum.

If the patient perspires heavily the rash may become macerated and ooze serum, which forms pale brown crusts.

The patient may present to a surgical clinic because of the changes in the scrotal skin, or you may notice the distinctive skin changes when examining the patient's scrotum for another complaint, such as a hernia.

Lymphoedema

Swelling of the penis and scrotum caused by excess fluid in the subcutaneous tissue commonly occurs in patients, sitting in bed, with heart failure or water retention. True lymphoedema of the genitalia – oedema due to retention of protein-rich lymph in the subcutaneous tissues – is uncommon. It may be associated with lymphoedema of one or both limbs.

The common cause is obstruction of the inguinal and iliac lymph pathways by secondary or primary tumour, or worms (*Wuchereria bancrofti*; filariasis). Primary genital lymphoedema is very rare and is due to hypoplastic lymphatics. It is not known if this is a congenital or an acquired condition.

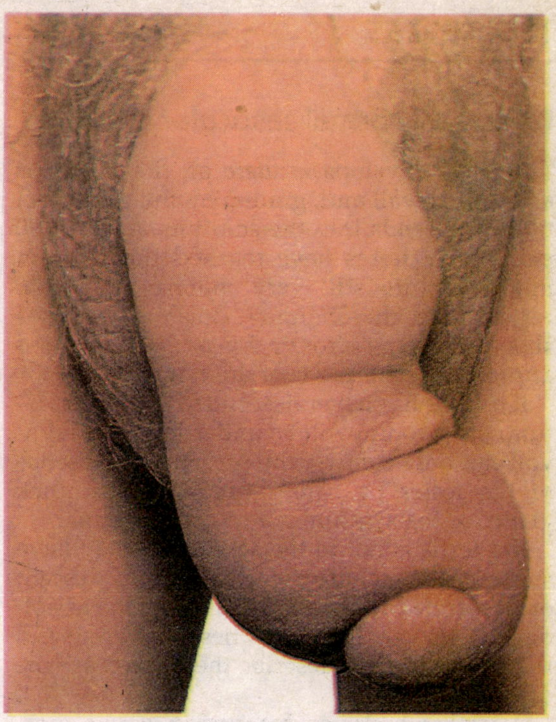

FIG. 14.12 Lymphoedema of the penis

Sinuses of the scrotum

Disease of the testis or epididymis may spread to the scrotal skin and form a sinus between the primary lesion and the skin surface.

Provided the testis is lying in the normal anatomical position, disease of the body of the testis tends to spread to the anterolateral aspect of the scrotum, and disease of the epididymis to the posterior aspect.

Thus an anterior sinus is likely to be secondary to a testicular tumour or a gumma, whereas a posterior sinus is likely to lead down to an epididymitis, usually tuberculous.

Remember to inspect the back of the scrotum for sinuses.

THE TESTES

Failure of normal testicular descent

The testis develops *in utero* on the posterior abdominal wall and, guided by the gubernaculum, descends into the scrotum. At birth 80 per cent of testes have reached the scrotum but many are still very mobile and often retract into the inguinal canal. The testes should be in the scrotum 1 year after birth but approximately 3 per cent are not.

If a testis has never descended into the scrotum, the scrotum will be underdeveloped, but you can only confirm the presence or absence of the testes by careful palpation; a quick glance at the scrotum is not good enough.

If a testis is not in the scrotum it may have stopped somewhere along its line of descent or descended to an abnormal site. The aetiology of these two abnormalities is different and the names used to describe them often are the cause of confusion.

A testis which has descended to an abnormal site is an ectopic testis. There is no confusion about this term. The testis may be in the superficial inguinal pouch, the femoral triangle or the perineum. The mechanism causing descent is normal but the guidance system is at fault.

A testis which is in its correct anatomical path but has failed to reach the scrotum is best called an **incompletely descended testis.**

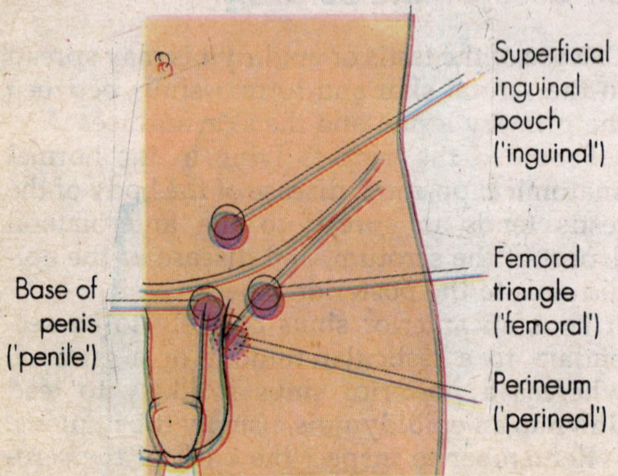

FIG. 14.13 The sites where you may find an ectopic testis

Although this is a cumbersome name it is better than 'undescended' or 'maldescended' because both these names could reasonably be used to describe both incompletely and ectopically descended testes.

The cause of incomplete descent is not known, but as there is a failure of the driving mechanism and the testis is often abnormal, it is most likely that the cause is an endocrine abnormality.

When a patient presents with the absence of a testis (or both) you must decide whether he has an ectopic or an incompletely descended testis. Ectopic testes are far less common than incompletely descended testes.

Absence of both testes from the scrotum is known as **cryptorchism.**

Ectopic testis

HISTORY

Age Not all parents notice that their infant child has one or both testes missing from his scrotum. If he is left to discover the abnormality himself the patient may not present until adolescence.

Symptoms **Absence of a testis** is the common presenting symptom, but the patient may also complain of **pain** or discomfort if the testis is in a site, such as the perineum, likely to be rubbed or compressed during normal physical activity.

Systemic effects If both testes are ectopic the patient may be sterile but rarely lacks secondary sex characteristics. Ectopic testes usually produce some spermatozoa and the patients are fertile.

EXAMINATION

The side of the scrotum without the testis will be poorly developed.

Site **An ectopic testis is always palpable. An incompletely descended testis lying in the inguinal canal or abdomen is not palpable. If the testis is not in the scrotum you must search for a smooth, sensitive, ovoid swelling in those sites where ectopic testes are known to settle.**

1 **Superficial inguinal pouch** Failure of the testis to descend into the scrotum may be caused by the presence of a dense layer of subcutaneous tissue at the neck of the scrotum. When this occurs, the testis turns upward to lie in a 'pouch' just above and superficial to the external inguinal ring. The testis can, therefore, be palpated in the subcutaneous tissue just above and lateral to the crest of the pubis and the pubic tubercle.

2 **Femoral triangle** If the testis moves laterally after leaving the external inguinal ring, it can come to rest in the upper medial corner of the femoral triangle. A testis in this site is easy to feel and may be confused with a lymph node or a femoral hernia.

3 **Base of the penis** If the testis moves medially, it will lie at the base of the penis where it can be easily felt against the underlying pubic bone.

4 **Perineum** Occasionally, the testis passes over the pubis and then backwards, instead of downwards, to lie in the perineum just to one side of the corpus cavernosum of the penis.

The lump An absent scrotal testis and a lump in one of the four sites described above make the diagnosis of ectopic testis very probable, but it is important to confirm that the lump has the features of a testis.

It should be ovoid, smooth, slightly tender, soft–solid in consistence and opaque. It should be mobile within the subcutaneous tissues, and firm pressure should cause the mild sickening sensation recognized by most males as testicular sensation.

It is unusual to be able to define the separate features of the body of the testis and the epididymis.

Any enlargement, irregularity or immobility should make you suspect the presence of malignant change in the testis.

Incompletely descended testis

HISTORY

Age Undescended testes are usually noticed in early life but are occasionally not noticed until adolescence.

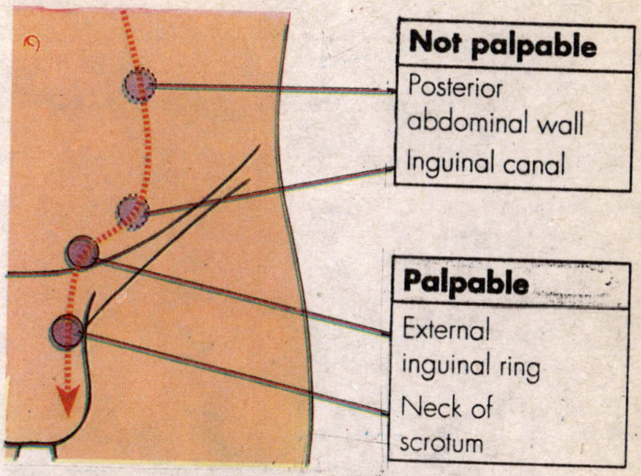

FIG. 14.14 The line of normal testicular descent. An incompletely decended testis may be found anywhere on this line. If it is above the external inguinal ring it will be impalpable

Symptoms **An absence of one or both testes** from the scrotum is the commonest presenting symptom. The patient may first notice that the **scrotum has not developed** – unaware of the absence of the testes. A small proportion of patients present in adult life with **infertility**. Although failure of testicular descent is invariably associated with abnormal spermatogenesis, the hormone-producing cells are usually normal so the boy has a normal puberty and secondary sex characteristics.

Many incompletely descended testes are associated with an **indirect inguinal hernia**, which may be the presenting complaint.

EXAMINATION

Site An incompletely descended testis should lie somewhere on the line of normal descent (i.e. at the neck of the scrotum over the external inguinal ring, in the inguinal canal or on the posterior abdominal wall).

The testis becomes palpable when it reaches, or is outside, the external inguinal ring.

A normal soft testis within the inguinal canal cannot be felt because the tense overlying external oblique aponeurosis conceals it. Thus, if you can feel a testis lateral to the inguinal ring, it must be superficial to the external oblique and therefore an ectopic testis not an incompletely descended testis.

Some testes which lie in the inguinal canal can be milked down to the external ring by gently stroking along the line of the canal.

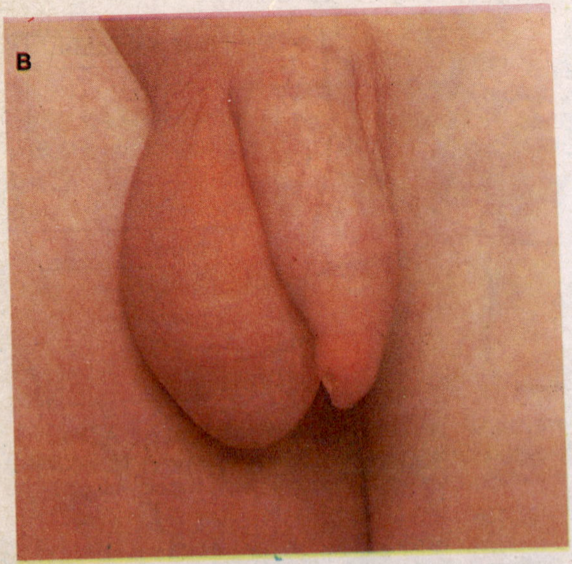

FIG. 14.15 A left undescended testis. Note the underdevelopment of the left side of the scrotum

The lump An incompletely descended testis is usually smaller than normal but otherwise has all the expected characteristics of a testis.

If the testis cannot be felt, press firmly along the line of the inguinal canal to see if there is a tender area or even a point where pressure evokes testicular sensations.

The appearance of a mass in the line of testicular descent, whether within the abdomen or the inguinal canal, and an empty scrotum should make you suspect malignant change. The risk of malignant change in an incompletely descended testis is 36 times greater than in a descended testis. Fixing the testis in the scrotum (orchidopexy) does not reduce this risk.

Revision Panel 14.3
The causes of hydrocele

Primary
- Idiopathic

Secondary
- Trauma
- Epididymo-orchitis
- Tumour
- Lymphatic obstruction

The scrotum When both testes are undescended the scrotum is small and hypoplastic. If only one testis has descended it is asymmetrical.

Retractile testes

A testis should only be classified as incompletely descended or ectopic if you cannot manipulate it into the scrotum.

The cremaster is a strong active muscle during childhood and the testes of many young children move feely up and down between the scrotum and the inguinal canal. A cold examining hand may be sufficient stimulus to cause retraction. If the patient is seen when the testis is retracted it may be misdiagnosed as an incompletely descended testis and surgical treatment advised. This will be an unnecessary operation because all retractile testes ultimately descend properly.

You should always attempt to manipulate the testis into the scrotum. If the testis is palpable, hold it gently between your thumb and index finger and try to draw it down into the scrotum. If it is a retracted testis it will move down easily.

If you cannot feel the testis, you should find out if it is in the inguinal canal by gently stroking along the line of the canal, from the lateral to the medial end, to 'milk' the testis, if present, through the external ring. The mid-inguinal testis is impalpable; the 'emergent' testis at the external ring is just palpable. If the testis becomes palpable, catch it gently with the thumb and index finger of your other hand and draw it down to the scrotum.

Any testis that can be manipulated into the scrotum is a retractile, not an undescended, testis.

When the testes are retractile the scrotum is normally developed.

Hydrocele

A hydrocele is an abnormal quantity of serous fluid within the tunica vaginalis. There are two varieties:

Primary – cause unknown.
Secondary – to trauma, infection or neoplasm.

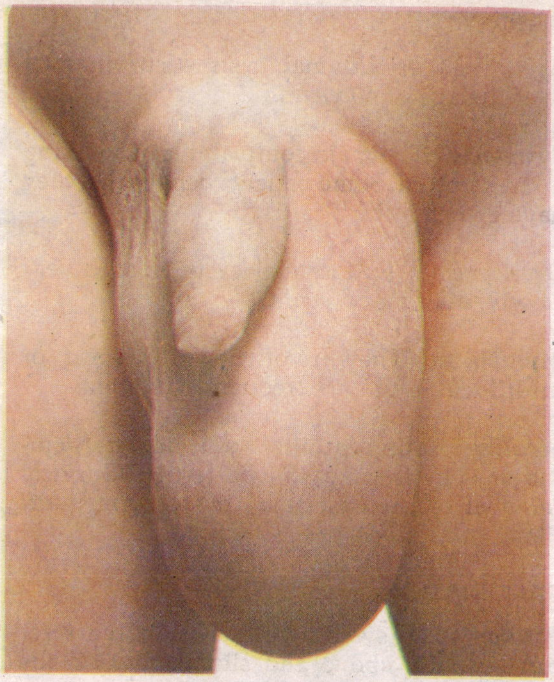

FIG. 14.16 A large hydrocele. The swelling is confined to the scrotum, not tender, fluctuant, translucent, and the testis is not palpable

Most secondary hydroceles appear rapidly in the presence of other symptoms associated with their cause, are not tense, and contain some altered blood. Primary (idiopathic) hydroceles develop slowly, and become large and tense.

HISTORY

Age Primary hydroceles are most common over the age of 40 years but can occur in children, when they usually have a patent connection with the peritoneal cavity via the processus vaginalis. Secondary hydroceles are more common between 20 and 40 years because trauma, infection and neoplasm are more common in this period.

Symptoms The patient complains of an increase in the size of the testis, or a **swelling** in the scrotum. There may be pain and discomfort if there is underlying testicular disease, but idiopathic hydroceles reach a considerable size without causing pain. The patient may complain of the social embarrassment of his large scrotum.

There may be urinary tract symptoms, such as frequent and painful micturition, if the hydrocele is secondary to epididymo-orchitis; or there may be malaise and weight loss if there is an underlying tumour with distant metastases.

Hydroceles do not affect fertility.

EXAMINATION

Position The swelling fills one side of the scrotum but is within the scrotum (i.e. you can feel the cord of the testis above the lump).

There is one exception to this statement. When the tunica vaginalis is patent up to the internal ring the hydrocele may extend up into the inguinal canal. This is called an infantile hydrocele and is uncommon.

Hydroceles are often bilateral.

Colour and temperature The colour and temperature of the overlying scrotal skin are normal.

Tenderness Idiopathic hydroceles are not tender. Secondary hydroceles may be tender if the underlying testis is tender.

Shape and size When the tunica vaginalis first fills with fluid the resulting hydrocele is just a little larger than the testis; but as time passes the volume of fluid increases and hydroceles can be 10–20 cm in diameter and contain 500 mL of fluid. They are ovoid.

Surface Their surface is smooth and well defined. Occasionally a weak spot in the wall gives way to form a small fluctuant bump – a hernia of the hydrocele through its coverings.

Composition Hydroceles are usually filled with a clear fluid. Therefore they are **fluctuant**; have a **fluid thrill** (if large enough); are **dull** to percussion; and – except when the fluid is turbulent – translucent.

They do not pulsate and are not compressible.

They may be **tense or lax** depending on the pressure of the contained fluid.

The wall of very old hydroceles may become calcified, making the mass hard and opaque.

Reducibility Hydroceles cannot be reduced.

Relations The fluid of a hydrocele **surrounds the body of the testis** making the **testis impalpable**. This is its most important relationship. If you can feel the testis separate from a scrotal swelling then the swelling cannot be a hydrocele. When a hydrocele is lax it is possible to feel the surface of the testis **through** the fluid, but this uncommon sign is easy to recognize.

The testis produces an opaque area in an otherwise highly translucent swelling.

The spermatic cord can be felt coming down to and running into the swelling. The skin of the scrotum is freely mobile over the swelling.

Lymph drainage The para-aortic lymph nodes, which receive lymph from the testis, should be carefully palpated if you think the swelling is a secondary hydrocele, because they may be enlarged if there is an underlying testicular tumour.

State of local tissues These should all be normal.

GENERAL EXAMINATION

Abdominal and **rectal** examination are important in case there is an underlying cause for the hydrocele.

Epididymal cysts

(Spermatoceles)

Epididymal cysts are fluid-filled swellings connected with the epididymis. Their aetiology has not been satisfactorily explained but they are believed to be derived from the collecting tubules of the epididymis.

An epididymal cyst contains clear fluid; a spermatocele contains slightly grey, opaque, 'barley-water' fluid and a few spermatozoa. This distinction can only be made after aspiration. There is no clinical way of differentiating between the two types of cyst, except when the fluid in a spermatocele becomes too dense to transmit light. As most cysts connected with the epididymis contain clear fluid it is best to call them all epididymal cysts and not use the term spermatocele.

HISTORY

Age Most epididymal cysts occur in men over the age of 40 years.

Symptoms The main complaint is of **swelling** in the scrotum. Some patients believe that they have grown a third testis.

Development Epididymal cysts enlarge very slowly, over many years.

Multiplicity They are often **multiple** and/or **multilocular** and are frequently **bilateral**.

Fertility Young adults with bilateral epididymal cysts may still be fertile. (Surgical removal of the cysts may make them infertile.)

EXAMINATION

Position The swelling lies **within** the scrotum, usually above and slightly behind the testis. The cord of the testis can be felt above it.

Tenderness Cysts of the epididymis are not tender.

Shape Because the cysts are usually multilocular the swelling is rarely a perfect sphere; it is usually elongated and bosselated, and individual loculi may be palpable.

Size These cysts may vary in size from a few millimetres to 5–10 cm diameter. They rarely reach the size of the large hydroceles.

Surface The surface is smooth but the contours of individual loculi may be palpable.

Composition These swellings are **fluctuant**; have a **fluid thrill**; are **translucent** if they contain clear fluid (but opaque if they are heavily contaminated with sperm); and are **dull** to percussion.

Epididymal cysts cannot be reduced.

All the signs mentioned in this section on composition are identical to those for hydrocele. The difference between a hydrocele and an epididymal cyst lies in the relation of the swelling to the testis.

Relations Epididymal cysts are separate from the testis; therefore **the testis is palpable.**

Most epididymal cysts are connected to the head of the epididymis and so lie above the testis with the spermatic cord descending into or behind them.

Lymph drainage The regional lymph nodes should not be palpable.

GENERAL EXAMINATION

This should be quite normal.

Varicocele

A varicocele is a bunch of dilated and tortuous veins in the pampiniform plexus (i.e. varicose veins in the spermatic cord).

Small symptomless varicoceles occur in 25 per cent of normal men, usually on the left side. When the veins become large they may cause a vague, dragging sensation and aching pain in the scrotum or groin.

The sudden appearance of a varicocele in middle or old age may be caused by a renal neoplasm spreading along the renal vein and obstructing the spermatic vein.

You cannot feel a varicocele when the patient is lying down because the veins are empty. This is one of the reasons why you must examine the scrotum with the patient standing up. The dilated, compressible veins above the testis are then palpable and often visible. They are said to feel like a 'bag of worms'. The testis below a large varicocele may be a little smaller and softer than the testis on the normal side.

Bilateral varicoceles may cause subfertility.

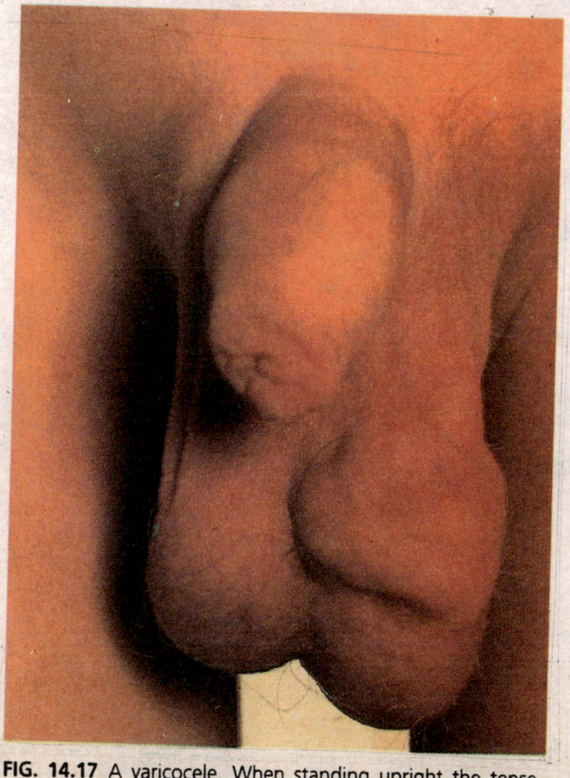

FIG. 14.17 A varicocele. When standing upright the tense, tortuous, distended veins are said to feel like 'a bag of worms'. When supine they collapse and are almost impalpable

Haematocele

An haematocele is a collection of blood within the tunica vaginalis. The bleeding is usually caused by trauma or underlying malignant disease.

In the acute phase the mass has the same physical signs as an hydrocele, except that it is not translucent and may be tender. When the blood clots, it contracts and forms a small hard mass which can cause diagnostic problems.

Acute haematocele

The patient usually gives a clear history of an injury, or of vague discomfort in the testis, followed by pain and rapid swelling of the testis.

The swelling, which is in one side of the scrotum, is tense, tender and fluctuant but does not transilluminate. **The testis cannot be felt** separate from the swelling.

Chronic haematocele

If the acute episode is ignored and not treated, or if the bleeding occurs without the patient's knowledge, the blood in the tunica vaginalis will clot. As time passes the clot which surrounds the testis contracts and hardens. The result is a hard mass which is not tender and not fluctuant. Normal testicular sensation may be lost if the contracting clot causes ischaemic necrosis of the testis.

A chronic haematocele is indistinguishable from a testicular tumour or a gumma (see below), and the testis may need to be explored before the final diagnosis can be made.

Torsion of the testis

The tunica vaginalis covers the sides and anterior aspect of the testis. The back of the epididymis and the posterior surface of the testis covered by the epididymis are not covered by the tunica vaginalis. A normal testis is, therefore, fixed within the tunica and cannot twist.

If the tunica vaginalis covers the whole of the testis, the testis is suspended in the tunica like 'a clapper in a bell', and can twist with ease, especially when aided by contraction of the spiral fibres of the cremaster muscle.

If the testis is separated from the epididymis by a long mesorchium, a twist can develop between them. Many textbooks claim that this is the common type of torsion, but in my own experience this variety of torsion is rare.

Extravaginal torsion (torsion of the cord) may occur in infants.

The abnormality that allows torsion is invariably bilateral.

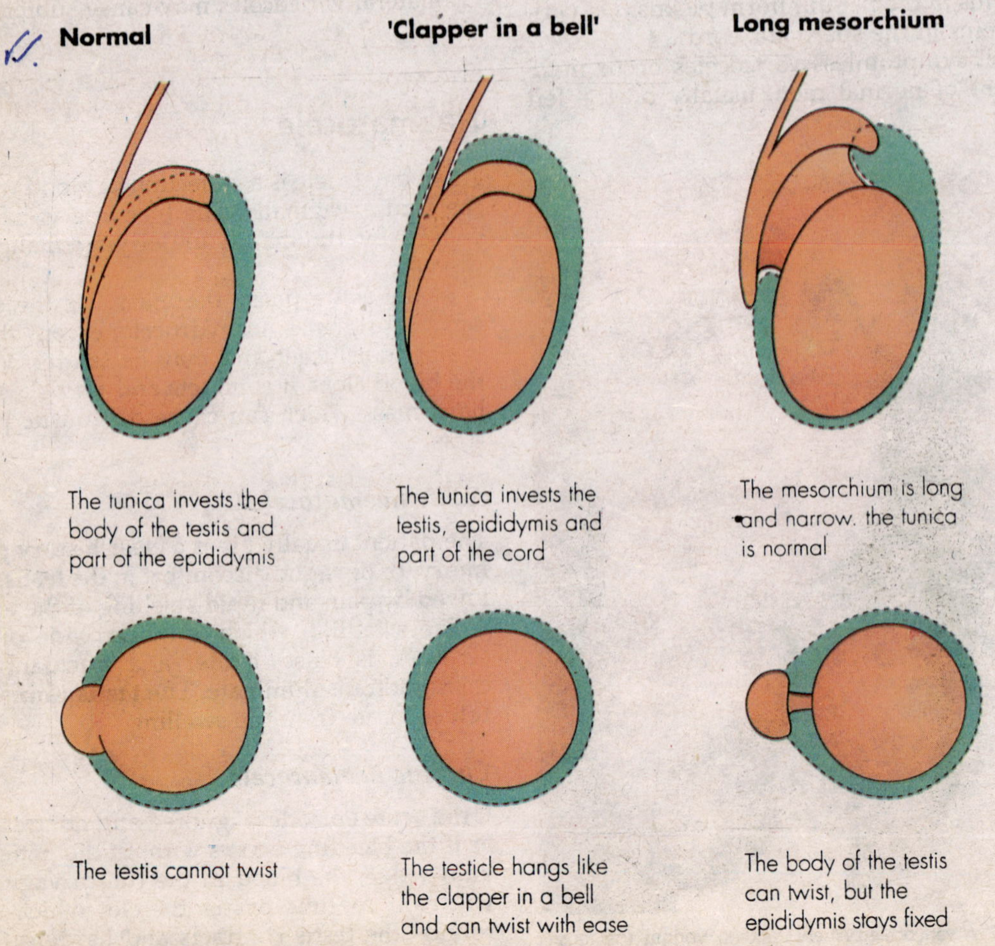

FIG. 14.18 The congenital anatomical abnormalities that permit torsion of the whole testicle or the body of the testis

HISTORY

Age The commonest age for torsion is between 10 and 15 years, but as the cause is a congenital abnormality it can occur in children, neonates and even *in utero*. It is very uncommon in men over 25 years of age.

Symptoms The principal symptom is **severe pain** in the testis and groin. The pain in the testis begins suddenly but may be preceded by a vague central abdominal pain.

Nausea and vomiting are common.

In a baby there may be restlessness and failure to eat.

Previous attacks The patient may have had similar mild attacks of pain which subsided spontaneously, or a severe attack on the other side which required treatment.

Cause Although the majority of torsions seem to occur spontaneously, often in the early hours of the morning, some follow minor trauma, one of the commonest being a blow on the scrotum as the boy jumps on his bicycle.

EXAMINATION

Position The swelling is confined to the scrotum. The affected testis hangs higher in the scrotum than the normal testis.

Colour The scrotal skin may be normal or red and oedematous. Although the latter changes are more commonly associated with epididymo-orchitis, their presence should not dissuade you from making a diagnosis of torsion.

Temperature The skin will be hot if it is red and hyperaemic.

Tenderness **The testis is exquisitely tender**, making palpation very difficult.

Shape The whole of the testis is swollen and it is usually impossible to distinguish the contours of the epididymis from those of the body of the testis.

Surface The surface of the testis is smooth but it may be obscured by testicular and scrotal oedema.

Composition It is usually impossible to elicit the signs which will reveal the composition of the mass in the scrotum because of the tenderness. The mass may be the testis, or the testis surrounded by an acute secondary hydrocele.

Reducibility The swelling will not reduce. This is an important sign if the testis is high in the scrotum, or incompletely descended, because in this position it is indistinguishable from a strangulated hernia.

Surrounding tissues Apart from the scrotal skin which may be red and oedematous, the other nearby tissues, including the other testis, should be normal.

DIFFERENTIAL DIAGNOSIS

A torsion of a testis within the scrotum may be indistinguishable from **acute epididymo-orchitis**, and a torsion of a testis in the inguinal canal or at the external inguinal ring indistinguishable from a **strangulated inguinal hernia**.

When in doubt, make a diagnosis of torsion, because failure to explore the testis and reduce the torsion will result in death of the testis. If the diagnosis is wrong and the patient has an epididymo-orchitis the surgical exploration will have done no harm.

Gumma of the testis

This is now a very rare condition in Europe. Congenital syphilis causes testicular atrophy, but in adult life the same interstitial inflammation turns the testis into a round, hard and insensitive mass – the 'billiard ball' testis.

A gumma of the testis is **painless** and therefore presents either as a lump felt on the surface of the testis or as an enlargement of the whole organ. It is usually indistinguishable from a tumour.

Orchitis

Acute orchitis, in the absence of epididymitis, is invariably due to a virus infection, commonly the mumps virus. The damage caused by a bilateral orchitis may leave the patient with a painful testis or, rarely, make him subfertile. Mumps orchitis may occur without enlargement of the salivary glands but there is usually a history of contact with mumps.

Acute epididymo-orchitis

This is primarily an infection of the epididymis, but some oedema and inflammatory changes spread into the testis. There may be an associated urinary tract infection. The common infecting organism in patients under 40 years old is *Chlamydia trachomatis*, and in older patients the *Gonococcus* and *Escherichia coli*.

HISTORY

Age This condition can affect all age groups but is commonest in young and middle-aged men.

Symptoms The patient complains of **severe pain and swelling** in one side of the scrotum. The pain usually comes on quite quickly – in 30–60 minutes. It can sometimes be relieved by supporting the scrotum. There may be the general signs of an infection – **malaise, sweating and loss of appetite**.

The signs of urinary tract infection may also be present – **frequency of micturition and painful micturition**.

EXAMINATION

Position The swelling is confined to one side of the scrotum.

Colour The scrotal skin is red and shiny. After a few days it turns a bronze colour and the superficial layers of skin desquamate.

Temperature The scrotal skin is hot.

Tenderness The scrotal skin is not tender but the testis and epididymis are **very tender**.

In many cases gentle and careful palpation will reveal that the **tenderness is in the epididymis** and that the body of the testis is not tender.

Shape and size The whole testicle may be enlarged and tender and you may be unable to distinguish epididymis from testis. This probably means that there is a small secondary hydrocele. If a hydrocele does not form, you should be able to distinguish the testis from the epididymis – the latter being two or three times the normal size.

In mild cases the inflammation may just affect the head or tail of the epididymis.

Surface The surface of the epididymis remains smooth.

Composition If there is a small hydrocele the swelling may be fluctuant, with the testis palpable through the fluid.

If there is no hydrocele the body of the testis feels a little more tense than normal. At first the epididymis feels boggy but, as the inflammation subsides, it becomes hard and craggy.

The para-aortic lymph nodes should not be palpable.

Relations and local tissues The skin over the involved testicle is oedematous and mobile except when the infection has spread beyond the epididymis to the surrounding tissues. In these circumstances the skin becomes fixed to the epididymis. If an abscess develops in the epididymis it may point to, and discharge through, the area of skin fixation. As the epididymis is normally behind the testis, epididymal disease involves the skin of the **back of the scrotum**, so always remember to examine the posterior aspect of the scrotum. The spermatic cord may be a little thickened. The other testis should feel normal.

GENERAL EXAMINATION

Pay particular attention to the urinary tract – kidney, bladder, prostate and **seminal vesicles** which may be enlarged and tender.

There may also be a fever and a tachycardia.

Tuberculous epididymo-orchitis

The tubercle bacillus reaches the epididymis via the blood stream or down the urinary tract. Its involvement of the epididymis is slow and surreptitious, quite different from acute epididymitis. Tuberculous epididymo-orchitis may pass unnoticed or cause very mild symptoms.

HISTORY

Age Tuberculous epididymo-orchitis commonly occurs between the ages of 15 and 40 years.

Symptoms Most patients complain of a **lump in the scrotum**, and an associated **dull aching pain**.

If the patient has systemic or renal tuberculosis he may have malaise, weight loss, a cough, haemoptysis and increased frequency of micturition.

The most noticeable feature of tuberculous epididymitis is the absence of acute pain and tenderness.

EXAMINATION

Position The swelling is confined to the scrotum.

Colour The scrotal skin is of normal colour, but is sometimes a little stretched and shiny.

Tenderness There is very little tenderness.

Shape In the absence of tenderness it is usually easy to discern the contours of the testis and epididymis and appreciate that the swelling is entirely confined to the epididymis, which is **hard, knobbly** and two or three times its normal size.

If there is a soft hydrocele the body of the testis is less easy to feel but the swelling of the epididymis is not usually obscured.

Surface The surface of the epididymis is a little rough and irregular but is clearly defined.

Composition The epididymis is **hard**, opaque and not fluctuant. If there is a secondary hydrocele, fluid may be palpable but the volume too small to transilluminate.

Local lymph nodes The para-aortic glands should not be enlarged.

Relations to nearby structures The whole **spermatic cord** is thickened. The vas deferens is often irregular and swollen and feels like a **string of beads**. This rare physical sign is diagnostic of tuberculosis.

The skin at the back of the scrotum may be adherent to the epididymis, and in long-standing untreated disease there may be a tuberculous sinus.

GENERAL EXAMINATION

Examine the chest and neck carefully for signs of pulmonary or cervical node tuberculosis.

Palpate the kidneys and try to feel the seminal vesicles when doing a rectal examination because they may be enlarged and hard.

Tumours of the testis

There are two main varieties of testicular tumour – seminoma (carcinoma of the seminiferous tubules) and teratoma (malignant change in totipotent cells) – but many tumours contain both types of cell and the final differentiation rests on histological, not clinical, evidence.

There are some clinical features which help differentiate between the two types, in particular the presence or absence of metastases in lymph nodes.

HISTORY

Age Teratoma commonly occurs between the ages of 20 and 30 years, and seminoma between the ages of 30 and 40 years, the maximum incidence being at 27 and 35 years, respectively.

Revision Panel 14.4

The causes of a solid single mass in one side of the scrotum

Tumour

Orchitis (mumps)

Haematocele

Gumma

Epididymo-orchitis (when the epididymis is large and the testis is small)

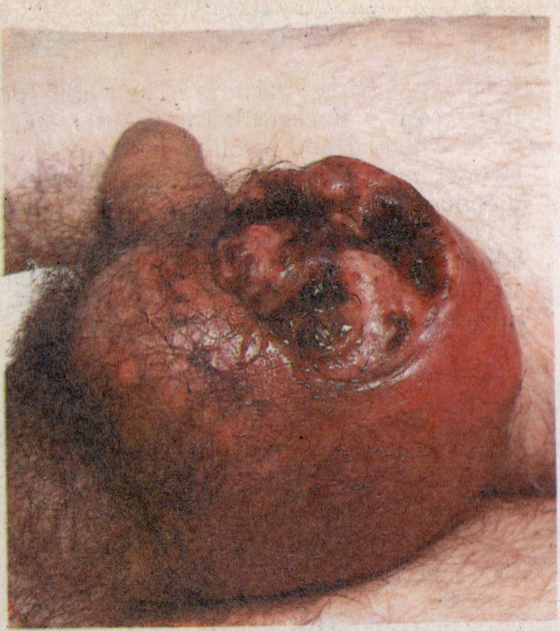

FIG. 14.19 A testicular tumour fungating through the anterior surface of the scrotum. Note that the edge of the scrotal skin is sloping and trying to heal

Symptoms The commonest presentation (80 per cent) is a **swelling** of the testis.

Acute pain and tenderness, similar to that of acute epididymo-orchitis, ocurs in 35–40 per cent of cases. In such cases the diagnosis can be very difficult.

Dull aching, dragging pains in the scrotum and groin occur in 40 per cent of patients, particularly if the testis becomes very large.

General malaise, wasting, loss of appetite, and other symptoms of diffuse secondary deposits may be the first indication that the patient has any disease.

There may be **abdominal pain** if the lymph nodes are enlarged, and **swelling of the legs** caused by lymphatic or venous obstruction.

Infertility and swelling caused by a secondary hydrocele are rare forms of presentation but should not be forgotten.

Cause Many patients will state that their symptoms followed an injury. Ignore this view and assume that the symptoms are unrelated to the injury. It is better to explore a testis and discover the correct diagnosis than miss a tumour.

There is a 36-fold increase in the incidence of malignant change in the incompletely descended testis. An absent testis or a history of an orchidopexy are highly significant symptoms.

Systemic effects A few testicular tumours secrete female sex hormones which can cause gynaecomastia and other mild feminizing symptoms.

EXAMINATION

Position The swelling is confined to the scrotum.

Temperature and colour If the tumour has spread beyond the testis into the adjacent scrotal skin, the skin may be hot and discoloured.

Tenderness Testicular tumours are not tender except when they are associated with acute pain.

In many instances normal testicular sensation is lost.

Shape The majority of testicular tumours start in the lower pole of the body of the testis but by the time they present they usually occupy the whole testis. They are **irregular** and variable in shape but basically spherical.

Size Some tumours are noticed by the patient when they are only a few millimetres in diameter; others reach a large size before the patient complains.

Surface The surface is usually smooth but can be irregular or nodular. In those places where it is beginning to spread outside the fibrous capsule of the testis (the tunica albuginea) the surface is indistinct.

Composition Testicular tumours are harder than a normal testis, dull to percussion, not fluctuant and not translucent.

Areas of cystic degeneration may feel soft.

Relations to surrounding tissues The other testis should be normal, but bilateral tumours occur in 2 per cent of cases. The spermatic cord may be thickened if it is infiltrated with tumour, but the vas deferens should be normal. Once the tumour breaks through the tunica albuginea it infiltrates the skin of the scrotum.

FIRST DECIDE THE ANSWERS TO THESE FOUR QUESTIONS

1 Can you get above the swelling?

2 Can you identified the testis and epididymis?

3 Is the swelling translucent?

4 Is the swelling tender?

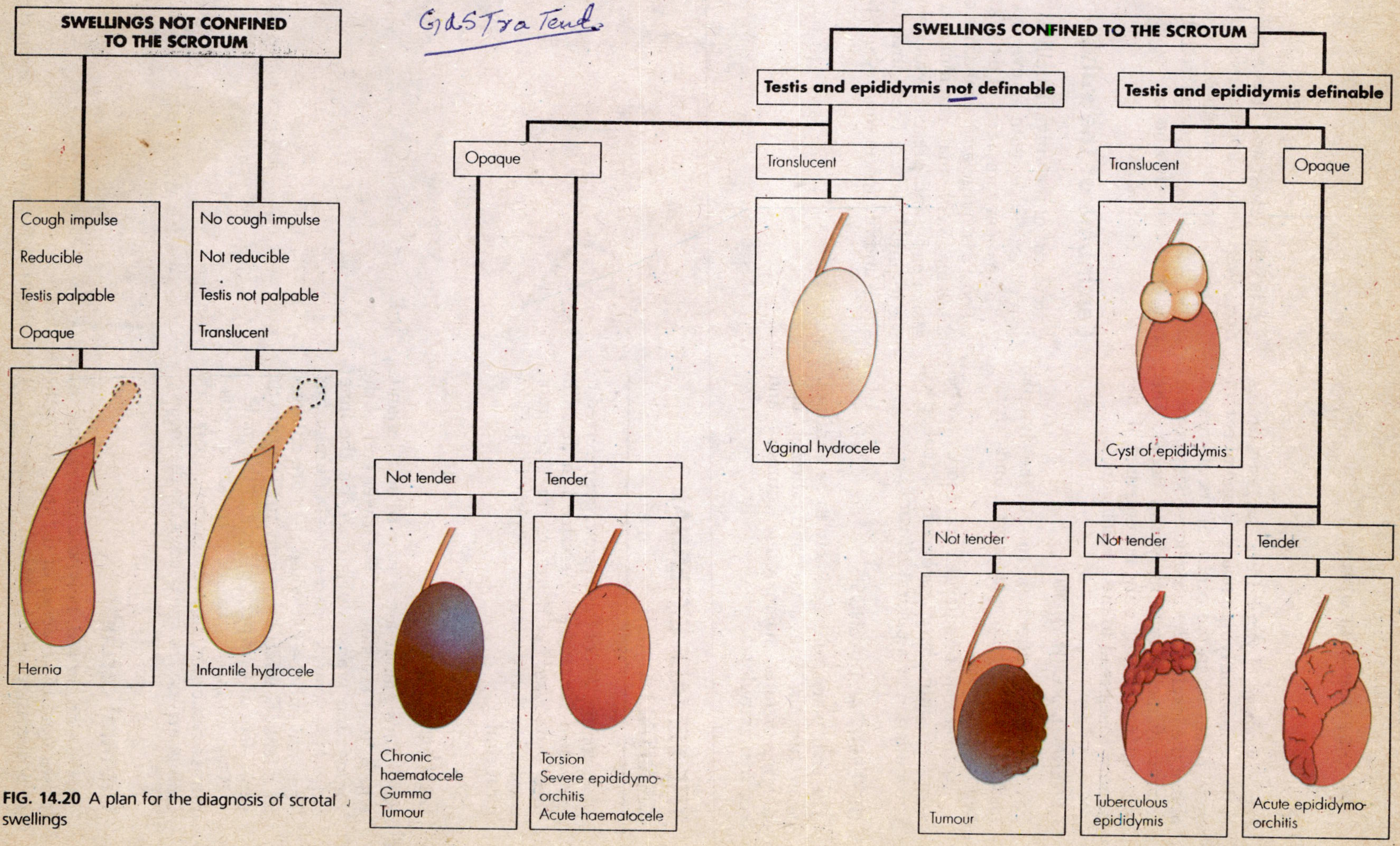

FIG. 14.20 A plan for the diagnosis of scrotal swellings

Lymph drainage Lymph from the testis drains to the para-aortic lymph nodes. Remember that these nodes lie in the centre of the abdomen **above** the level of the umbilicus. Seminomata commonly metastasize to lymph nodes. The inguinal nodes will only be enlarged if the tumour has spread to the scrotal skin.

GENERAL EXAMINATION

Pay particular attention to all the lymph nodes, especially the para-aortic and supraclavicular groups.

The liver may be enlarged and there may be signs of pulmonary secondaries (collapse, consolidation or a pleural effusion).

DIFFERENTIAL DIAGNOSIS

The testicular swellings likely to be confused with tumours are acute and chronic epididymo-orchitis, haematocele, gumma and seminal granuloma.

THE FEMALE EXTERNAL GENITALIA

Most complaints of this system get referred to gynaecologists and are described in detail in their textbooks, but there are three common conditions that quite often appear in the surgical clinic.

Bartholin cyst

Bartholin's glands are a pair of small glands which lie at the sides of the lower end of the vagina, and whose ducts open on the inner side of the posterior part of the **labium minus**. They can only be felt when they are enlarged by retention, infection or tumour. They are the equivalent of Cowper's glands in the male.

When a gland is full of secretion or pus it forms a cystic swelling in the posterior part of the **labium majus**. The site betrays the diagnosis.

Urethral caruncle

This is a bright red, polypoid granuloma that arises from the mucosa of the urethral orifice in post-menopausal women.

It is very tender and causes painful micturition, dyspareunia and occasional bleeding.

The differential diagnosis is urethral prolapse, which is purple in colour and not so tender, and carcinoma.

Carcinoma of the vulva

Carcinoma of the vulva usually takes the form of a chronic ulcer with an everted edge.

The patient complains of **pain**, a purulent or bloody **discharge** and sometimes of a **lump** in the labia. Very small carcinomata can metastasize early and present with enlargement of the inguinal glands. The primary ulcer can be small and hidden in the folds of the labia.

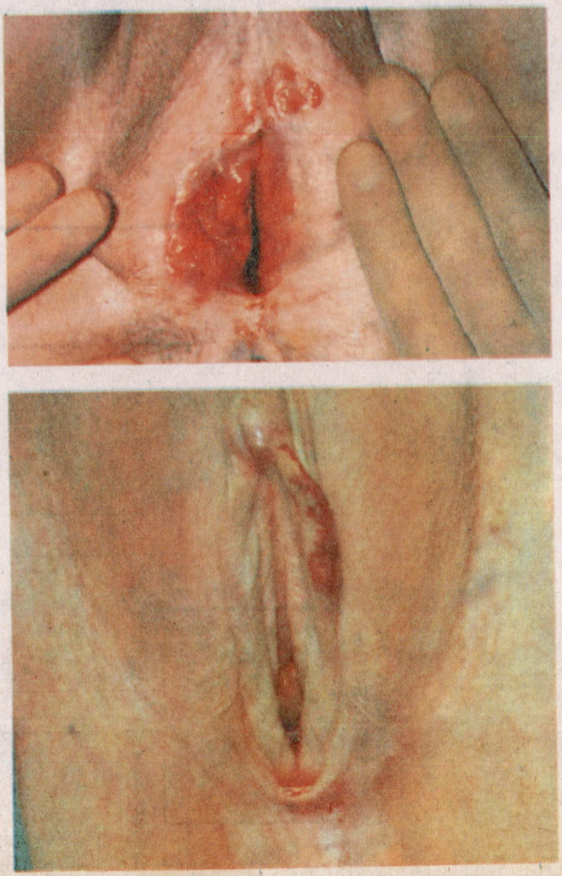

FIG. 14.21 Two examples of carcinoma of the vulva

The abdominal wall and umbilicus

15

THE ABDOMINAL WALL

The abdominal wall is afflicted by many of the common skin, subcutaneous, fascial and muscle tissue lesions described in the earlier chapters of this book. They are no more difficult to diagnose when they arise in the abdominal wall than when they appear in other sites. However, it is most important to decide whether any abdominal lump is **deep to, or in, the abdominal wall.**

This is done by palpating the lump with the abdominal wall relaxed and then with it tense. A lump deep to the abdominal wall becomes impalpable when the abdominal muscles contract. A lump superficial to the muscles becomes more prominent. Most medical students forget to apply this simple test to abdominal lumps.

Contracting the abdominal muscles

If you ask a patient to lift up his head and shoulders off the couch, he will contract his abdominal muscles – provided he does not lever himself up with his elbows, which is what most elderly patients do. The most effective way to make a patient contract his abdominal muscles is to put your hand beneath both heels, lift them up 30 cm, and then ask him to hold his legs straight, in that elevated position, by himself. This makes the rectus abdominis muscle rock hard and any mass deep to it completely impalpable (Fig. 15.1).

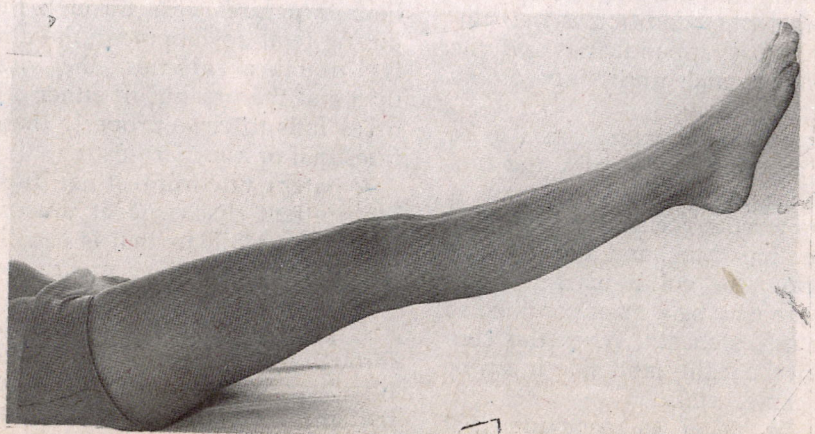

FIG. 15.1 Examination of the abdominal wall. To tense the abdominal muscles, ask the patient to hold their legs elevated and straight

Frail elderly patients who cannot lift their legs will also be unable to raise their head and shoulders. In these circumstances you cannot do the test properly.

Ruptured epigastric arteries

The inferior and superior epigastric arteries lie deep to, or within, the rectus abdominis muscles. If these muscles contract suddenly and violently the epigastric arteries may be torn. The haematoma which then develops within the muscle causes pain and swelling.

Rupture of the **inferior epigastric artery** occurs in athletes and during coughing in elderly chronic bronchitics. The blood spreads within the muscle, but as there is no posterior rectus sheath below the arcuate line (the lower edge of the rectus sheath, mid-way between the pubis and the umbilicus) it spreads out into the extraperitoneal tissues of the iliac fossa.

The patient complains of pain and tenderness in the iliac fossa. The pain is made worse by contracting the abdominal muscles. Examination reveals a diffuse, tender mass in the iliac fossa, deep to the abdominal wall. Sometimes the skin becomes discoloured 6–12 hours after the onset of the pain.

If the pain is not made worse by contracting the rectus abdominis muscle, and if there is no bruise in the skin, this condition is indistinguishable from acute appendicitis, and the diagnosis may not be made until a laparotomy is performed.

The **superior epigastric artery** can also be torn by coughing. This causes pain and tenderness in the upper abdomen. The pain is made worse by tensing the abdominal muscles and by deep breathing, and a bruise may appear just below the costal margin 12–24 hours later. There may be a mass confined to the area of the rectus sheath. When this condition occurs on the right-hand side it can be confused with cholecystitis.

Although it is usual to conclude that haematomata in the rectus sheath arise from tears of the epigastric arteries, they may also be caused by **tears of the muscle fibres** with damage to very small nutrient vessels.

THE UMBILICUS

The commonest abnormality of the umbilicus is an umbilical hernia. The varieties and presentation of umbilical herniae are described on page 332.

The important congenital abnormalities of the umbilicus are exomphalos and fistula, and the common acquired conditions (apart from herniae) are inflammation and invasion by tumour.

Exomphalos

This condition, which is **present at birth**, represents an intrauterine failure of the intestine to return to the abdomen. The intestines protrude **through a defect in all layers of the abdominal wall** at the centre of the abdomen. Their only covering is a thin transparent membrane formed from the remnant of the coverings of the yolk sac. Once this membrane is exposed to the air it rapidly loses its thin transparent appearance. It becomes thicker and covered with an opaque fibrinous exudate. It may rupture and the infant die of peritonitis.

Umbilical fistulae

Four structures pass through the umbilicus during fetal development: the umbilical vein, the umbilical arteries, the vitellointestinal duct and the urachus. If either of the last two tubes fails to close properly there will be an intestinal or a urinary fistula.

A **patent vitellointestinal duct** permits an intermittent discharge of mucus and faeces from the umbilicus that is usually noticed in the first few weeks or months of life. It is a very rare abnormality.

A **patent urachus** permits a leak of urine through the umbilicus. This condition does not usually present until **adult** life because in a child the strong contractions of the bladder during micturition close the mouth of the fistula.

The patient complains of a watery discharge from the umbilicus. Although this complaint is nearly always caused by an infection, not a

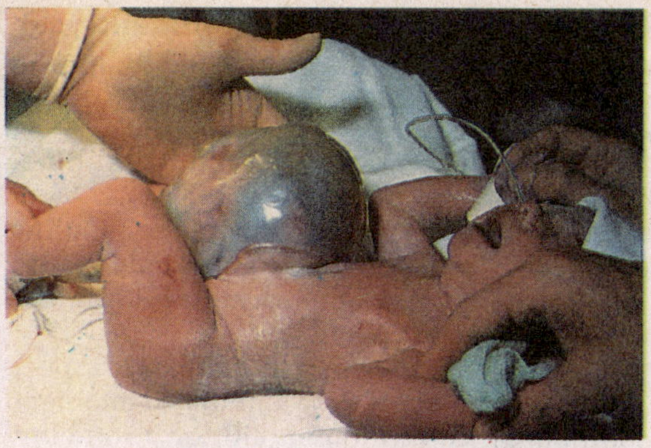

In this example the bowel can be seen through the thin membrane

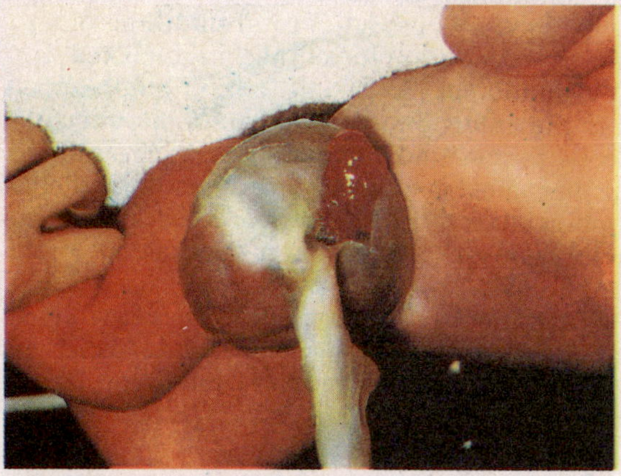

In this example the thin membrane is covered with fibrin but has nevertheless ruptured. The umbilical cord is still present

FIG. 15.2 TWO EXAMPLES OF EXOMPHALOS

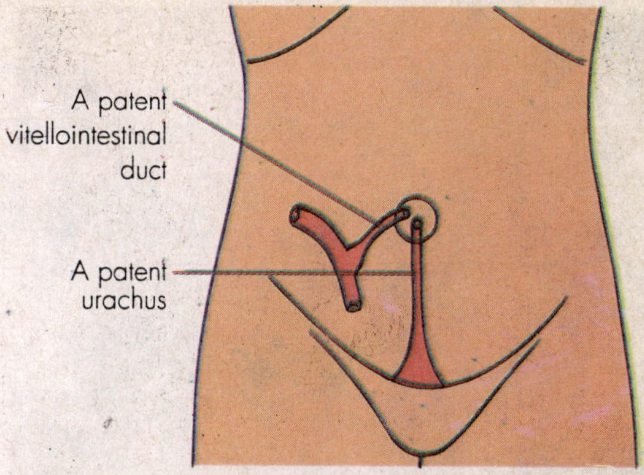

FIG. 15.3 A persistent vitellointestinal duct or a patent urachus can become an intestinal or urinary fistula, respectively

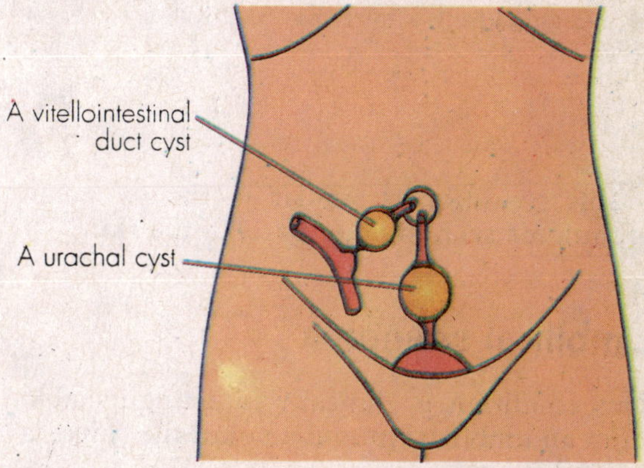

FIG. 15.4 If the vitellointestinal duct or urachus are not completely obliterated they may turn into cysts

fistula, the possibility of a urachal fistula should always be at the back of your mind.

Both these tracts may partially close, leaving a patent segment that becomes a cyst.

A **vitellointestinal duct cyst** is a small, spherical, mobile swelling deep to the umbilicus that is tethered to the umbilicus and to the small bowel.

A **urachal cyst** is an immobile swelling in the hypogastrium deep to the abdominal muscles. It may become large enough to fluctuate and have a fluid thrill. If it is still connected to the bladder it may vary in size. If it becomes infected it may present with a throbbing lower abdominal pain and a tender mass.

Umbilical granuloma

After the umbilical cord has been severed and tied, the small remnant shrivels and falls off. The area of chronic inflammation at the line of demarcation is then quickly covered by epithelium. If the inflammatory process becomes florid – commonly because of infection – excess granulation tissue is formed which prevents the raw area becoming epithelialized.

The baby presents with a pouting umbilicus surmounted by a **bright red, moist, friable, sometimes hemispherical mass of bleeding granulation tissue.**

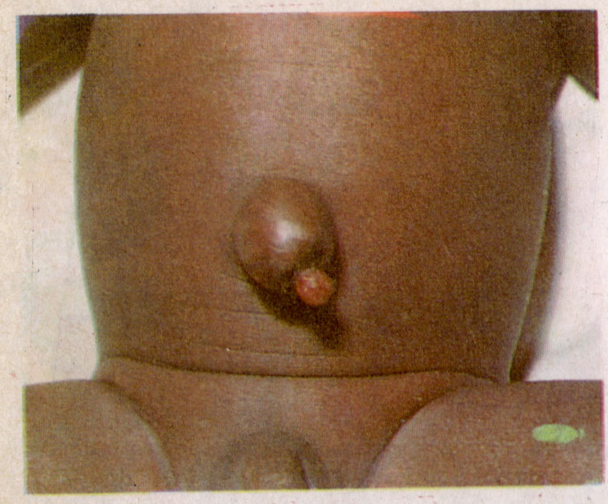

FIG. 15.5 An umbilical granuloma. This is an excessive amount of granulation tissue at the point where the umbilical cord separated. It is often associated with an umbilical hernia

This condition is similar to the pyogenic granuloma seen in other parts of the skin.

Umbilical adenoma

This condition is clinically indistinguishable from an umbilical granuloma but the cause is quite different.

An umbilical adenoma is a patch of **intestinal epithelium** left behind when the vitellointestinal duct closed. It may form in a deep sinus in the depths of the umbilicus, but commonly protrudes from it and looks like a raspberry.

The mother complains that the baby has a lump at the umbilicus and a mucous discharge.

Umbilical dermatitis

(Omphalitis)

Infection within the umbilicus is common in adults. It is usually associated with inadequate hygiene and deepening of the umbilicus caused by obesity. The condition is really a **dermatitis** and analogous to the intertrigo that often occurs between folds of skin. Although it is primarily a 'seborrhoeic' dermatitis, it frequently becomes secondarily infected with skin organisms.

The patient complains of an umbilical **discharge, pain and soreness.**

On examination, the skin in and around the umbilicus is found to be **red and tender**, and a **seropurulent discharge** is visible which has a most unpleasant smell.

The whole umbilicus may feel hard, especially if the discharge is secondary to another condition such as an ompholith or a tumour deposit.

Although a primary skin infection is by far the commonest cause of a discharge from the umbilicus, it is essential to exclude the other causes of an umbilical discharge, listed in Revision Panel 15.1.

If the infection spreads into the subcutaneous tissues and the opening of the umbilicus becomes narrowed by oedema, the whole umbilicus can turn into an **abscess**. Most umbilical abscesses are associated with ompholiths.

The patient complains of a painful swollen umbilicus that discharges pus and throbs at night. The clinical diagnosis rests upon finding a red, hot, tender swelling in and around the umbilicus that exudes pus.

True omphalitis is infection of the stump of the **umbilical cord** following improper or inadequate maternal care.

Ompholiths

When the sebaceous secretions, which accumulate in the umbilicus, are mixed with the hairs and fluff from clothing that are sucked into the umbilicus, the mixture can form a hard lump, worthy of the name umbilical stone or ompholith.

Obviously these events can only happen if the patient does not keep his umbilicus clean. This is not as simple as it sounds, for the umbilicus can be very deep and narrow in fat people.

Small concretions are common and cause no trouble. When they enlarge they rub and damage the skin, which then becomes infected, and the infection will not subside until the concretions are removed.

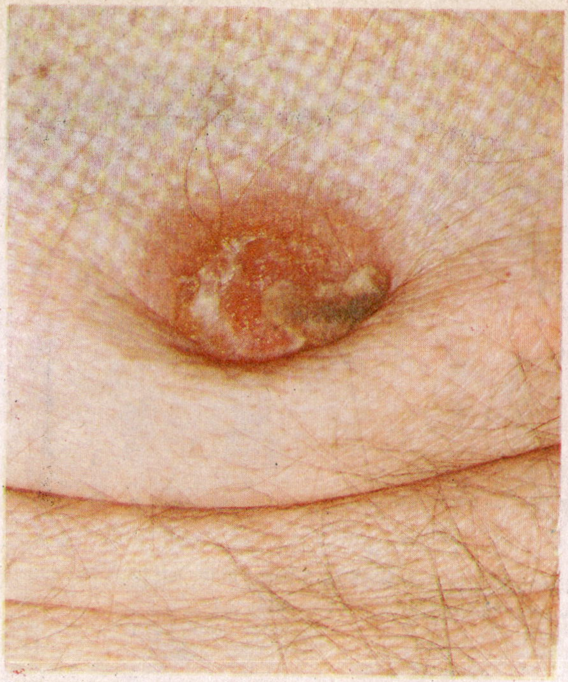

FIG. 15.6 Omphalitis. A protruding mass of infected granulation tissue caused by a large ompholith, the brown tip of which is just visible

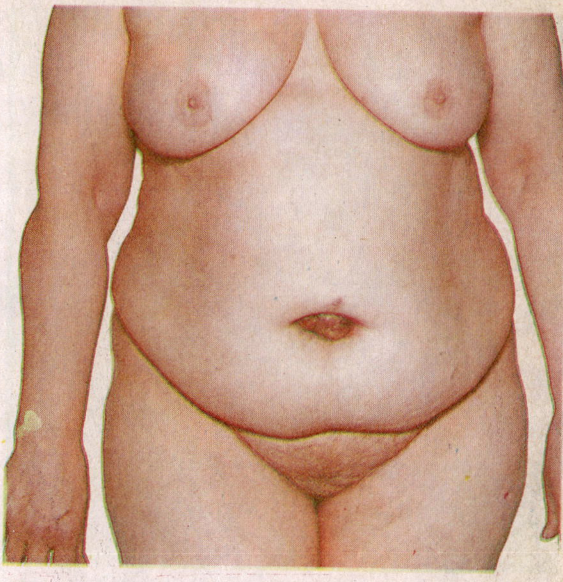

FIG. 15.7 A nodule of metastatic carcinoma bulging through the umbilicus causing a serosanguinous discharge. This is known as Sister Joseph's nodule

If the infection spreads through the skin, an umbilical abscess or periumbilical cellulitis will develop.

The diagnosis can be made on inspection if the grey–brown surface of the stone is visible. On palpation the whole umbilicus feels swollen and **hard**.

Umbilical concretions are not stony hard and a probe can be pushed into them with ease.

Secondary carcinoma

A nodule bulging into the umbilicus, in a patient who is losing weight and feels ill, is very likely to be a nodule of metastatic tumour. This presentation always indicates advanced, widespread disease and the primary tumour is commonly in the abdomen.

The tumour cells reach the umbilicus via the lymphatics that run in the edge of the falciform ligament alongside the obliterated umbilical vein, or by transperitoneal spread. Umbilical metastases are usually associated with multiple peritoneal metastases.

Nodules of secondary carcinoma usually ulcerate, bleed and become infected.

Metastases at the umbilicus may become attached to and infiltrate the underlying bowel. Necrosis of the tumour tissue may then cause an acquired **umbilical–intestinal fistula**.

Endometrioma

If the umbilicus enlarges, becomes painful and discharges blood at the same time as the patient menstruates, she may have a patch of ectopic endometrial glands in the umbilicus.

Discolouration of the umbilicus

The following physical signs are *rare*, but the diseases that cause them are common and serious.

A **blue tinge**, around the umbilicus, caused by dilated, tortuous, sometimes visible, veins, is a **caput medusae**. The dilated veins are collateral vessels which have developed to circumvent a **portal vein obstruction**.

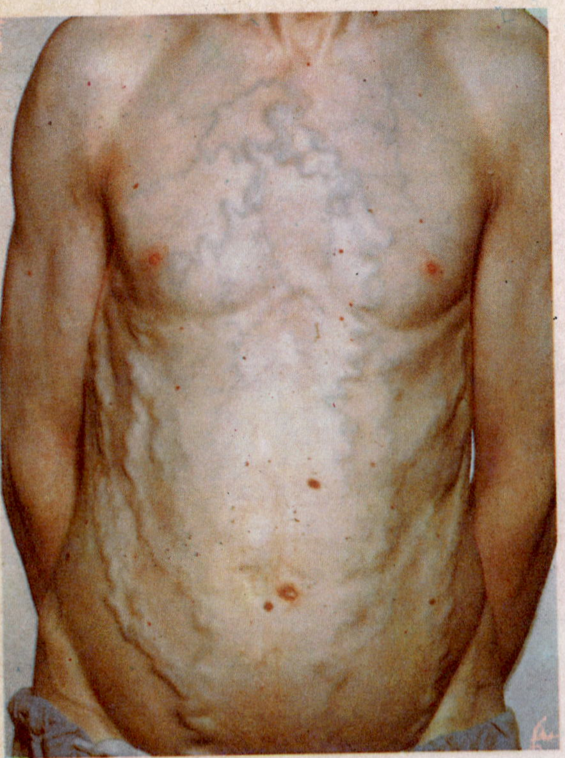

FIG. 15.8 Inferior vena caval obstruction may present with dilated subcutaneous veins in the abdominal and chest wall

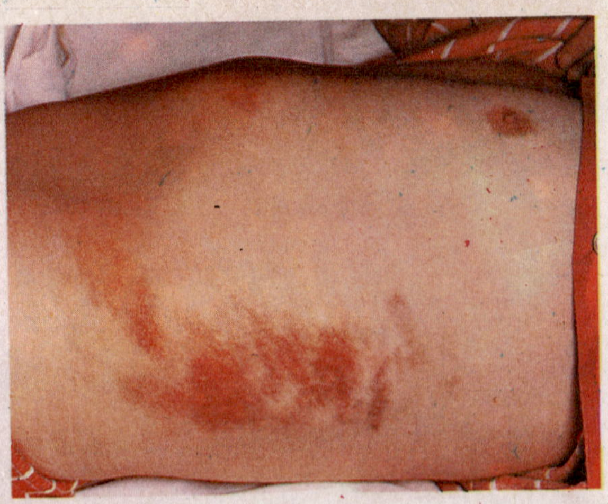

FIG. 15.9 Grey–Turner's sign. Bruising in the left flank caused by acute haemorrhagic pancreatitis

Yellow–blue bruising around the umbilicus (Cullen's sign) is caused by pancreatic enzymes which have tracked along the falciform ligament and digested the subcutaneous tissues around the umbilicus. It is a sign of **severe acute pancreatitis**.

Bruising at the umbilicus can also be caused by a massive long-standing **haemoperitoneum**, such as that which may accompany a ruptured ectopic pregnancy.

Revision Panel 15.1

The causes of a discharge from the umbilicus

Congenital
- Intestinal fistula
- Patent urachus
- Umbilical adenoma

Acquired
- Umbilical granuloma
- Dermatitis (intertrigo)
- Ompholith (umbilical concretion)
- Fistula (intestinal)
- Secondary carcinoma
- Endometriosis

The abdomen

16

TECHNIQUE FOR EXAMINATION OF THE ABDOMEN

The abdomen contains the stomach, duodenum, small and large bowel, liver, pancreas, kidneys, bladder, aorta, vena cava, . . . ; a large number of different structures within a relatively small cavity, all susceptible to disease or malfunction and capable of producing symptoms. It is not surprising, therefore, that the diagnosis of abdominal complaints is extremely difficult.

Because the abdominal organs are so close to each other the brain cannot distinguish with any accuracy which of them is the source of a pain. This means that the patient's description of a pain may not be specific, although other symptoms may clearly indicate the organ involved, and the diagnosis of the source of the pain will depend on physical examination.

But here the examiner meets with another problem. Many of the contents of the abdominal cavity are inaccessible to palpation. The abdomen stretches from the dome of the diaphragm, just below the level of the nipples, to the bottom of the pelvis, a few inches above the anal canal. The top part is covered by the lower ribs; the lower part is in the pelvis; and the posterior aspect is hidden and protected by the spinal column.

Figure 16.1 shows the extent of the abdominal cavity and the area available for direct palpation. Fortunately, it is possible to feel beneath the costal margin, and to reach into the pelvis per rectum or vaginam; nevertheless, many of the abdominal contents are difficult to palpate, especially if the patient is

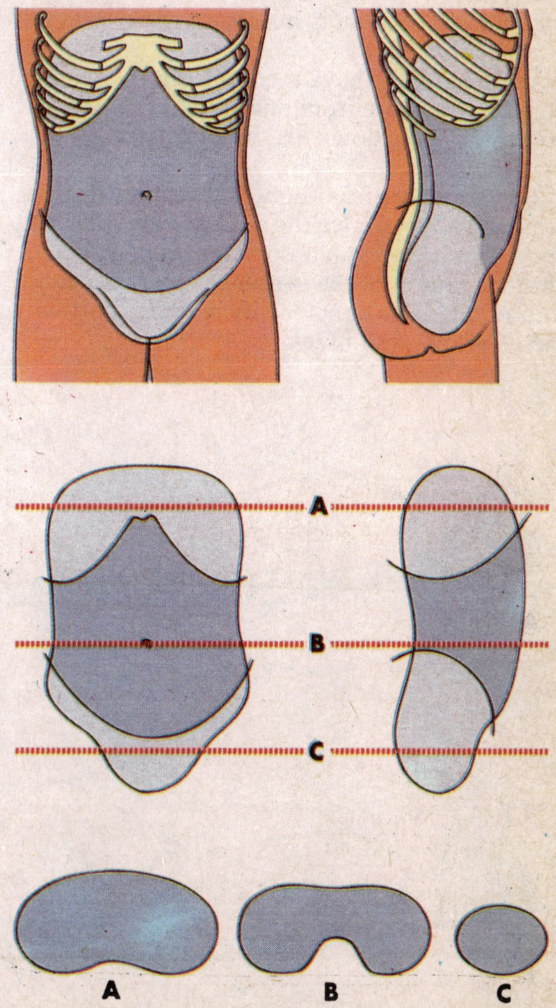

FIG. 16.1 These figures show the extent of the abdominal cavity. The paler lavender areas indicate the parts of the abdomen protected by the ribs and the pelvis. The levels of the three cross-sections are indicated on the central diagram

protecting himself by tensing his muscles. Because of these anatomical restrictions the position of the patient and the technique of examination are of paramount importance if you wish to obtain the maximum information.

Preparation

The environment

The examination room must be **warm** and **private** if you want your patient to lie undressed and relaxed. A cold couch, in a draught, in view of other patients makes a proper examination impossible.

You must also have a **good light**. Daylight, coming obliquely from one side of the patient so that the shadows are emphasized, is the best light.

Beware of artificial light. If it comes from a source directly above the patient you will lose the soft shadows that so often give you the first indication of the presence of asymmetry; and many neon lights falsify colours, particularly yellows and blues.

The examination couch or bed

You must strike a compromise between the very hard, flat couch which, by making the patient lie absolutely flat, opens the gap between the pubis and xiphisternum but stretches and tightens the abdominal muscles, and the soft bed which lets the lumbar spine sink into a deep curve and closes the gap between pubis and ribs

The best compromise in an outpatient situation is a hard couch with a backrest that can be raised by 15–20°. The hard couch makes the patient maintain most of his lumbar lordosis, so opening the access to the abdomen and pushing the central contents anteriorly, but the elevation of the thoracic cage relaxes the anterior abdominal muscles.

This type of couch is, in fact, essential, because some patients with orthopnoea or musculoskeletal deformities cannot lie flat.

Exposure

You must see the full extent of the abdomen. Therefore you must uncover the patient from **nipples to knees**.

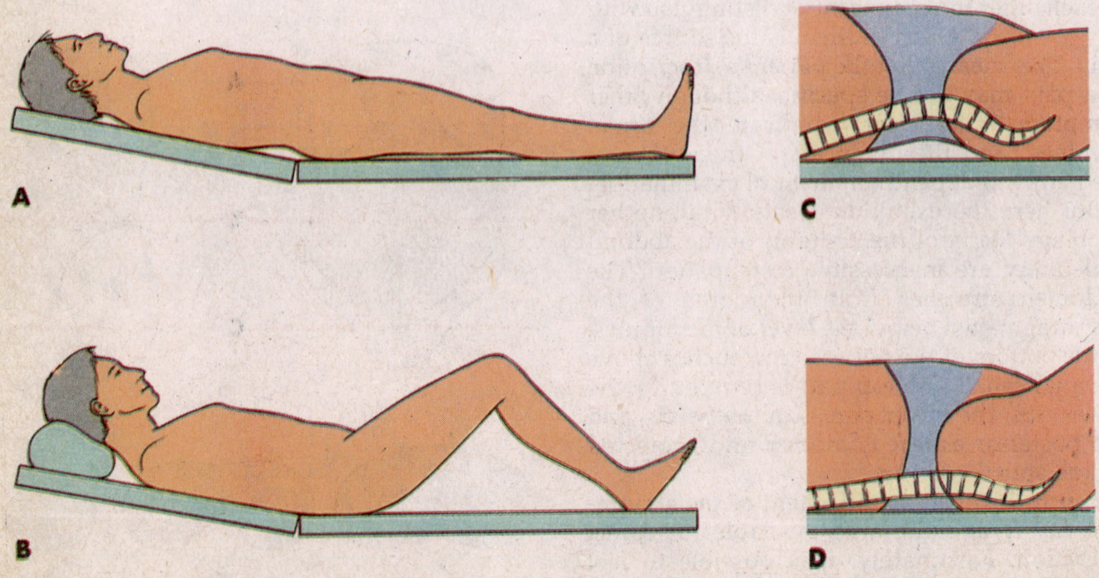

FIG. 16.2 Examination of the abdomen. **A**: Examine the abdomen with the patient on a firm couch or bed with just sufficient support beneath the shoulders and head to stop the anterior abdominal wall being stretched tight. **B**: If the abdominal wall is tight, raise the head and flex the hips. **C & D**: These figures show the reduction in the area of abdomen available for palpation if the patient lies on a soft bed that allows the lumbar lordosis to straighten

Many patients find this embarrassing, but if you do not do it then you will easily forget to examine the areas that are not uncovered, such as the genitalia and hernial orifices. It will relieve the patient's embarrassment if you begin by examining the genitalia and then cover them with a sheet or blanket before examining the rest of the abdomen.

Get the patient to relax

If the patient is tense you will not be able to feel anything within the abdomen. There are a number of ways by which you can encourage relaxation:

- First ask the patient to rest his head on the couch or pillow. If he keeps lifting it up he will tense his rectus abdominis muscles.
- Ask him to rest his arms by his side, not to hold them up behind his head.
- Suggest that he lets his back sink into the couch.
- Ask him to breathe regularly and slowly, and only press your hand into the abdomen during expiration, when the abdominal muscles relax.

If these manoeuvres do not succeed then flex the hips to 45° and the knees to 90° and put an extra pillow behind the head. Although this tips up the pelvis and reduces your area of access to the abdomen, it usually relaxes the abdominal muscles.

The position of the examiner

Your hands must be clean and warm and your nails short. You cannot palpate deeply with long nails, and **it is an insult to the patient to have dirty hands.**

Your whole hand must rest on the abdomen. The only comfortable way to achieve this is by keeping your **hand and forearm horizontal** in the same plane as the front of the abdomen. This means that you must sit or kneel beside the patient. If you stand up your forearm will not be horizontal, your wrist will be extended and gentle palpation much more difficult.

Sitting beside the patient with your forearm level with the front of the abdomen puts your eyes about 50 cm above your hand. This is the ideal level for seeing the soft shadows caused by lumps and bumps.

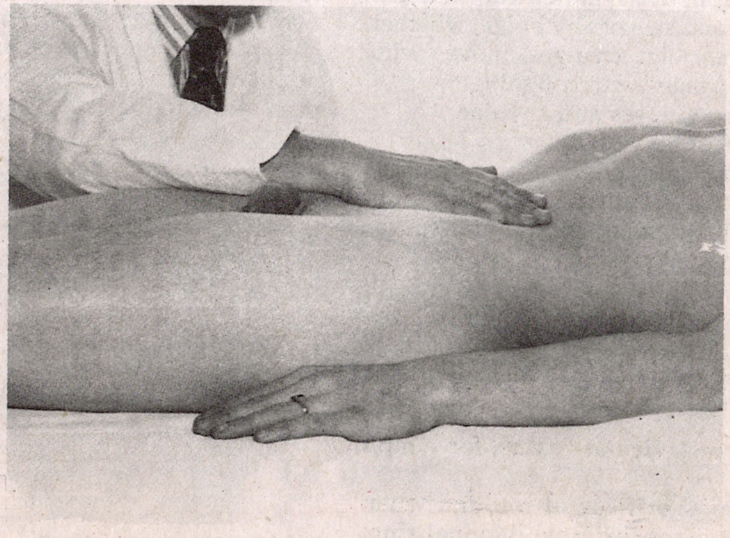

FIG. 16.3 When you palpate the abdomen, sit or kneel so that your forearm is horizontal and level with the anterior abdominal wall, and your eyes are 50 cm above this level. If you are higher, your wrist will be extended and you will not be able to palpate comfortably and firmly

Palpate **gently but deliberately;** that is to say, firmly and with purpose. Rapid, jerky or circular movements that look as though you are kneading dough are distressing for the patient, make him lose confidence in your ability and yield no information. You will learn much more by **keeping your hand still** and feeling the structures moving beneath it.

The routine of examination

Follow the standard routine – inspection, palpation, percussion and auscultation.

Inspection

Look at the whole patient. You will have done this already when examining the head, neck and chest, but look again for general abnormalities particularly relevant to intra-abdominal disease, such as cachexia, pallor and jaundice.

Look at the abdomen. Asymmetry is often easier to detect if you stand at the foot of the couch, or bed, and look along the length of the patient.

Note the **shape** of the abdomen. Is it **symmetrical** – flat, distended, or hollow (scaphoid) – or **asymmetrical**? If asymmetrical, note the position, shape and size of any bulge, whether the shape of the bulge changes, moves with respiration or changes with coughing.

Look for **scars, sinuses** and **fistulae.**

Look for **distended veins.**

Watch for the reaction of the patient to coughing or moving. Patients with peritonitis find movement extremely painful and consequently tend to lie very still.

Palpation

Begin by feeling the areas that you might otherwise forget:

1 Feel the **supraclavicular fossae,** for lymph nodes.
2 Feel the **hernial orifices,** at rest and when the patient coughs (external inguinal ring, femoral canal and umbilicus).
3 Feel the **femoral pulses.**
4 Examine the **external genitalia** (described in detail in Chapter 14).

Two other vital procedures are easily forgotten – **auscultation** for bowel sounds and bruits, and the **rectal examination** – but it is more convenient to do these later.

General light palpation for tenderness

This should be done by gently resting the hand on the abdomen and pressing lightly. Move your hand systematically over all areas of the abdomen.

If the patient has a pain, ask him to point to its site so that you can begin palpation in a non-tender area and move towards the tender spot.

Determine the *area* of tenderness so that you can depict it as a hatched area on a drawing of the abdomen in your notes (see Fig. 16.4).

Try to **assess the degree of tenderness.** Palpation over an area of mild tenderness just causes pain. If the area is **moderately** tender the patient's abdominal muscles tighten as you press – this is **guarding. Severe** tenderness is also associated with guarding but, in addition, the sudden withdrawal of the manual pressure causes a sharp exacerbation of the pain – this is known as **rebound** or **release tenderness**. The elicitation of release tenderness is usually distressing to the patient, so the technique should not be used routinely. Light percussion is just as accurate a method of detecting tenderness.

Sometimes release of pressure on a distant non-tender part of the abdomen may cause pain in the tender area.

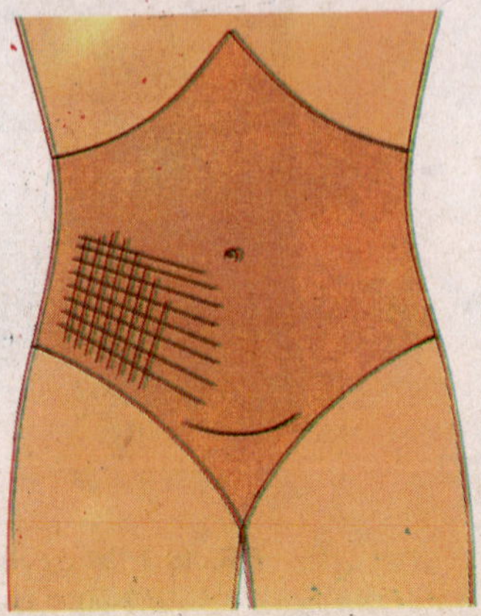

FIG. 16.4 Indicate areas of tenderness by oblique lines on a sketch like this. Masses are depicted by outlining their shape

Although these signs indicate increasingly severe tenderness, it is usual to describe their presence or absence rather than grade the tenderness because pain sensitivity varies so much from patient to patient.

General deep palpation for tenderness

If systematic light palpation over the whole abdomen elicits no pain, repeat the process, pressing firmly and deeply to see if there is deep tenderness.

Palpate for masses

Although your initial palpation for tenderness might have detected some other abnormalities, you must feel firmly over the whole abdomen, specifically searching for masses. If you find a mass you must elicit all its physical signs – position, shape, size, surface, edge, and composition (consistence, fluctuation, fluid thrill, resonance, and pulsatility).

Tender masses in the abdomen are very difficult to assess because of the protective guarding of the abdominal wall muscles. If you let your hand rest gently on the tender area and gradually press it a little deeper during each expiration, you will find that you will be able to overcome guarding and feel tender masses well enough to get some idea of their surface and size. If you just push hard you will feel nothing because the abdominal muscles will become iron hard.

Palpate the normal solid viscera

Liver With your hand resting transversely and flat, on the right side of the abdomen, at the level of the umbilicus, ask the patient to take a deep breath. If the liver is grossly enlarged its lower edge may move downwards and bump against the radial side of your index finger.

If you feel nothing abnormal, repeat the process with your hand a little higher, inch by inch, until you reach the costal margin.

The liver edge may be straight or irregular, thin and sharp, or thick and rounded.

If you begin palpation just below the costal margin you will miss a big liver. Gross hepatomegaly may fill the whole abdomen, so if in doubt begin your palpation in the left iliac fossa.

Spleen An enlarged spleen appears below the tip of the 10th rib along a line heading for the umbilicus. A normal spleen is not palpable.

Begin palpating for the spleen with your finger tips to the *right* of *and below* the umbilicus, because a very large spleen may extend across the abdomen into the right iliac fossa. Then ask the patient to take a deep breath. If you feel nothing, move your hand, in stages, towards the tip of the left 10th rib. When you reach the costal margin put your left hand around the lower left rib cage and lift it forwards as the patient inspires. This manoeuvre occasionally lifts a slightly enlarged spleen far enough forwards to make it palpable.

The spleen is recognizable from its shape and site and, when present, the notch on its superomedial edge.

Kidneys The kidneys are often impalpable, but both lumbar regions should always be carefully examined.

To feel the right kidney, put your left hand behind the patient's right loin, between the 12th rib and the iliac crest, and lift the loin and kidney forwards. Put your right hand on the right side of the abdomen just above the level of the anterior superior iliac spine and, as the patient breathes in and out, palpate deeply into the loin.

You will often feel the lower pole of a normal kidney at the height of inspiration. If the kidney is very easy to feel, it is either enlarged or abnormally low.

To feel the left kidney, lean across the patient, put your left hand round the flank into the left loin to lift it forwards, and your right hand on the abdomen.

Percussion

Percuss over the whole abdomen and particularly over any masses.

Sometimes you will find a dull area, and with further palpation feel a mass that you had missed, so percussion is important.

If there is a circumscribed mass, tap it on one side while feeling the other side with the other hand to see if it conducts a fluid thrill.

Any area of dullness should be outlined by percussion with the abdomen in two positions

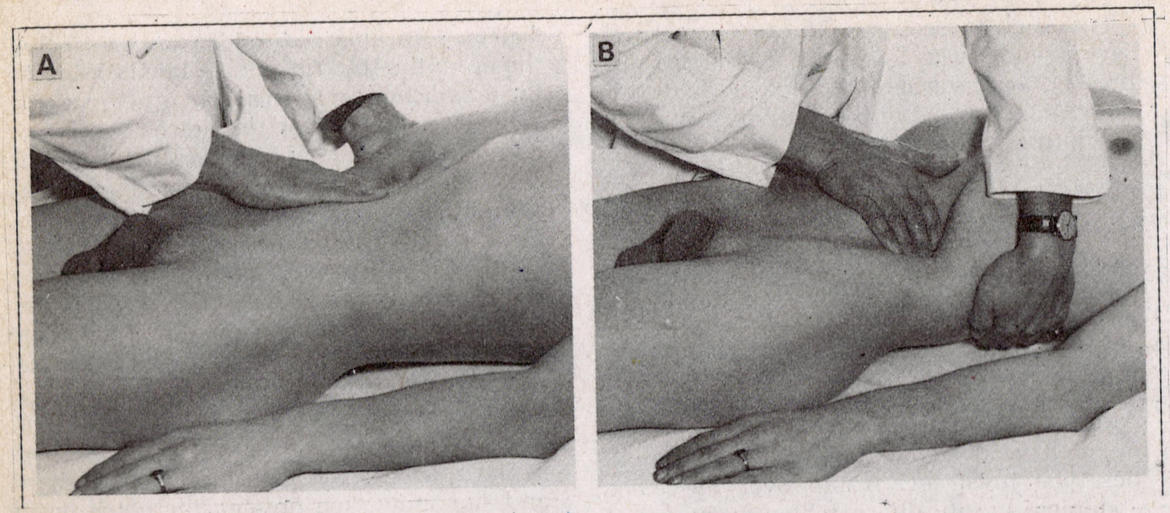

Palpate the liver by resting your fingers on the abdomen almost parallel to the right costal margin and asking the patient to breathe in. The liver edge can be made more prominent by putting your left hand under the lower ribs and lifting them forwards

Palpate the spleen with your fingers lying transversely across the abdomen so that its tip will hit the tips of your index and middle fingers when the patient breathes in. Make the spleen more prominent by lifting the lower ribs forwards with your left hand

FIG. 16.5 PALPATING THE ABDOMEN

to see if it moves or changes shape. Free fluid (ascites) changes shape and moves (**shifting dullness**) if the patient is turned on his side.

Percussion will cause pain if there is underlying peritonitis and is therefore a useful method for determining the extent of a tender area.

Auscultation

First listen for bowel sounds. Bowel can only produce gurgling noises if it contains a mixture of fluid and gas. The pitch of the noise depends upon the distension of the bowel and the proportions of gas and fluid. Normal bowel sounds are low-pitched gurgles occurring every few seconds. If there are no bowel sounds then there is probably no peristalsis, which may be a primary or secondary phenomenon. If you can hear the heart and breath sounds but no bowel sounds over a 15–30 second period, the patient probably has a paralytic ileus. Increased peristalsis increases the volume and frequency of the sounds. Distension of the bowel caused by mechanical intestinal obstruction makes the sounds high pitched, best described as 'tinkling sounds'.

Second, listen along the course of the aorta and the iliac arteries for systolic bruits.

When part, or the whole, of the abdomen is distended, or if you suspect pyloric obstruction, hold the patient at the hips and shake the abdomen from side to side. Splashing sounds (a **succussion splash**) indicate that there is an intra-abdominal viscus, usually the stomach, distended with fluid and gas.

Revision Panel 16.1

Never forget to examine:

- Supraclavicular lymph nodes
- Hernial orifices
- Femoral pulses
- Genitalia
- Bowel sounds
- Anal canal and rectum

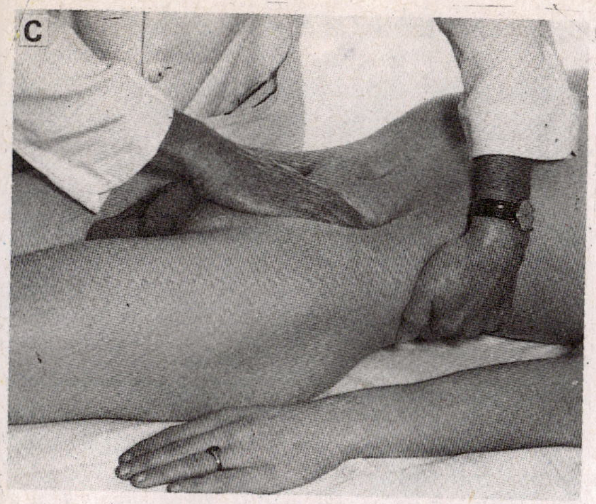

Palpate the kidneys by pressing firmly into the lumbar region during inspiration while lifting the kidney forwards with your other hand in the loin

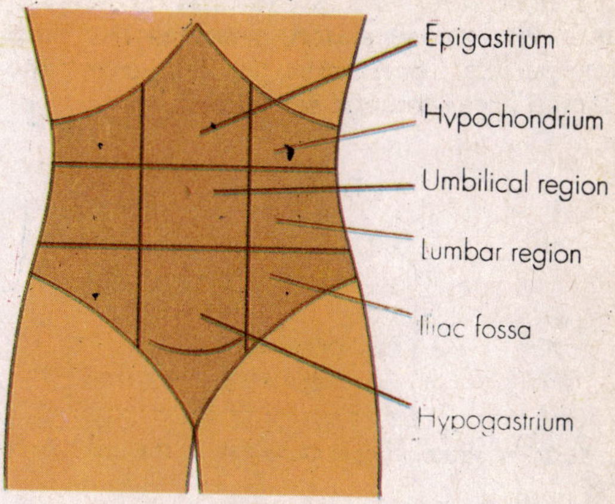

FIG. 16.6 The names of the regions of the abdomen

ABDOMINAL PAIN

The features of pain have been discussed fully in Chapter 1. Being so important they deserve repeating – see Revision Panel 16.2.

So many intra-abdominal diseases present with pain alone that time spent taking a careful history of all its features is never wasted.

The two most significant properties of an abdominal pain are its **site** and its **nature**. If you know about these features, you have a good chance of making the correct diagnosis.

The significance of the site of abdominal pain

The abdomen can be divided into three horizontal zones – upper, central and lower; and each of these can be divided into three regions – central, right and left lateral. The anatomical names of these nine regions are:

- Epigastrium, and right and left hypochondrium.
- Umbilical, and right and left lumbar.
- Hypogastrium, and right and left iliac fossa.

The localization of pain to the upper, middle and lower zones is often more significant than localization to right or left, except for the right hypochondrium, and right and left iliac fossae.

In general, colicky pain is referred to the centre of the abdomen, whatever its source, as

Revision Panel 16.2

The features in the history of a pain that must be elicited

Site

Time and nature of onset

Severity

Nature
(burning, throbbing, stabbing, constricting, colicky, aching)

Progression

End

Duration

Relieving factors

Exacerbating factors

Radiation

Cause

it is a visceral sensation; whereas the pain from parietal peritonitis is felt over the inflamed area (somatic sensation).

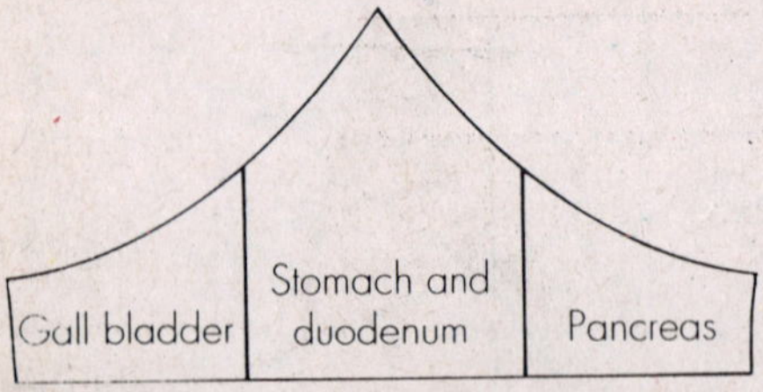

FIG. 16.7 The structures that cause pain in the upper three zones

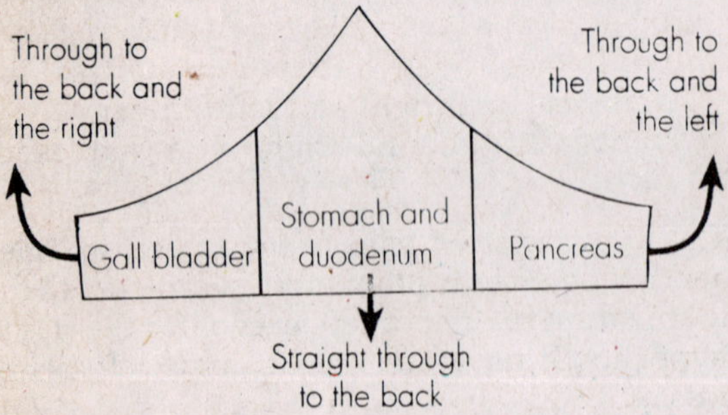

FIG. 16.8 The radiation of pain in the upper zones

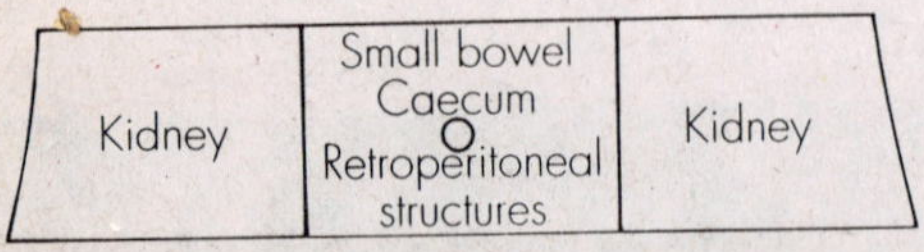

FIG. 16.9 The structures that cause pain in the central three zones

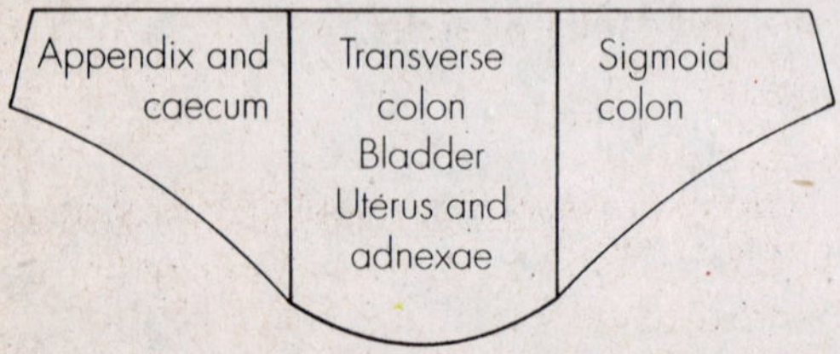

FIG. 16.10 The structures that cause pain in the lower three zones

Upper abdominal pain

Pain is most likely to come from the biliary tree, stomach and duodenum, or pancreas.

In general terms, and with a great deal of overlap, these structures produce right-sided, central and left-sided pain, respectively.

The pain from these three sites also **radiates** in different directions.

Gall bladder pain may radiate through to the back and to the right, to reach the **tip of the shoulder blade**; but more often it is referred to this area and consequently seems, to the patient, to be a separate and independent pain at this site.

Stomach and duodenal pain goes straight through **to the back**.

Pancreatic pain tends to go through to the **back but to the left**.

Central abdominal pain

This is likely to come from the small bowel and caecum, or from mid-line retroperitoneal structures such as the aorta.

Pain in the lateral zones of the central region is most likely to come from the kidneys.

Pain from the kidney is also felt in the loin and may radiate down into the groin.

Small-bowel pain does not usually radiate but may **move** when somatic as well as visceral nerves become irritated.

Lower abdominal pain

This comes from the appendix and caecum, colon, bladder, uterus, ovaries and fallopian tubes.

Pain felt in the hypogastrium usually arises in the transverse or descending colon, bladder, uterus and adnexae. Right iliac fossa pain comes from the caecum and appendix, and left iliac fossa pain from the sigmoid colon.

Lower abdominal pains rarely radiate. The pain from structures deep in the pelvis may be referred to the lower back or perineum.

The significance of the nature of abdominal pain

It is possible to subdivide almost all the painful conditions that occur within the abdomen into two large categories: conditions associated with inflammation, and conditions associated with obstruction of a muscular conducting tube such as the bowel or the ureter. Included in the latter are pains from muscular dysfunction (i.e. disorders of gastrointestinal motility, such as the irritable bowel syndrome), as opposed to true colic secondary to obstruction.

These two conditions cause different types of pain. Inflammation, whether it be the mild inflammatory response around a chronic peptic ulcer or the acute response to a perforated appendix, causes a constant pain made worse by any local or general disturbance, which persists until the inflammation subsides. The patient describes it as 'a pain', of varying severity. Inflammation within the abdomen does not throb or burn in the same way that inflammatory pains often do elsewhere.

Obstruction to a muscular conducting tube produces a colic. A colic is a pain which fluctuates in severity at frequent intervals and feels 'griping' in nature. Although the peaks of pain are short and intermittent the pain seldom goes away completely between exacerbations.

Prolonged obstruction to the outflow of any hollow viscus ultimately causes distension of the viscus. This produces a constant stretching pain, different from the ache of inflammation, but not colicky.

A similar pain can come from retroperitoneal conditions stretching the tissues.

The significance of radiation

When a pain radiates this signifies that other structures are becoming involved. For example, when the pain from a duodenal ulcer radiates through to the back it indicates that the inflammation has spread beyond the duodenum into the structures of the posterior abdominal wall, such as the pancreas. Thus radiation not only indicates the source of the pain but also the extent of the disease.

CONDITIONS PRESENTING WITH ABDOMINAL PAIN

Peptic ulceration

Benign gastric and duodenal ulcers are best classified together as peptic ulcers, even though their aetiology is different, because the substance that ultimately digests the mucosa and causes the ulcer is acid pepsin. Duodenal ulcer is more common than gastric ulcer.

HISTORY

Age The majority of patients with duodenal ulcers are between 20 and 60 years old.

The majority of patients with gastric ulcers are between 40 and 80 years old – a slightly older age group. Thus duodenal ulcers are more common than gastric ulcers in patients under the age of 40 years.

Sex Both types of ulcer are more common in men than women. In women the incidence of both types of ulcer is approximately the same.

Ethnic groups The relative incidence of duodenal to gastric ulcer varies throughout the world. In Great Britain the ratio of DU to GU is approximately 2:1, whereas in the Indian subcontinent it is more than 20:1.

Occupation There is a higher incidence of peptic ulcer amongst professional men and executives, perhaps caused by the greater stresses, strains and responsibilities they carry.

Symptoms The main symptom is **epigastric discomfort or pain**, commonly recognized by the patient as indigestion. It can vary from a vague and mild discomfort, which the patient ignores, to a very severe pain that makes him lie down. The history of the pain helps to distinguish the duodenal from the gastric ulcer in about half the cases. In the others it is not possible to make a clinical diagnosis more specific than peptic ulcer. (See Revision Panel 16.3.)

Patients with gastric ulcers are **afraid to eat** because it causes pain. Patients with duodenal ulcers usually have a good appetite and rarely lose weight because they eat frequently to relieve their pain.

The patient with a gastric ulcer may **lose a little weight** because eating seems to cause the pain.

Acid brash, water brash and heartburn are symptoms common to both types of ulcer, but occur slightly more often in patients with duodenal ulcers.

Revision Panel 16.3

The distinguishing features of the pains of duodenal and gastric ulcers

Feature	*Gastric ulcer*	*Duodenal ulcer*
Site	Epigastrium	Epigastrium
Onset	Soon after eating (15–30 minutes)	2–3 hours after eating; therefore often described by the patient as starting *before* a meal. Also comes on in the middle of the night
Relieving factors	Vomiting	Eating. Patient keeps milk and biscuits at bedside
Precipitating factors	Eating	Missing a meal Anxiety and stress
Periodicity	Comes and goes in a 2–3 month cycle	4–6 month cycle; often worse in spring and autumn
Duration of attack	A few weeks	A month or two

Vomiting relieves the pain of a gastric ulcer and some patients force themselves to vomit after eating to relieve symptoms. Vomiting is an uncommon symptom of duodenal ulceration, unless complications supervene.

Haematemesis and **melaena** may complicate all forms of peptic ulcer.

Drugs Take a careful drug history because many drugs irritate the gastric mucosa and exacerbate the ulcer.

Social history In past years patients with duodenal ulcers were more likely to belong to social classes I and II, and have business and domestic worries, but these factors are always changing.

A large proportion smoke.

EXAMINATION

General examination is likely to be normal. There is usually no more than mild to moderate epigastric tenderness.

If there are complications such as bleeding, pyloric stenosis, or malignant change, there may be anaemia, visible peristalsis and a succussion splash, or wasting, respectively.

The clinical diagnosis is made from the history and confirmed by special investigations.

Perforated peptic ulcer

If a peptic ulcer erodes the wall of the stomach or duodenum at a point where it is covered by visceral peritoneum, the lumen of the gut becomes connected to the peritoneal cavity. The subsequent escape of gastric acid or alkaline bile into the peritoneal cavity causes a chemical, later followed by a bacterial, peritonitis, both of which are acutely painful.

HISTORY

Age Perforated peptic ulcers are most common between the ages of 40 and 60 years, but can occur in the very young and the very old.

All the factors relevant to the incidence of peptic ulcer are obviously also applicable to the incidence of perforated ulcers.

Symptoms The only symptom that concerns the patient is **pain**. This is **severe and constant**. It usually begins very **suddenly**, in the **epigastrium**, reaches its maximum intensity quickly and remains severe for many hours. All movements, including respiration, make the pain worse, so the patient lies immobile on his bed.

Other gastric symptoms such as nausea and vomiting are uncommon.

Previous history The majority of patients give a history of indigestion or epigastric pain typical of a duodenal or gastric ulcer. Some patients have no history of dyspepsia. They may have a perforation of an acute ulcer, a mild ulcer exacerbated by drug therapy, or simply just an ordinary peptic ulcer that has given no symptoms.

Drug history It is important to enquire whether the patient has taken any steroids, non-steroidal anti-inflammatory drugs or aspirin because these drugs can cause ulcers and exacerbate old ulcers to the point of perforation.

EXAMINATION

General appearance The patient looks ill, and is obviously in pain, lying unusually still. There is a **tachycardia**, and respiration is shallow, but the temperature is normal.

Abdomen: Inspection The abdomen is flat, and does not rise and fall with respiration. In thin people the muscles can be seen to be contracted.

Palpation The abdomen is very **tender** and there is intense guarding, often described as **board-like rigidity**. No intra-abdominal viscus or masses can be felt because of the guarding. In the early stages the tenderness and guarding may be confined to the epigastrium and right side, but once the whole peritoneal cavity is contaminated the full-blown clinical picture quickly appears.

Percussion If air has escaped into the peritoneal cavity, the area of **liver dullness may be absent** or diminished.

Percussion is usually painful.

Auscultation The bowel sounds do not disappear until the peritonitis is well established, 6–12 hours after the onset of pain.

Rectal examination Movement of the finger in the pelvis causes pain.

BEWARE. The above description applies to a perforation seen in the first 6–12 hours. After 4–6 hours the acid in the peritoneal cavity becomes diluted and the pain and guarding **decrease**. The patient thinks he is getting better. He is not; he is getting worse. His peritonitis is progressing and he is becoming hypovolaemic. The most valuable signs indicating these circumstances are an **increasing tachycardia** and **absent bowel sounds**.

Carcinoma of the stomach

Carcinoma of the stomach is a common cause of death in men. Pernicious anaemia, gastric polyps and chronic gastric ulcers are known to be premalignant conditions, but the majority of gastric cancers arise spontaneously. There is much speculation but no proof about the role of diet and foodstuffs in the aetiology of this condition.

HISTORY

Age The incidence of gastric carcinoma reaches its peak between the ages of 50 and 70 years, but young adults and old men are often afflicted.

Sex Gastric cancer is two to three times more common in **men**.

Geography There are unexplained variations in the incidence of this disease between countries and within countries.

Symptoms The onset of **indigestion** or **epigastric pain** in a patient over 40 years old, however vague, should always be treated very seriously. The pain may be so mild that the patient ignores it or goes and buys himself some indigestion tablets, **but antacids do not usually relieve the pain**.

Many people think it is usual to have indigestion; it is not.

Unlike the indigestion and pain of a peptic ulcer, the pain of a gastric cancer is not periodic and not solely started by eating. It is often exacerbated by eating but can begin at any time. It is not usually relieved by eating or vomiting.

If the patient has had the symptoms of a benign gastric ulcer for many years he is usually aware that the **nature of the pain has changed.**

Loss of appetite is a cardinal symptom of gastric cancer. Patients with benign ulcers may be frightened to eat because eating causes pain but they still want to eat. Patients with stomach cancer do not want to eat.

The inevitable consequence of the loss of appetite is **loss of weight**. The patient may lose 10–20 kg in 1–2 months. The loss of appetite and weight may occur long before any other symptoms appear to indicate the site of the tumour.

Carcinomata near the cardia may cause oesophagogastric obstruction. The patient may complain of **difficulty in swallowing** because he feels the food sticking behind the lower sternum. As the dysphagia increases, food may be **regurgitated** from the oesophagus.

Cancer of the pylorus often obstructs the outflow tract of the stomach. The patient then has the symptoms of **pyloric stenosis** – the vomiting of large quantities of undigested food, epigastric discomfort and distension. Eructations of gas may be frequent and foul smelling.

Some cancers grow to a considerable size without producing symptoms except mild weight loss. An unsuspecting patient may accidentally feel his **epigastric mass** or **enlarged liver** and present with this finding as his main complaint.

Systematic questions The systematic review of the other systems may reveal evidence of distant metastases, such as weakness and tiredness; dyspnoea and chest pains from pulmonary and pleural deposits; and neurological disturbances from cerebral secondaries and **peripheral neuritis**.

Cancer of the stomach is one of the tumours that sometimes presents with **recurrent superficial thrombophlebitis**.

Previous history The patient may have a long history of benign gastric ulceration, or have had an ulcer some years ago which was 'cured' with medicine.

He may know that he has pernicious anaemia and be taking vitamin B_{12}.

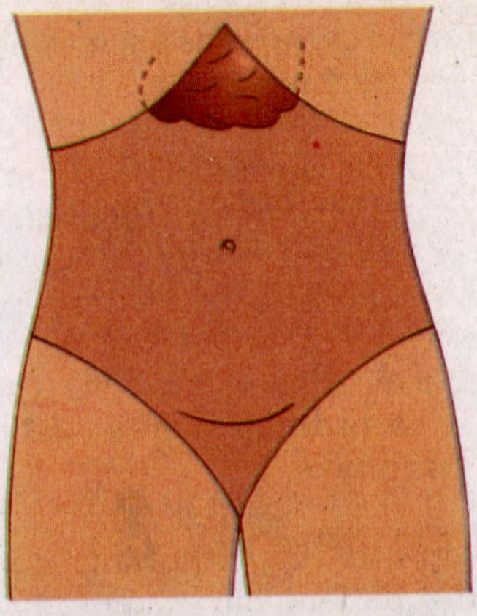

FIG. 16.11 Some cancers of the stomach may present as a palpable mass in the epigastrium but the majority are impalpable

EXAMINATION

General appearance The most noticeable features are **wasting and pallor**. The wasting is obvious in the face and hands. The anaemia may be caused by chronic bleeding from the carcinoma or lack of protein and iron in the diet.

Many patients present at an advanced stage when multiple hepatic metastases have affected liver function, or metastases in the lymph nodes around the porta hepatis have caused biliary obstruction. The resulting **jaundice** is at first mild and may be difficult to detect.

The neck Feel the supraclavicular fossae with great care. Secondary deposits in the supraclavicular nodes are common. A palpable left supraclavicular node is often called **Virchow's node**, or its presence referred to as **Troisier's sign**.

The lungs If the tumour has spread to the lungs there may be pleural effusions. Direct spread of the tumour through the left side of the diaphragm will cause a left-sided effusion and basal consolidation.

Abdomen: Inspection The abdomen is **scaphoid** and the skin wrinkled and inelastic.

Paradoxically, there may be generalized abdominal distension if there is ascites.

There may be **epigastric distension** and visible peristalsis if there is pyloric obstruction, or an irregular fullness in the epigastrium which moves with respiration.

These physical signs can only be seen in very thin patients; in the majority the mass is too high and too deep to be seen.

Palpation In the majority of patients the only physical sign will be **epigastric tenderness**. Deep palpation at full inspiration may reveal an **epigastric mass**.

In a thin patient with advanced disease there may be a **hard, irregular, dull epigastric mass** which moves with respiration. The liver **may be palpable**, and its edge and surface knobbly and irregular.

If there is pyloric obstruction the epigastrium may be distended but soft, and there may be a **succussion splash**.

Percussion Percuss the whole abdomen with care, not only to delineate any palpable masses, but also to see if there is **shifting dullness** in the flanks, caused by ascites.

Auscultation The bowel sounds should be normal.

Rectal examination Metastatic **nodules** may be felt **in the pelvis**. The ovaries may be enlarged by secondary deposits (Krukenberg's tumours).

The limbs Look for evidence of superficial thrombophlebitis and peripheral neuropathy.

Chronic cholecystitis

Chronic or recurrent infection in the gall bladder is commonly associated with **gallstones**. Indeed, in some instances the gallstone may *precede* the infection.

The combination of infection and stones may present a variety of clinical pictures: indigestion (flatulent dyspepsia, chronic cholecystitis), acute pain (acute cholecystitis), gallstone colic, obstructive jaundice, and less common presentations such as ascending cholangitis, pancreatitis and intestinal obstruction. All these presentations may be associated with abdominal pain.

HISTORY

Age Gallstones can form at all ages. The majority of patients with symptoms are between 30 and 60 years old, but you will see a number of young women between the ages of 15 and 25 years with gallstone symptoms.

Sex Gallstones and their complications are far more common in women.

Ethnic group Some races, such as the North American Indian, are particularly liable to develop gallstones.

Symptoms The common complaint is **indigestion or pain** after eating, but not so closely related to eating as the symptoms of peptic ulcer. The pain begins gradually 15–30 minutes after the meal and lasts for 30–90 minutes. It is not relieved by anything except analgesic drugs.

The patient often notices that the pain is worse **after eating fatty foods**.

The attacks of pain are irregular, lasting for weeks or months, with pain-free intervals of varying length.

There is often postprandial **belching**, hence the description 'flatulent dyspepsia'.

The patient's appetite remains good and her weight is steady, or increases.

Nausea and vomiting are uncommon but the patient may develop an intense distaste for fatty foods, akin to nausea.

Previous history Apart from previous episodes of dyspepsia the patient may have been jaundiced or noticed that her stool was pale, offensive and floated on the water in the lavatory pan.

EXAMINATION

General appearance It is the firm belief of all medical students that almost every patient with gallstones is **female, fair, fat, fertile** and **forty**. Many are, but enough are male, thin, dark and of any age to make one pay scant attention to the five 'Fs' as an aid to diagnosis.

The skin should be normal colour, but might be yellow if the patient has obstructive jaundice as well as chronic cholecystitis.

Abdomen: Inspection The abdomen usually looks normal:

Palpation The patient is tender in the right hypochondrium, just below the tip of the ninth rib where the edge of the rectus abdominis muscle crosses the costal margin. It may be necessary to palpate deeply beneath the costal margin, as the patient takes a deep breath, to detect mild tenderness. If the tenderness is acute the right rectus muscle will be tense.

There should be no masses in the abdomen except when the chronic infection is associated with a stone obstructing the cystic duct, and has consequently caused the development of a mucocele, empyema or chronic inflammatory mass.

Percussion, auscultation and rectal examination These should all be normal.

The diagnosis of chronic cholecystitis is usually based on the history and special investigations. The clinical signs are minimal and usually not much help.

Acute cholecystitis

Acute inflammation of the gall bladder is commonly caused by obstruction of the cystic duct by a small stone, with proximal distension, stasis and secondary infection.

HISTORY

Age, sex and ethnic group These factors are similar to those described for chronic cholecystitis.

Symptoms The main symptom is **pain**. It may be of sudden onset or superimposed on the pain of chronic cholecystitis. It is felt in the right **hypochondrium** and often radiates through the trunk to the **tip of the right shoulder blade**.

The pain is continuous and is **exacerbated by movement and breathing**. Nothing, except analgesic drugs, relieves it. The patient often recognizes it as a severe version of her chronic indigestion pain.

The patient always feels **nauseated** and often **vomits**. The abdomen often feels **distended**.

The **appetite** is completely **lost**, but the bowel habit is unchanged.

Previous history There may be a history of flatulent dyspepsia, other acute attacks, or jaundice.

EXAMINATION

General appearance The patient is distressed by the pain and lies quietly, breathing shallowly. She may be sweating. There is a **tachycardia** (90–100 beats/minute) and a **pyrexia** 38–39°C (100–102°F). There may be **rigors**.

Abdomen: Inspection The movement of the abdomen with respiration is diminished.

Palpation There is **tenderness** and **guarding** in the right hypochondrium. If the patient is asked to take a deep breath while you are palpating the tender area, the downward movement of the gall bladder striking the palpating hand may cause a sharp pain that prevents further inspiration. This is called **Murphy's sign**. In severe cases there may be an inflammatory mass around the gall bladder, which can be felt, through the guarding, as a soft indistinct mass bulging down below the edge of the liver. It is exquisitely tender and moves a little with respiration. It can be so large that it reaches down to the level of the umbilicus.

When the pain radiates through to the tip of the scapula there may be an area of skin below the scapula which is hyperaesthetic. This is called **Boas' sign**.

Percussion An inflammatory mass may be detectable by percussion when guarding prevents its palpation.

Auscultation The bowel sounds should be present unless the infection has spread beyond the gall bladder to cause a general peritonitis.

Rectal examination The rectum and contents of the pelvis are normal.

The diagnosis of acute cholecystitis is based upon the site and nature of the pain, fever, tachycardia and tenderness in the right hypochondrium.

Gallstone colic (biliary pain)

Gallstone colic is a severe pain caused by spasm of the gall bladder as it tries to force a stone down the cystic duct. It is called a colic because it is intermittent but the patient seldom describes it as a griping pain. The common bile duct has very little smooth muscle in its wall and probably cannot be the source of a severe colicky pain.

About one-fifth of the patients who present with biliary pain become jaundiced.

HISTORY

Symptoms Gallstone colic begins suddenly across the upper abdomen. The patient is often unable to indicate which side of the abdomen is most affected. It is a **very severe**, constant pain, with excruciating exacerbations. Gallstone colic is **not a true colic**. The patient describes it as a severe pain, not griping in nature, which does not remit between exacerbations. In spite of these facts, the pain is by common usage called gallstone, or biliary, colic because its different features help differentiate it from the pains of acute and chronic cholecystitis.

The severe pain seldom lasts longer than 2 hours. Nothing, except strong analgesia, relieves it.

There is often **nausea** and occasional **vomiting**.

Previous history Many patients give a history of flatulent dyspepsia, previous, less severe episodes of biliary colic, and jaundice.

EXAMINATION

General appearance The patient is frightened and made restless by the intensity of the pain and so has a mild **tachycardia**, but in the early stages the temperature is normal. There may be the beginning of a tinge of jaundice.

Abdomen The abdomen is often too tender to allow deep palpation. Even when the patient lies quietly enough to be examined there is intense guarding in the upper abdomen.

The rectum and pelvis are normal.

Obstructive jaundice

The differential diagnosis of jaundice is discussed in Chapter 8, page 196, but is mentioned here because it is such an important symptom of biliary tract disease.

The principal features of jaundice caused by gallstones are:

1 A history of dyspepsia, pain or biliary colic.
2 No premonitory period of malaise and loss of appetite.
3 A sudden onset.
4 A simultaneous appearance of pale faeces and dark urine.
5 Itching of the skin.

These are the features that help to differentiate obstructive from hepatic and prehepatic jaundice.

Acute pancreatitis

Acute pancreatitis is a condition in which activated pancreatic enzymes leak into the substance of the pancreas and initiate the autodigestion of the gland. One obvious cause of such an event is obstruction of the pancreatic duct, but pancreatitis is also commonly associated with the alcohol ingestion, virus infections and trauma. The mechanism by which alcohol causes pancreatitis is not known, but it is a serious problem in countries with a high incidence of alcoholism.

One-third of the cases of pancreatitis have no association with alcohol, no biliary tract disease and no pancreatic duct obstruction. These cases are labelled idiopathic pancreatitis; one day we may understand their aetiology.

Pancreatitis can vary from a very mild inflammation to an acute haemorrhagic destruction of the whole gland which is fatal in 50 per cent of cases.

HISTORY

Sex Pancreatitis occurs equally in men and women, in spite of the common association with gallstones which are more common in females.

Age The peak incidence is in the fourth and fifth decades of life but pancreatitis can occur at any age.

Symptoms The common presenting symptom is **pain**. It begins suddenly, high in the epigastrium, and steadily increases in severity until it is **very severe** and makes the patient lie still and breathe shallowly.

Nothing relieves it. Movements exacerbate it. It may radiate through to the back, a little to the left of the mid-line.

Frequent vomiting and retching are common symptoms. Most acute abdominal conditions cause nausea and an occasional vomit. Pancreatitis is usually associated with frequent vomiting and retching. This is a very important and valuable clue when considering the diagnosis.

There is persistent **nausea** between the bouts of vomiting but the patient is not nauseated before the attack begins.

Many patients have eaten an unusually large meal or drunk some alcohol an hour or so before the pain began.

When the pain is severe, any movement of the lower chest wall and abdomen causes more pain. This makes the patient breathe rapidly and shallowly and he may complain of difficulty with breathing (dyspnoea).

In severe and advanced pancreatitis the patient may notice **muscle twitches, cramps and spasms.** This is tetany and is caused by the hypocalcaemia which develops if there is extensive intra-abdominal fat necrosis.

Previous history In Great Britain nearly half of the patients who present with pancreatitis have biliary tract disease. Thus there is a high possibility that the patient will have a history of flatulent dyspepsia or other gall bladder symptoms.

Social history Take a careful history of the patient's **alcohol intake**. If in doubt ask a relative. Some alcoholics will not reveal the true extent of their drinking habits.

Also ask about any contact, within and outside the family, with **mumps.**

EXAMINATION

General appearance The severity of the pain makes the patient lie still and causes fear and worry.

As the condition progresses the patient becomes hypovolaemic. This makes him pale and sweaty. If the pain is interfering with respiration he may be dyspnoeic and cyanosed, or grey and very apprehensive.

The sclera may reveal a slight tinge of jaundice if the pancreatitis is secondary to a stone in the lower end of the bile duct. Mild jaundice may appear on the second or third day of the illness if the oedema in the head of the pancreas compresses the bile duct.

Abdomen: Inspection If the pain is severe the tone of the abdominal muscles will be increased and prevent the abdomen moving with respiration.

A paralytic ileus may develop, causing **mild abdominal distension.**

Severe, advanced cases may develop bruising and discolouration in the left flank (Grey Turner's sign) and around the umbilicus (Cullen's sign). These are rare and **late** signs of extensive destruction of the pancreas.

Palpation After listening to the patient's description of his symptoms you will expect to find a very tender, rigid abdomen, but in fact excessive guarding is unusual because the peritonitis is caused by a mild chemical irritation and is not severe.

There is always **tenderness** and **guarding** in the upper abdomen, but the guarding is never as intense as you expect. Thus in any patient with severe pain but surprisingly weak abdominal signs, think of pancreatitis.

If there is a collection of inflammatory exudate in the lesser sac, there may be **epigastric fullness** which may, over the following 5–10 days, become more prominent if it turns into a **pseudocyst** or **lesser sac abscess.**

Percussion The abdomen is slightly distended and resonant with gas collecting in the bowel as the paralytic ileus develops. A pseudocyst in the epigastrium will be dull to percussion.

Auscultation The bowel sounds will be present in the first 12–24 hours of the disease but disappear when the bowel movement becomes paralysed.

Pancreatitis is diagnosed on the history and examination. Measurements of the serum amylase can be misleading and should only be used to confirm your clinical suspicions.

Pancreatitis can be extremely difficult to diagnose and, as it has no distinctive clinical features, is often forgotten and missed. Whenever you see an acute abdomen remember to ask yourself, 'Could it be pancreatitis, a mesenteric vascular accident, or a leaking aneurysm?'

Abdominal aortic aneurysm

Remember that the aorta lies on the posterior abdominal wall, in the upper half of the abdomen, and can cause abdominal pain.

The pain may come from the wall of a stretching or rupturing fusiform aneurysm, or from a circumferential split in the wall of the aorta – an aortic dissection. Fusiform aneurysms commonly begin just below the renal arteries. Aortic dissections begin in the arch of the aorta but can extend down as far as the femoral arteries. Aneurysms caused by atherosclerosis rarely dissect; they just leak or rupture.

When an aneurysm has leaked or ruptured the patient has the general signs of massive blood loss – pallor, sweating, stertorous breathing, tachycardia and hypotension, together with abdominal tenderness and guarding. The aneurysm is palpable but the reduced blood pressure and the haematoma make it less clearly defined. Some of the mass may be haematoma and not pulsate.

The femoral pulses are usually present but weak.

HISTORY

Age Abdominal aneurysms become more frequent with increasing age. The majority of patients are more than 60 years old.

Sex Aneurysms are less common in women.

Symptoms The common symptom is **an aching pain** in the epigastrium and central abdomen. It is a persistent pain, present throughout the day and less noticeable when resting at night, but not relieved or exacerbated by anything. The patient often thinks that he has indigestion even though his pain has no relation to eating.

The abdominal pain is often associated with **backache**. Sometimes backache is the only symptom and it may radiate down to the buttock or leg and be mistaken for **sciatica**.

If the aneurysm enlarges, leaks or ruptures the patient experiences a **severe abdominal pain**. This pain is constant, in the centre of the abdomen, and radiates through to the back.

The patient may feel **a pulsatile mass** in his abdomen or just be aware of a throbbing or pulsating sensation in his abdomen.

Other symptoms, caused by complications such as arterial emboli and thrombosis, present as vascular problems and are described in Chapter 7.

Systematic questions The direct questions often reveal the presence of other cardiovascular symptoms such as angina pectoris, intermittent claudication and the aftermath of previous strokes.

Previous history The patient may have had other aneurysms treated, and may have had previous myocardial and cerebral infarctions.

Family history Arterial disease is often familial.

EXAMINATION

General appearance There is no special facies associated with atherosclerotic vascular disease. Many patients are fat but a significant number are thin and have xanthomata and arcus senilis.

Neck There may be bruits over the carotid arteries.

Heart The blood pressure is often elevated and the heart slightly enlarged.

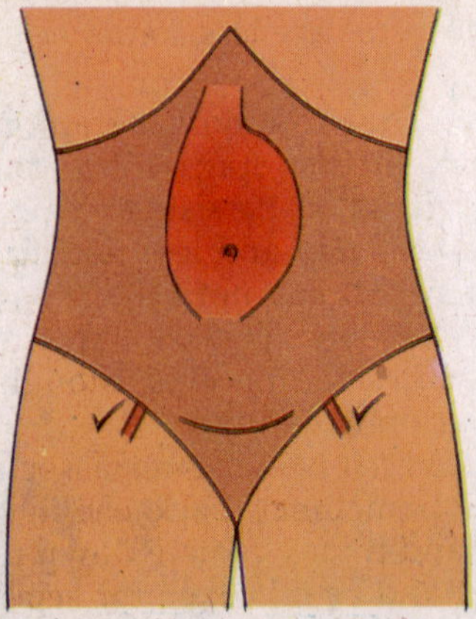

FIG. 16.12 An abdominal aortic aneurysm. The femoral pulses are usually palpable

Abdomen: Inspection A pulsation may be visible in the epigastrium or umbilical region. If the aneurysm is large it will be visible as a pulsating mass.

Palpation If the aneurysm is causing pain it will be tender to firm pressure but there will only be guarding and generalized tenderness if the aneurysm has leaked.

The mass is usually fusiform. If the iliac arteries are involved it may feel bilobed.

The mass has an **expansile pulsation**. Put your hands on either side of the mass and make quite sure that they are being pushed apart, not up and down. Many carcinomata present with vague abdominal pain and an epigastric mass which **transmits** aortic pulsations. You may diagnose an aneurysm only if you can feel an **expansile** pulse.

Abdominal aortic aneurysms are tethered above and below by the renal and iliac arteries. As the artery distends and elongates it arches forwards. This means that aneurysms can often be **moved from side to side** but not up and down.

If you can feel the upper limit of the aneurysm it must begin below the origin of the renal arteries.

The femoral pulses and the limb pulses are usually present. Indeed these vessels often feel dilated and may be aneurysmal.

Percussion The aneurysm will be dull to percussion if it is large enough to displace the bowel laterally and reach the anterior abdominal wall.

Auscultation There are often bruits over aneurysms caused by stenoses at their ends.

Rectal examination This may reveal pulsatile aneurysmal internal iliac arteries.

Renal pain

The symptoms and signs of urinary tract disease are discussed in Chapter 17.

Pain from the kidneys is felt mainly in the loins, but it may radiate anteriorly to the lumbar regions and cause the patient to complain of abdominal pain.

When a patient complains of a kidney pain he usually puts his hands on his waist, thumb forwards and fingers spreading backwards between the 12th rib and the iliac crest. Such a demonstration by the patient of the site of his pain is almost diagnostic of renal pain.

Renal pain is constant, aching or severe, relieved only by analgesic drugs, and exacerbated by movement.

It does not usually radiate unless it is ureteric colic (see page 414).

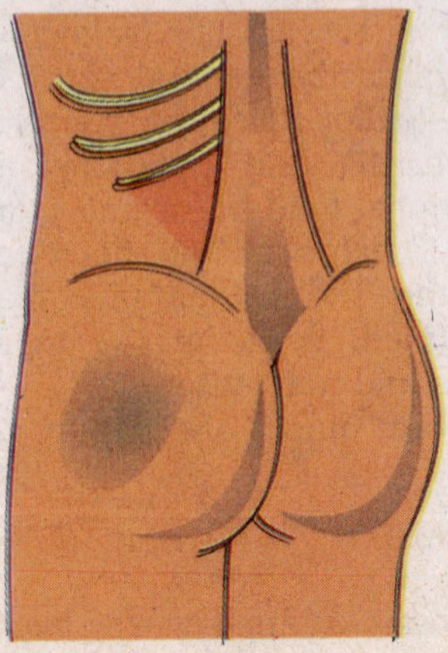

FIG. 16.13 The renal angle is between the 12th rib and the edge of the erector spinae muscle

It is important to ascertain the exact site of the pain by asking the patient to point to it, and then palpate the area for tenderness.

It is easier to feel the renal angle with the patient sitting up and leaning slightly forwards. If the pain is severe he may be unwilling to do this and you will have to get him to roll over onto his side.

Palpation of the abdomen, especially the kidney area, is essential. The kidneys may be tender or enlarged.

Make sure that the bladder is not enlarged.

Examination of the external genitalia and a rectal examination are mandatory as these organs may be affected by the same disease process that is causing the renal pain.

Acute appendicitis

Acute appendicitis is one of the commonest causes of an acute abdomen in the Western world. In 9 cases out of 10 the infection develops in the appendix because its lumen is obstructed by a faecolith or a lesion in the caecum such as a carcinoma.

HISTORY

Age Appendicitis can, and does, occur at all ages.

Sex There is no difference in incidence between the two sexes.

Race, diet and social status These factors may be associated with the incidence of appendicitis, but their role is not yet clearly defined.

Symptoms The principal symptom is **pain**. It commonly begins as a **vague, central** abdominal pain, often thought to be indigestion and ignored. After a varying period, usually a few hours but sometimes 2 or 3 days, the pain **shifts to the right iliac fossa and becomes intense.**

Such a history is almost diagnostic of appendicitis but it only occurs in about half of the patients. The other half present a variety of patterns of pain. It may begin and remain in the right iliac fossa, or may be felt only in the centre of the abdomen. There may be pain in both places simultaneously and a few unfortunate patients have no pain at all.

The central pain is a **referred** pain. The visceral innervation of the appendix comes from the 10th thoracic spinal segment; the corresponding dermatome encircles the abdomen at the umbilicus. If the visceral innervation is higher the mid-line pain will be higher. Some patients have retrosternal pain that shifts to the iliac fossa. Therefore the important feature of the initial pain is its **central location**, not its precise level.

Acute appendicitis may also present with **colic** and abdominal **distention** if part of the small bowel becomes involved in the inflammatory process.

If the inflammation has spread to the bladder or large bowel the patient may present with misleading bladder or large bowel symptoms.

There is a **loss of appetite** which precedes the pain by a few hours.

Most patients feel slightly **nauseated**. Frequent vomiting is uncommon but many patients vomit once or twice.

The majority of patients with appendicitis state that they have been **constipated** for a few days before the attack of pain. A few have diarrhoea, and this may lead to a mistaken diagnosis of gastroenteritis, especially in children.

If the initial stages of the disease are silent the patient may present with the symptoms of general peritonitis: generalized abdominal pain, nausea and vomiting, sweating and sometimes rigors.

EXAMINATION

General appearance Children with appendicitis often look pale and have flushed cheeks. Their skin feels hot but pyrexia is **not** a feature of appendicitis; the oral temperature is seldom above 38°C (100°F).

The tongue is **white** and **furred** and there is a distinctive **foetor oris**.

The pulse rate is elevated by 10 or 20 beats/minute, a change which increases as the infection spreads.

Neck Palpate the neck glands and look at the tonsils. If they are enlarged the diagnosis may be mesenteric adenitis, not appendicitis.

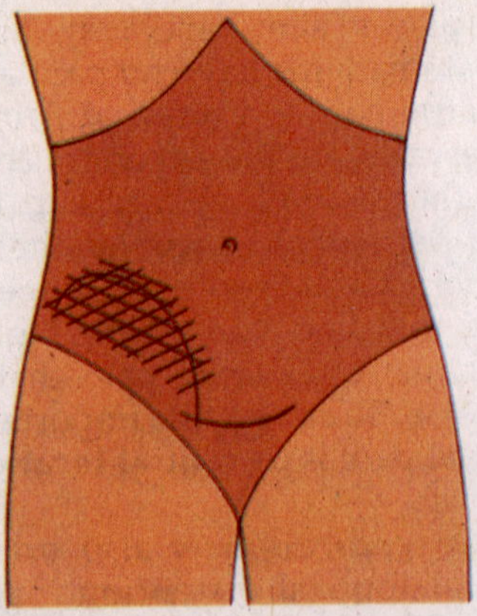

FIG. 16.14 An appendix mass or abscess. The continuous line indicates the edge of the mass; the hatching is the area of tenderness

Chest Examine the lungs carefully. A right-sided basal pneumonia can cause right-sided abdominal pain and mimic appendicitis, especially in children.

Abdomen: Inspection The abdomen looks normal, and moves gently with respiration. If the appendix is lying upon and irritating the psoas major muscle the right hip may be kept slightly flexed. Coughing and sudden movements cause pain.

Palpation **The right iliac fossa is tender** and the overlying muscles guard.

Palpate the tender area very carefully because there may be an underlying inflammatory mass.

Three other physical signs will indicate the degree of tenderness and thus the severity of the peritonitis:

1 There may be release (rebound) tenderness in the right iliac fossa.
2 Pressure on the left iliac fossa may cause pain on the right.
3 Release of pressure on the left may cause pain on the right.

All these manoeuvres cause pain because they move the appendix, as it lies in the right iliac fossa, by varying degrees and so indicate the extent of its inflammation.

When the appendix is retrocaecal the tenderness may be well out in the lateral part of the lumbar region.

A subhepatic appendix produces pain and tenderness below the right costal margin.

The features and differential diagnosis of an appendix mass and appendix abscess are described on page 406.

Percussion This will cause pain if the patient is very tender but it can also help you to detect the presence and limits of any mass that is being obscured by the tenderness and guarding.

Check that the liver dullness is present.

Auscultation Bowel sounds will be present provided the infection is localized to the right iliac fossa.

Rectal examination This usually causes pain, rather than the expected discomfort, deep in the pelvis if the finger is pushed high up to the right. If the appendix is in the pelvis, rectal examination will be very painful. If it is, you should consider the possible alternative diagnosis of salpingitis.

Hip movements Extension of the right hip joint may cause abdominal pain. This sign is often noticed in children because the abdominal pain caused by walking makes them limp.

Diverticular disease

Acquired diverticula appear in the colon, especially the **sigmoid colon**, probably as a result of changes in bowel motility and the consistence of the faeces. Many believe that the condition is caused solely by the Western diet with its low roughage content.

Diverticula are often present without symptoms.

When they cause vague abdominal symptoms the syndrome is called **painful diverticular disease**. When the diverticula become acutely inflamed the condition is called **diverticulitis**.

HISTORY

Age The symptoms from diverticula commonly appear between the ages of 50 and 70 years.

Sex This condition is more common in women.

Ethnic group It is rare in native Africans and Asians.

Symptoms The commonest symptom is **pain/indigestion**. It may be very mild, or severe enough to make the patient lie down. It is a persistent ache with colicky exacerbations.

The pain is usually felt in the **left-hand side of the lower abdomen** but may spread across the whole of the lower abdomen. On rare occasions the pain is felt in the central region of the lower zone of the abdomen. The pain of diverticular disease does not radiate and is not precipitated by eating.

Although the patients do not notice any direct relationship between the time of eating and the appearance of the pain, they often observe that certain foods make their attacks of pain worse. The type of food which does this varies enormously from patient to patient.

When the pain begins there is often gaseous **distension, flatulence and belching**. This is probably due to mild colonic obstruction caused by the smooth muscle hypertrophy of the bowel wall.

Most patients with diverticular disease are **constipated**; that is to say, they have infrequent bowel actions and hard stool. Their appetite and weight remain **normal**.

EXAMINATION

There may be nothing abnormal to find on examination and the diagnosis is made by the appearance of the bowel on a barium enema. However, in most patients the sigmoid colon is easily **palpable** and slightly tender. During an attack of pain the whole of the left iliac fossa is tender.

Acute diverticulitis

HISTORY

Age, sex and ethnic group These features are similar to those described above for painless diverticular disease.

Symptoms The patient develops a **severe pain** in the left iliac fossa or the whole of the lower abdomen. The pain begins suddenly, is constant and is exacerbated by movement. Occasionally the pain begins in the centre of the lower abdomen and then moves to the left side, in a manner (and for the same reasons) similar to appendicitis.

The abdomen usually feels a little **distended**. If the inflammation spreads, peritonitis and (sometimes) intestinal obstruction may develop and the distension increase.

The patient is **nauseated, loses her appetite**, but does not usually vomit.

Most patients are constipated; a few have diarrhoea.

The inflammation may cause the patient to feel hot, feverish and sweaty.

If the inflamed colon is lying on the vault of the bladder it may cause an increased frequency of micturition and painful micturition.

Previous history The patient often has a long history of painful diverticular disease: flatulence, distension and left iliac fossa pain.

EXAMINATION

General appearance The patient lies still because of the pain. She looks flushed and feverish. The temperature is often 38–39°C (100–102°F) and the pulse rate over 100 beats/minute.

Abdomen: Inspection The abdomen moves with respiration because the inflamed bowel is

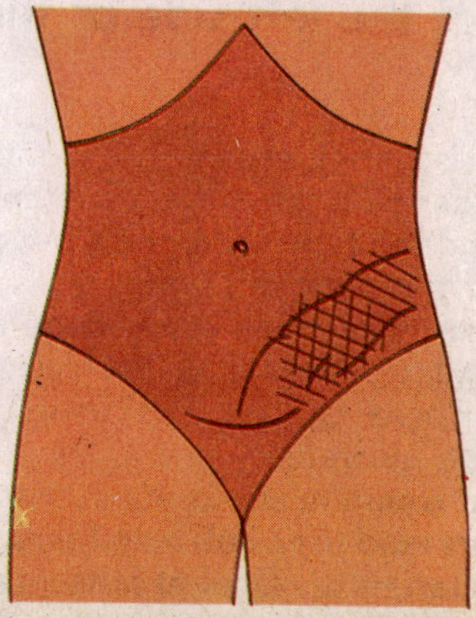

FIG. 16.15 The mass and tenderness of acute diverticul

confined to its lower half. It is slightly distended.

Palpation The left iliac fossa is tender and protected by spasm of the overlying muscles. Careful palpation may detect a palpable tender **sausage-shaped mass** in the left iliac fossa. There may be rebound tenderness and left-sided pain during pressure on the right side of the abdomen.

Percussion If there is a palpable mass in the left iliac fossa, it should be dull to percussion.

Auscultation The bowel sounds are normal or hyperactive until a general peritonitis develops and causes a paralytic ileus.

Rectal examination The patient feels pain when the finger is pushed high into the left side of the pelvis. If the inflamed colon is lying in the pelvis, rectal examination is very painful.

The clinical diagnosis of diverticulitis rests solely on the site of the pain, the tenderness and, when present, the mass.

The symptoms and signs of some of the complications of diverticulitis – diverticular abscess, intestinal obstruction and general peritonitis – are described later in this chapter.

Cancer of the left side of the colon

The colon is a long organ. The symptoms of cancer of the colon differ according to the part affected and the type of tumour, but pain is a common symptom of all types.

The majority of colon cancers are found in ` sigmoid colon and at the rectosigmoid 'on. These cancers are usually small, and ulcerated.

common site is the caecum, where end to be bulky and papilliferous. rters of all colon cancers are distal nic flexure.

HISTORY

Age The majority of patients are over 50 years old, but colon cancer can occur in young adults and children, because it can complicate ulcerative colitis and familial polyposis coli.

Sex Both sexes are equally affected.

Symptoms **Pain is not the commonest symptom**. When present it is usually a mild lower abdominal colic or ache which, after some weeks or months, becomes a persistent pain in the left lower abdomen, with severe colicky exacerbations.

The commonest symptom is a **change of bowel habit**. The initial change is **constipation**, meaning the infrequent passage of hard faeces. Suddenly, often following an episode of colic, the patient passes a number of loose stools – **diarrhoea**. The constipation then returns. Alternating constipation and diarrhoea is typical of annular carcinomata of the left colon. The constipation is caused by the intestinal obstruction, the diarrhoea by the liquefaction of faeces above the obstruction, helped by inflammation of the colonic mucosa and excess secretion of mucus.

The episodes of colicky pain are accompanied by distension.

Loss of weight and appetite are not very common symptoms. When they do occur the weight loss often precedes the anorexia.

The patient may feel a lump in his abdomen.

Rectal bleeding is not a common symptom of sigmoid or descending colon tumours because these tumours only bleed a little and the blood becomes intimately mixed with the faeces.

When the tumour is at the rectosigmoid junction it may prolapse into the rectum and cause tenesmus, but this symptom is much more frequently associated with rectal carcinoma.

Painful, frequent micturition indicates involvement of the bladder.

EXAMINATION

General appearance The weight loss may be apparent. The patient may be pale if chronic blood loss has caused anaemia.

Neck The left supraclavicular lymph nodes may be enlarged.

Abdomen: Inspection In a thin patient there may be a swelling in the left iliac fossa. The colon, especially the caecum, may be visibly distended with faeces.

Palpation If the tumour is small and lying in the paravertebral gutter the abdomen will feel normal, but it may form a palpable mass on the left-hand side, usually in the left iliac fossa. Part of this mass may be hard **faeces** above the tumour, not the tumour itself. If this is the case the mass should be **indentable**.

The mass will be tender if there is any surrounding inflammation.

The liver may be palpable, with an irregular surface and edge.

Percussion The mass in the left iliac fossa will be dull to percussion.

Auscultation If there is any chronic intestinal obstruction the bowel sounds will be hyperactive. During an attack of colic, loud, high-pitched, continuous gurglings can be heard.

Rectal examination A tumour in the apex of the loop of the sigmoid colon, hanging down into the pelvis, may be felt on bimanual examination of the pelvis.

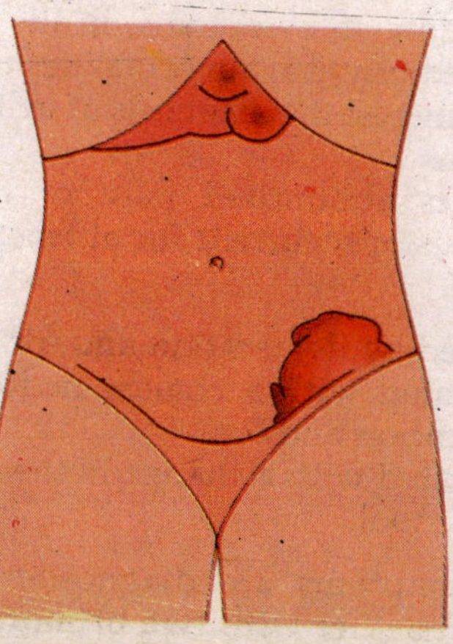

FIG. 16.16 The mass of a carcinoma of the sigmoid colon, with metastases in the liver

There may be secondary nodules on the pelvic peritoneum.

Test the faeces for **blood**. The stool is often dark brown and the test positive.

Cancer of the caecum

Carcinoma of the caecum has a deserved reputation for being 'silent' until it has grown to a considerable size. The majority of patients with this disease ultimately present with abdominal pain, but many have had other symptoms for much longer which they have ignored or which have been misdiagnosed.

HISTORY

Symptoms The commonest type of **pain** is a dull ache in the right iliac fossa, but this is a **late** symptom. If the growth occludes the ileocaecal valve the patient will have **intestinal colic** and intestinal obstruction.

Loss of weight followed by anorexia is common.

Large tumours in the caecum bleed continually and the patient gets anaemic. This causes **pallor, debility and breathlessness** but the blood loss is not sufficient to colour the faeces.

A **change in bowel habit** is not such a prominent symptom as with left-sided tumours, but it does occur. Sometimes there is constipation, sometimes diarrhoea, but these symptoms do not alternate.

The patient may feel **a lump** in the right iliac fossa.

If the tumour blocks the mouth of the appendix, the appendix will distend and become acutely inflamed. The possibility that the inflammation is caused by a carcinoma of the caecum should always be remembered in anyone over 40 years old who gets **acute appendicitis**.

EXAMINATION

General appearance The patient may be pale and thin.

Neck The supraclavicular lymph nodes may be palpable.

Abdomen: Inspection The abdomen may be generally distended or 'full' in the right iliac fossa.

Palpation The right iliac fossa is often tender with some guarding of the covering muscles.

There may be a firm irregular mass in the right iliac fossa, which may be fixed or freely mobile. When it is mobile it tends to slip up into the paravertebral gutter or medially and downwards into the pelvis.

The liver may be palpable and irregular.

Percussion The mass will be dull to percussion.

Auscultation The bowel sounds should be normal but if there is any obstruction of the ileocaecal valve they will be hyperactive.

Rectal examination The rectum is normal, but the faeces may contain blood.

When the tumour causes **appendicitis** the physical signs are indistinguishable from those of simple acute appendicitis. Even when a mass is palpable it is rarely possible to be certain that it is not an inflammatory mass. If the mass is very hard, discrete, knobbly and not very tender you should suspect that it is not just caused by inflammation.

Inflammatory bowel disease

Crohn's disease and ulcerative colitis may present with acute or chronic abdominal pain together with a variety of other gastrointestinal symptoms.

Acute Crohn's disease presents with symptoms and signs similar to those of appendicitis. The thickened, tender terminal ileum may be palpable in the right iliac fossa. The symptom that helps distinguish acute Crohn's disease from appendicitis is the occurrence of episodes of diarrhoea before the acute attack.

Chonic Crohn's disease is associated with a long history of attacks of diarrhoea over months or years, accompanied by intestinal colic. A tender mass may be palpable in the right iliac fossa.

Acute fulminating ulcerative colitis may present with acute abdominal pain caused by toxic dilatation of the colon or even a perforation of the colon but such symptoms are invariably preceded by severe incessant diarrhoea with the passage of blood, mucus and pus.

Chronic ulcerative colitis rarely presents with severe abdominal pain but the frequent episodes of diarrhoea may be accompanied by intestinal colic.

Irritable bowel syndrome

Irritable bowel syndrome is a functional disorder of the bowel, of unknown aetiology, which causes chronic abdominal pain, changes in bowel habit and defaecation, and abdominal distention.

Mixtures of these symptoms occur in at least 10 per cent of the population, so it is feasible that irritable bowel syndrome is simply a variant of the normal, not a disease.

Many aetiological factors have been postulated – the quantity of fibre in the diet, food allergies, disorders of bowel motility, abnormalities of visceral perception, psychological disorders, and social and behavioural problems.

The diagnosis is based solely on the history and physical examination, so it is essential to enquire about any symptoms or signs that might indicate the presence of organic disease, such as anaemia, bleeding, weight loss, fever, or the recent development of abdominal pain or change in bowel habit.

The following symptoms, in the absence of any related physical abnormalities upon examination, suggest the diagnosis of irritable bowel syndrome.

There is **abdominal pain or discomfort**, continuous or recurrent **for at least 3 months**, which is:

- relieved by defaecation and/or
- associated with a change in frequency of defaecation and/or
- associated with a change in the consistence of the stool.

These symptoms are diagnostic when presenting **together with two or more** of the following complaints not associated with the pain:

An altered frequency of defaecation.
An altered consistence of the stool (hard or watery).
Problems with defaecation (straining, incomplete evacuation).
The passage of mucus.
'Bloated' feelings of abdominal distension.

Acute salpingitis

This is an infection of the fallopian tubes. It is usually bilateral and the common infecting organisms are the gonococcus and *Streptococcus*. These organisms reach the fallopian tubes by direct spread through the vagina and uterus, or by the blood stream. Bacteria can also spread into the fallopian tubes across the peritoneal cavity from an inflamed appendix or sigmoid diverticulum.

HISTORY

Age Salpingitis occurs most often between the ages of 15 and 40 years, but can occur in children.

Symptoms The patient complains of the gradual onset (a few hours) of **lower abdominal pain**. It is constant and can become severe. It is not affected by movement or relieved by anything but analgesic drugs. It may radiate to the lower part of the back. The abdominal pain is sometimes preceded by low backache.

The woman has often noticed a purulent, yellow–white **vaginal discharge** a few days before the pain begins.

Menstruation may have been irregular over the previous months. These patients often have a history of dysmenorrhoea.

Salpingitis is a recognized complication of the **puerperium** and abortion.

Although the patient complains of abdominal pain there is usually **no nausea, vomiting** or change in bowel habit.

By contrast, urinary tract symptoms such as **painful, frequent micturition** are common because the urinary tract is often infected.

Sweating and rigors occur if the temperature is elevated.

Previous history The patient may have had previous attacks of salpingitis or know that she has had gonorrhoea, or been exposed to it.

EXAMINATION

General appearance The patient looks flushed and feverish. There is no distinctive foetor oris. The oral temperature may be 38–39.5°C (101–103°F).

Abdomen: Inspection The abdomen moves with respiration, and looks normal.

Palpation There is tenderness, with some guarding, across the lower abdomen. The tenderness will be asymmetrical if one fallopian tube is more inflamed than the other.

The tenderness is lower and nearer the midline than the tenderness of appendicitis.

No masses can be felt.

Percussion This is normal.

Auscultation The bowel sounds are normal. The peritonitis is usually confined to the pelvis and rarely causes a paralytic ileus.

Rectal and vaginal examination There is a yellow–white vaginal discharge, a specimen of which should be sent for culture.

The cervix and uterus are of normal size, but bimanual palpation of the adnexae is very painful, and movement of the cervix also causes pain.

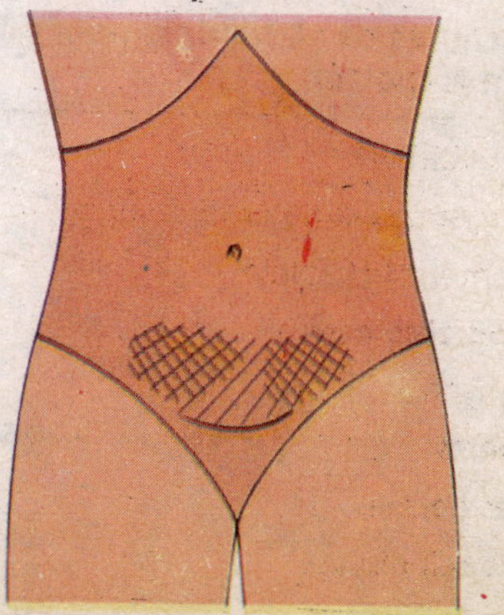

FIG. 16.17 The areas of tenderness associated with salpingitis

If there is a pyosalpinx or tubo-ovarian abscess there will be a palpable mass at the side of the uterus.

Rectal examination will confirm the tenderness on either side of the uterus. The inside of the rectum often feels hot.

Acute retention of urine

Acute retention of urine is very painful. The patient therefore presents with abdominal pain but the diagnosis is made easy by his knowledge that he has not and cannot pass urine in spite of a desperate desire to do so.

The varieties of retention are discussed in Chapter 17. The significant physical sign is a palpable bladder, pressure on which increases the desire to micturate.

> **Revision Panel 16.4**
>
> **The causes of haematemesis and melaena**
>
> Chronic peptic ulceration
> - Idiopathic
> - Steroids
>
> Acute erosions
> - Aspirin
> - Phenylbutazone
> - Steroids
> - Trauma, especially burns
>
> Carcinoma of the stomach
>
> Oesophageal varices
>
> Mallory–Weiss syndrome
>
> Purpura
>
> Haemophilia

> **Revision Panel 16.5**
>
> **The causes of abdominal pain which are often forgotten**
>
> Pancreatitis
>
> Aneurysm (leaking or dissecting)
>
> Mesenteric ischaemia
>
> Herpes zoster (shingles)
>
> Porphyria
>
> Diabetes
>
> Tabes dorsalis
>
> Sickle-cell disease
>
> Pneumonia

ALIMENTARY CONDITIONS PRESENTING WITH DYSPHAGIA OR VOMITING

Some serious alimentary diseases do not cause abdominal pain but do affect swallowing and may cause retrosternal pain.

Carcinoma of the oesophagus rarely produces any physical signs apart from wasting and perhaps a palpable supraclavicular lymph node. The diagnosis is suspected when the patient complains of **dysphagia**. At first he cannot swallow large pieces of food, but ultimately he cannot swallow fluids. Patients are often able to locate the level of the obstruction in their oesophagus quite accurately. For example, a carcinoma in the lower third of the oesophagus causes a block which the patient feels to be behind the lower part of the sternum.

Reflux oesophagitis causes a retrosternal burning sensation, described by the patient as **heartburn**. If the oesophagus becomes very inflamed the patient will also have dysphagia. Apart from the nature of the pain, the clue to the diagnosis of reflux oesophagitis is its relationship to posture. Bending, stooping, heavy lifting and tight clothes all force acid up into the oesophagus and cause heartburn.

Reflux oesophagitis is sometimes the only symptom of **hiatus hernia**.

Pyloric stenosis occurs in neonates with **congenital hypertrophic pyloric stenosis** and adults with cicatrizing benign ulceration of their pylorus or duodenum, or **carcinoma of the antrum** of the stomach. The last two conditions may be associated with the symptoms of benign peptic ulcer or carcinoma of the stomach, previously described in this chapter.

An adult with pyloric stenosis presents with **vomiting**. The vomit is usually large in volume, not bile-stained and, if the condition is long-standing, not acidic because gastric acid secretion is reduced. The stomach contents are therefore not digested and the patient may recognize food that he ate 24 or 48 hours previously. Apart from epigastric distension, visible gastric peristalsis and a **succussion splash**, there may be no other abnormal physical signs.

The neonate with congenital hypertrophic pyloric stenosis vomits large quantities of curdled and unpleasant-smelling milk. The vomit is forcefully ejected, justifying the adjective **projectile**. The baby becomes thin and dehydrated but has a good appetite.

Careful examination may reveal the distended stomach and a **smooth ovoid mass just below the right costal margin**. This is the hypertrophic pylorus. You can only be certain of the diagnosis if you can feel the pyloric mass.

CONDITIONS PRESENTING WITH DIARRHOEA

Some diseases of the large bowel cause diarrhoea and no other symptoms. The nature of the diarrhoea sometimes suggests the diagnosis, but its proof usually rests on the results of endoscopy, biopsy, barium enema and stool cultures.

The common causes of severe diarrhoea are as follows (see also Revision Panel 18.5).

Infections in food, such as typhoid and staphylococcal toxins, are often lumped together as 'food poisoning'.

The stool is watery, brown and passed with great frequency. There is abdominal colic, nausea, vomiting and thirst.

Typhoid may present as a surgical problem with abdominal pain from the perforation of the ulcers in the small bowel.

In tropical countries the most likely causes of diarrhoea are bacillary dysentery, amoebic dysentery, malignant tertian malaria, kala-azar and schistosomiasis.

Ulcerative (and Crohn's) colitis. The patient complains of the sudden onset of frequent diarrhoea. Some of the motions are watery brown fluid, others are just mucus. Both contain dark altered blood and flecks of fresh red blood. The patient may have to evacuate the rectum 20 or 30 times a day. Abdominal pain is uncommon unless complications such as colonic distension and perforation occur. The patient is dehydrated, thin, ill and feverish.

Cholera presents with vomiting, cramps and severe diarrhoea. The diarrhoea lasts up to 3–4 days. The patient passes colourless opaque stools, known as **rice-water stools**, which consist of an inflammatory exudate, mucus, flakes of epithelium, the casts of villi and the infecting organism.

Rectal villous tumours. Most carcinomata on the left-hand side of the colon cause a change in bowel habit, pain and bleeding. Persistent copious diarrhoea is not a prominent feature, but may occur.

One rectal tumour, the **villous papilloma**, causes excessive mucus secretion and the patient frequently passes stools of pure mucus. He may become dehydrated and sodium depleted. This is a rare tumour.

ACUTE PERITONITIS

Many of the conditions mentioned in this chapter cause localized or general acute peritonitis. When you can determine the cause of peritonitis it is easy to formulate a plan of treatment, but if you cannot make a specific diagnosis you must decide whether the patient needs a laparotomy. There are two circumstances in which a laparotomy is essential:

1 If there is evidence of ischaemia of the bowel (caused by strangulation or a vascular occlusion).
2 If there is an unexplained general peritonitis where laparotomy is needed to make the diagnosis.

Both conditions produce similar physical signs. The severity of the pain is not an indication of the degree of inflammation; the diagnosis of peritonitis must be based on the physical signs. The clinical features of peritonitis are as follows.

An increasing tachycardia If the pulse rate increases gradually during 1–2 hours of observation, there is likely to be serious disease within the abdomen.

Pyrexia The temperature rises only when the peritoneal cavity becomes heavily infected. Remember that steroids damp down the inflammatory response. Patients on corticosteroids with a severe peritonitis may have a normal temperature.

Tenderness and guarding Guarding is an excellent indication of the severity of the tenderness. If the whole abdomen is tense there is likely to be general peritonitis.

Rebound tenderness This is just another way of showing that the abdomen is very tender. It can be a valuable sign because the patient is not expecting pain as you suddenly remove your hand, so the apprehension which can cause guarding during direct palpation is absent. However, it causes considerable discomfort and should be used sparingly.

Localized pain during distant palpation If a tender spot hurts when you press a distant non-tender part of the abdomen, the structures in the painful area are likely to be very inflamed.

Absence of bowel sounds The absence of bowel sounds *per se* does not indicate peritonitis, but their absence in a tender, rigid abdomen makes it highly likely that there is generalized peritonitis.

Revision Panel 16.6

The cardinal symptoms of intestinal obstruction

Vomiting

Colic

Distension

Absolute constipation

INTESTINAL OBSTRUCTION

The causes of intestinal obstruction are legion. Some are listed in Revision Panel 16.7.

The clinician must be able to answer two questions:

1 Is there intestinal obstruction?
2 Is the bowel strangulated?

The signs of strangulation are the same as the signs of local peritoneal inflammation – pain, tenderness, guarding and rebound tenderness – discussed above.

The cardinal symptoms of intestinal obstruction are pain, vomiting, distension and absolute constipation, but the severity and time of onset of each of these symptoms will depend upon the level of the obstruction.

Revision Panel 16.7

Age, and the common causes of alimentary tract obstruction

Birth
- Atresia (duodenum, ileum)
- Meconium obstruction
- Volvulus neonatorum

3 weeks
- Congenital hypertrophic pyloric stenosis

6–9 months
- Intussusception

Teenage
- Inflammatory masses (appendicitis)
- Intussusception of Meckel's diverticulum or polyp

Young adult
- Hernia
- Adhesions

Adult
- Hernia
- Adhesions
- Inflammation (appendicitis, Crohn's disease)
- Carcinoma

Elderly
- Carcinoma
- Inflammation (diverticulitis)
- Sigmoid volvulus

Pain

The pain of intestinal obstruction is a true colic. There are severe gripping exacerbations, interspersed with periods of little or no pain.

Colic is uncommon with obstructions above the pylorus. Small-bowel colic is felt in the central part of the abdomen, large-bowel colic in the lower third of the abdomen.

Vomiting

Intestinal obstruction causes frequent vomiting. The nature of the vomitus depends upon the level of the obstruction. With pyloric obstruction the vomitus is watery and acid. High small-bowel obstruction gives a greenish-blue bile-stained vomit. Obstruction below the middle of the small bowel is associated with a brown vomit which becomes increasingly foul smelling as the obstruction persists. It becomes so thick, brown and foul that it is often called 'faeculent' vomit, but this is a misnomer; it is not faeces, just stagnant lower small-bowel and caecal contents.

Distension

The lower down the gut the obstruction, the more bowel there is available to distend and so ultimately the greater the distension. High obstruction is not associated with much distension, particularly if the patient is vomiting frequently.

An obstruction in the left side of the colon first causes the colon to distend. The distension extends into the small bowel only if the ileocaecal valve is incompetent. If this valve remains closed the right side of the colon, especially the caecum, can become grossly distended, causing a visible asymmetry. The right iliac fossa bulges outwards and is hyper-resonant.

Absolute constipation

Once an obstruction is complete and the bowel below it is empty there is **absolute** constipation; that is to say, *no* defaecation. This takes a varying time to develop, depending upon the level of the obstruction.

The foregoing cardinal symptoms present in a different sequence according to the level of the obstruction. A high small-bowel obstruction starts with pain and vomiting, the distension is slight and the absolute constipation is the last symptom to appear. A left-sided large-bowel obstruction starts with pain and absolute constipation, followed quite quickly by distension, and vomiting is the last symptom to appear.

The **bowel sounds** of a mechanical intestinal obstruction are at first **hyperactive**, loud and frequent. As the bowel distends, the sounds become **resonant** and **high pitched**, and eventually **tinkling**.

THE ABDOMINAL MASS: CAUSES AND SIGNS

The techniques for palpating the liver, spleen and kidneys are described on page 375.

Hepatomegaly

The causes of enlargement of the liver, classified according to their clinical presentation, are listed below.

Smooth generalized enlargement, without jaundice

- Congestion from heart failure.
- Cirrhosis.
- Reticuloses.
- Hepatic vein obstruction (Budd–Chiari syndrome).
- Amyloid disease.

Revision Panel 16.8
Causes of hepatomegaly

Infection
Congestion
Bile duct distension
Cellular infiltration
Cellular proliferation
Space-occupying lesions

Smooth generalized enlargement, with jaundice

Infective hepatitis.
Biliary tract obstruction (gallstones, carcinoma of pancreas).
Cholangitis.
Portal pyaemia.

Knobbly generalized enlargement, without jaundice

Secondary carcinoma.
Macronodular cirrhosis.
Polycystic disease.
Primary liver carcinoma.

Knobbly generalized enlargement, with jaundice

Extensive secondary carcinoma.
Cirrhosis.

Localized swellings

Riedel's lobe.
Secondary carcinoma.
Hydatid cyst.
Liver abscess.
Primary liver carcinoma.

The physical signs of an enlarged liver area are:

1 It descends from below the right costal margin and costal angle.
2 You cannot get above it.
3 It moves with respiration.
4 It is dull to percussion up to the level of the eighth rib in the mid-axillary line.
5 Its edge can be sharp or rounded and its surface smooth or irregular.

Remember Riedel's lobe. This is an extension of the right lobe of the liver down below the costal margin, along the anterior axillary line. It is often mistaken for a pathological enlargement of the liver or gall bladder. It is a **normal anatomical variation**.

Splenomegaly

The spleen is almost always uniformly enlarged, so concealing the cause of its

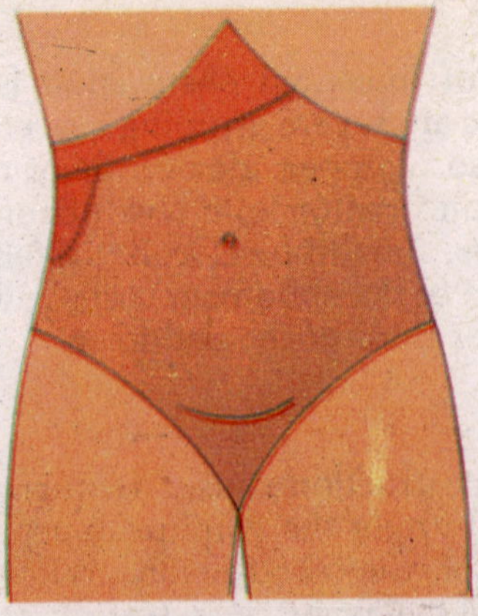

FIG. 16.18 Hepatomegaly. The dotted line indicates the site of Riedel's lobe – a normal anatomical variation

enlargement. The causes of splenomegaly are best classified according to the underlying disease.

Infection

Bacterial

Typhoid.
Typhus.
Tuberculosis.
General septicaemia.

Spirochaetal

Syphilis.
Leptospirosis (Weil's disease).

Revision Panel 16.9
Causes of splenomegaly

Infection
Cellular proliferation
Congestion
Infarction
Cellular infiltration
Collagen diseases
Space-occupying lesions

Viral

Glandular fever.

Protozoal.

Malaria.
Kala-azar.

Cellular proliferation

Myeloid and lymphatic leukaemia.
Pernicious anaemia.
Polycythaemia rubra vera.
Spherocytosis.
Thrombocytopenic purpura.
Myelosclerosis.
Mediterranean anaemia.

Congestion

Portal hypertension (cirrhosis, portal vein thrombosis).
Hepatic vein obstruction.
Congestive heart failure (cor pulmonale, constrictive pericarditis).

Infarction

Emboli from bacterial endocarditis, emboli from the left atrium during atrial fibrillation associated with mitral stenosis, emboli from the left ventricle after myocardial infarction.
Splenic artery or vein thrombosis in polycythaemia and retroperitoneal malignancy.

Cellular infiltration

Amyloidosis.
Gaucher's disease.

Collagen diseases

Felty's syndrome.
Still's disease.

Space-occupying lesions

True solitary cysts.
Polycystic disease.
Hydatid cysts.
Angioma.
Lymphosarcoma.
Lymphoma.

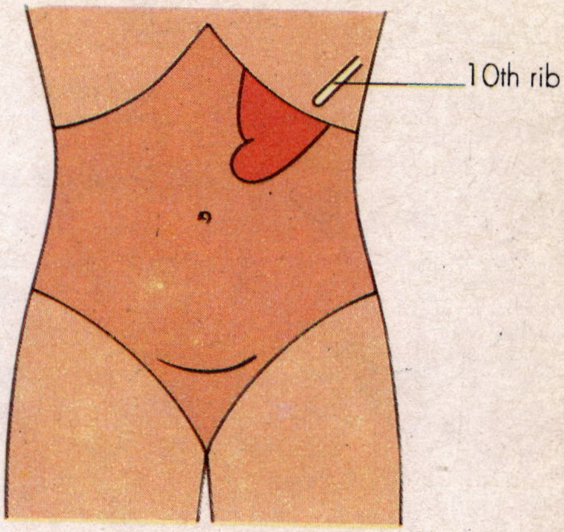

FIG. 16.19 Splenomegaly. The notch is not always palpable

The physical signs of an enlarged spleen are:

1 It appears from below the tip of the left 10th rib and enlarges along the line of the rib towards the umbilicus.
2 It is firm, smooth, and usually spleen shaped. It often has a definite notch on its upper edge.
3 You cannot get above it.
4 It moves with respiration.
5 It is dull to percussion.
6 Although it may be possible to bring it forwards by lifting the left lower ribs forwards, it cannot be felt bimanually or be ballotted.

Enlargement of the kidney

One or both kidneys may be enlarged. The common causes of enlargement of the kidney are:

Hydronephrosis.
Pyonephrosis.
Perinephric abscess.
Malignant disease: carcinoma of the kidney and nephroblastoma.
Solitary cysts.
Polycystic disease.
Hypertrophy.

A mobile or low-lying kidney may be easily palpable and so seem to be enlarged.

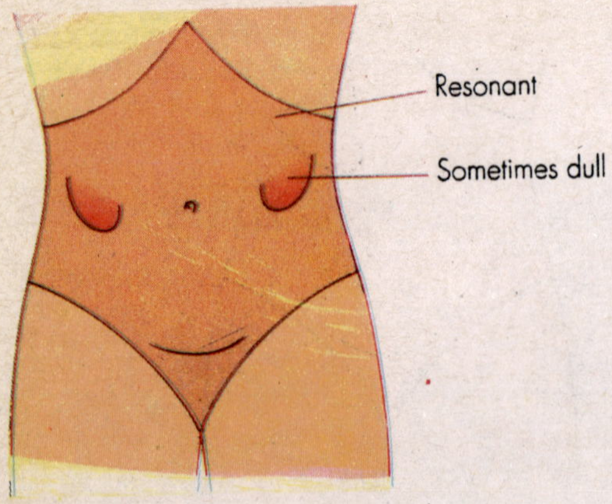

FIG. 16.20 Bilateral enlargement of the kidneys

Polycystic disease is very likely to affect both kidneys.

Hydronephrosis may be bilateral if the obstructing lesion is in or distal to the neck of the bladder.

Nephroblastoma is occasionally bilateral.

The physical signs of an enlarged kidney are:

1 It lies in the paracolic gutter or can be pushed back into this gutter; that is to say, it can be **reduced into the loin**.
2 It is usually only possible to feel the lower pole, which is smooth and hemi-ovoid.
3 It moves with respiration.
4 It is **not** dull to percussion because it is covered by the colon. Even when a large kidney reaches the anterior abdominal wall it has a band of resonance across it.

Revision Panel 16.10

Causes of enlargement of the kidney

Distension of the pelvi-calyceal system

Space-occupying lesions
- Single:
  - Cyst
  - Abscess
  - Tumour
- Multiple:
  - Polycystic disease

Compensatory hypertrophy

5 It can be felt **bimanually**.
6 It can be **ballotted**. This means that it can be bounced between your two hands, one on the anterior abdominal wall and the other behind the renal angle, rather like a ball being patted between the hands. This sign is diagnostic of a renal mass and depends upon the mass reducing into the loin.

Pancreatic pseudocyst

This is a collection of pancreatic secretion, caused by pancreatitis, on the surface of the pancreas or in part or the whole of the lesser sac.

The patient may give a history of acute pancreatitis (see page 385) or present with epigastric fullness, pain, nausea and, sometimes, vomiting.

If the cyst becomes infected the patient will develop severe pain, sweating and rigors.

The physical characteristics of a pancreatic pseudocyst are:

1 The epigastrium contains a firm, sometimes tender, mass with an indistinct lower edge. The upper limit is not palpable.
2 It is usually resonant to percussion because it is covered by the stomach.
3 It moves very slightly with respiration.
4 It is not possible to elicit fluctuation or a fluid thrill.

These swellings can be very difficult to feel as most of their bulk is beneath the costal margin.

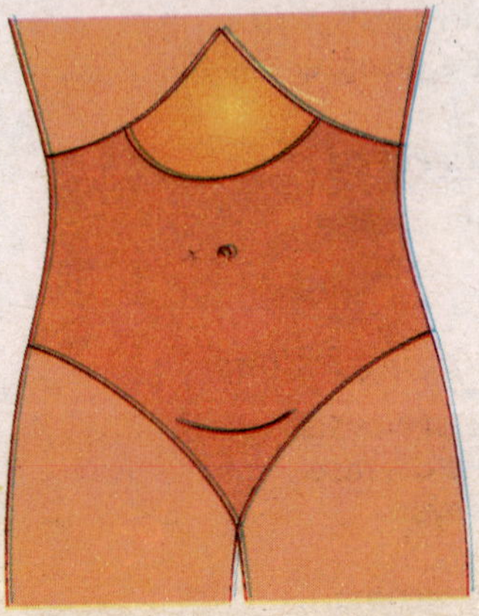

FIG. 16.21 A pancreatic, lesser sac, pseudocyst

Mesenteric cysts

These are cysts of clear fluid found in the mesentery. They arise from the vestigial remnants of reduplicated bowel.

They may be found by chance, being symptomless, or cause abdominal distension or recurrent colicky pain.

Like all cysts they can rupture, twist and have intraluminal bleeding. Twisting is rare because they are fixed within the small bowel mesentery.

The physical characteristics of a mesenteric cyst are:

1 The cyst forms a smooth, mobile, spherical swelling in the centre of the abdomen.
2 It moves freely at right-angles to the line of the root of the mesentery, but only slightly along a line parallel to the root of the mesentery.
3 It is dull to percussion.
4 If it can be fixed, it can be felt to **fluctuate** and have a **fluid thrill**.

It is difficult to discriminate between a very large cyst and a tight ascites.

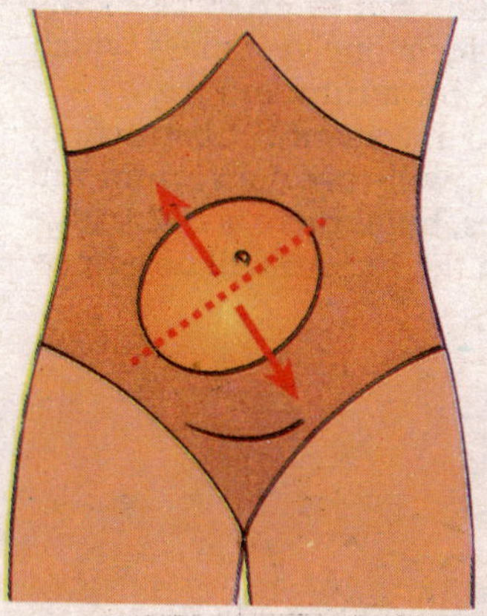

FIG. 16.22 A mesenteric cyst

Retroperitoneal tumours

Retroperitoneal tumours, excepting primary and secondary tumours of the lymph nodes, are rare; the commonest variety is the liposarcoma. They grow slowly and silently and are usually quite large before they are noticed by the patient or become palpable. The patient complains of distension, a vague abdominal pain, and sometimes anorexia and loss of weight.

They produce the following physical signs:

1 Abdominal distension.
2 A smooth or bosselated mass with an indistinct edge and a soft-to-firm consistence.
3 While they are covered with bowel they are resonant, but when they reach the anterior abdominal wall and push the bowel out to the flanks they become dull to percussion.
4 They move very little with respiration.
5 They may transmit aortic pulsations or occlude the vena cava.

Carcinoma of the stomach

The symptoms of carcinoma of the stomach are described on page 381.

Although stomach cancers are often large, hard masses, they are notoriously difficult to feel because they are high in the abdomen, beneath the costal margin. If there is a palpable mass it will be hard and irregular, disappear beneath the costal margin so you cannot get above it, and move with respiration.

The symptoms – abdominal pain or indigestion with loss of appetite and weight – are far more significant than the physical signs. The common finding in a patient with carcinoma of the stomach is a normal or slightly tender epigastrium. Thus although carcinoma of the stomach can present with an abdominal mass, the message of this section is **do not expect to feel a mass in a patient with carcinoma of the stomach.**

The gall bladder

The gall bladder is usually easy to recognize from its shape and position. The causes of enlargement of the gall bladder are:

- **Obstruction of the cystic duct**, usually by a gallstone, rarely by an intrinsic or extrinsic carcinoma. The patient is not jaundiced and the gall bladder will contain bile, mucus (a mucocele) or pus (an empyema).
- **Obstruction of the common bile duct**, usually by a stone or a carcinoma of the head of the pancreas. The patient will be **jaundiced.**

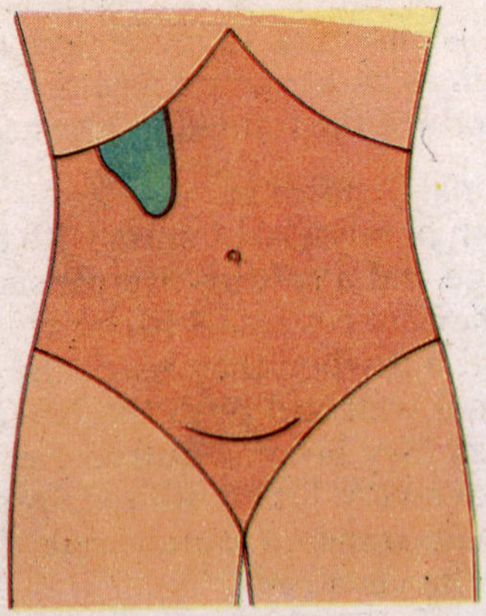

FIG. 16.23 An enlarged gall bladder

Courvoisier's law states: 'When the gall bladder is palpable and the patient is jaundiced the obstruction of the bile duct causing the jaundice is unlikely to be a stone because previous inflammation will have made the gall bladder thick and non-distensible.' This is a very useful clinical rule but there are a number of exceptions to it:

1 Stones can form in the bile duct and obstruct it in the presence of a normal distensible gall bladder.
2 There may be a double pathology: a stone in the cystic duct causing gall bladder distension and a carcinoma or a stone blocking the lower end of the bile duct.
3 The converse of the law, jaundice without a palpable gall bladder, does **not** mean that the jaundice is caused by stones. In such cases the obstruction may be caused by a cancer of the head of the pancreas, and the gall bladder distension be insufficient to be palpable, or the jaundice may be caused by a carcinoma of the biliary tree above the entry of the cystic duct.

The physical features of an enlarged gall bladder are:

1 It appears from beneath the tip of the right ninth rib.
2 It is smooth and hemi-ovoid.
3 It moves with respiration.
4 You cannot feel a space between the lump and the edge of the liver.
5 It is dull to percussion.

If the gall bladder is acutely inflamed it becomes surrounded by adherent omentum and bowel and loses some of its characteristics. **A gall bladder mass** is diffuse, and tender, lies in the right hypochondrium, and does not move much with respiration.

As the infection subsides it becomes more discrete and mobile, and less tender.

Faeces

The colon can become grossly distended with faeces as a result of a mechanical obstruction or chronic constipation. The patient may complain of diarrhoea, but this is actually mucus and a little watery faeces leaking out around the main mass of faeces.

The physical characteristics of faeces are:

1 The masses lie in that part of the abdomen occupied by the colon – the flanks and across the lower part of the epigastrium.
2 Faeces feel firm or hard but are **indentable**. This means that they can be dented by firm pressure with the fingers and this dent persists after releasing the pressure.
3 There may be multiple separate masses in the line of the colon, but in gross cases the faeces coalesce to form one vast mass which is easy to mistake for a tumour.
4 When there is no mechanical obstruction, rectal examination will reveal a rectum full of rock-hard faeces, but if there is a blockage in the lower colon the rectum will be empty.

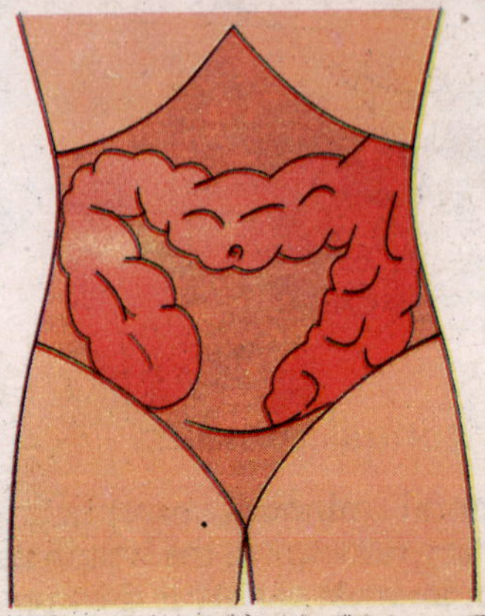

FIG. 16.24 A colon distended with faeces. The masses are indentable. Faecal impaction of this degree is likely to be caused by Hirschsprung's disease or gross constipation

The urinary bladder

The causes of retention of urine are listed on page 421. The bladder may be tense and painful – acute retention; or enlarged and painless – chronic retention.

The physical features of an enlarged bladder are:

1 It arises out of the pelvis and so it has no lower edge.
2 It is hemi-ovoid in shape, usually deviated a little to one side.
3 It may vary in size; a very large bladder can extend up above the umbilicus.
4 It is not mobile.
5 It is dull to percussion.
6 If it is large enough to permit the necessary simultaneous percussion and palpation it will have a fluid thrill.
7 Direct pressure on the swelling often produces a desire to micturate.
8 It does not bulge into the pelvis and can only be felt indistinctly on bimanual (rectal and abdominal) examination.

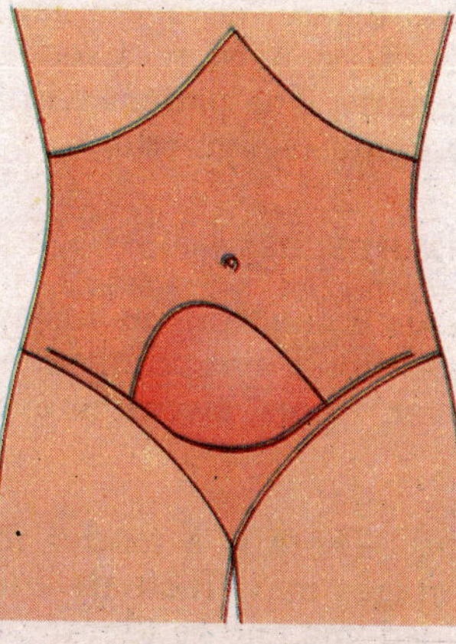

FIG. 16.25 A distended urinary bladder

Ovarian cyst

Small ovarian cysts are common and are not palpable. When they enlarge they rise up out of the pelvis into the lower abdomen and become palpable.

The physical features of a large ovarian cyst are:

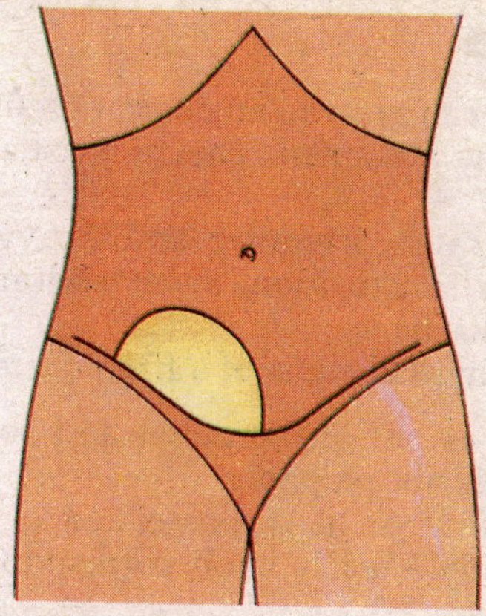

FIG. 16.26 A large ovarian cyst

1 Like all cysts, it is smooth and spherical, with distinct edges.
2 It arises from the pelvis so its lower limit is not palpable; i.e. you cannot 'get below it'.
3 It may be mobile from side to side but cannot be moved up and down.
4 It is dull to percussion.
5 It has a fluid thrill.
6 Its lower extremity may be palpable in the pelvis during rectal or vaginal examination, and movement of the cyst may produce some movement of the uterus.

The pregnant uterus

Never forget that **pregnancy** is the commonest cause of enlargement of the uterus, and of abdominal distension.

The uterus enlarges to the xiphisternum by the 36th week of pregnancy. At this stage the fetus is palpable and jumping about.

The diagnosis of pregnancy is more difficult in the first 20 weeks, when the uterus is smaller and there are no fetal movements.

A pregnant uterus is a smooth, firm, dull swelling, arising out of the pelvis.

The diagnosis is made with a bimanual examination which reveals that the mass cannot be moved independently of the cervix and that the cervix is soft and patulous.

Never squeeze an enlarged uterus during a bimanual examination – you might cause an abortion.

Fibroids

Fibroids can grow to an enormous size and fill the whole abdomen. They are usually multiple.

They cause irregular and heavy periods, disturbed micturition, lower abdominal pain and backache.

The physical signs of a fibroid uterus are:

1 It arises out of the pelvis and so its lower edge is not palpable.
2 It is firm or hard, bosselated or distinctly knobbly – each knob corresponding to a fibroid.
3 The mass moves slightly in a transverse direction and any movement of the abdominal mass moves the cervix.
4 It is dull to percussion.
5 It is palpable bimanually. A moderately enlarged uterus can be pushed down into the pelvis.

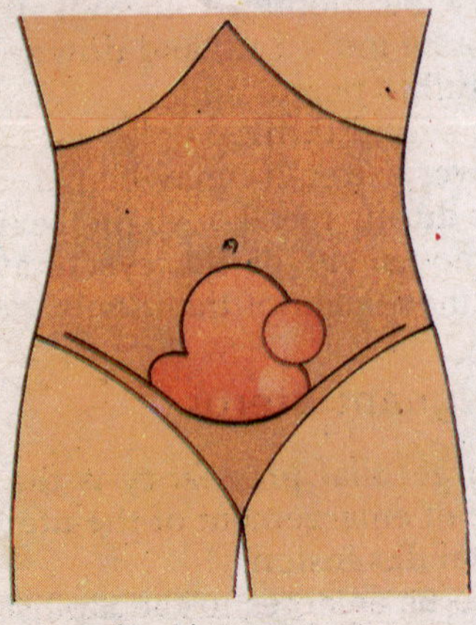

FIG. 16.27 A large fibroid uterus

CAUSES OF A MASS IN THE RIGHT ILIAC FOSSA

A mass in the right iliac fossa is a common physical finding and there are many possible causes to remember when you are considering the diagnosis. This section describes the important features in the history and examination of each cause.

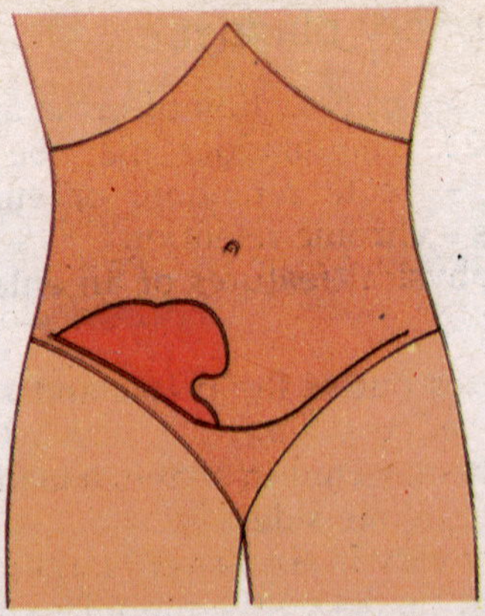

FIG. 16.28 A common diagnostic problem: a mass in the right iliac fossa

Appendix mass

History The patient complains of a period of central abdominal pain followed by a pain in the right iliac fossa, with malaise, loss of appetite and a slight change of bowel habit.

Examination There is a tender, indistinct mass, dull to percussion, fixed to the iliac fossa posteriorly. The patient will have a persistent fever and tachycardia.

Appendix abscess

History This is the same as for appendicitis, with the additional symptoms of an abscess – such as fever, rigors, sweating and increased local pain.

Examination There is a tender mass, which in its late stages may fluctuate and be associated with oedema and reddening of the overlying skin. The patient will have a swinging, intermittent fever and an increasing tachycardia.

Tuberculosis

In many parts of the world tuberculosis is more often the cause of an inflammatory mass in the right iliac fossa than is appendicitis. The mass consists of the inflamed ileocaecal lymph nodes and parts of the caecum and terminal ileum that are also inflamed.

History The patient often has a vague central pain for months, with general ill-health and loss of weight, and changes in bowel habit. The pain then becomes intense and settles in the iliac fossa. An acute episode of central abdominal pain moving to the right iliac fossa, similar to appendicitis, is uncommon.

Examination The mass is firm, tender and very indistinct. The surface and the edge are difficult to define. If there is a tuberculous peritonitis the abdomen will be swollen and less flexible – often described as a 'doughy' abdomen.

Carcinoma of the caecum

History Often there is no acute pain, just a dull discomfort in the right iliac fossa. Some patients present with anaemia, diarrhoea, or intestinal obstruction.

Examination The mass is firm, distinct and hard. Sometimes it is fixed to the posterior abdominal wall but sometimes it is mobile. It is not tender and does not resolve with observation. The patient's temperature and pulse are normal.

Crohn's disease (Terminal ileitis)

History The patient experiences recurrent episodes of pain in the right iliac fossa, general malaise, loss of weight and, sometimes, episodes of diarrhoea and melaena.

Examination The swollen terminal ileum forms an elongated sausage-shaped mass which is rubbery and tender. It lies in a transverse position and often slips up and down the abdomen during examination.

Iliac lymph nodes

History The symptoms depend on the cause of the lymphadenopathy. There may be a generalized disease, or local disease in the limb, perineum or genitalia.

Examination Enlarged iliac lymph nodes form an indistinct mass, with no clear contours, which follows the line of the iliac vessels. The mass can bulge forwards just above the inguinal ligament and be easy to feel, or be no more than a fullness in the depths of the iliac fossa.

Examine all other lymph nodes, and the lower limb for the cause of the lymphadenopathy.

Iliac artery aneurysm

History The patient may have noticed a pulsating mass or felt an aching pain in the right iliac fossa.

Examination The common iliac artery dilates more often than the external iliac artery, so the smooth, distinct mass with an expansile pulsation is usually in the upper medial corner of the iliac fossa.

Psoas abscess

History The patient is likely to have felt ill for some months and had night sweats and loss of weight. He may also complain of back pain and abdominal pain.

Examination The iliac fossa is filled with a soft, tender, dull, compressible mass. There may be a fullness in the lumbar region which

Revision Panel 16.11

The causes of a mass in the right iliac fossa *

- Appendicitis
- Tuberculosis
- Carcinoma of caecum
- Crohn's disease (terminal ileitis)
- Ilial lymphadenopathy
- Iliac artery aneurysm
- Psoas abscess
- Chondrosarcoma of the ilium
- Tumour in an undescended testis
- Actinomycosis
- Ruptured epigastric artery

* For left iliac fossa delete the first three causes and insert *diverticulitis* and *carcinoma of the colon.*

is accentuated by pressing on the mass in the iliac fossa. The swelling may extend below the groin and it may be possible to empty the swelling below the groin into the swelling above, and vice versa.

Back movements may be painful and limited.

Chondroma of the ilium

Chondromata and chondrosarcomata occur in the iliac bones. They grow slowly and may bulge into the iliac fossa. They are large, hard, not tender and clearly fixed to the skeleton. They often lie out in the lateral part of the iliac fossa, more so than the intra-abdominal causes of a right iliac fossa mass.

Actinomycosis

This invariably develops as a complication of appendicitis, but may present *de novo* as a mass in the iliac fossa with a number of discharging sinuses. It is rare.

Ruptured epigastric artery

This occurs as a result of straining or coughing. The haematoma tracks beneath the abdominal wall, extraperitoneally, to produce a mass in the iliac fossa. It is diffuse and there may be discolouration of the skin. This is the only right iliac fossa mass which is always attached to the anterior abdominal wall, but as it is on its deep surface it becomes impalpable when the muscles contract, like all the other intra-abdominal masses. Contraction of the abdominal muscles is usually painful.

Malignant change in an undescended testis

This is a rarity but is easily suspected provided you remember to examine the scrotum whenever you examine the abdomen.

CAUSES OF A MASS IN THE LEFT ILIAC FOSSA

The causes of a mass in the left iliac fossa are identical to those of a mass in the right iliac fossa, with the exception of appendicitis, carcinoma of the caecum and tuberculosis, which are replaced by diverticulitis and carcinoma of the colon.

It must be remembered that the normal sigmoid colon is palpable in one out of three of all patients.

Diverticulitis

Diverticular disease presents in many ways, but when the diverticula become inflamed it can present as an inflammatory mass.

History The patient may have suffered from recurrent lower abdominal pains and chronic constipation for years. The acute episode starts suddenly with a severe left iliac fossa pain, nausea, loss of appetite and constipation.

Examination The left iliac fossa contains a very tender, indistinct mass whose long axis lies parallel to the inguinal ligament. There may be a general or a local peritonitis, and intestinal obstruction. The diagnosis depends upon the site of the tenderness. There are very few acute inflammatory conditions which present with a mass in the left iliac fossa.

Carcinoma of the sigmoid colon

History The patient may present with lower abdominal pain, abdominal colic, intestinal obstruction, a change in bowel habit, rectal bleeding and general cachexia.

Examination The mass is hard, easily palpable and not tender. It may be mobile or fixed. The colon above the mass may be distended with indentable faeces.

CAUSES OF A LUMP IN THE GROIN

The inguinal region is part of the iliac fossa, and swellings in it, and just below it in the groin, can be confused with iliac fossa masses.

Hernia (inguinal or femoral)

The diagnosis is made from its site and shape and, if present, reducibility and an expansile cough impulse.

Lymph nodes

Inguinal lymph nodes present as hard or firm discrete nodules, or an indistinct mass, spreading across the groin, down the thigh along the line of the long saphenous vein, and up into the iliac fossa. Look for a local cause of lymphadenopathy and examine all the other lymph glands.

Saphena varix

A saphena varix is a soft, compressible dilatation at the top of the saphenous vein. It has an expansile cough impulse. A fluid thrill will be felt when the saphenous vein lower down the leg is percussed.

Psoas abscess

A psoas abscess may pass down beneath the inguinal ligament and present in the upper part of the femoral triangle as a soft, fluctuant, compressible mass. It is possible to elicit fluctuation between the parts of the abscess above and below the inguinal ligament, and empty one part into the other.

Psoas bursa

The psoas bursa lies between the psoas tendon and the lesser trochanter of the femur. If it becomes distended or inflamed it bulges into the upper outer corner of the femoral triangle, lateral to the femoral vessels, where it causes a diffuse swelling. It is too deep to have a distinct shape or to fluctuate. It is painful when the hip joint is moved.

Femoral aneurysm

This presents as a mass with an **expansile pulsation** lying in the line of the femoral artery.

Hydrocele of a femoral hernial sac

See page 330.

Hydrocele of the cord, or canal of Nück

See page 338.

Ectopic testis

See page 352.

ABDOMINAL DISTENSION

The causes of abdominal distension can be remembered by using the letter 'F' six times: fetus, flatus, faeces, fat, fluid (free and encysted), and fibroids and other solid tumours.

Fetus

Pregnancy is the most common cause of abdominal distension. The features of a pregnant uterus are described on page 405.

Flatus (also known as tympanites)

Gas in the intestine can cause considerable abdominal distension.

In the early stages the distension may be localized to that part of the abdomen containing the

Revision Panel 16.12

The causes of abdominal distension

Fetus
Flatus
Faeces
Fat
Fluid
- Free (ascites)
- Encysted

Large solid tumours such as:
- Fibroids
- Enlarged liver
- Enlarged spleen
- Polycystic kidneys
- Retroperitoneal sarcomata

Fat
Fluid
Foetus
Flatus
Faeces
Food
Fibroids
Foreign body
Full bladder
[illegible]

distended gut, such as the epigastrium when the stomach is distended or the right iliac fossa when the caecum is distended, but as the distension progresses through the gut the whole abdomen swells.

The distension will remain localized if the bowel twists into a volvulus. This is a common complication of a long sigmoid colon combined with a narrow base of the mesocolon.

Distended bowel has no palpable surface or edge. The only diagnostic feature is **hyperresonance** and, when there is obstruction, **visible peristalsis**. The bowel sounds may be hyperactive. Shaking the patient causes a splashing sound as the thin layer of fluid in the distended bowel splashes about. This is known as a **succussion splash** and is particularly common in gastric distension secondary to pyloric stenosis.

The causes of tympanites are aerophagy, acute dilatation of the stomach, mechanical intenstinal obstruction and paralytic ileus.

Faeces

Faecal impaction may present as abdominal distension or an abdominal mass. The physical features of faecal masses in the abdomen are described on page 404. The diagnosis can usually be suspected from the history of the patient's bowel habits. The common causes are Hirschsprung's disease, acquired megacolon, chronic intestinal obstruction and chronic constipation.

Fat

Fat rarely causes distension, but frequently makes the patient **pot-bellied**.

A large fat abdomen may be caused by a thick layer of subcutaneous fat, or by excess fat in the omentum and mesentery. These two sites of fat deposition do not necessarily enlarge together. The protuberant, round abdomen often has a thin layer of subcutaneous fat but contains a heavy, thick omentum.

Fluid: ascites

Fluid that is free in the peritoneal cavity is called ascites.

It is caused by a variety of conditions but they all fall into one of four groups: those which raise the portal venous pressure, those which lower the plasma proteins, those which cause a peritonitis, and those which allow a direct leak of lymph into the peritoneal cavity.

Causes of an increased portal venous pressure

Prehepatic

- Portal vein thrombosis.
- Compression of the portal vein by lymph nodes.

Hepatic

- Cirrhosis.
- Multiple hepatic metastases.

Post-hepatic

- Budd–Chiari syndrome.

Cardiac

- Constrictive pericarditis.
- Right heart failure caused by mitral stenosis or tricuspid incompetence.

Pulmonary

- Pulmonary hypertension and right heart failure.

Causes of hypoproteinaemia

- Kidney disease associated with albuminuria.
- Cirrhosis of the liver.
- The cachexia of wasting diseases, malignancy and starvation.
- Protein-losing enteropathies.

Causes of chronic peritonitis

Physical

- Post irradiation.
- Talc granuloma.

Infection

- Tuberculous peritonitis.

Neoplasms

- Secondary peritoneal deposits of carcinoma.
- 'Mucus'-forming tumours (pseudomyxoma peritonei).

Causes of chylous ascites

Chylous ascites is caused by the leakage of lymph from the lacteals or the cisterna chyli as a result of congenital abnormalities, trauma, and primary or secondary lymph gland disease.

Physical signs of ascites:

1 A fluid thrill.
2 Shifting dullness.

A **fluid thrill** is elicited by flicking one side of the abdomen with your index finger and feeling the vibrations, when they reach the other side of the abdomen, with your other hand. Before doing this you must place the edge of the patient's (or an assistant's) hand on the abdomen at the umbilicus to prevent the percussion wave being transmitted in the abdominal wall.

A fluid thrill is present in any fluid-filled cavity so that the difference between free and encysted fluid depends upon the recognition of shifting dullness.

Shifting dullness is a dull area which moves or changes shape when the patient changes position. The dullness of ascites is found in the flanks and across the lower abdomen.

Percuss the medial limits of the flank dullness carefully. Then ask the patient to turn on his side to an angle of approximately 45°. Wait a few seconds and percuss again. If there is free fluid moving under the influence of gravity, the medial limit of dullness will have extended towards the mid-line on the lower side of the abdomen and retracted on the upper side.

Fluid: encysted

Fluid trapped in a cyst, or in the renal pelvis, or between adhesions, will have a fluid thrill, be dull to percussion, but **not shift**.

The position and features of a cyst depend upon its anatomical origin. The following cysts

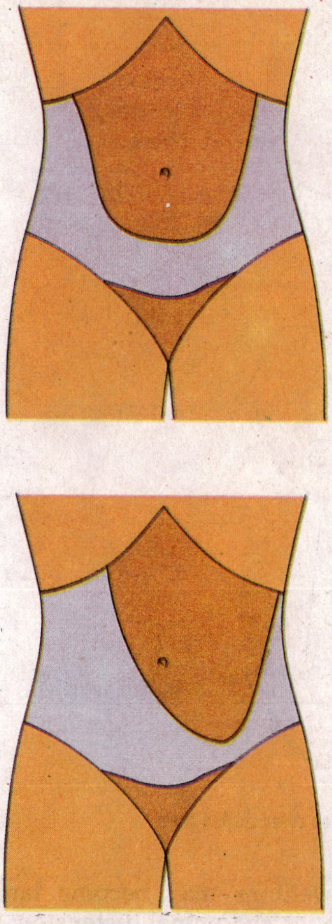

FIG. 16.29 Shifing dullness is diagnostic of free intraperitoneal fluid (ascites).

> Revision Panel 16.13
> **Aetiology of ascites**
>
> *Raised portal venous pressure*
> Pre-, intra- and post-hepatic
> Cardiac
> Pulmonary
>
> *Hypoproteinaemia*
> Renal
> Hepatic
> General
>
> *Peritonitis*
> Acute and chronic
> Traumatic, chemical, infective, neoplastic
>
> *Lymphatic obstruction*
> (Chylous ascites)

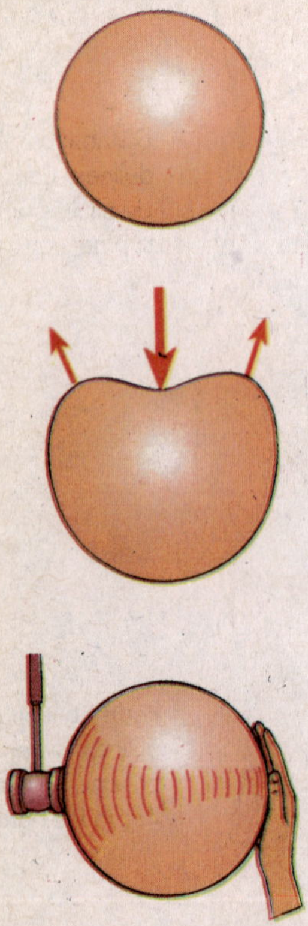

FIG. 16.30 The features of encysted fluid

or fluid-filled swellings may become large enough to present as abdominal distension:

- Ovarian cysts.
- Hydronephrosis.
- Polycystic kidney.
- Urinary bladder.
- Pancreatic cysts.
- Mesenteric cysts.
- Hydatid cysts.

A large **aortic aneurysm** can also distend the abdomen, but although an aneurysm is full of fluid it does not have a detectable fluid thrill because it is being subjected to repeated intrinsic percussion – the pulse. It is diagnosed by the presence of an **expansile pulsation**.

Solid tumours

The solid tumours which can become so large that they may cause abdominal distension are, in approximate order of frequency:

- Hepatomegaly.
- Fibroids.
- Splenomegaly.
- Large cancers of the colon.
- Carcinoma of the pancreas.
- Polycystic kidney.
- Retroperitoneal lymphadenopathy.
- Carcinoma of the kidney.
- Primary carcinoma of the liver.
- Perinephric abscess.
- Retroperitoneal sarcoma.
- Ganglioneuroma (in children).
- Nephroblastoma (in children).

The physical signs of most of these tumours are described in the preceding parts of this chapter.

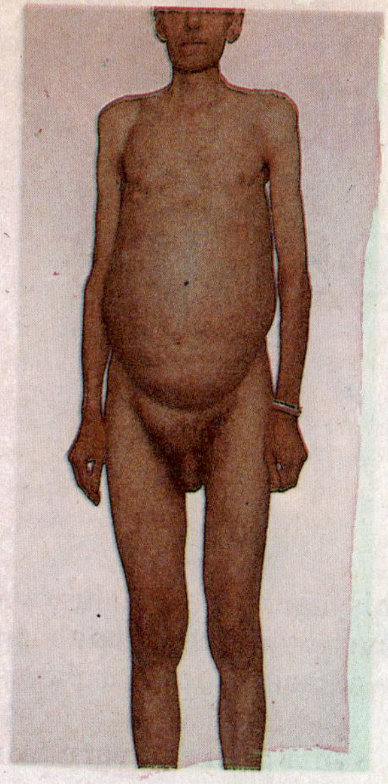

Ascites secondary to carcinoma of the stomach. Note the wasting and the right inguinal hernia full of ascitic fluid

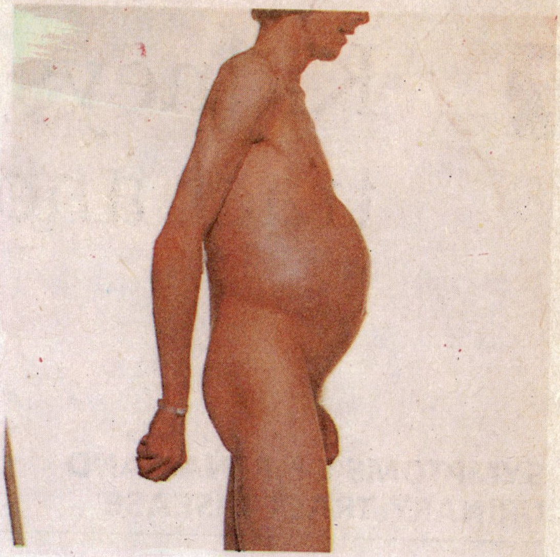

Abdominal distension caused by a retroperitoneal liposarcoma in a young man

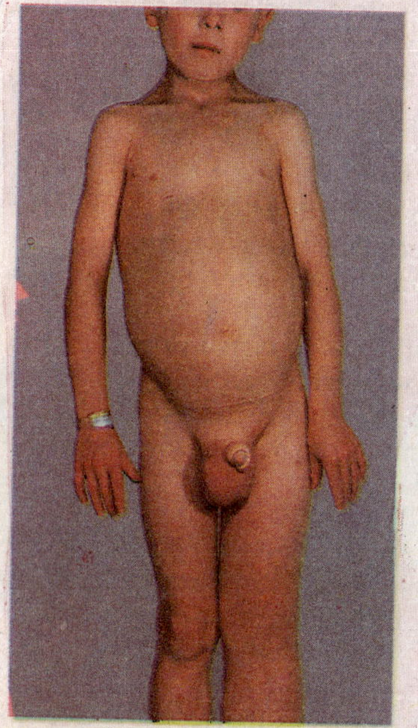

Congenital chylous ascites. Note the lymphoedema of the genitalia and left leg, and the right hydrocele

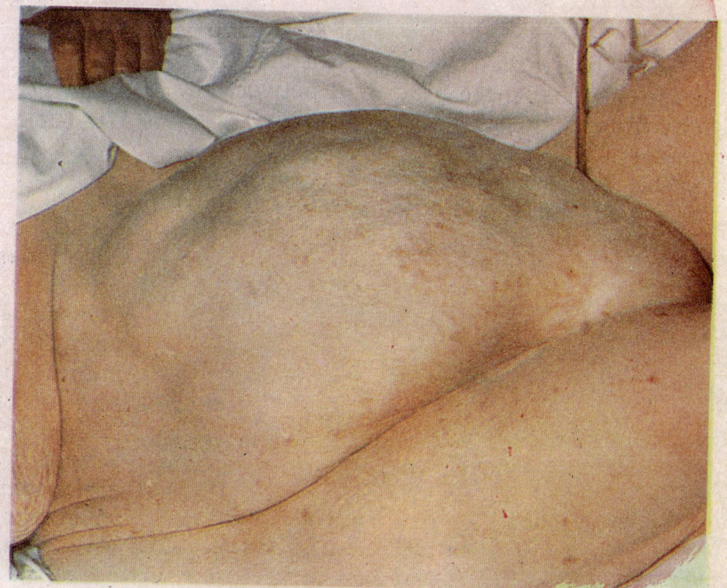

Abdominal distension caused by intestinal obstruction. The obstruction was caused by the large right inguinal hernia. The distended loops of bowel can be seen because the abdominal wall is very thin. Peristaltic waves were clearly visible

17

Kidneys, urinary tract and prostate

SYMPTOMS OF RENAL AND URINARY TRACT DISEASE

It is very important to obtain an exact history of the symptoms of renal and urinary tract disease because the kidney, ureter and bladder are not accessible for close physical examination.

Renal pain

Site Pain from the kidney is felt in the **loin** – the space below the 12th rib and the iliac crest; and in the renal **angle** – the angle between the 12th rib and the edge of the erector spinae muscles.

When you ask a patient with renal pain to show you the site of the pain, he usually spreads his hand around his waist with his fingers covering the renal angle and his thumb above the anterior superior iliac spine.

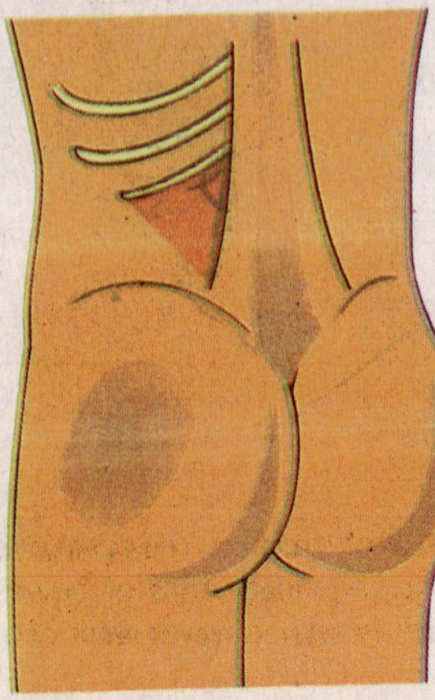

FIG. 17.1 The renal angle is the area in the loin between the 12th rib and the edge of the erector spinae muscle

Severity Renal pain can vary from a constant dull ache to a very severe pain.

Nature Do not use the term 'renal colic'. True colic can only come from an obstructed muscular conducting tube such as the ureter. Because the severity of renal pain often fluctuates rapidly it gets called renal colic, but it rarely has a 'gripping' nature, and never disappears completely between exacerbations.

Ureteric colic

Site Colic from the ureter is felt along the line of the ureter. The point where it begins usually corresponds to the level of the obstruction.

In most cases the pain starts in the loin and then radiates downwards, around the waist, obliquely across the abdomen just above the inguinal ligament, to the base of the penis, the scrotum or the labia.

Severity The exacerbations of ureteric colic are extremely severe. The patient tries to relieve the pain by rolling around the bed or walking about.

Nature Ureteric colic is a true colic. It is **gripping** in nature and comes in waves, with pain-free periods between each attack.

Cause The patient may notice that his attacks of colic follow episodes of jolting or unusual

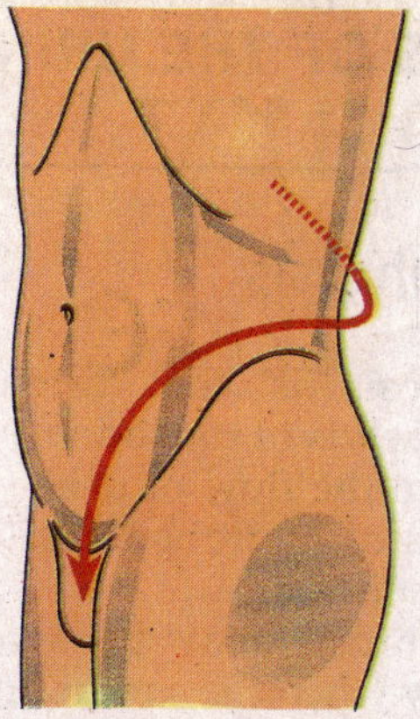

FIG. 17.2 Ureteric colic radiates down from the renal angle, along a line parallel to the inguinal ligament, into the base of the penis, the scrotum or the labium majus

physical activity. Such a history suggests that he has a stone in the ureter, which is being moved by the jolting.

Haematuria

The patient may notice blood in the urine during or after micturition. A few red cells have no visible effect on urine colour, but if there is heavy bleeding the urine may look like pure blood.

If the blood is coming from the lower part of the bladder it may appear only at the end of micturition.

The causes of haematuria are listed in Revision Panel 17.1.

Make quite sure that female patients have not mistaken menstrual bleeding for haematuria.

Check that other causes of discolouration of the urine are not present, such as:

Excess beetroot eating.
Paroxysmal haemoglobinuria.
Porphyria.

Vesical pain

Pain from the bladder is usually a dull, suprapubic ache, made worse by micturition.

A painful desire to micturate, which starts in the bladder and radiates into the urethra, is called **strangury**. When the patient tries to

Revision Panel 17.1
The causes of haematuria

Kidney
- Congenital
  - Polycystic kidney
- Traumatic
  - Ruptured kidney
  - Stone
- Inflammatory
  - Tuberculosis
- Neoplastic
  - Carcinoma of the kidney
  - Carcinoma of the renal pelvis
- Blood disorders
  - Anticoagulant drugs
  - Purpura
  - Sickle-cell disease
  - Haemophilia
  - Scurvy
  - Malaria
- Congestion
  - Right heart failure
  - Renal vein thrombosis
- Infarction
  - Arterial emboli from:
  - a myocardial infarct
  - or
  - subacute bacterial endocarditis

Ureter
- Stone
- Neoplasm

Bladder
- Traumatic
  - Stone
- Inflammatory
  - Non-specific cystitis or ulceration
  - Tuberculosis
  - Schistosomiasis (bilharzia)
- Neoplastic
  - Carcinoma

Prostate
- Benign and malignant enlargement

Urethra
- Traumatic
  - Rupture
  - Stone
- Inflammatory
  - Acute urethritis
- Neoplastic
  - Transitional cell carcinoma

micturate he cannot produce any urine and fails to relieve the pain.

Frequency of micturition

Retention of urine in the bladder following inadequate emptying increases the frequency of micturition. This is first noticed at night, so remember to ask about the frequency of nocturnal micturition and record the 24-hour frequency as a day/night ratio.

'Dysuria' is a meaningless and misused word – **do not use it**. Describe each facet of micturition, the pain, the nature of the stream and the frequency.

Prostatic pain

Pain from the prostate gland is felt deep inside the pelvis and between the legs in the perineum. It cannot be clearly defined and the patient often thinks the pain is coming from the rectum.

Revision Panel 17.2

The causes of hydronephrosis

Unilateral hydronephrosis

Pelviureteric obstruction
- Congenital pelvi-ureteric junction stenosis
- Pressure from aberrant arteries
- Stones and tumours in the renal pelvis, occluding the opening into the ureter

Ureteric obstruction
- Stones
- Tumour infiltrating the ureter from the cervix, rectum, colon, or prostate
- Tumours of the ureter
- Ureterocele
- Schistosomiasis
- Bladder tumour

Bilateral hydronephrosis
- Retroperitoneal fibrosis
- Prostatic enlargement – benign or malignant
- Carcinoma of the bladder
- Schistosomiasis
- Urethral strictures and valves
- Phimosis

DISEASES OF THE URINARY TRACT

Hydronephrosis

Hydronephrosis is the distension of the calyces and pelvis of the kidney, caused by an obstruction to the flow of urine.

The causes of hydronephrosis are listed in Revision Panel 17.2.

Hydronephrosis may be symptomless or detected only when the condition which is creating the obstruction to the flow of urine causes symptoms of its own.

HISTORY

Age Hydronephrosis occurs at all ages.

Symptoms The commonest symptom is **pain in the loin**. This is a dull, persistent ache which can be so mild that it is accepted by the patient as mild backache and ignored.

If the hydronephrosis develops quickly the pain can be severe. The pain is sometimes referred to the epigastrium and mistaken for the pain of duodenal ulceration.

Sometimes the pain is severe and colicky.

The pain may be exacerbated by drinking an excessive amount of water or alcohol, or by taking any drug which causes a diuresis.

If the hydronephrosis becomes very large the abdomen may be distended.

There are usually no general symptoms unless both kidneys are so badly damaged that **uraemia** is developing.

EXAMINATION

The kidney will be enlarged and should be palpable. The features of an enlarged kidney are described in detail in Chapter 16.

A hydronephrosis should:

1 Arise from the loin.
2 Be reducible into the loin.
3 Be palpable bimanually.
4 Ballotte.

Acute pyelitis

(Pyelonephritis)

Acute pyelonephritis, or pyelitis, is an infection, in the upper part of the urinary tract, by bacteria which have come from the blood stream or up the ureter from the urethra or bladder. Pyelitis is common in women because the shortness of their urethra makes it easy for bacteria to get into the bladder.

HISTORY

Sex Pyelitis is much more common in females.

Age It is common in children, and in women soon after marriage as a complication of 'honeymoon cystitis', and during pregnancy.

Symptoms The patient complains of the sudden onset of a **severe pain in one or both loins**. The pain may also be felt anteriorly, and when it is on the right-hand side can be mistaken for the pains of cholecystitis.

At approximately the same time as the onset of loin pain, **micturition becomes frequent and painful**. Although there may be a vague suprapubic ache, the main pain during micturition is a burning sensation along the length of the urethra, which persists after micturition. The patient may also complain of **strangury**, a painful but fruitless desire to micturate.

Headache, nausea and vomiting often begin a few hours before the pain.

The **urine** may become cloudy and blood-stained. The patient feels ill, **hot and sweaty** and, in severe cases, may suffer **rigors**.

Cause The patient may have had similar attacks and know of their relationship to sexual intercourse or pregnancy.

EXAMINATION

General features The patient looks ill. She may be flushed and sweating. The tongue is dry and furred. The temperature is usually between 39 and 40°C (102 and 104°F) and there is a marked tachycardia.

Abdomen One or both kidneys are tender when palpated through the abdomen, and the renal angle is very tender. The degree of guarding depends upon the tenderness.

The kidneys are not enlarged unless the infection has arisen in a previously hydronephrotic kidney.

There may be mild suprapubic tenderness.

Urine The urine looks cloudy and blood-stained. Red blood cells and pus cells will be seen if the sediment is inspected with a microscope.

Carcinoma of the kidney

This tumour is also called a hypernephroma, because of its macroscopic appearance and common site of occurrence.

HISTORY

Age Carcinoma of the kidney is uncommon below the age of 50 years.

Sex It is twice as common in males than females.

Symptoms It can present in many ways, but there are four common forms of presentation.

Haematuria This is the most common symptom. It is usually sufficient to stain the urine a pale red colour and appears intermittently. Occasionally, the haematuria is profuse and the patient gets **ureteric colic** as blood clots pass down the ureter (clot colic).

General debility More than one-quarter of the patients with renal carcinomata have no symptoms until the secondary deposits, or the size of the primary growth, cause **general malaise, loss of energy and loss of weight**. Some patients present with **bone pain** and **pathological fractures**.

Pain in the loin This is also a common symptom, especially when the tumour breaks through its false capsule and invades nearby structures.

A mass A mass may frequently be felt by chance at a routine examination, or by the patient, or it may cause abdominal distension.

Because of the seriousness of the underlying disease it is also important to know the rarer symptoms.

Pyrexia of unknown origin (PUO), often associated with night sweats, suggests a clinical diagnosis of an infection such as tuberculosis or a lymphoma, but every patient who presents with a PUO should have an intravenous pyelogram.

Some kidney diseases are associated with an increased production of erythropoietin and **erythrocythaemia**. This causes redness of the face and hands, dyspnoea, heart failure, and spontaneous venous and arterial thromboses.

Occlusion of the left renal and testicular vein by direct spread of the tumour along the renal vein can cause a **varicocele** (see page 357). If the tumour spreads into the vena cava, the patient may present with **oedema of both legs** and the abdominal wall.

A **sudden severe abdominal pain** may indicate haemorrhage into the tumour, or, if there is acute abdominal tenderness, rupture of the tumour in the peritoneal cavity.

Hypertension, which is a common presentation of other forms of renal disease, is rarely a complication of renal carcinoma.

EXAMINATION

General features The patient usually shows signs of recent **weight loss**. If the haematuria has caused anaemia he will be **pale**.

Abdomen Large tumours are palpable and have all the signs of an enlarged kidney, described on page 401.

A small tumour in the upper pole of the kidney may push the whole kidney downwards and make the lower pole easier to feel.

There is not usually any tenderness or guarding.

Skeleton There may be areas of swelling and tenderness in the bones, caused by secondary deposits. Secondary deposits of renal carcinoma can be very vascular and may feel soft, pulsatile and compressible, and have an audible bruit.

Chest There may be a pleural effusion on the side of the tumour if it has spread up through the diaphragm.

Carcinoma of the kidney is one of the tumours which can cause a solitary pulmonary metastasis worthy of resection.

Transitional cell carcinoma of the renal pelvis

These tumours present with **haematuria**. The urine is coloured pale pink or red. Occasionally the patient has **clot colic** and passes 'stringy' blood clots. If the lesions are obstructing the pelvi-ureteric junction and causing a hydronephrosis the patient may have a vague **loin pain** or a loin mass.

The causes of transitional cell carcinoma of the uroepithelium are discussed on page 420.

The symptoms and signs of these tumours are non-specific. Their presence must be proved by cystoscopy and intravenous pyelography.

Renal and ureteric calculi

Stones in the renal pelvis may lie silent for years and not present until complications such as infection or renal parenchymal damage occur. Stones in the ureter invariably cause pain.

HISTORY

Age Renal and ureteric calculi are most often found between the ages of 30 and 50 years.

Sex They are slightly more common in men than women.

Symptoms The predominant symptoms caused by the stone are **pain and haematuria**. The **pain** is either a constant pain in the loin, or a **ureteric colic**. The patient notices a dull ache in the loin which becomes a severe colic, radiating down along the line of the ureter. The pain is so severe that he has to walk or roll about. Although this movement helps ease the acute colic, it often makes the constant loin pain worse. The loin pain is caused by the acute hydronephrosis which follows obstruction of the ureter.

If the stone impacts in the lower ureter, the ureteric colic precedes the loin pain.

A patient with ureteric colic invariably has microscopic haematuria, but rarely visible haematuria. Sometimes stones can ulcerate through the uroepithelium without causing pain, yet cause heavy haematuria.

The first indication of the presence of a stone may be the symptoms of **acute pyelitis** – fever, loin pain and scalding micturition.

Large bilateral staghorn calculi and small bilateral stones blocking both ureters may cause **uraemia**. The symptoms of uraemia are headache, **restlessness, twitching, fits, convulsions, drowsiness and coma.**

EXAMINATION

Abdomen It is not possible to examine the abdomen properly when a patient is having an attack of ureteric colic because he is rolling around and holding his muscles tense. Between these attacks the abdomen feels normal unless there is a secondary pyelitis or hydronephrosis causing tenderness and/or enlargement of the kidney.

The confirmation of the diagnosis rests on special investigations which reveal the presence of the stone.

Bladder calculi

Stones may form in the bladder in association with stasis, infection or tumours, or come into the bladder from the ureter.

HISTORY

Age Bladder stones are most common in middle-aged adults, but they are also quite common in malnourished children in countries that are hot and dry.

Sex Males are affected more than females.

Symptoms The most common symptom is an **increased frequency** of micturition, usually related to posture. When the patient stands up the stone falls onto the trigone and initiates a desire to micturate. During the night the stone rolls off the trigone and the frequent desires to micturate abate.

As the stone moves around the bladder it causes a suprapubic, stabbing **pain** which is exacerbated by standing and any **sudden, jolting movement.**

Haematuria at the end of micturition is also a common symptom which is made worse by exercise.

The presence of the stone increases the chances of developing **cystitis**, which causes burning, frequent micturition and suprapubic pain.

The symptoms caused by the stone are often preceded by the symptoms of its cause – prostatism, infection and bladder tumours.

EXAMINATION

There may be slight suprapubic tenderness but there are rarely any other physical signs.

Very large stones can sometimes be felt on bimanual examination of the pelvis.

Cystitis

Cystitis is an infection of the urine within the bladder, with a concomitant inflammatory reaction in the bladder wall. The common predisposing factors of cystitis are incomplete emptying of the bladder, abnormalities within the bladder and, in women, ascending infection.

HISTORY

Age Cystitis occurs often in young and middle-aged women, in young men with urethritis and in elderly men with prostatism and bladder tumours.

Symptoms The most common symptom is an **increased frequency** of micturition. It begins suddenly and persists through the night as well as the day. The patient often wants to micturate every few minutes.

Passing urine causes a **burning or scalding pain** along the length of the urethra. It is often so bad that the patient does her utmost to avoid passing water. There is also a mild **suprapubic ache.**

Haematuria is common. It is usually a few drops of bloody urine at the end of micturition but it may turn the urine mahogany brown.

The urine is usually **cloudy** and often foul smelling.

EXAMINATION

Apart from mild suprapubic tenderness there are rarely any other abnormal physical signs.

Remember to look at the urine and examine the sediment for pus cells.

Carcinoma of the bladder

Bladder cancer can be formed of transitional cells or squamous cells. It rarely produces any physical signs so the diagnosis must be suspected from the history.

HISTORY

Age Bladder cancer occurs throughout adult life but the peak incidence is between the ages of 60 and 70 years.

Sex Males are afflicted more than females.

Occupation Some chemicals are excreted in the urine and can stimulate malignant change in the uroepithelium. The better known ones are **alpha- and beta-naphthylamine, benzidine** and **xylenamine**, and artificial sweeteners such as cyclamates. The industries which use these chemicals are the rubber and cable industries, printers and dyers.

Predisposing conditions **Bilharzia** and squamous cell carcinoma are so often found together that it is believed that the chronic irritation caused by this infection stimulates neoplastic change.

> **Revision Panel 17.3**
> **Bladder carcinogens**
>
> Aniline dyes
> 2 –Naphthylamine
> Xylenamine
> Benzidine
>
> *Occupations associated with exposure to bladder carcinogens*
> Dry cleaners
> Leather workers
> Painters and decorators
> Paper and rubber manufacturers
> Dental technicians

Symptoms In 95 per cent of cases carcinoma of the bladder presents with **haematuria**, which turns the urine bright red and may be passed intermittently or every time the bladder is emptied. The passage of blood clots may cause **pain** and **difficulty** during micturition.

If the urine becomes infected the patient will experience a suprapubic ache, burning micturition and strangury.

Pain in the loin is a common presenting symptom because bladder tumours often begin near the ureteric orifice and obstruct the lower end of the ureter.

Pain in the pelvis and lower abdomen, and nerve root pain down the legs, can occur if the tumour spreads through the wall of the bladder into the pelvis.

EXAMINATION

It is unusual to find any abnormality. If the tumour is large it may be felt bimanually and if it has spread beyond the bladder the floor of the pelvis may be indurated.

RETENTION OF URINE

There are two forms of retention of urine – acute and chronic – and they are usually easy to distinguish. **Acute retention is painful. Chronic retention is painless.** This simple differentiation fails when infection supervenes on chronic retention because this makes the bladder painful. In some textbooks this is called acute-on-chronic retention. This is not a good expression. The term 'infection-on-chronic retention' is better.

Acute retention in the presence of a normal bladder is rare and occurs only after a surgical operation, anaesthesia or an injury to the urethra. In all other circumstances there has usually been some mild, symptomless, chronic retention before the acute attack. These cases could also be called acute-on-chronic and so it is better not to use the expression. I suggest that you use the following definitions.

Acute retention is the sudden inability to micturate in the presence of a **painful bladder** (whatever its size).

Chronic retention is an **enlarged painless bladder**, whether or not the patient is having difficulty with micturition.

CINDAMVTO.

The causes of retention are presented in Revision Panel 17.4. It is a long list. The common causes are pregnancy, pelvic and lower abdominal operations and prostatic enlargement. Although the other causes are important they are far less common.

Acute retention

HISTORY

Symptoms The patient is likely to have some symptoms related to one of the causes listed in Revision Panel 17.4, as well as **pain and an inability to pass urine.** The pain is severe and feels like a grossly exaggerated desire to micturate. The patient knows that his bladder is overdistended.

EXAMINATION

Even if the bladder was completely normal before the onset of the retention it will have enlarged sufficiently to become a palpable, tense, dull, rounded mass arising out of the pelvis. Pressure on the swelling exacerbates the patient's desire to micturate.

A rectal examination will reveal that the prostate or uterus is pushed backwards and downwards, and the cystic mass of the bladder will be felt filling the front half of the pelvis. **You cannot assess the size of the prostate gland when the bladder is full.**

If the patient has had chronic retention before the acute episode, the bladder may reach up to, or above, the umbilicus. The physical signs of the underlying chronic retention may be present.

Remember to examine the prostate, the urethra and the contents of the pelvis as well as

Revision Panel 17.4

The causes of retention of urine

1 ***Mechanical***

In the lumen of the urethra, or overlying the internal urethral orifice:
- Congenital valves
- Foreign bodies
- Tumour
- Blood clot
- Stones

In the wall of the bladder or the urethra:
- Phimosis
- Trauma (rupture of the urethra)
- Urethral stricture
- Urethritis
- Meatal ulcer
- Tumour
- Prostatic enlargement (benign and malignant)

Outside the wall
- Pregnancy (retroverted gravid uterus)
- Fibroids
- Ovarian cyst
- Faecal impaction
- Paraphimosis

2 ***Neurogenic***
- Postoperative retention
- Spinal cord injuries
- Spinal cord disease
  - Disseminated sclerosis
  - Tabes dorsalis
- Hysteria
- Drugs
  - Anticholinergics, antihistamines, smooth-muscle relaxants, some tranquillizers

Revision Panel 17.5

Symptoms of bladder outflow obstruction

- Hesitancy
- Poor flow
- Intermittent flow
- Postmicturition dribbling
- Pis-en-deux

Revision Panel 17.6

Symptoms of bladder and bladder neck irritation

- Increased frequency of micturition
- Urgency
- Nocturia
- Urge incontinence

the sensory, motor and reflex functions of the nerves of the perineum and lower limbs.

Chronic retention

HISTORY

Age and sex Chronic retention is most common in elderly men.

Symptoms The patient may be unaware of his chronic retention but complains of symptoms related to the cause of the retention, such as an **increased frequency** of micturition, **and difficulty with micturition** (i.e. delays on starting, a poor stream and a dribbling finish).

If the urethral sphincters fail the patient will become incontinent. **Overflow incontinence** is an uncontrollable leakage and dribbling of urine from the urethra. The patient may still be able to void a normal volume of urine but after having done so feels that his bladder is not empty, and the leak continues.

Chronic retention is painless.

EXAMINATION

The bladder will be palpable. It is likely to reach at least halfway up to the umbilicus. It is not tense or tender, and suprapubic pressure may not induce a desire to micturate.

The palpable bladder of chronic retention is dull to percussion, and will fluctuate and have a fluid thrill if the patient is thin enough to enable you to perform the manoeuvres necessary to elicit these signs.

Look for the signs of the cause of the retention in the pelvis, prostate, urethra and nervous system.

THE PROSTATE GLAND

Benign hypertrophy of the prostate gland

The inner portion of the prostate gland hypertrophies during late adult life. As it grows it compresses the outer layers into a false capsule, and bulges centrally into the urethra and the base of the bladder. The cause of this hypertrophy is not known. The popular theory is that it is an involutional hypertrophy in response to a changing hormone environment.

The majority of the symptoms result from a mechanical interference with the act of micturition.

HISTORY

Age The prostate starts enlarging at the age of 40 years but the symptoms commonly appear between ages 50 and 70 years.

Ethnic group There are variations in the prevalence of prostatic hypertrophy. It is rare in Far Eastern races.

Symptoms The commonest, and usually the first symptom, is an **increased frequency** of micturition. This is first noticed by the patient when he finds that he has to pass urine in the middle of the night. It is caused by inadequate emptying of the bladder. In addition to the increased frequency of micturition, the patient finds that he must pass water as soon as the desire arises. This is **urgency** and is caused by urine leaking into the prostatic urethra.

Difficulty with micturition is very common. The patient has **to wait** before the stream starts, the **stream is weak** and **dribbles** down to nothing as it finishes. Straining does not help; it prolongs the waiting time before the stream starts.

Haematuria, in the form of a little dark blood at the end of micturition, is not an uncommon symptom.

Some patients present with **acute retention** (i.e. **severe suprapubic pain** and an inability to pass water).

Conversely, others present with overflow **incontinence**.

The symptoms of **uraemia** may be present – headaches, fits and drowsiness.

EXAMINATION

Abdomen The bladder will be palpable if there is acute or chronic retention.

Rectal examination The normal features of the prostate gland are described on page 428. Benign hypertrophy causes a diffuse enlargement. The gland bulges into the rectum, its surface is smooth but the enlargement is often slightly asymmetrical and the surface bosselated. The consistence of the gland is firm, rubbery and **homogeneous**.

The median sulcus usually remains palpable even when the gland is grossly enlarged, and the rectal mucosa moves freely over the gland. The gland is not tender.

The floor of the pelvis is normal.

Remember that a full bladder pushes the prostate downwards and makes it feel bigger.

Carcinoma of the prostate

Cancer of the prostate begins in the outer part of the prostate gland, so it does not develop a false capsule and can easily spread into the floor of the pelvis. It is usually quite advanced before it causes symptoms.

HISTORY

Age Carcinoma of the prostate is common in old men, 65–75 years old.

Symptoms The commonest symptoms are similar to those caused by benign prostatic hypertrophy – **frequency, urgency and difficulty** of micturition, which are collectively called **prostatism**. The only difference is that these symptoms often appear suddenly and get worse rapidly.

Nearly half the patients with carcinoma of the prostate present with some form of **retention of urine** – acute or chronic – the symptoms of which are described on page 420.

If the tumour spreads into the floor of the pelvis it may cause **pain** in the lower abdomen and perineum.

General debility and loss of weight are common presenting symptoms, because this tumour often spreads throughout the body before causing local symptoms. Metastases in the bones of the pelvis and the lumbosacral spine often cause **bone pains and pathological fractures**. When **sciatica** develops in an elderly man it may well be caused by bony metastases from a malignant prostate gland.

EXAMINATION

The bladder will be palpable if there is retention of urine.

Rectal examination The prostate gland is asymmetrically enlarged or distorted. It is **irregular** in contour and **heterogeneous** in texture. Some areas are hard and knobbly, others are soft. The median sulcus may be absent and the rectal mucosa may be tethered to the gland.

The tissues of the pelvis, lateral to the gland and around the rectum, may be infiltrated by tumour. This is known as 'winging' of the prostate. Nine out of ten prostatic carcinomata are diagnosed by rectal examination.

The only other physical signs will be those caused by any metastases. Carcinoma of the prostate gland sometimes gives rise to metastases in the skin. If the spread around the rectum is extensive the tumour may spread along the lymphatics of the anal canal to the inguinal lymph nodes.

THE URETHRA

Urethral stricture

Urethral strictures follow damage or destruction of the urethral mucosa. The common causes of urethral stricture are given in Revision Panel 17.7.

Revision Panel 17.7

The causes of urethral stricture

Congenital
- Pinhole meatus
- Urethral valves (not a true stricture)

Traumatic
- Instrumentation (catheterization)
- Foreign bodies
- Prostatectomy
- Amputation of the penis
- Direct injuries

Inflammatory
- Gonorrhoea
- Meatal ulceration

Neoplastic
- Primary and secondary neoplasms

HISTORY

Age Urethral strictures occur at all ages. The most common cause is gonorrhoea, which is a disease of the sexually active, so the strictures that follow it appear in young and middle-aged men.

Symptoms The commonest symptom is **difficulty with micturition** but, in contrast to the difficulty which occurs with benign prostatic hypertrophy, the difficulty of passing urine caused by a stricture can be partly **overcome by straining**. The **stream is thin** and dribbles at its end. Attacks of **cystitis** and **acute retention** are common.

There may be a slight glairy **urethral discharge** which is particularly noticeable in the morning.

An increasing frequency of micturition indicates the development of retention of urine.

Revision Panel 17.8

Causes of a urethral discharge

Infection (urethritis) by:
- Gonorrhoea
- Chlamydia
- Coliforms
- Trichomonas
- Candida

Lesions in the urethra
- Warts
- Herpes

Foreign bodies

EXAMINATION

The bladder will be palpable. In long-standing cases both kidneys may be hydronephrotic and palpable.

The penis and urethra usually feel normal because the commonest site for stricture is where the urethra passes through the perineal membrane, but a stricture caused by scarring of the penile urethra can sometimes be felt as an area of induration. Meatal strictures can be seen.

The rectum and anal canal

The principal symptoms of rectal and anal conditions are bleeding, pain, tenesmus, change of bowel habit, changes in the stool, discharge and pruritis. These have been mentioned in Chapter 1, but deserve more detailed consideration.

SYMPTOMS OF ANORECTAL DISEASE

Bleeding

Blood passed per rectum may be fresh or altered. When blood is degraded by intestinal enzymes and bacteria it becomes black. A black tarry stool is called **melaena**. The blood must come from high in the intestinal tract to have time to turn black before it reaches the rectum.

Recognizable blood may appear in four ways:

1. Mixed with the faeces.
2. On the surface of the faeces.
3. Separate from the faeces, either after or unrelated to defaecation.
4. On the toilet paper after cleaning.

Blood mixed with the faeces This must have come from bowel higher than the sigmoid colon, where the softness of the stool and the time left for transit is still sufficient for mixing.

Blood on the surface of the faeces This has usually come from the lower sigmoid colon, rectum or anal canal.

Blood separate from the faeces If the bleeding follows defaecation then it is probably from an anal condition such as haemorrhoids. If the blood is passed by itself then either it has accumulated in the rectum so as to give a desire to defaecate and is from a rapidly bleeding carcinoma, inflammatory bowel disease or diverticulitis, or it has passed down rapidly from high up in the gut from a bleeding Meckel's diverticulum or a peptic ulcer.

Blood on the toilet paper This is usually caused by minor bleeding left on the anal skin from anal conditions such as fissures or haemorrhoids.

Colour of recognizable blood Bright red blood is likely to have come from an anal or low rectal condition. Dark blood (like red wine) has usually come from a more proximal lesion in the large bowel.

Pain

Pain from the anal canal is protracted, cramp-like and distressing. Its presence is extremely significant because haemorrhoids and rectal cancer are *not* usually painful.

An annular lesion high in the rectum may obstruct the lumen of the bowel and cause lower abdominal colic. Excessive stretching of the anal canal during defaecation may cause a sharp, splitting pain.

Pruritis

Incontinence and soiling

Tenesmus

This is an intense, painful but fruitless desire to defaecate. The rectum feels full, but when the patient tries to empty it, nothing appears. Tenesmus is caused by a space-occupying lesion in the lumen or wall of the rectum which mimics the presence of faeces.

Bowel habit

Beware of the terms 'diarrhoea' and 'constipation'. Make sure that you find out what the patient means when he uses them. It is better to record the frequency of bowel action and the consistence of the stool than to use these lay terms. What is 'constipation' to one patient may be 'diarrhoea' to another.

TECHNIQUE FOR ANORECTAL EXAMINATION

This is commonly called a rectal examination, but I have added the prefix 'ano' to remind you to look at and feel the anal canal as well as the rectum.

Preparation

Position of the patient

Ensure adequate privacy and uncover the patient from the waist to the knees.

The patient should lie in the left lateral position with his neck and shoulders rounded so that his chin rests on his chest, hips flexed to 90° or more, but knees flexed to slightly less than 90°. If the knees are flexed more than 90° the patient's ankles will get in your way.

If the patient is lying on a soft bed make him move towards you so that his buttocks are up on the edge of the bed. This makes inspection easier and tips the abdominal contents forwards, which helps the bimanual examination.

You should never omit the rectal examination from your routine examination.

Equipment

You need a plastic glove or finger stall, an inert lubricating jelly and a good light. If you do not have a finger cot, lubricate your index finger with soap lather and fill the space under your nail with hard soap to keep it clean. Faeces on your finger will do you no harm and wash off easily.

Proctoscopy and sigmoidoscopy are also part of the routine examination in an outpatient department, so ensure that the necessary equipment is prepared. (These techniques are not described in this book.)

Tell the patient what you are going to do

Tell him that you are going to examine the 'back passage' and the inside of the abdomen. Tell him it will be uncomfortable but not painful, and ask him to relax by breathing deeply and letting his knees go loose.

Inspection

Lift up the uppermost buttock with your left hand so that you can see the anus, perianal skin and perineum clearly. Look for:

- Skin rashes and excoriation.
- Faecal soiling, blood or mucus.
- Scars or fistula openings.
- Lumps and bumps (e.g. polyps, papillomata, condylomata, perianal haematomata, prolapsed piles, or carcinomata).
- Ulcers, especially fissures.

Palpation

Place the **pulp** of your right index finger (suitably gloved) on the centre of the anus, with the finger parallel to the skin of the perineum and in the mid-line. Then press gently into the anal canal but at the same time press backwards against the skin of the posterior wall of the anal canal and the underlying sling of puborectalis muscle. This overcomes most of the tone in the anal sphincter and allows the finger to straighten and slip into the rectum. Never thrust the tip of your finger straight in.

Look at your finger, when you remove it from the rectum, to note the colour of the faeces and the presence of blood or mucus.

The anal canal As the finger goes through the anal canal, note the tone of the sphincter, and any pain or tenderness, any thickening or masses.

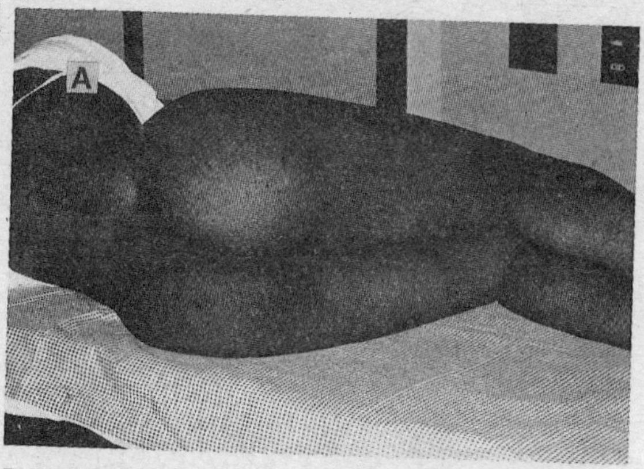

Place the patient in the left lateral position, hips flexed to 90°, knees less flexed to 110°.

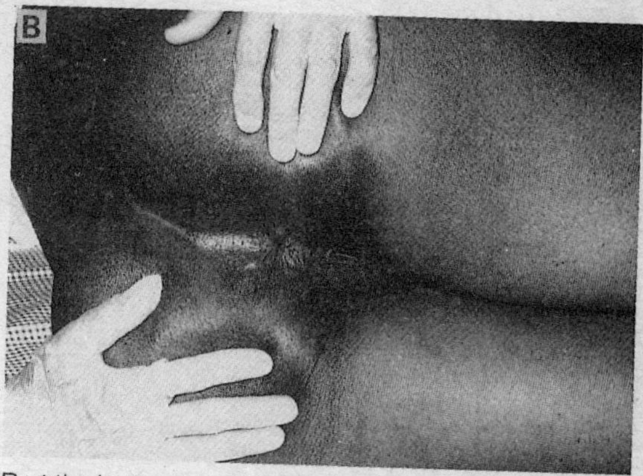

Part the buttocks and inspect the anus and perineum.

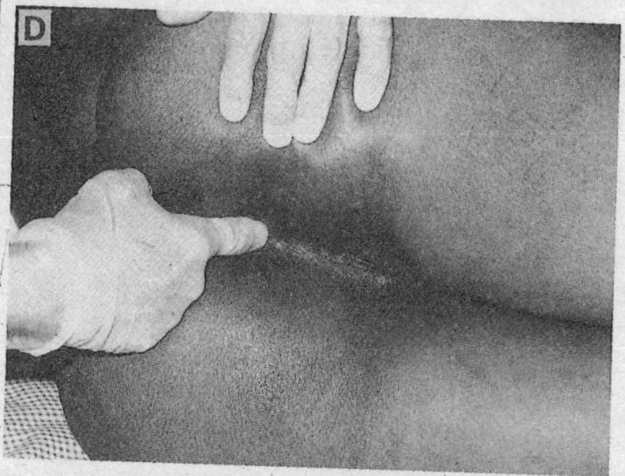

Place the pulp of your finger on the anus.

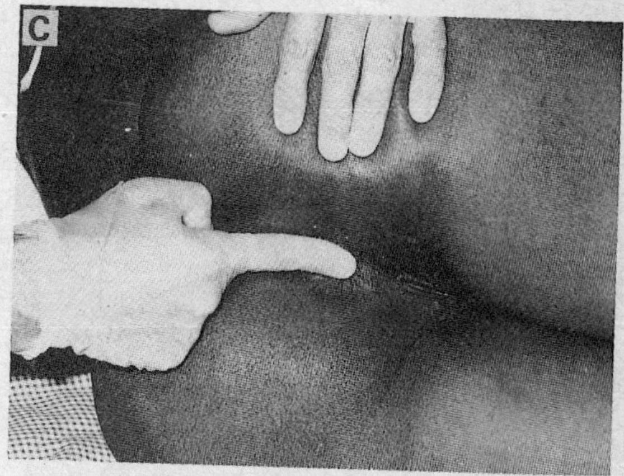

As you insert your finger pull backwards to counteract the tone in the puborectalis muscle.

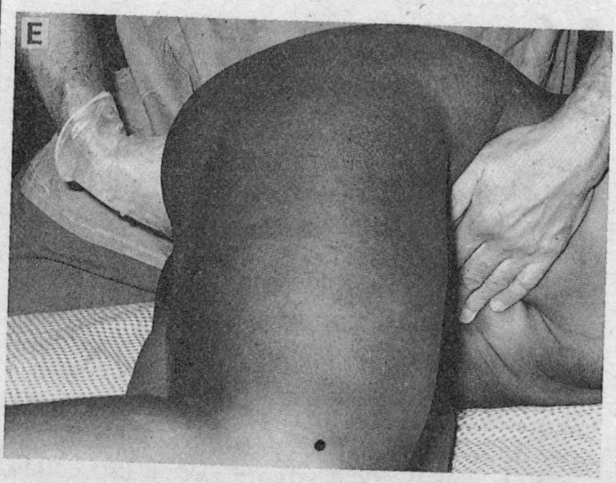

After examining the anal canal and rectum, place your hand on the abdomen and examine the contents of the pelvis bimanually

FIG. 18.1 THE TECHNIQUE OF ANORECTAL EXAMINATION

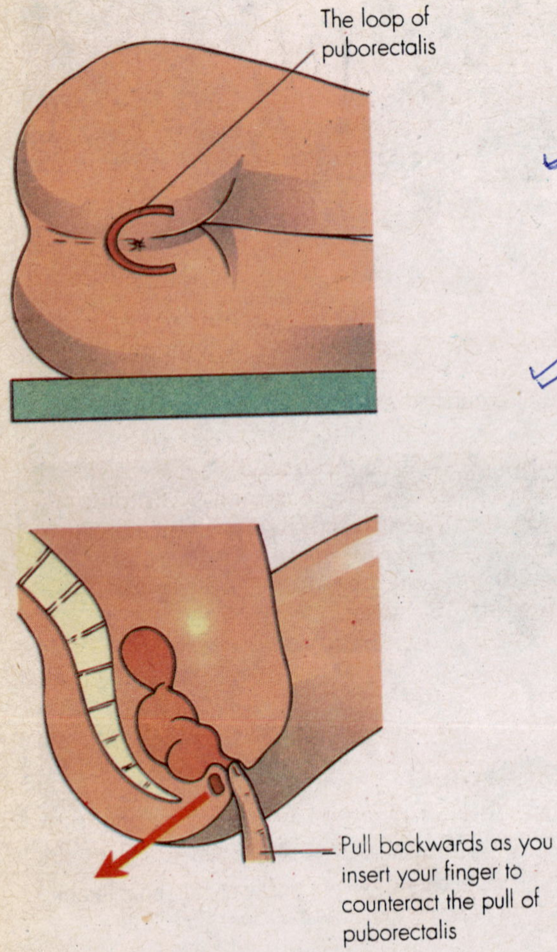

FIG. 18.2 The puborectalis muscle forms a loop which helps to keep the anal canal closed. As you insert your finger into the anal canal you must oppose this tone by pressing your finger backwards

Patients with fissures or abscesses may have so much spasm and pain that rectal examination is extremely difficult. In these circumstances you should *not* try to pass a finger. If the pain is so severe, then the patient will need treatment, and your rectal examination can be postponed until the patient is anaesthetized.

The rectum Feel all around the rectum as high as possible. You may have to push quite hard in a fat patient. Note the texture of the wall of the rectum and the presence of any masses or ulcers. If you feel a mass, try to decide if it is within or outside the wall of the rectum by testing the mobility of the mucosa over it.

Note the contents of the rectum. The rectum may be full of faeces (hard or soft), empty and collapsed, or empty but 'ballooned out'. Faeces may feel like a tumour but are indentable; no other mass is indentable.

If you can feel a mass at your finger tip ask the patient to strain down. This will often move the mass down 2 cm or so and bring it within your reach.

The rectovesico/rectouterine pouch Turn your finger round so that the pulp feels forwards and can detect any masses outside the rectum in the peritoneal pouch between the rectum and the bladder or uterus.

Bimanual examination

The examination of the contents of the pelvis is helped if you place your left hand on the abdomen and feel bimanually. This gives you a much better idea of the size, shape and nature of any pelvic mass.

The cervix and uterus These structures are easy to feel per rectum, and with the help of bimanual palpation you should be able to define the shape and size of the uterus and any ovarian masses. Do not call the hard mass that you can feel in the anterior rectal wall a carcinoma until you are sure that it is neither the cervix nor a **tampon**.

The prostate and seminal vesicles The normal prostate gland is firm, rubbery, bilobed and 2–3 cm across. Its surface should be smooth, with a shallow central sulcus, and the rectal mucosa should move freely over it. The seminal vesicles may be palpable just above the upper lateral edges of the gland.

Benign hypertrophy of the prostate causes enlargement of the whole gland but the central sulcus is one of the last features to disappear. The hypertrophy affects the whole gland, which bulges backwards into the rectum. The gland may feel lobulated. The overlying rectal mucosa remains uninvolved and mobile.

Carcinoma of the prostate causes an irregular, **hard** enlargement which is often unilateral. The edge of the enlarged area is indistinct.

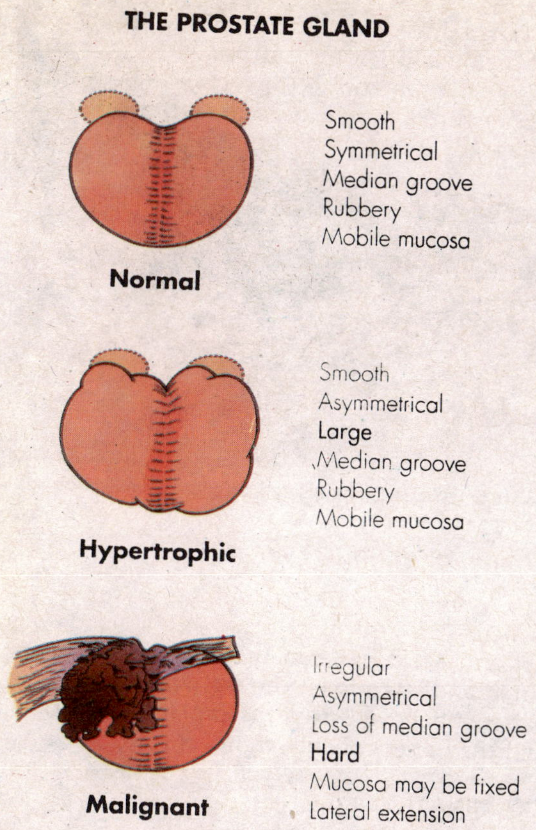

FIG. 18.3

If the tumour has spread out into the floor of the pelvis you will feel thickening either side of the gland, which can sometimes encircle the rectum. This lateral thickening is described as 'winging' of the prostate.

The central sulcus may be distorted or obliterated at an early stage of the disease and the rectal mucosa fixed to the underlying gland.

CONDITIONS PRESENTING WITH RECTAL BLEEDING

Haemorrhoids

Haemorrhoids, commonly called 'piles', are enlarged congested patches of the mucosa and submucosa at the level of the anorectal junction.

The normal vascular plexus of the submucosa is expanded at the anorectal junction to form three anal 'cushions'. These cushions help close the anal canal, but if they enlarge they can prolapse, be damaged, bleed, and even become pedunculated – that is to say, turn into piles.

HISTORY

Age Piles occur at all ages but are uncommon below the age of 20 years. When they occur in children they are often secondary to vascular malformations in the pelvis.

Symptoms **Uncomplicated piles do not cause pain.** The two common symptoms they cause are **bleeding** and a palpable **lump** (or prolapse) after defaecation. They may also cause perianal discomfort and **pruritis**, and a **mucous discharge**.

The bleeding occurs after defaecation. If it is a small quantity it may just stain the toilet paper or streak the faeces, but if it is copious it may **splash around the lavatory pan** and cause **anaemia**.

The patient notices the lump when cleaning himself after defaecation. It may return to the rectum spontaneously or need to be pushed back.

Piles are categorized into three degrees on the basis of the history:

First-degree piles bleed but do not prolapse.
Second-degree piles prolapse but reduce spontaneously.
Third-degree piles prolapse and must be reduced manually.

Although it is worthwhile classifying piles in this way as it helps decide the form of treatment, it is an artificial classification. All piles are prolapsed **during** defaecation and this is when they bleed. If they return to their proper place when the anal sphincter closes they are never felt by the patient and are, therefore, called first-degree piles. Second-degree piles are vascular pads which remain down below the sphincter when it contracts and then return slowly but spontaneously, while third-degree piles are so big and pendulous that they have to be pushed back.

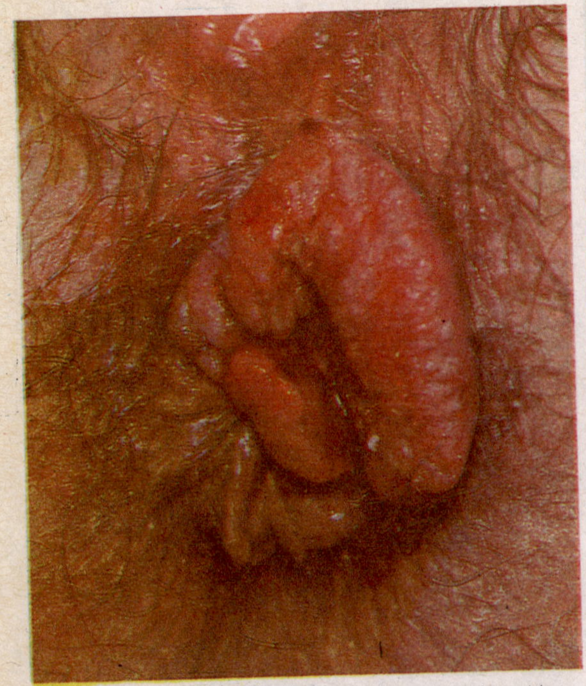

FIG. 18.4 Third-degree (prolapsed) haemorrhoids. The epithelium covering the 3 o'clock pile is becoming thick and white. The 7 o'clock pile is bleeding

Revision Panel 18.1

Diagnosis of conditions which present with rectal bleeding

Bleeding but **no pain**:

Blood mixed with stool	=	Carcinoma of colon*
Blood streaked on stool	=	Carcinoma of rectum*
Blood after defaecation	=	Haemorrhoids*
Blood and mucus	=	Colitis*
Blood alone	=	Diverticular disease
Melaena	=	Peptic ulceration
Bleeding + **pain**	=	Fissure (or carcinoma of anal canal)

* Also proctitis caused by specific infections (e.g. schistosomiasis)

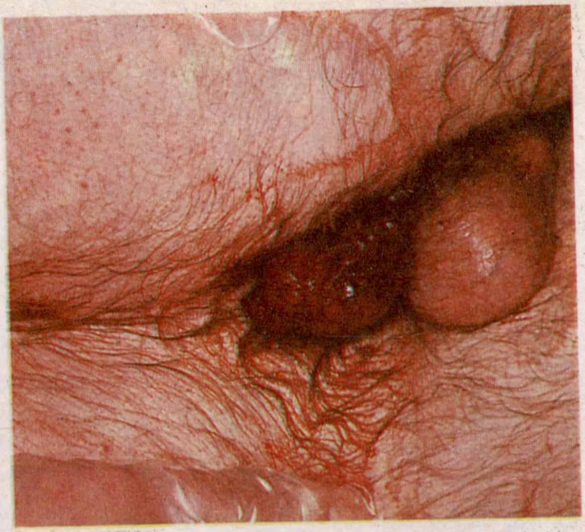

FIG. 18.5 Prolapsed, strangulated, thrombosed haemorrhoids. Note the bloody serous discharge

Cause Many patients with piles are constipated and strain a lot during defaecation. The patients believe this is the cause of their piles and they are probably right.

EXAMINATION

First- and second-degree piles Piles which are not prolapsed **cannot be felt with the finger.** They are indistinguishable from normal mucosa, and can only be diagnosed with a **proctoscope**.

When a proctoscope is withdrawn through a normal anal canal the red–blue mucosa can be seen collapsing over the end of the proctoscope. Piles are purple and bulge so much that they protrude into the end of the proctoscope. The multiple longitudinal corrugations are lost and three deep clefts appear between the bulging piles.

The three common primary piles are at 3, 7 and 11 o'clock (when the patient is in the lithotomy position); these are the sites of the three anal cushions.

Do not forget – **you cannot diagnose haemorrhoids with your finger**.

Third-degree piles If you are fortunate (and the patient unfortunate!) you may see the piles prolapsed. They are bluish-purple swellings, usually 0.5–1 cm in diameter, in the 3, 7 or 11

A

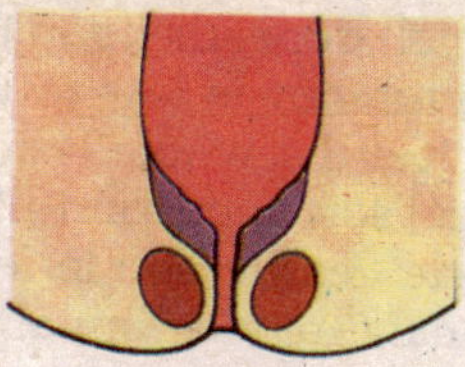

The vascular pads which become haemorrhoids close the anorectal junction.

B

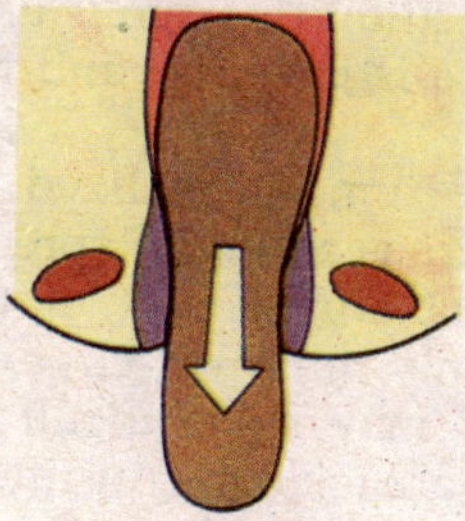

During defaecation the sphincter relaxes, the anal canal everts and the haemorrhoids are compressed by the faeces. The faeces scratch the mucosa.

C

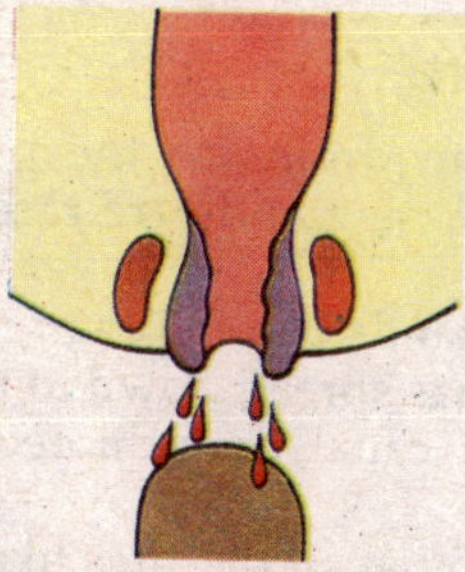

After the faeces have passed, the haemorrhoids are left scratched and unsupported so they drip blood onto the faeces.

D

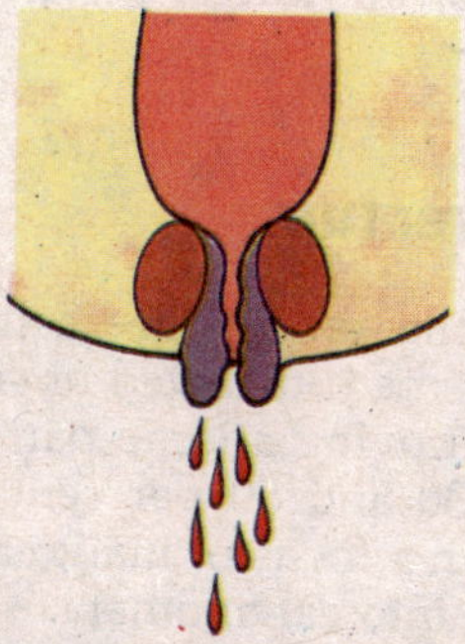

If they do not retract when the sphincter begins to close their venous drainage is obstructed and the bleeding is made worse so that it splashes into the pan.

FIG. 18.6 The way in which haemorrhoids are caused to bleed

o'clock positions. Their distinguishing and diagnostic feature is their mucosal covering, recognized by its soft, velvety, mucus-producing surface.

The other common cause of a localized anal swelling is the perianal haematoma. This lesion is always covered by skin, which distinguishes it from a mucosa-covered prolapsed haemorrhoid.

If piles remain prolapsed they ulcerate and bleed. If the submucous veins thrombose, the pile becomes tense, hard and oedematous. Palpation and rectal examination in these circumstances is painful and difficult because of spasm.

Piles are painful only when such complications occur.

Carcinoma of the rectum

Carcinoma of the rectum is diagnosed on the history, the findings on rectal examination and sigmoidoscopy, and finally by biopsy.

Seventy-five per cent of carcinomata of the rectum occur in the lower part of the rectal ampulla, where they tend to be papilliferous or a simple ulcer with an everted edge. The remaining 25 per cent are in the upper part of the rectum and often have an annular ('cotton reel') shape.

About 90 per cent of rectal cancers can be felt with your finger.

Every patient with any rectal complaint must have a rectal examination. You are being negligent if you fail to perform a rectal examination on a patient complaining of rectal bleeding.

HISTORY

Age Rectal carcinoma is common in middle and old age but can occur in young adults.

Sex It is common in both sexes.

Symptoms The commonest symptom is rectal bleeding, usually a **small amount of red blood streaked on the stool.** Sometimes enough blood accumulates in the rectum to be passed by itself, but this is uncommon. **Mucus** may also be passed.

Low rectal cancers cause a vague **change in bowel habit**, usually a little constipation.

High cancers of the annular variety may cause partial obstruction which presents as **alternating episodes of diarrhoea and constipation**. The constipation is caused by the obstruction. The diarrhoea follows irritation of the colon above the obstruction by the impacted faeces, which gradually liquefy and, when they are fluid, pass through the carcinomatous stenosis and appear as diarrhoea.

Tenesmus occurs when a tumour in the lower part of the rectum reaches a size large enough to be mistaken by the patient's rectal sensory mechanisms for faeces. The patient has a persistent, sometimes painful, desire to empty his rectum but cannot do so.

Even small, symptomless, primary lesions may be associated with multiple metastases and cause **general debility and malaise**. The preaortic lymph nodes and the liver are the first sites to be invaded by metastases.

Pain is an uncommon symptom of carcinoma of the rectum. It can be of three types:

1 **Colic, with distension and vomiting,** caused by annular tumours obstructing the lumen of the bowel.
2 **Local pain** in the rectum, perineum or lower abdomen, caused by direct spread of the tumour to surrounding structures, especially the sacral nerves.
3 **Pain during defaecation**; this is uncommon but can occur if the tumour has spread downwards into the sensitive anal canal.

Previous history Long-standing ulcerative colitis increases the chance of malignant change in the colon and rectum fortyfold. Always ask about any previous large-bowel symptoms, particularly recurrent episodes of diarrhoea associated with the passage of mucus and blood. The fact that the ulcerative colitis has been quiescent for many years does not reduce the increased chance of malignant change.

Family history Polyposis coli is a rare but definitely premalignant condition. The family history may reveal that the patient's parents or siblings have had rectal bleeding, abdominal pain caused by their polyps, or even surgical excision of their colon for carcinoma.

EXAMINATION

Rectal examination There is usually nothing abnormal to see around the anus, but in 90 per cent of cases rectal examination reveals the carcinoma. What can be felt depends upon the site of the lesion. If the tumour is low in the ampulla the finger can feel the whole lesion. Papilliferous tumours feel soft and frond-like, and have a narrow pedicle. Sessile, soft lesions such as villous carcinomata may be impalpable.

A carcinomatous ulcer feels hard and bulges into the lumen of the rectum. Its edge is usually everted and its base is irregular and friable.

Try to decide if the tumour is fixed or mobile and whether there is any local spread.

If the cancer is in the upper part of the rectum you may feel only its lower edge. In these circumstances it may be difficult to decide if the lesion you are feeling is inside or outside the rectum. This question is answered by inspecting it through a sigmoidoscope.

GENERAL EXAMINATION

Lymph from the rectum drains to the preaortic lymph glands. These glands are rarely palpable.

The inguinal lymph glands become enlarged only when the tumour has spread down to the lymphatics of the anal canal or ischiorectal fossa.

It is important to examine all the sites likely to contain metastases, particularly the supraclavicular lymph nodes, the lungs, the liver and the skin.

Adenoma of the rectum

Benign neoplasms of the rectum are called adenomas. They may be pedunculated or sessile, small or large (occupying a large part of the rectum). Between 30 and 50 per cent of large adenomata contain a focus of malignant invasion, making them into carcinomata.

There is **bleeding, mucous discharge** and **diarrhoea**.

Adenomata are soft and often difficult to feel on rectal examination.

Diverticular disease

Diverticular disease usually presents with chronic left-sided abdominal pain and constipation, or acute abdominal symptoms. These are discussed in Chapter 16.

However, the disease may present with rectal bleeding, hence its appearance in this chapter. The bleeding is typically **acute, massive**, and **fresh**. The patient feels a little faint, gets lower abdominal pain, and then has a desire to defaecate. When he empties his rectum he passes 100–500 mL of fresh blood.

This type of bleeding is uncommon and the wise clinician accepts diverticular disease as the cause of a patient's rectal bleeding only after he has excluded all other possible causes, such as carcinoma, adenoma and vascular abnormalities.

CONDITIONS PRESENTING WITH ANAL PAIN

Perianal 'haematoma'

The name of this condition is well established, but most authorities no longer believe that it is an extravascular haematoma. It is probably a large thrombus in a vein of the subcutaneous perianal plexus, caused by excessive stretching of the anus when passing a very bulky hard stool, or the sudden changes in sphincter tone and rectal pressure that occur during the precipitous emptying of the rectum in acute diarrhoea.

Perianal haematomata are also common after childbirth, following the straining and stretching of the perineum during the second stage of labour.

The thrombus causes a surrounding inflammatory reaction of pain and oedema.

HISTORY

Age Perianal haematomata occur at all ages.

Sex Excepting the postpartum variety, they are equally common in men and women.

Symptoms The dominant symptom is a **pain**, which begins gradually, increases in severity over a few hours or days and then subsides spontaneously over a period of 4–5 days. It is a continuous discomfort, made worse by sitting, moving and defaecation, but it is clearly localized to the lump by the patient.

The lump appears at the same time as the pain. At first it is small and spherical but may gradually enlarge and become more painful.

Bleeding occurs if the lump bursts through the skin or if the skin over the lump ulcerates.

The patient often notices that the perianal skin is moist and itchy. This is caused by an increased secretion from the anal glands onto the surrounding skin.

Perianal haematomata are often multiple and the patient has often had a previous 'attack'

Cause The patient may remember that the symptoms began after an uncomfortable defaecation, but as the haematoma may take a few hours to form the connection is not always obvious.

The patient always thinks that he has an attack of 'piles'. Do not be misled by his belief. Perianal haematomata are *not* piles.

EXAMINATION

Position The lump may be anywhere around the anal margin. More than one may be present.

Colour When it is close to the skin and the skin is not oedematous, the lump has a deep red–purple colour. If the skin becomes oedematous the redness of the underlying blood clot cannot be seen.

Tenderness The lump is tender, but disproportionately less than you would expect from the pain felt by the patient; but it becomes very tender if it becomes oedematous and ulcerated.

Shape and size The initial lump is spherical, and 0.3–1.0 cm in diameter. If the anal skin is lax the lump may become polypoid. This invariably happens when it becomes oedematous.

Surface Perianal haematomata are covered by **skin**. The skin may be normal or oedematous but it is always clearly recognizable as skin. That part of the lump which rubs against the skin of the buttocks may be rubbed raw.

The surface of the lump beneath the skin is smooth.

Composition The central lump can be felt as a hard, hemispherical mass. A cluster of many small haematomata feels like a small bunch of grapes. Individual lumps are too small to feel fluctuant.

Relations The mass is under the perianal skin, and superficial to the external sphincter.

It is not fixed to the skin or the deep structures and **cannot be reduced** into the anal canal.

State of local tissues The remainder of the anal skin and anal canal is usually normal but there may be a palpable cord running up the anal canal from the haematoma. This is probably caused by thrombosis in the vein that has been damaged.

Lymph drainage The inguinal nodes should not be enlarged.

Fissure-in-ano

An anal fissure is a longitudinal split in the skin of the anal canal.

An acute tear is quite a common event and usually heals quickly. If the tear is reopened every time the patient defaecates, because he is constipated and has a high sphincter tone, its base becomes fibrous and does not heal. It becomes, in fact, a chronic ulcer.

HISTORY

Age Acute fissures are quite common in children who often pass bulky stools very quickly.

Chronic fissures are most common in patients between the ages of 20 and 40 years. They frequently begin in women after childbirth.

Sex Fissure-in-ano is a little more common in men than women.

Symptoms Both acute and chronic fissures are very painful. The pain begins during defaecation and **persists for minutes or hours** afterwards. The pain can be so severe that the patient becomes frightened to defaecate. This makes him more constipated, which makes the pain still worse when he eventually evacuates his rectum. A vicious circle is established.

Acute fissures bleed sufficiently to **streak the stool with blood** and stain the toilet paper. Chronic fissures bleed less and usually cause just a little blood-staining of the toilet paper.

A small skin tag (called a sentinel tag) which the patient can feel, may form at the lower end of a chronic fissure.

The patient complains of **constipation** and realizes that it is the hard bulky stool which causes the pain.

Persistence The symptoms of fissure are slow to develop and long-standing. They hardly

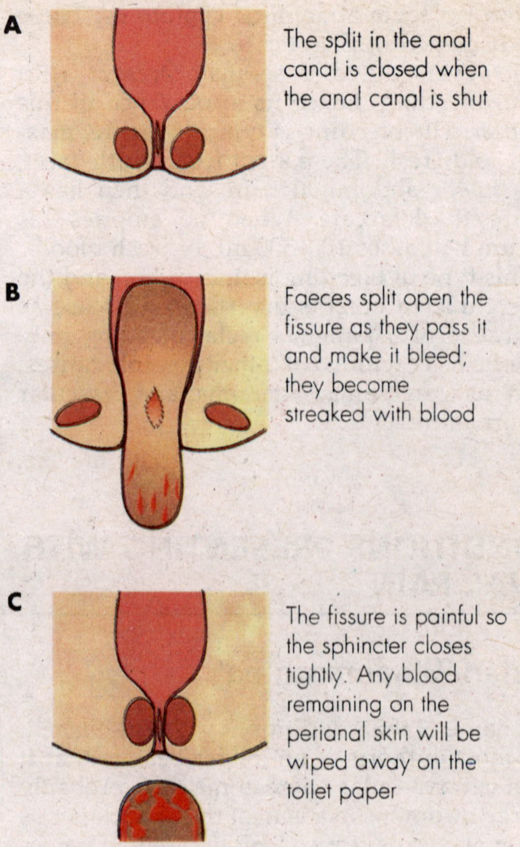

FIG. 18.7 The way in which a fissure is caused to bleed

ever disappear spontaneously, but often vary in severity from week to week. Many patients suffer for months before going to see their doctor.

Cause The patients either believe that their symptoms are caused by constipation or think that their distressing pain must indicate some dreadful, incurable disease.

EXAMINATION

Position The majority of fissures are in the mid-line, posteriorly, but some are anterior and a few are lateral.

The diagnosis is made by gently parting the skin of the anus and looking for a split in the anal skin. This may be all that you will be allowed to do, because further examination is often prevented by pain.

Tenderness The anal sphincter is usually in spasm, and any attempt to open the sphincter by firm traction on the buttocks or inserting a finger into the rectum is exquisitely painful. In these circumstances rectal examination is contraindicated.

Rectal examination If the pain and tenderness are not severe you may be able to perform a rectal examination and feel the defect in the anal canal skin and also some surrounding induration. There will often be a streak of fresh blood on the finger stall when it is withdrawn.

Proctoscopy It is most unlikely that this will be possible, but when it is you will see the open, raw base of the fissure as the instrument is withdrawn through the anal canal.

Fistula-in-ano

A fistula is a track, lined with epithelium or granulation tissue, connecting two epithelial surfaces such as those in two body cavities or one cavity and the body's external surface.

A fistula-in-ano connects the lumen of the rectum or anal canal with the external surface. It is usually lined with granulation tissue. In most instances it is caused by an anorectal abscess in the intersphincteric space bursting in two directions – internally into the anal canal, and externally into the skin.

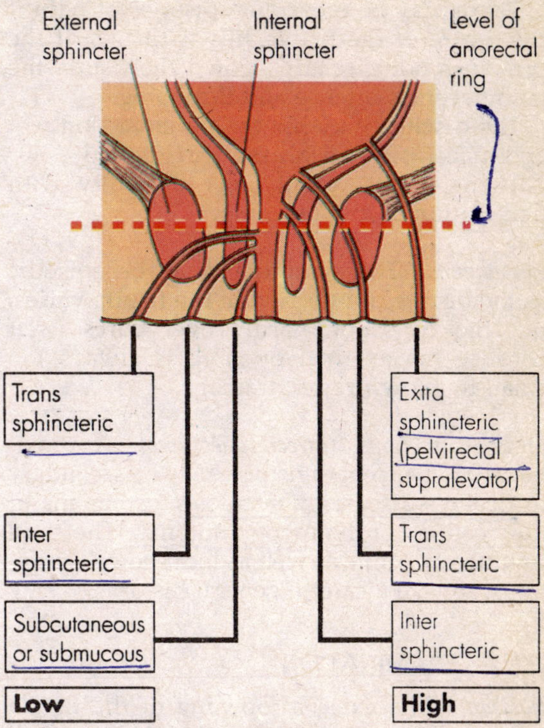

FIG. 18.8 The varieties of fistula-in-ano

The abscess may be secondary to another rectal inflammatory disease such as ulcerative colitis or Crohn's disease.

Some fistulae are caused by direct infiltration and necrosis of a tumour. The rectal neoplasm most likely to present with a fistula-in-ano is the colloid carcinoma.

Fistulae-in-ano can run through a variety of anatomical planes subcutaneous, submucous, between the sphincter muscles, or above the sphincter.

HISTORY

Age Fistula-in-ano can occur at any time during adult life.

Symptoms The commonest symptom is a watery or purulent **discharge** from the external opening of the fistula.

There may be recurrent episodes of **pain** if the centre of the fistula fills with pus. If the pus does not discharge down the fistula the pain becomes intense and throbbing.

The discharge makes the perianal skin wet and macerated and causes **pruritus ani**.

There is not usually any difficulty with defaecation or any bleeding.

Persistence The symptoms may be episodic as the degree of infection in the fistula varies, but the condition hardly ever cures itself because the external opening is always too small to allow proper drainage.

Other symptoms (direct questions) Approximately 50 per cent of fistulae may be secondary to Crohn's disease, tuberculosis, carcinoma of the rectum, or lymphogranuloma. These all produce systemic as well as local bowel symptoms, so take a careful general history.

LOCAL EXAMINATION

Position The external opening of the fistula will be visible as a puckered scar or a small tuft of granulation tissue, within 2–4 cm of the anal canal.

Fistulae can open anywhere around the anus, but the majority of openings are in the posterolateral area. There may be more than one opening.

Tenderness The opening of the fistula is not tender but the tissues deep to it may be thickened and tender.

Discharge The discharge, which can be serous or purulent, may be visible on the skin.

Rectal examination Rectal examination is not painful. The internal opening of the fistula can usually be identified as an area of induration under the mucosa. Two-thirds are posterior, one-third anterior.

The indurated track of the fistula between the internal and external openings can be felt by palpating the wall of the anus between your index finger in the rectum, and your thumb (or other hand) on the perianal skin.

Take care to perform a full rectal examination. Look for other diseases, such as a carcinoma, which might be the cause of the fistula. **Proctoscopy and sigmoidoscopy** are essential to exclude underlying diseases such as Crohn's disease, carcinoma and tuberculosis.

Revision Panel 18.2

Diagnosis of anal conditions which present with pain

Pain alone
- Fissure (pain after defaecation)
- Proctalgia fugax (pain spontaneously at night)
- Anorectal abscess

Pain and bleeding
- Fissure

Pain and a lump
- Perianal haematoma
- Anorectal abscess

Pain, a lump and bleeding
- Prolapsed haemorrhoids
- Carcinoma of the anal canal
- Prolapsed rectal polyp or carcinoma
- Prolapsed rectum

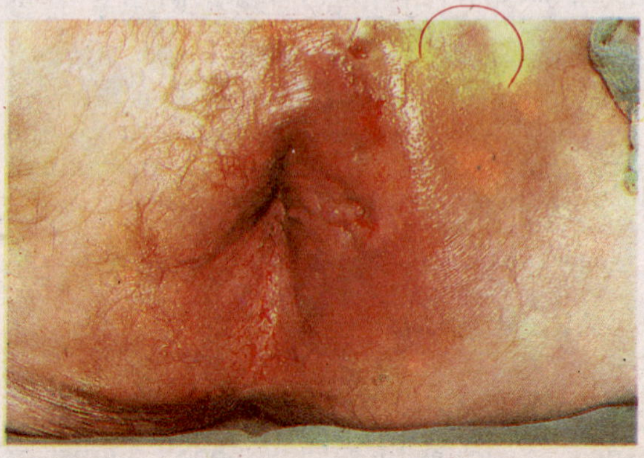

FIG. 18.9 Fistula-in-ano. Multiple openings behind and to the left of the anus. Although the opening looks as if it is healing there is a track leading through the muscles to the anal canal

It is not a good idea for students to pass probes into fistulae; leave that for the consultant.

Local lymph glands The inguinal lymph glands which receive lymph from the anal canal should not be enlarged unless the fistula is acutely inflamed or secondary to an infiltrating carcinoma. Inguinal lymphadenopathy is a prominent feature of fistulae caused by lymphogranuloma.

State of local tissues It cannot be repeated too often that the anus and rectum must be carefully examined to exclude serious causes of the fistula. If the fistula was solely caused by a simple intersphincteric or ischiorectal abscess, the rest of the anus and rectum is likely to be normal.

GENERAL EXAMINATION

Many of the diseases mentioned above may have associated abdominal and general clinical signs, so *never* confine your examination to the patient's perineum.

Anorectal abscess

Anorectal abscesses occur in the space between the internal and external sphincters (intersphincteric or perianal abscess) or in the ischiorectal fossa (ischiorectal abscess). The infection probably begins in an anal gland from which pus either tracks down to the perineum between the sphincters or penetrates the external sphincter to reach the ischiorectal fossa.

HISTORY

Age Anorectal abscess is common between the ages of 20 and 50 years.

Sex It is seen more often in men than women.

Symptoms The main symptom is a severe, throbbing pain which makes sitting, moving and defaecation difficult and is exacerbated by them all.

The patient may have felt a tender swelling close by the anus.

Systemic effects The general symptoms of an abscess – malaise, loss of appetite, sweating and even rigors – may be present.

EXAMINATION

Position The painful area lies lateral to the anus in the soft tissues between the anus and the ischial tuberosity, but it may encircle the whole of the posterior half of the anus.

Tenderness The whole area is *very* tender.

Colour and temperature The overlying skin eventually becomes hot and red, but the abscess has to be quite big before these skin changes appear.

Shape, size and composition It is not usually possible to define the features of the mass. Its surface is indistinct. Its size can be crudely assessed (when it is large) by bimanual palpation with a finger in the rectum and one on the overlying skin. It is usually too tender to test for fluctuation.

Rectal examination This is possible but very painful and best deferred until the patient is anaesthetized. The abscess may bulge into the side of the lower part of the rectum, and the rectum on the side of the abscess feels **hot**.

Lymph drainage The inguinal glands are sometimes enlarged and tender.

Local tissues The nearby structures – the anus, the rectum and the contents of the pelvis – may show evidence of previous abscesses and fistulae, such as scars and sinuses.

GENERAL EXAMINATION

There is likely to be a tachycardia, pyrexia, sweating, a dry, furred tongue and foetor oris.

Pilonidal sinus

The word 'pilonidal' means a nest of hairs. A pilonidal sinus is a sinus which contains a tuft of hairs. These sinuses are commonly found i[illegible] the skin covering the sacrum and coccyx[illegible] can occur between the fingers, particul[illegible] hairdressers, and at the umbilicus.

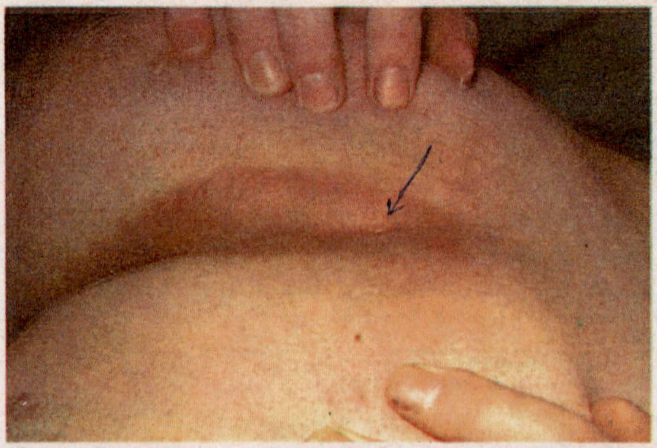

The patient is lying on his right side with buttocks held apart to expose the bottom of the natal cleft. The sinus, which is difficult to see, is the small pale central pit. The stiff black hair which commonly covers the buttocks of these patients has been shaved off

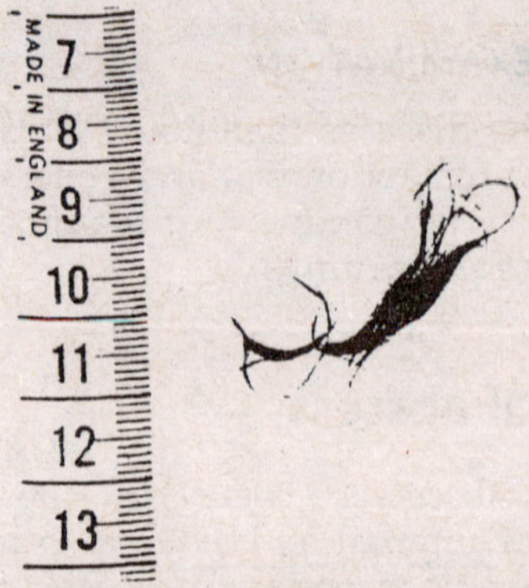

The hairs that were removed from the sinus shown in (**A**)

FIG. 18.10 PILONIDAL SINUS

There is a continual argument about the source of the hairs. A pilonidal sinus is not lined by skin and there are no hairs growing within it. In fact, the hairs in the sinus are short, broken pieces of hair that either get sucked into a pre-existing dimple in the skin or actually pierce the normal skin in the gluteal cleft and then, by acting as foreign bodies, aid and support the development and persistence of chronic infection. The result is a chronic abscess which contains hair and which flares up at frequent intervals into an acute abscess.

HISTORY

Age Pilonidal sinus is rare before puberty and in people over 40 years of age. This suggests that it is a self-limiting condition. Perhaps the strength of the hairs and the likelihood of their pricking into the skin varies with age.

Sex It is more common in men than women.

Ethnic group Pilonidal sinuses are more common in dark-haired, hirsute men. This description does not define an ethnic group but certain ethnic groups have more men with these characteristics.

Occupation Short hairs are very strong and easily pierce the skin. Men's hairdressers sometimes get pilonidal sinuses in the webs between their fingers.

Symptoms The common symptoms are **pain and a discharge**, which develop when an abscess forms in the sinus. The pain may vary from a dull ache to an acute throbbing pain and the discharge will vary from a little serum to a sudden gush of pus.

In between the acute exacerbations the sinus produces few symptoms and the patient often thinks it has disappeared.

The acute exacerbations occur at irregular intervals. If a sinus becomes chronically inflamed it may discharge continually.

EXAMINATION

Position Pilonidal sinuses are often misdiagnosed as anal fistulae because of their proximity to the anus, but this misdiagnosis should not occur because pilonidal sinuses are always in the **mid-line of the natal cleft and lie over the lowest part of the sacrum and coccyx** (whereas the opening of a fistula can be anywhere around the anus). It is very rare for a pilonidal sinus or a pilonidal abscess to involve the tissues between the tip of the coccyx and the anus, or the ischiorectal fossa; these are the common sites of fistulae.

There may be one or many sinuses, some with a smooth epithelialized edge, others with a puckered scarred edge and some with pouting granulation tissue. The latter are usually the sinuses which are discharging pus and the orifices of the most recent abscesses.

Temperature and tenderness The skin around a pilonidal sinus is normal except when the sinus is acutely infected, when it becomes red and tender.

The sinus The actual sinus (or sinuses) is usually easy to see. It is a small mid-line pit with epithelialized edges. Gentle pressure may produce a small quantity of serous discharge and reveal the tips of a few hairs.

When a sinus is infected it becomes indistinguishable from any other form of subcutaneous abscess.

Palpation of the skin and subcutaneous tissues around the sinus reveals areas of subcutaneous induration which correspond to the ramifications of the sinus beneath the skin. There may be scars well away from the mid-line, as high as the first sacral vertebra, where previous abscesses have discharged or been incised.

Lymph drainage The inguinal lymph nodes do not enlarge because the infection is mostly mild and chronic.

Local tissues The underlying sacrum, the skin of the perineum, the anal canal and the ischiorectal fossa should be normal.

Perianal warts

(Condylomata acuminata)

Perianal warts are multiple, pedunculated, papilliferous lesions that are easy to recognize. They are often spread over the whole perineum, including the labia majora and the back of the scrotum.

They are caused by a virus which is a variant of the papilloma virus responsible for skin warts, and can be transmitted by sexual contact. Consequently they are often associated with other sexually transmitted diseases such as herpes genitalis, AIDS, gonorrhoea and syphilis.

They are also seen in patients whose immune response has been depressed with steroids and other forms of chemotherapy.

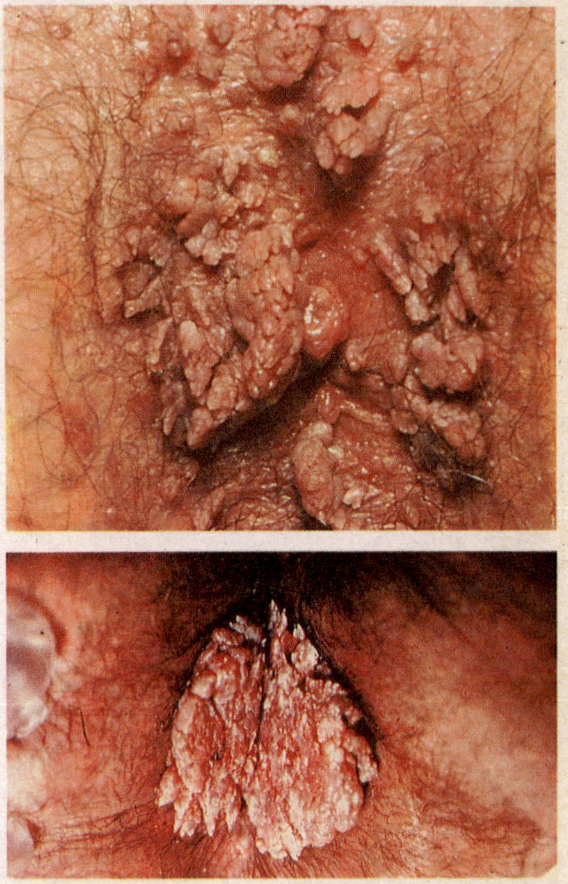

FIG. 18.11 Two examples of multiple perianal warts (condylomata)

Condylomata lata also occur as a manifestation of secondary syphilis, but these are broad-based, flat-topped papules. They are highly contagious.

All condylomata cause irritation, discomfort and pain from rubbing, and may ulcerate and become infected.

Proctalgia fugax

This is an uncommon condition but is mentioned because the patient presents to the doctor complaining of severe rectal pain.

The pain comes on suddenly, often at night, is cramp-like and deep inside the anal canal.

Nothing relieves it and it passes off spontaneously within minutes or hours.

General and rectal examination are normal. Its cause is unknown, but there is some evidence to suggest that it is caused by spasm (cramp) of the muscles of the pelvic floor.

CONDITIONS PRESENTING AS AN ANAL LUMP WITH OR WITHOUT PAIN

A number of the conditions already described present with pain and a lump but in the majority the pain is the dominant symptom. The following conditions are not necessarily painless but the lump is the dominant symptom.

Prolapsed haemorrhoids

The symptoms of haemorrhoids have already been described because their commonest symptom is rectal bleeding; but some piles do not bleed (or the patient does not observe the bleeding) and are therefore not noticed until the patient feels them when cleaning himself after defaecation. He often observes that the lumps retract spontaneously or can be pushed back into the anal canal.

Piles which only prolapse during defaecation are **not painful**, but if they become permanently prolapsed, strangulated, thrombosed, or ulcerated they become very painful and tender.

Examination then reveals two or three tense, tender, red–purple **mucosa-covered** swellings protruding from the anal canal. The covering of purple mucosa and the disposition of swellings at the 3, 7 and 11 o'clock positions (12 o'clock is anterior) make the diagnosis easy.

If the piles have been prolapsed and thrombosed for a long time they may be so ulcerated and infected that they are difficult to distinguish from a prolapsing carcinoma.

Tags

Small tags of skin, with narrow pedicles, are commonly found on the lax perianal skin. They follow minor trauma or small perianal haematomata and are usually symptomless. If

> Revision Panel 18.3
>
> **Diagnosis of anal conditions which present with a lump**
>
> *A lump and no other symptoms*
> Anal warts
> Skin tags
>
> *A lump and pain*
> Perianal haematoma
>
> *A lump, pain and bleeding*
> Prolapsed haemorrhoids
> Carcinoma of anal canal
> Prolapsed rectal polyp or carcinoma
> Prolapsed rectum

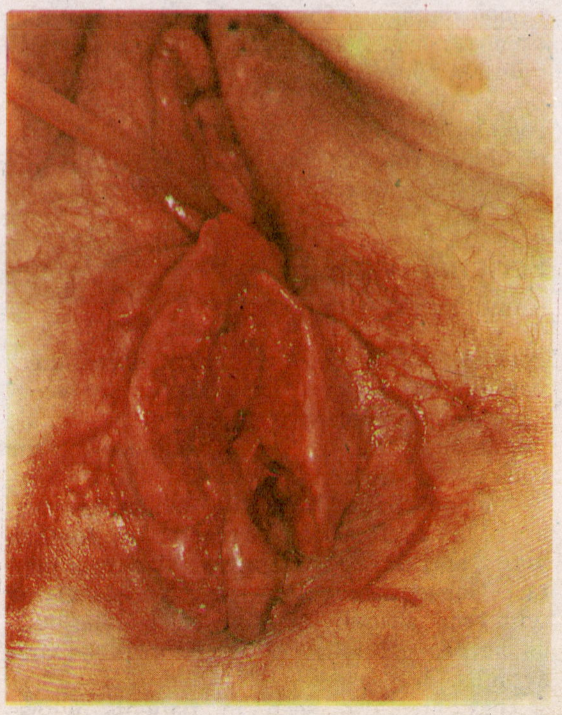

FIG. 18.12 A carcinoma of the anal canal which has spread into the skin of the perineum. The patient was still able to defaecate. The patient is in the lithotomy position

they rub, catch or itch they may cause enough symptoms to warrant removal.

Sometimes part of the lining of the lower anal canal may develop into a papilla which prolapses (a fibrosed anal polyp).

A tag may develop at the lower end of an anal fissure – the 'sentinel tag'.

Carcinoma

A carcinoma of the rectum or the anal canal can present as an anal lump if it prolapses through the anus or spreads directly down the wall of the anal canal to the perianal skin.

When the anal canal is invaded by tumour the patient usually has pain on defaecation, as well as a lump. This is one of the few circumstances in which a low rectal carcinoma presents with pain.

Squamous cell **carcinoma of the anal canal** is rare. It presents with pain on defaecation and streaks of blood on the faeces and the toilet paper, but ultimately causes a palpable lump.

Prolapse of the rectum

This is an eversion of the whole thickness of the lower part of the rectum and the anal canal. It occurs when the structures in the floor of the pelvis that normally hold the rectum in the curve of the sacrum become weak and lax.

HISTORY

Age Prolapse of the rectum is common in the elderly. The majority of patients requiring treatment are over 65, many being in their 80s and 90s.

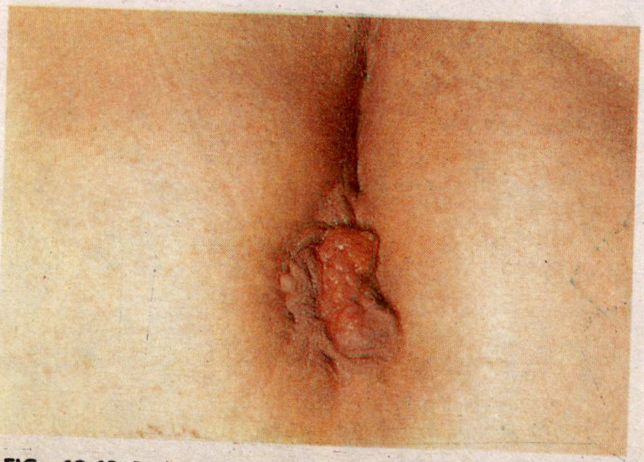

FIG. 18.13 Prolapsing rectal mucosa which has become fibrosed and papillomatous – a 'fibrosed anal polyp'. The patient is in the lithotomy position

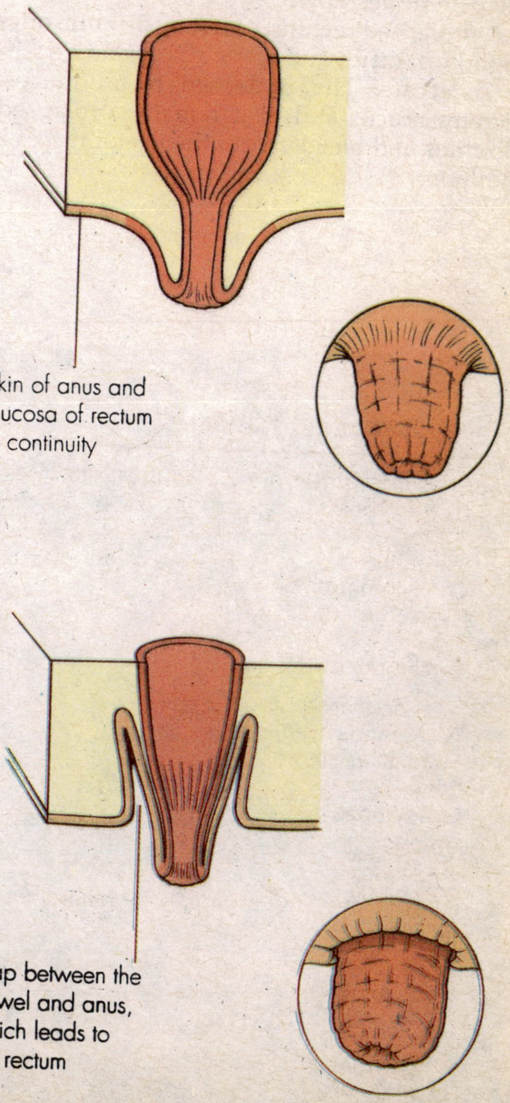

FIG. 18.14 The difference between a rectal prolapse (A) and an intussusception presenting through the anus (B)

Sex Prolapse is much more common in women because the female perineum is weakened by the presence of the vagina and the trauma of childbirth.

Symptoms The patient complains of a **large lump** which appears at the anus after defaecation, or sometimes spontaneously when standing, walking or coughing.

The lump can usually be pushed back into the rectum or may return spontaneously when the patient lies down.

A prolapsed rectum is **uncomfortable**, often slightly **painful**, and gives a persistent desire to defaecate. The prolapsed rectal mucosa secretes mucus and, if it remains prolapsed, ulcerates and bleeds. Incontinence of faeces is common.

EXAMINATION

Colour and shape The prolapsed rectum forms a long tubular mass protruding symmetrically through the anus. The exposed mucosa is red, and thrown into circumferential **concentric** folds around a central pit, which is the lumen of the rectum.

Sometimes it is necessary to ask the patient to strain down to produce the prolapse. The

Revision Panel 18.4
The causes of pruritus ani

Mucous discharge from the anus caused by:
- Haemorrhoids
- Polyps
- Skin tags
- Condylomata
- Fissure
- Fistula
- Carcinoma of the anus

Vaginal discharge caused by:
- Trichomonas vaginitis
- Monilial vaginitis
- Cervicitis
- Gonorrhoea

Skin diseases
- Tinea cruris
- Fungal infections, especially monilial infections in diabetics

Parasites
- Threadworm

Faecal soiling
- Poor hygiene
- Incontinence
- Diarrhoea

Psychoneuroses

Revision Panel 18.5
Some common causes of diarrhoea

Intestinal
- Enteritis:
  - Non-specific
  - Staphyloccocal
  - Typhoid
  - Bacillary dysentery
  - Amoebic
  - Cholera
- Worms
- Ulcerative colitis
- Crohn's disease
- Carcinoma
- Irritable colon
- Faecal impaction (spurious diarrhoea)
- Tropical sprue

Gastric
- Post gastrectomy
- Post vagotomy
- Gastrocolic fistula

Pancreatic
- Pancreatitis
- Carcinoma

Pelvic abscess

Drugs
- Digitalis
- Antibiotics
- Laxatives

Endocrine
- Uraemia
- Thyrotoxicosis
- Carcinoid syndrome
- Zollinger–Ellison syndrome
- Medullary carcinoma of thyroid
- Hypoparathyroidism
- Diet

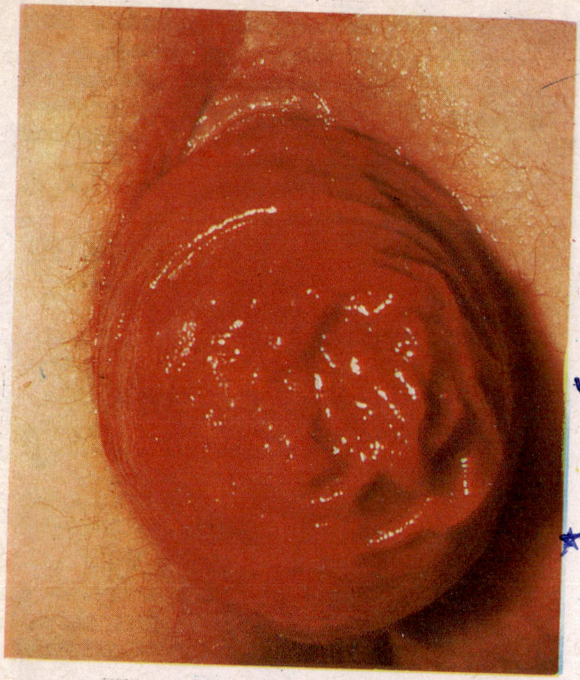

FIG. 18.15 A rectal prolapse

diagnosis is made by inspection and may be missed if this essential manoeuvre is omitted.

The prolapse may vary from 2–3 cm to 20 cm in length.

The prolapsed bowel is not tender and can be handled without causing the patient discomfort.

The important area to examine is the junction of the mass with the anal canal. If the lump is a rectal prolapse, its mucosal covering and the anal skin will be continuous. If the lump is an intussusception there will be a gap between the mucosa covering the lump and the anal skin. If you put your finger into this gap it will pass through the anal canal, into the rectum, alongside the intussusception.

Reducibility It is usually possible to reduce a prolapse with gentle compression and upward pressure.

Local tissues The rectum and anal canal are normal but the anal sphincter is very lax.

GENERAL EXAMINATION

The patient is usually a thin, small, elderly woman with a weak pelvic floor.

Intussusception

It is rare for an ileocolic or caecocolic intussusception in a child to present at the anus, but when it does it forms a sausage-shaped lump, covered with red–purple mucosa, similar to a rectal prolapse. The only way to distinguish it from a prolapse is by finding, on rectal examination, that the anal canal is normal and that a finger can be passed into it, alongside the intussusception (see Fig. 18.14).

The history will give a clue to the diagnosis. Intussusception usually occurs in children between the ages of 9 months and 2 years, and is associated with colicky abdominal pain, distension, vomiting and (rarely) the passage of blood-stained mucus – 'redcurrant jelly'.

Intussusception of the sigmoid colon and upper rectum occurs in adults when a polyp or carcinoma acts as the head of the intussusception. The causative lesion will be visible on the apex of the intussusception.

Revision Panel 18.6

Causes of pericoccygeal swellings

- Pilonidal sinus
- Postanal dermoid cyst
- Chordoma
- Sacrococcygeal teratoma

Revision Panel 18.7

Causes of faecal incontinence

- Diarrhoea
- Faecal impaction
- Nerve damage
- Sphincter muscle damage
- Dementia

Index

Page numbers in **bold** refer to Revision Panels